RADIOLOGY TODAY
A Multinational Series

Radiology Today 1

Edited by

M. W. Donner and F. H. W. Heuck

With 290 Figures and 61 Tables

Springer-Verlag
Berlin Heidelberg New York 1981

Proceedings of the Multinational Postgraduate Course,
held in Salzburg, June 12 – 15, 1980

Editors

Professor Dr. Martin W. Donner
Department of Radiology and Radiological Sciences,
The Johns Hopkins Medical Institutions,
Baltimore, MA 21205 (USA)

Professor Dr. Friedrich H. W. Heuck
Radiologisches Institut im Zentrum Radiologie
des Katharinenhospitals der Stadt Stuttgart,
D-7000 Stuttgart 1

Organization of the Salzburg Symposium

Professor Dr. H. H. Ellegast
Röntgendiagnostisches Zentralinstitut,
Landeskrankenanstalten, A-5020 Salzburg

ISBN 3-540-10099-7 Springer-Verlag Berlin Heidelberg New York
ISBN 0-387-10099-7 Springer-Verlag New York Heidelberg Berlin

Printing: Beltz, Offsetdruck, Hemsbach/Bergstr.
Binding: J. Schäffer OHG, Grünstadt

2121/3140-543210

Preface

This book encompasses the proceedings of a very successful post-graduate course entitled "Radiology Today" held in Salzburg in June 1980. It was organised by Dr. Martin W. Donner of Baltimore and Dr. F. H. W. Heuck of Stuttgart. It was attended by 230 radiologists from 17 countries. The aim was to select a certain number of subjects in diagnostic radiology and in each to have a broad spectrum overview reviewing recent advances presented by an acknowledged expert, followed by a series of rather more detailed papers on various aspects of that field, again given by acknowledged experts drawn from countries throughout Europe and also from the United States of America. This series of presentations on a theme was then followed later the same day by a "workshop" discussion at which the speakers, sometimes joined by other experts from collateral fields of interest, acted as a panel for discussion with the over-view speaker acting as moderator.

The whole concept of this course, ranging from the selection of subjects for presentation, through the high calibre of speakers and their presentations, to the enthusiasm with which participants joined in the workshop discussions, was an enormous success. Presentations were enhanced by the use of triple projection a new feature to the majority of European speakers, but with which they grappled masterfully and successfully. The conference hall specifically designed for such occasions was the ideal venue for a meeting of this sort, and provided all that the participants and speakers required. The attendance at the course was large enough to be viable and small enough to be friendly so that the participants combined into a group that was cohesive and was able to indulge fully in the most educational of all pursuits – open discussion with peers and teachers taking part.

The course was sponsored by the European Association of Radiology (EAR), which is more and more taking part in guiding and supporting educational activities throughout Europe, and by the College d'Enseignement Post-Universitaire de Radiologie (C. E. P. U. R.). With the increasing interest in and the increasing number of candidates coming forward for the examination for the Diploma in Radiology of the European Association it is to be hoped that the organisers will continue their efforts and establish this course as a regular event. They are to be congratulated on their efforts and encouraged to repeat it regularly. Both the concept and the putting of it into practice were ideal. A social programme was arranged successfully by Dr. H. H. Ellegast of Salzburg. In the very lovely city of Salzburg and the surrounding country it was well conceived, beautifully executed and kept the participants and their wives fully occupied.

I commend these proceedings to you.

J. H. Middlemiss, C. M. G.
President, Commission on Education
European Association of Radiology

Introduction

Recent advances in medical imaging have led to an unprecedented accumulation of new knowledge. Information previously in accessible by any imaging technique has become available, as in computerized tomography of the brain. Furthermore, ultrasound and computerized tomography have led to the replacement of a number of invasive X-ray procedures, such as pneumencephalography and in some cases arteriography.

In terms of patient management as well, radiologists have assumed a major role in the field of interventional radiology. Radiologic procedures are successful in certain peripheral vascular lesions and biliary tract problems, thereby providing an alternative to surgical procedures involving high risk because of patient age or concurrent disease.

At a time of such profound change in our specialty it seemed appropriate that radiologists from different countries should participate in a review of radiology of today. Hence, a multinational symposium was held in Salzburg, Austria, in June 1980, bringing together experts from Europe and the North American continent. They discussed the important and practical advances of diagnostic radiology, nuclear medicine, and ultrasound as they contribute to gastrointestinal, urologic, skeletal, cardiovascular, pediatric and neuroradiology.

These contributions were presented in the format of overviews, single subject presentations, and workshops. We feel that this material lends itself well to the publication of a yearbook, updating our knowledge to the year 1980. It is hoped that "Radiology Today" will convey to our readership the significant advances in radiology at a truly revolutionary time.

It is with much gratitude that we acknowledge the assistance of Mrs. Brigitte Bast in preparing the symposium and the publication of this book. The social-program in Salzburg was selected and arranged by Mrs. Pauli Ellegast. Her contribution provided a delightful frame for all participants in "Radiology Today" Salzburg 1980.

Martin W. Donner
Friedrich H. W. Heuck

Contents

List of Contributors

Archer, R.
St. Louis University, School of Medicine, Department of Radiology,
510 South Kingshighway Boulevard, St. Louis, MO 63110 (USA)

Aronberg, D. J.
St. Louis University, School of Medicine, Department of Radiology,
510 South Kingshighway Boulevard, St. Louis, MO 63110 (USA)

Atzinger, A.
Städtisches Krankenhaus, Radiologische Abteilung,
Bischof-Pilgrim-Strasse 1, D-8390 Passau

Baert, A. L.
Katholieke Universiteit Leuven, Universitaire Ziekenhuizen,
Diagnostische Radiologie, Capucijnenvoer 35, B-3000 Leuven

Baleriaux, D.
Institut Bordet, Service de Radiodiagnostic, B-1000 Bruxelles

Beyer, D.
Radiologisches Institut, Radiologisches Institut,
Joseph-Stelzmann-Strasse 9, D-5000 Köln 41

Böttger, E.
Klinikum der Stadt Mannheim, Institut für Klinische Radiologie,
Fakultät für Klinische Medizin,
Theodor-Kutzer-Ufer, D-6800 Mannheim 1

Bollaert, A.
Hôpital Universitaire Saint-Pierre, Service de Radiodiagnostic,
Rue Haute, 322, B-1000 Bruxelles

Borcke, E.
AGFA-GEVAERT-Technikum, Anwendungstechnik Röntgen,
Kistlerhofstrasse 75, D-8000 München 70

Bosniak, M. A.
New York University Medical Center,
550 First Avenue, New York, NY 10016 (USA)

Breit, A.
Städtisches Krankenhaus, Radiologische Abteilung,
Bischof-Pilgrim-Strasse 1, D-8390 Passau

Buchmann, F.
c/o C. H. F. Müller Unternehmensbereich der Philips GmbH,
Alexanderstrasse 1, D-2000 Hamburg 1

Clauss, W.
Schering AG, Fachbereich Medizin, Department Radiologie,
Müllerstrasse 170–178, D-1000 Berlin 65

Cleare, H. M.
Eastman Kodak Company, Receiving Department Kodak Park,
66 Eastman Avenue, Rochester, NY 14650 (USA)

Deininger, H. K.
Strahleninstitut der Städtischen Kliniken,
Grafenstrasse 9, D-6100 Darmstadt

Döhring, W.
Medizinische Hochschule Hannover, Institut für Klinische Radiologie,
Karl-Wiechert-Allee 9, D-3000 Hannover 61

Doppmann, J.
Diagnostic Radiology Department, NIH, The Clinical Center,
Building 10, Room 6S211, Bethesda, MD 20205 (USA)

Ekelund, L.
University Hospital, Department of Diagnostic Radiology,
S-22185 Lund

Feifel, G.
Ludwig-Maximilians-Universität, Klinikum Grosshadern,
Chirurgische Klinik, Marchioninistrasse 15, D-8000 München 70

Feser, J.-A.
c/o C. H. F. Müller, Unternehmensbereich der Philips GmbH,
Abteilung Nuklearmedizin, Alexanderstrasse 1, D-2000 Hamburg 1

Fraser, R. G.
The University of Alabama in Birmingham, School of Medicine,
Department of Diagnostic Radiology,
619 South 19th Street, Birmingham, AL 35233 (USA)

Freiberger, R. H.
Cornell University Medical College, Department of Radiology,
535 East 70th Street, New York, NY 10021 (USA)

Friedrich, M.
Klinikum Steglitz, Abteilung für Röntgendiagnostik,
Hindenburgdamm 30, D-1000 Berlin 45

Frommhold, W.
Universität Tübingen, Medizinisches Strahleninstitut,
Röntgenweg 11, D-7400 Tübingen

Fürste, H. O.
Universitäts-Kinderklinik, Abteilung Pädiatrische Kardiologie,
Mathildenstrasse 1, D-7800 Freiburg/Brsg.

Gebauer, A.
Ludwig-Maximilians-Universität, Klinikum Grosshadern,
Radiologische Klinik und Poliklinik,
Marchioninistrasse 15, D-8000 München 70

Georgi, M.
Klinikum der Stadt Mannheim, Institut für Klinische Radiologie,
Fakultät für Klinische Medizin,
Theodor-Kutzer-Ufer, D-6800 Mannheim 1

Haap, K.
Universitäts-Kinderklinik, Abteilung Pädiatrische Kardiologie,
Mathildenstrasse 1, D-7800 Freiburg

Hauke, R.
Firma CGR Koch & Sterzel, Kruppstrasse 82–96, D-4300 Essen 1

Auf der Heide, J. F.
St. Louis University, School of Medicine, Department of Radiology,
510 South Kingshighway Boulevard, St. Louis, MO 63110 (USA)

Hotton, F.
Hôpital Universitaire Saint-Pierre, Service de Radiodiagnostic,
Rue Haute, 322, B-1000 Bruxelles

Jacobson, H. G.
Montefiore Hospital and Medical Center,
Albert Einstein College of Medicine, Department of Radiology,
111 East 210th Street, Bronx, NY 10467 (USA)

Jaschke, W.
Klinikum der Stadt Mannheim, Institut für Klinische Radiologie,
Fakultät für Klinische Medizin,
Theodor-Kutzer-Ufer, D-6800 Mannheim 1

Kempmann, G.
Klinikum der Stadt Mannheim, Institut für Klinische Radiologie,
Fakultät für Klinische Medizin,
Theodor-Kutzer-Ufer, D-6800 Mannheim 1

Kessler, M.
Ludwig-Maximilians-Universität, Klinikum Grosshadern,
Radiologische Klinik und Poliklinik,
Marchioninistrasse 15, D-8000 München 70

Khouri, N. F.
Johns Hopkins Medical Institutions,
Department of Radiology and Radiological Science,
601 N. Broadway, Baltimore, MD 21205 (USA)

Kröpelin, T.
Albert-Ludwigs-Universität, Zentrum Radiologie der Universität
Freiburg, Abteilung Röntgendiagnostik, Sektion Innere Medizin IV,
Hermann-Herder-Strasse 6, D-7800 Freiburg/Brsg.

Laufer, I.
Hospital of the University of Pennsylvania,
3400 Spruce Street, Philadelphia, PA 19104 (USA)

Leo, F. P.
Johns Hopkins Medical Institutions, Department of Radiology and
Radiological Science, 601 N. Broadway, Baltimore, MD 21205 (USA)

Linke, G.
Siemens AG, Bereich Medizinische Technik,
Henkestrasse 127, D-8520 Erlangen

Lissner, J.
Ludwig-Maximilians-Universität, Klinikum Grosshadern,
Radiologische Klinik, Marchioninistrasse 15, D-8000 München 70

Mannesmann, G.
Schering AG, Pharma Forschung,
Abteilung Herz-Kreislauf-Pharmakologie,
Müllerstrasse 170 – 178, 1000 Berlin 65

Marchal, G.
Katholieke Universiteit Leuven, Universitaire Ziekenhuizen,
Diagnostische Radiologie, Capucijnenvoer 35, B-3000 Leuven

Mayr, B.
Ludwig-Maximilians-Universität, Klinikum Grosshadern,
Klinik für Radiologie, Röntgen A,
Marchioninistrasse 15, D-8000 München 70

Meyers, M. A.
State University of New York at Stony Brook,
Health Sciences Center, Department of Radiology,
Stony Brook, NY 11794 (USA)

Meyers, P. H.
401 Emerald Street, New Orleans, LA 70124 (USA)

Middlemiss, J. H.
University of Bristol, The Medical School,
Department of Radiodiagnosis,
University Walk, GB-Bristol BS8 1TD

Miklautz, H.
Schering AG, Fachbereich Physikochemie und Informatik,
Department Allgemeine Physikochemie,
Müllerstrasse 170 – 178, D-1000 Berlin 65

Miller, R. E.
Indiana University Medical Center, Department of Radiology,
1100 West Michigan Street, Indianapolis, IN 46223 (USA)

Moseley, I. F.
The National Hospital, Lysholm Radiological Department,
Queen Square, GB-London WC1N 3BG

Mützel, W.
Schering AG, Pharma Forschung, Abteilung Biodynamik,
Müllerstrasse 170 – 178, D-1000 Berlin 65

Nadjmi, M.
Universität Würzburg, Kopfklinik, Abteilung für Neuroradiologie,
Josef-Schneider-Strasse 11, D-8700 Würzburg

Nickel, O.
Städtisches Krankenhaus, Radiologische Abteilung,
Bischof-Pilgrim-Strasse 1, D-8390 Passau

Nickoloff, E. L.
John Hopkins Medical Institutions,
Department of Radiology and Radiological Science,
601 N. Broadway, Baltimore, MD 21205 (USA)

Paulin, S.
Harvard Medical School, Beth Israel Hospital,
Department of Radiology,
330 Brookline Avenue, Boston, MA 02215 (USA)

Peters, P. E.
Universität Köln, Radiologisches Institut,
Joseph-Stelzmann-Strasse 9, D-5000 Köln 41

Pfeiler, M.
Siemens AG, Unternehmensbereich Medizinische Technik,
Henkestrasse 127, D-8520 Erlangen

Piepgras, U.
Universität des Saarlandes, Medizinische Fakultät,
Abteilung für Neuroradiologie, D-6650 Homburg/Saar

Piroth, D.
Marienhospital, Onkologische- und Radiologische Abteilung,
Rochusstrasse 2, D-4000 Düsseldorf 30

Pokieser, H.
Universität Wien, Zentrales Institut für Radiodiagnostik,
Allgemeines Krankenhaus, Alser Strasse 4, A-1090 Wien

Ponette, E.
Katholieke Universiteit Leuven, Universitaire Ziekenhuizen,
Diagnostische Radiologie, Capucijnenvoer 35, B-3000 Leuven

Pullicino, P.
525 Goler House, Rochester, NY 14620 (USA)

Rohde, U.
Städtisches Krankenhaus, Radiologische Abteilung,
Bischof-Pilgrim-Strasse 1, D-8390 Passau

Sagel, S. S.
Washington University, School of Medicine,
The Edward Mallinkrodt Institute of Radiology,
510 South Kingshighway, St. Louis, MO 63110 (USA)

Sanders, R. C.
Johns Hopkins Medical Institutions,
Department of Radiology and Radiological Science
601 N. Broadway, Baltimore, MD 21205 (USA)

Schad, N.
Städtisches Krankenhaus, Radiologische Abteilung,
Bischof-Pilgrim-Strasse 1, D-8390 Passau

Scherer, U.
Ludwig-Maximilians-Universität, Klinikum Grosshadern,
Radiologische Klinik, Marchioninistrasse 15, D-8000 München 70

Schmidt-Redemann, B.
Universitäts-Kinderklinik, Abteilung für Pädiatrische Kardiologie,
Mathildenstrasse 1, D-7800 Freiburg

Schmiedel, E.
Byk Gulden Lomberg, Chemische Fabrik GmbH,
Gyk-Gulden-Strasse 2, D-7750 Konstanz

Schöbel, C.
Schering AG, Fachbereich Vorklinische Entwicklung,
Department Experimentelle Toxikologie,
Müllerstrasse 170 – 178, D-1000 Berlin 65

Schröder, G.
Schering AG, Pharma Forschung,
Abteilung Herz-Kreislauf-Pharmakologie,
Müllerstrasse 170 – 178, D-1000 Berlin 65

Sellink, J. L.
Rijnsburgerweg 17, NL-2334 BC Leiden

Siefert, H.-M.
Schering AG, Fachbereich Vorklinische Entwicklung,
Department Röntgenkontrastmittel,
Müllerstrasse 170 – 178, D-1000 Berlin 65

Siegelman, S. S.
Johns Hopkins Medical Institutions,
Department of Radiology and Radiological Science,
601 N. Broadway, Baltimore, MD 21205 (USA)

Siegmund, F.
Schering AG, Fachbereich Vorklinische Entwicklung,
Department Experimentelle Toxikologie,
Müllerstrasse 170 – 178, D-1000 Berlin 65

Smedt de, E.
Akademisch Ziekenhuis VUB, Bosstraat, B-1090 Bruxelles

Sommer, B.
Ludwig-Maximilians-Universität, Klinikum Grosshadern,
Radiologische Klinik, Marchioninistrasse 15, D-8000 München 70

Speck, U.
Schering AG, Pharma-Forschung, Abteilung Biodynamik,
Müllerstrasse 170 – 178, D-1000 Berlin 65

Stanley, R. J.
St. Louis University, School of Medicine, Department of Radiology,
510 South Kingshighway Boulevard, St. Louis, MO 63110 (USA)

Stender, H.-St.
Medizinische Hochschule Hannover, Institut für Klinische Radiologie,
Karl-Wiechert-Allee 9, D-3000 Hannover 61

Stitik, F. P.
Johns Hopkins Medical Institutions,
Department of Radiology and Radiological Science,
601 N. Broadway, Baltimore, MD 21205 (USA)

Voigt, K.
Medizinisches Strahleninstitut der Universität,
Abteilung für Neuroradiologie, Oslandstrasse 22, D-7400 Tübingen

Wagner, H. N.
Johns Hopkins Medical Institutions,
Department of Radiology and Radiological Science,
601 N. Broadway, Baltimore, MD 21205 (USA)

Wegelius, U.
The University Central Hospital of Turku, Department of Radiology,
SF-20520 Turku 52

Weinmann, H. J.
Schering AG, Pharma-Forschung, Abteilung Biodynamik,
Müllerstrasse 170 – 178, D-1000 Berlin 65

Weiss, H.
Philips Forschungslaboratorium,
Vogt-Kölln-Strasse 30, D-2000 Hamburg 34

Wende, S.
Neurochirurgische Universitätsklinik, Abteilung für Neuroradiologie,
Langenbeckstrasse 1, D-6500 Mainz

Wenzel-Hora, B. I.
Schering AG, Fachbereich Medizin, Department Radiologie,
Müllerstrasse 170 – 178, D-1000 Berlin 65

Wetzel, E.
Klinikum der Stadt Mannheim, Institut für Klinische Radiologie,
Fakultät für Klinische Medizin,
Theodor-Kutzer-Ufer, D-6800 Mannheim 1

White, R. I.
Johns Hopkins Medical Institutions,
Department of Radiology and Radiological Science,
601 N. Broadway, Baltimore, MD 21205 (USA)

Wozney, P.
General Electric Company, Medical Systems Division,
Post Office Box 414, Milwaukee, WI 53201 (USA)

Zeitler, E.
Klinikum Nürnberg, Radiologisches Zentrum,
Flurstrasse 17, D-8500 Nürnberg

Zerhouni, E. A.
Johns Hopkins Medical Institutions,
Department of Radiology and Radiological Science,
601 N. Broadway, Baltimore, MD 21205 (USA)

Cardiovascular Radiology

Cardiovascular Radiology: Overview

S. Paulin

Harvard Medical School, Beth Israel Hospital, Department of Radiology,
330 Brookline Avenue, Boston, MA 02215 (USA)

The impact of modern development in imaging technology and computer sciences on the practice of clinical medicine has been profound. Undoubtedly, this development has increased our medical diagnostic and therapeutic potentials. However, it also caused a spiraling increase of costs because of advanced complexity of the procedures as well as greater demand for their use. Experts in health care planning, whose primary goal at present is cost containment, begin to speak of the so-called technology crisis in medicine. Recent developments in the field of cardiac imaging, the topic of this presentation, have not been free from these troubles, and it will be in order for me to include appropriate comments on the subject in this overview.

For didactic reasons, I have grouped the major modalities of radiologic imaging:

1. Plain film radiography
2. Angiography
3. Emission Imaging
4. Computerized tomography.

Plain film radiography of the chest is still one of the most widely practiced examinations and, although limited in its ability to render specific cardiac diagnoses, it improves significantly the accuracy with which the patient's degree of cardiovascular impairment can be judged. Radiologic findings such as cardiac size and changes in pulmonary vascular pattern, proven in the past to be valuable and reproducible parameters, have again been tested on initially obtained chest X-rays from patients hospitalized for an acute myocardial infarction and were found to provide much information about early and late prognosis, allowing definition of low- and high-risk groups [1], as clearly supported by the figures in Table 1. It is interesting to note that this work was accomplished on radiographs obtained at the patient's bedside in order to meet the requirements for convenient examination of the critically ill patients. Apparently the practical limitations for technical standardization did not detract significantly from the diagnostic value of these films.

The performance of the so-called radiographic-cardiac series, which includes teleradiographs in frontal, lateral, and the two major oblique projections and which usually is combined with a performance of cardiac fluoroscopy by an experienced examiner, has lost much of its attractiveness, not least because of strong competition from other noninvasive diagnostic tests such as echocardiography and radioisotope examinations of the cardiovascular system. The number of requests for cardiac-radiographic examinations with plain films and fluoroscopy has declined significantly over the years as judged from my own experience in my

Table 1. Initial chest X-rays [1]

Radiologic findings	Survival		
	30 days	6 months	1 year
Normal	98%	97%	94%
Enlarged heart no congestion	86%	81%	79%
No enlarged heart pulm. congestion	62%	53%	45%
Enlarged heart pulm. congestion	58%	47%	39%
Severe pulmonary edema	18%	9%	0%

Radiology Today 1. Ed. by M. W. Donner and F. H. W. Heuck

Table 2. Cinefluoroscopy vs left ventricular angiography [2]

	Observer 1	Observer 2	Observer agreement
Correct	44%	46%	52%
False (−)	41%	24%	
False (+)	24%	29%	

Total material = 113 cases
Of 16 left ventricular aneurysms — Obs. 1 identified 3 cases; Obs. 2 identified 7 cases

department, and the final and perhaps mortal blow to this examination came when Sos and colleagues evaluated the capability of cinefluoroscopy to detect left ventricular contraction abnormalities or aneurysms in comparison with selective left ventriculography [2]. Two experienced observers were asked to identify areas of motions abnormality on cine films of the heart and these findings were related to the presence of aneurysms and hypo- or akinetic portions of the left ventricular wall as demonstrated in selective left ventriculography. As obvious from Table 2, the results were very discouraging, indicating not only an unacceptably high percentage of false negative and false positive diagnoses, but also poor agreement between the two expert observers. Most remarkable was that out of the angiographically documented 16 left ventricular aneurysms, one observer identified three and the other seven cases only. These results lead to the statement by the authors that cinefluoroscopy for evaluation of left ventricular contractility is grossly inaccurate and that it should not be performed.

Remaining indications for fluoroscopy would then be the detection and localization of intracardiac calcifications. In this respect, cineradiographic recordings are more sensitive than ultrasonic examinations in the detection of abnormal calcium deposits in abnormal heart valves. The increasing availability of high definition cesium-iodide image intensifiers increased also the interest to explore the possible predictive value of coronary calcification as detected by fluoroscopy. In an extensive study based on the examination of 360 patients, Bartel and co-workers [3] claimed as strong relationship between detectable coronary calcium and the presence of significant coronary artery disease as demonstrated on the subsequently performed coronary arteriograms. Although many patients with significant coronary stenosis had no detectable coronary calcifications by fluoroscopy (false negatives, 44%), the authors were impressed by the high specificity of a positive coronary calcification since only 3% false positives were found in their material. It has, however, to be emphasized that the original material used for this study consisted of a largely symptomatic population; all, indeed, were found to have a symptomatology strong enough to submit them to the angiographic test. Thus, it is likely that the frequency of coronary calcification in an asymptomatic or outpatient population would be much lower. This, again, raises questions as to the authors' recommendation that fluoroscopy should become a widely applicable technique for screening large patient populations. Obviously, this recommendation omitted considerations concerning radiation exposure which, parenthetically, are quite appreciable in fluoroscopic examinations.

Most recently a technical refinement of the old slit-kymography applicable to chest radiographs has been developed and introduced in the market under the name of "Interlaced ECG-Gated Radiography" [4]. A movable mask consisting of an array of parallel 3 mm wide lead strips is interposed between the patient and the film cassettes. The mask and the X-ray exposures are controlled by a physiologic synchronizer. Following a first exposure triggered to occur in diastole, the mask is advanced to its second position in which the lead strips shield the previously exposed film and a second exposure occurs during the systolic heart phase. The film shows an interlacing or interdigitation of the two sequential exposures in which stationary anatomic structures appear substantially as they would in ordinary films. Moving structures, such as the border of heart and great vessels, have a serrated appearance that allows the measurement of the amplitude of pulsation. The technique differs from conventional slit-kymography inasmuch as it only displays the end systolic and end-diastolic position of the cardiac contours. It does not record the motion pattern continuously during the entire heart cycle

Table 3. Ventriculography [4]

Interlaced radiography	Normal	Hypokinesis	Severe hypokinesis	Paradoxical motion
Paradoxical	1			3
Akinesis			17	1
0 – 1.5 mm	1	4	4	
> 1.5 mm	47	1	1	

as is, for example, accomplished by conventional slit- or electrokymography. On the other hand, the authors [4] are of the opinion that this new "intergated" technique has a much less detrimental effect on the quality of chest X-ray and suggest that it may substitute for the widely performed standard chest X-ray. Initial experience with this technique has shown that it is capable of documenting cardiovascular motion abnormalities as they occur in conjunction with valve lesions, for example, aortic insufficiency, and of documenting their subsequent normalization following surgical correction. Comparative studies between interlaced ECG-gated radiographs on which amplitude measurements of 0.5 mm accuracy were performed with calipers and left ventricular angiography have shown a strong positive correlation (Table 3). Again, these initial results were obtained from a relatively small and selected patient material, and further studies are required to explore the reliability and practicality of this technique.

Cardiac angiography has solidified its position as the most definitive and accurate diagnostic method for anatomic evaluation of cardiac abnormalities and certain functional parameters as well. It has been estimated that several hundred thousand coronary angiograms and left ventricular angiograms are performed per year in the United States alone. The recording technique of preference is cinematography, the quality of which has improved significantly over the past decade due to the introduction of certain technical innovations, of which the cesium-iodide image intensifier deserves to be mentioned specifically. The need for large size film series has almost disappeared completely.

A more recent technical innovation is the design of X-ray stands that allow a more flexible radiographic examination of the heart in multidirectional views, responding to a general request from angiographers who felt limited by the rather rigid arrangement of X-ray equipment in the older conventional designs. In particular, proper evaluation of the coronary arteries posed difficulties when certain critical segments could not be projected in reasonable perpendicular views or without significant overlapping by other simultaneously filled vascular structures. A number of different stands allowing for oblique, caudal, and cranial X-ray beam angulation are available on the market and are widely used in the performance of selective coronary arteriography [5, 6]. With the availability of these devices, projectional improvements for angiographic delineation of cardiac chambers and large vessels have also been accomplished. Incorporation of the so-called half-axial left anterior oblique view to biplane angiography of the left ventricle significantly improved the statistical correlation between cardiac output determined by thermodilution technique and the angiographic volumetry of the left ventricular cavity (Fig. 1) [7]. This technique also improved, by increasing the surface contour of the septal and lateral wall of the left ventricle, the ability to detect wall motion abnormalities related to septal and lateral myocardial infarctions which otherwise would have remained undetected. This modified biplane technique also opens the possibility for more precise wall motion analysis since measurement of systolic shortening of diameters can be performed at equal distance from the left ventricular apex in both projections (Fig. 2). The tilted view has also been found useful for the evaluation of certain congenital abnormalities such as differentiation of subtypes of ventricular septal defects, better definition of aortic over-riding, and the delineation of segmental stenosis of the pulmonary artery bifurcation [8].

The concept of arterial spasm as the cause of angina pectoris, myocardial ischemia, and infarction has reentered the medical arena and at present dominates clinical and experimental research efforts [9, 10, 11, 12]. Dr. Wegelius addresses himself to this subject in his presentation, in which he also presents the present status of transluminal angioplasty of the coronary arteries, a method which has invoked great attention, both inducing optimistic hopes and cautious words of reservation.

Angiographers, cardiologists, or radiologists became increasingly more cognizant of the subjectivity inherent in the conventional angiographic

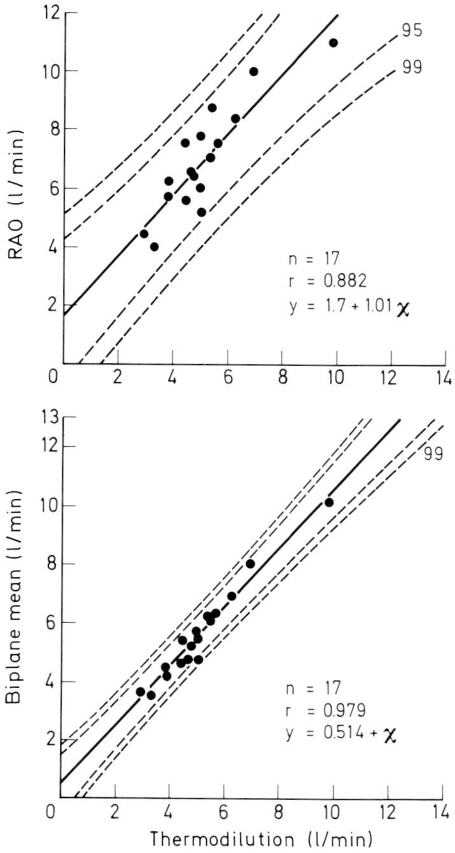

Fig. 1. *Above:* Single plane RAO cardiac output vs thermodilution cardiac output. *Below:* Angiographic cardiac output determined with biplane technique including LAO cranial tilt view vs thermodilution cardiac output. Note the significantly improved correlation between the two methods [27]

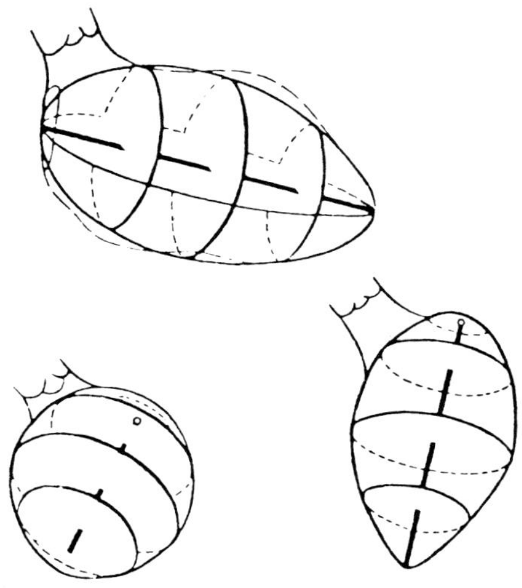

Fig. 2. Schematic drawing of left ventricle also illustrating three equidistant planes located perpendicularly to the long axis. *Above:* As seen in RAO view. *Right below:* As seen in cranial tilt view. The largest diameters of the planes can be identified in both views. The marked foreshortened display of the left ventricle in the conventional LAO projection precludes identification of the diameter's endpoints and thus proper measurements of circumferential shortening [27]

interpretations and the thereto related shortcomings that arise in comparative studies between angiographic findings and other parameters that are presented quantitatively. With regard to coronary arteriography, there are basically two different approaches. One aims at the determination of contrast edges that occur at the vascular borders and distance measurements between them [13]. The other determines densitometric profiles extracted from cine films that have been submitted to high precision densitometry with an electrooptical scanner, the density distribution of which has been fed into a computer [14]. Although both approaches decrease significantly the intraobserver error (Table 4), it has to be recognized that the angiographic determination of the degree of vascular narrowing cannot simply be translated in resistance and flow reduction. It also has to be remembered that the selective coronary angiogram is usually performed with the patient in resting condition, during which time regional flow deficits are unlikely to occur. Efforts have also been made to measure the intensity of contrast accumulation in the periphery of the coronary circulation. Experimental and a few preliminary clinical studies on selective coronary arteriograms have demonstrated that densitometric techniques have the potential to depict the so-called peripheral myocardial contrast blush; however, studies on the isolated heart have also shown that significant alterations in blush intensity can be observed following different contrast agents and when injections are performed repetitively [15, 16].

Table 4. Analysis of intraobserver error [14]

Observer	Slope	Standard error of estimate
1	-0.219 ± 0.044	2.63
2	-0.228 ± 0.034	2.35
3	-0.158 ± 0.036	2.34
1 + 2 + 3	-0.205 ± 0.023	2.54

Improvements in roentgenographic contrast agents have been made continuously and Dr. Speck presents some of the most recent research results within this book. With regard to clinically performed angiocardiography and selective coronary angiography, contrast side-effects have played a relatively small role as a cause of severe complications. Calcium-ameliorated contrast agents, widely used in European centers during the last decade, were not available to cardiac angiographers in the United States. In the experimental laboratory using the isolated heart model, we observed that this beneficial effect did not apply to conditions of underperfusion, i.e., simulating the presence of myocardial ischemia. Thus, we were warned not to use this contrast preparation when examining patients in critical conditions and suffering from regional myocardial ischemia at the time of the examination [17].

Under the term emission imgaging. I have listed the different varieties of radioisotope procedures that are used increasingly in the diagnostic workup of cardiac patients:

1. Radionuclide angiocardiography
   Anatomy, transit times, cardiac output shunts – detection and quantitation
2. Radionuclide ventriculography
   Global function, regional function relative chamber size, changes with stress
3. Myocardial perfusion scintigraphy
   Myocardial ischemia, myocardial infarction
4. Pyrophosphates scintigraphy
   Acute stages of myocardial injury
5. Myocardial metabolic studies
   Fractional oxygen extraction'
   Fatty acid uptake
6. Lung Scan
   Regional lung perfusion and ventilation

In my personal opinion as an angiographer, these techniques have made startling progress in becoming increasingly refined and sensitive, allowing the detection not only of global, but also of regional functional abnormalities of the left ventricle. The considerably less invasive nature of these tests also permits their sequential use and, not least important, their performance during the resting conditions as well as under cardiac stress. These techniques have the great potential to become the most valuable complementary study to the coronary arteriogram, particularly in those instances where the translation of topographic changes in the coronary arteries into hemodynamic parameters cannot be accomplished. Dr. Wagner brings us up to the present state of the art in his presentation.

Finally, a few comments should be made concerning the most recent research development that will probably influence the future practice of cardiac radiology. CT scanning has not yet made a significant impact on clinical cardiac diagnosis, a fact which is related to the present scanning equipment's inability to generate images fast enough to demonstrate the rapidly moving heart. Electrocardiographic gating of the exposures over several heart beats have overcome some of these problems and, for example, allowed the determination of left ventricular wall thickness [17] or identification of the patency of coronary artery bypass graft merely requiring intravenous injection of moderate amounts of contrast agents [18]. Practical work is being undertaken to develop cardiac CT scanners using exposures of millisecond duration [19] which should allow the precise and three-dimensional delineation of heart structures. The radiographic contrast agent itself may find a use as a direct tracer for the localization of ischemic cardiac tissue [20]. Only a few weeks ago, the first prototype of a dynamic-three dimensional reconstructor was installed at the Mayo Clinic as a result of the many years of intense research efforts by Dr. Earl Wood and his associates [21]. The potentials of this equipment with regard to image reconstruction and enhancement appear to be unlimited. However, the enthusiasm of an angiographer may be dampened slightly when considering the dimensions and complexity of this equipment weighing 17 tons, including 28 X-ray tubes and image intensifiers in a 6 m long aluminum gantry and being coupled to a very large computer for data storage and analysis.

Still another innovated form of medical imaging has been described recently, which is based on the principle of nuclear magnetic resonance (NMR) [22]. Images of small animals and portions of extremities of the human body were produced with this technique with amazing detail and clarity [23]. Most recently NMR images of the chest including mediastinal structures and the heart of humans were successfully produced using this principle (Fig. 3). As can be seen from the illustrated sample, this noninvasive and nonradiation generating system is able to identify the gross structures of the chest and to differentiate between chest wall, spine, lungs, and heart, and may possibly even discriminate between the different cardiac cavities and the myocardium. It is difficult to predict how long it will take for NMR imaging technology to become commercially available on a

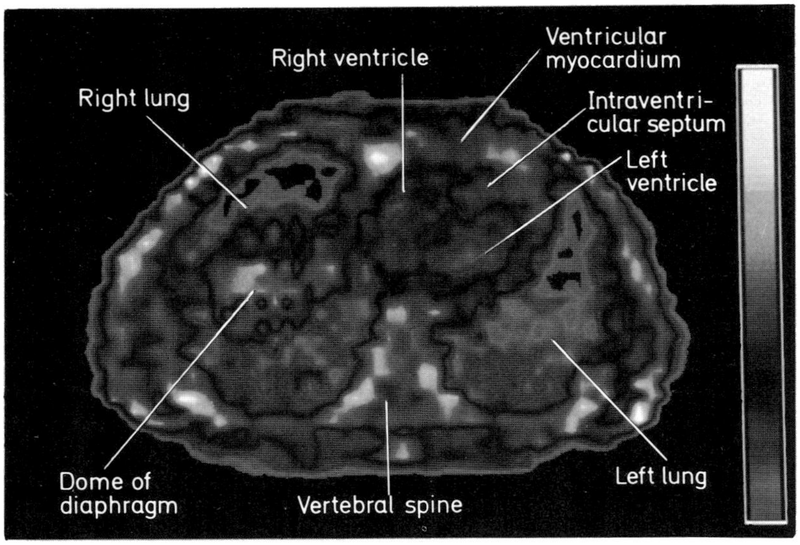

Fig. 3. NMR image of human thorax at level of the dome clearly illustrating structures such as the chest wall, spine, lungs, dome of diaphragm, heart, ventricular myocardium, interventricular septum, and cardiac chambers. This picture was obtained on QED-80 whole body scanner and reproduced with the permission of Fonar Corporation, Melville, New York

larger scale, and it is also difficult to calculate the cost of such equipment once it has reached the stage where it becomes an important and useful tool for clinical cardiologic diagnosis.

A less costly technique aiming at a similar goal, i.e., to allow imaging of cardiac chambers following intravenous injection of relatively small amounts of contrast agents, consists of so-called computerized fluoroscopy, which essentially is based on the principle of subtraction radiography [24]. The problem of patient immobilization for the entire period of contrast transit was in part overcome by developing the presentation of a so-called time interval difference imaging, subtracting, for example, the systolic left ventricular image from the most previously occurring diastolic image. An example of such subtraction generates an area of positive density in regions of ordinary inward motion, no contours in areas of akinesis, and images of negative density in areas of paradoxical motion [25]. Results from early experience appears to be encouraging, at least in the minds of the authors. The practicality of these approaches to clinical medicine and cardiology will have to await further testing.

References

1. Battler A, Karliner JS, Higgins CB, Slutsky R, Gilpin EA, Froelicher VF, Ross J Jr. (1980) The initial chest X-ray in acute myocardial infarction: prediction of early and late mortality and survival. Circulation 61/5:1004 – 1009
2. Sos T, Sniderman KW, Levin DC, Buckmann CF (1979) Cinefluoroscopy in evaluating left ventricular contractility and aneurysms. Radiology 133:31 – 39
3. Bartel AG, Chen JT, Peter RH, Behar VS, Kong K, Lester RG (1974) The significance of coronary calcification detected by fluoroscopy. Circulation 49:1247 – 1252
4. Dinsmore RE, Wernikoff RE, Miller SW, Pohost GM, Blick PC, Potsaid MS (1979) Evaluation of left ventricular free wall asynergy due to coronary artery disease: use of an interlaced ECG-gated radiography system. AJR 132:909 – 914
5. Bunnell IL, Green DG, Tandon RN, Arani DT (1973) The half-axial projection – a new look at the proximal left coronary artery. Circulation 48: 1151 – 1156
6. Eldh P, Silverman JF (1974) Methods of studying the proximal left anterior descending coronary artery. Radiology 113:738 – 740
7. Als AV, Paulin S, Aroesty J (1978) Biplane angiographic volumetry using the right anterior oblique and half-axila left anterior oblique technique. Radiology 126/2:511 – 514
8. Fellows KE, Kean JF, Freed MD (1977) Angled views in cine angiocardiography of congenital heart disease. Circulation 56:485 – 490
9. Maseri A, L'Abbate A, Chierchia S et al. (1979) Significance of spasm in the pathogenesis of ischemic heart disease. Am J Cardiol 44(5):788
10. Oliva P, Potts D, Pluss R (1974) Coronary arterial spasm in Prinzmetal angina: documentation by coronary arteriography. N Engl J Med 288:746
11. Cipriano PR, Guthaner DF, Orlick AE, Ricci DR, Wexler L, Silverman JF (1979) The effects of ergonovine maleate on coronary arterial size. Circulation 59:82

12. Heupler F, Proudfit W, Razavi M, Shirey EK, Greenstreet R, Sheldon WC (1978) Ergonovine maleate provocative test for coronary arterial spasm. Am J Cardiol 41:631
13. Brown BF, Bolson E, Fimer M, Dodge HT (1977) Quantitative coronary arteriography. Circulation 55: 329 – 337
14. Sandor T, Als AV, Paulin S (1979) Cine-densitometric measurement of coronary arterial stenosis. Cathet Cardiovasc Diagn 5:229 – 245
15. Paulin S, Sandor T, Serur JR, Als AV (1980) Densitometric analysis of myocardial contrast blush: preliminary results from experiments in isolated dog hearts. Annual Meeting of the North American Society for Cardiac Angiography, April 24 – 25, 1980, San Francisco, California
16. Sandor T, Paulin S, Sridhar B (1977) Densitometric evaluation of myocardial contrast accumulation. SPIE 127, Optical Instrumentation in Medicine VI: 349 – 352
17. Als AV, Serur JR, LaRaia PJ, Paulin S (1978) Differential effects of sodium meglumine calcium metrizoate on the inotropic state of normal and ischemic myocardium. Radiology 128:499 – 501
18. Skioldebrand CG, Ovenfors C, Mavroudis C, Lipton MS (1980) Assessment of ventricular wall thickness in vivo by computer transmission tomography. Circulation 61/5:960 – 965
19. Brundage BH, Lipton MH, Herfkens RJ, Berninger WH, Redington RW, Chatterjee K, Carlsson E (1980) Detection of patent coronary bypass grafts by computed tomography: a preliminary report. Circulation 61/4:826 – 831
20. Boyd D: Physics of cardiac computerized tomography gating versus millisecond scan acquisition. Annual Meeting of the North American Society for Cardiac Angiography, April 24 – 25, 1980, San Francisco, California
21. Higgins C: The detection and quantification of ischemic cardiac tissue by computerized tomography. Annual Meeting of the North American Society for Cardiac Angiography, April 24 – 25, 1980, San Francisco, California
24. Ritman E: Dynamic three dimensional reconstruction of the heart. Annual Meeting of the North American Society for Cardiac Angiography, April 24 – 25, 1980, San Francisco, California
25. Kruger RA, Mistretta CA et al. (1979) Computerized fluoroscopy in real time for noninvasive visualization of the cardiovascular system. Radiology 130:49 – 57
26. Kruger RA, Mistretta CA et al. (1979) Computerized fluoroscopy techniques for intravenous study of cardiac chamber dynamics. Investigative Radiol. 14:279 – 287
27. Paulin S (1979) Tilted views in cardiac angiography. Medicamundi 24/1:2 – 9
22. Lauterbur PC (1973) Image formation by induced local interactions: examples employing nuclear magnetic resonance. Nature 242:190 – 191
23. Hinshaw WS, Boltomly PA, Holland GN (1977) Radiographic thin-section image of the human wrist by nuclear magnetic resonance. Nature 270:722 – 723

Nuclear Cardiology

H. N. Wagner, Jr.

Johns Hopkins Medical Institutions, Divisions of Nuclear Medicine and Radiation Health Sciences, Radiology and Environmental Health Sciences, 615 North Wolfe Street, Baltimore, MD 21205 (USA)

Progress in medicine has followed advances in our perception of bodily structure and function as well as in our concept of disease processes. In 1806 with the publication of Corvisart's book *Diseases of the Heart,* "observation" of patients became "examination." Corvisart describes pericarditis, dilation and hypertrophy of the heart, and diseases of the heart muscle, valves, and aorta. His use of perfusion allowed him to surpass all his predecessors in clinical skills, and his book is full of excellent case histories and autopsy correlations. He propagated Auenbrugger's invention until, by 1825, it was used generally in Paris and had spread everywhere from there. With the use of percussion, medicine became less "conjectural." Corvisart was the inventor of the heart function test. His student René Laennec invented the stethoscope and then described it in his 1819 *Treatise on Mediate Auscultation and on the Diseases of the Lung and Heart.* Together, auscultation and percussion made possible a kind of living pathologic anatomy of anatomic pathology.

Einthoven developed the string galvanometer to record the electrical changes accompanying each heart beat. Soon, Sir Thomas Lewis began to use the instrument in England and to correlate resulting data with clinical observations. Today, the electrocardiogram is an indispensable aid to modern cardiologists. Electrocardiography and with it, modern cardiology, evolved from Einthoven's original development. The next major technical advance was the development of cardiac catheterization and contrast angiography, both essential to the growth of modern cardiovascular surgery.

Few persons realize that the first diagnostic uses of radioactive tracers were not in the study of the thyroid, but in the study of the heart. Blumgart and Weiss saw the potential of radioactive tracers in diagnosis and began their studies only a few years after Einthoven won the Nobel Prize. In 1927 they described their studies of normal persons and patients with heart disease. When we think about their use of radium salt solution as a tracer and a cloud chamber as a detector, we can appreciate the enormous advances made over the last half century. The prospect of using radioactive tracers to study the heart has now become a reality with the invention of suitable instruments and radioactive tracers.

The growth of the field of nuclear cardiology over the past few years can be seen in Fig. 1, which shows the increase in number of the two most common nuclear cardiology studies performed today in the Johns Hopkins Hospital, the thallium-201 myocardial perfusion study and the ventricular function test. Initially these studies were used primarily in the diagnosis of the cause of chest pain. They are also used in the differential

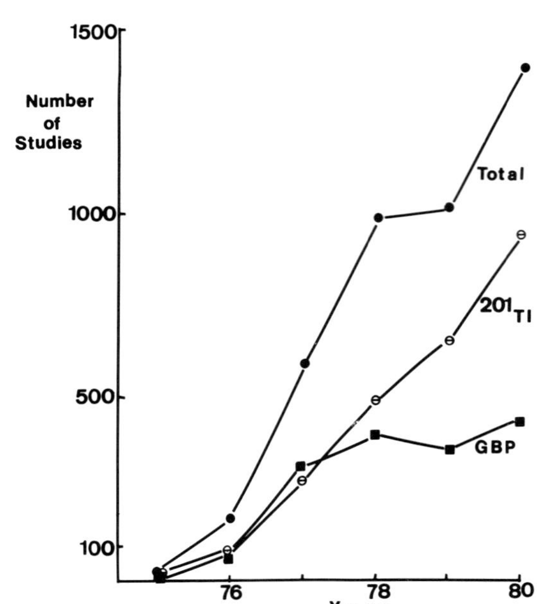

Fig. 1. Nuclear cardiovascular studies performed at the Johns Hopkins Hospital between 1975 and 1980

Radiology Today 1. Ed. by M. W. Donner and F. H. W. Heuck

diagnosis of patients with dyspnea, in patients with unexplained heart murmurs, and in children with cyanosis.

Measurements that can now be made with intravenous injection of radioactive tracers include:

1. Right and left ventricular volumes
2. Right and left ventricular hypertrophy
3. Cardiac output at rest and exercise
4. Mitral and aortic valvular regurgitation
5. Right-to-left and left-to-right shunt quantification
6. Global and regional wall motion of the right and left ventricle
7. Regional myocardial blood flow
8. Left ventricular work and power.

It will take years of further research to refine these measurements and define their precision, accuracy, indications, and utility, but even today we can conclude that they will probably continue to play a major role in clinical cardiology and cardiovascular research. For example, among the questions now being asked of these studies are the following:

1. What is the cause of the patient's chest pain?
2. What is the hemodynamic significance of electrocardiographic abnormalities such as premature ventricular beats and atrial fibrillation?
3. Has the patient had myocardial infarction?
4. How much of the left ventricular muscle is involved?
5. How recent is the infarction?
6. What is the patient's right and left ventricular function at rest, during exercise, or after drugs?
7. Does the patient have a ventricular aneurysm?
8. Does the patient have a complication of infarction such as mitral regurgitation or a ruptured septum?
9. Is the right ventricle affected by infarction?
10. Does the patient have transient ischemia in addition to fixed perfusion defects at rest?

In patients with dyspnea, the questions being asked include:

1. Does the patient have predominantly lung disease with normal cardiac function?
2. What is the relative involvement of perfusion and ventilation?
3. Does the patient have cor pulmonale as evidenced by right ventricular ejection fraction?
4. What is the relative involvement of the right ventricle, lungs, and left ventricle?

Although nuclear cardiology has been used for nearly a decade in the diagnosis of congenital heart disease, for example in differentiating cardiac from noncardiac causes of cyanosis, the use of these studies has not increased as dramatically as the use of those used to evaluate coronary heart disease. Echocardiography has become the screening procedure of choice in these patients. Nevertheless, in the detection of intracardiac shunts and complicated congenital diseases, the tracer studies are probably the most sensitive and accurate methods to quantitate left-to-right shunts.

Of course, the nuclear studies will never replace cardiac catheterization and contrast angiography. This is seen clearly in Fig. 2, which shows the concomitant increase in patients studied by cardiac catheterization at Johns Hopkins Hospital during the period of rapid growth of the nuclear studies (and echocardiography). Since each of the modalities – history, physical examination, electrocardiography, echocardiography, nuclear cardiology, cardiac catheterization, and contrast angiocardiography – provides a different type of information, that is, each assesses something different, it seems unlikely that one will replace the other. For many patients the noninvasive tests will replace the invasive studies. For example, it is no longer necessary to perform coronary angiography to exclude a diagnosis of coronary heart disease with 90% certainty in an airline pilot who had an abnormal electrocardiogram on routine examination, or to perform ventriculography to exclude aneurysm in patients with demonstrably diffuse hypokinesis. Noninvasive testing is also being used in patients for whom invasive studies are not

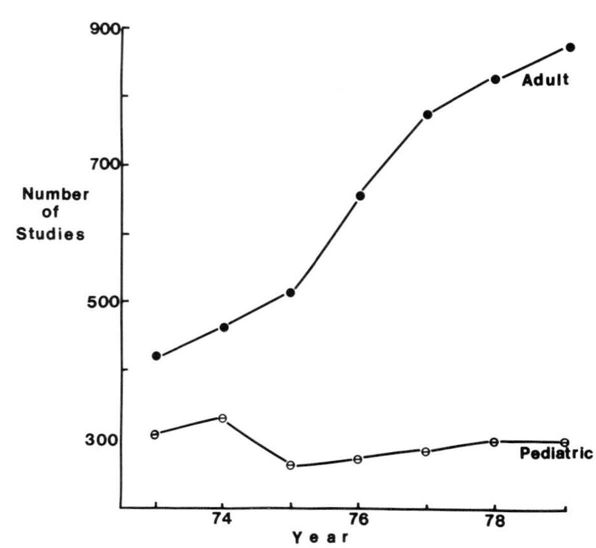

Fig. 2. Cardiac catheterizations performed at the Johns Hopkins Hospital

thought justified as a screening test. At times the noninvasive techniques reveal abnormalities at early stages when corrective measures can still reverse or arrest the disease process. Assessment of ventricular function in patients with left-to-right shunts is an example of such a use. Another example is the finding of abnormal ventricular function in patients with hypothyroidism. Finally, in patients with noncoronary cardiomyopathies, such as sarcoidosis, involvement of the myocardium can be diagnosed early by noninvasive techniques.

Much of the research in nuclear cardiology today is concerned with trying to answer these questions:

1. What are the relative advantages and disadvantages of the various nuclear cardiology procedures, e.g., thallium-201 imaging of regional myocardial perfusion and technetium-99m albumin or red blood cell imaging of ventricular function?
2. When should first transit of ECG-synchronized studies be performed?
3. Which is more accurate in the detection of coronary artery disease, thallium-201 exercise studies or gated blood pool studies during exercise?
4. Will the Anger camera remain the predominant imaging device?
5. How quantitative can the results be?
6. Will tomography improve detection of lesions such as subendocardial infarction where sensitivity is still troublesome today?
7. Can the 10% – 20% false negative rate for thallium-201 exercise tests be decreased?
8. Will simpler special purpose devices become widespread, for example, in monitoring patients in conjunction with electrocardiography?
9. Will Swan-Ganz monitoring be replaced by ventricular function monitoring?

As recently as 40 years ago assessment of left ventricular function was limited to the appearance of congestion or shock. Subsequently, methods were developed for cardiac diagnosis that clearly showed that clinical signs are insensitive and that dysfunctional changes precede clinical signs. The invention and application of nuclear and echocardiographic methods have allowed measurement of regional as well as of global function. As with other organs, regional changes in the heart are often found before overall function falls outside the wide range of normal global function. This has been called the "homogeneity principle" and provides the basis for early diagnosis. The function of one part of the heart is compared to that of other parts, as in measurement of ventricular wall motion or the distribution of myocardial blood flow.

In addition to their usefulness in the differential diagnosis of chest pain, dyspnea, and fatigue, nuclear methods can also serve in prognosis and planning treatment. For example, severely impaired left ventricular function can pose a relative contraindication to valvular or coronary artery surgery, while early ventricular failure may indicate the need for cardiac surgery in patients with intracardiac shunts. Drugs such as propranolol or adriamycin can be used more effectively if their effect on ventricular function can be monitored.

Perhaps the greatest appeal of nuclear cardiology is the visual display of function. Human beings derive nearly all of their sensory input through their eyes. People are better at perception than conception, and therefore nuclear and echocardiographic images, especially when they are displayed as motion pictures are very convincing. The greatest limitation of the nuclear studies at the present time is quantification, although this is improving.

The radiation dose is low and decades of experience with exposures at the level of nuclear cardiology studies have not revealed any deleterious effects. The quality of today's images has improved greatly over the first lung scans or myocardial perfusion studies performed with potassium-43. Computers are now commonplace and are considered necessary for first-class cardiovascular nuclear medicine studies. Cinematic display on color television is now widely used. New collimators are being introduced. Tomography is providing important improvements in sensitivity and quantification. Sixteen new tomographic systems were reported at the last Society of Nuclear Medicine meeting, together with four special purpose systems that are much simpler than scintillation camera systems. At present, spatial resolution in imaging systems is limited to about 2 cm^3 with a precision of about 90% in quantitative assays done with tomography. It is likely that this figure will improve. Problems remain, but the future is bright.

In summary, the knowledge now being accumulated on radionuclide cardiovascular procedures has direct applications to the care of cardiac patients.

Noninvasive Assessment of Left Ventricular Function

N. Schad and O. Nickel*

Städtisches Krankenhaus, Radiologische Abteilung, Bischof-Pilgrim-Strasse 1, D-8390 Passau

Assessment of left ventricular (LV) function is important in the evaluation of patients with known or suspected coronary artery disease. The rapid deterioration in contractility in myocardial territories with inadequate coronary blood flow leads to regional abnormalities of ventricular wall contraction and to diminished regional ejection of blood. Overall ventricular performance is deprived of the contribution of the involved myocardium.
Impaired global and regional LV function influence the prognosis in coronary artery disease with either medical treatment or coronary artery bypass surgery. Therefore, a noninvasive assessment of global and regional ventricular function should precede coronary angiography. At present, radionuclide angiocardiography is probably the most promising technique for the noninvasive assessment of LV function.

First-Pass vs Equilibrium Technique

Two basic approaches can be used for imaging of the heart cavities: (1) cumulative imaging with high temporal resolution (10 – 20 ms) using multiple gated acquisition after technetium-99m-labeled serum albumin or red blood cells have equilibrated in the blood pool, and (2) recording of the first pass of a ^{99m}Tc-pertechnetate bolus through the heart at a rate of 20 – 50 frames/s.
The main advantage of the equilibrium technique is that it allows sequential measurements of global function to be obtained. For example, changes in ejection fraction (EF) during exercise can be measured with only one tracer injection. Frontal and left anterior oblique views can be recorded, but with all other projections there is a significant overlap of right and left heart chambers, which precludes regional analysis. With the first-pass technique, the right anterior oblique view can be used, as in invasive angiocardiography, for regional evaluation of wall motion and ejection. The first-pass technique also allows compartmental analysis of right and left heart chamber function and lung function, such as evaluation of transit times, indicator dilution curves, and shunt ratios. Repeated measurements require tracer reinjection. Both techniques provide reliable information about global ventricular function, particularly the LV EF [1, 2, 3]. When regional information is important, however, the first-pass technique is generally preferred, since the usable RAO view produces the maximum extension of the left ventricle and the best separation of the vascular territories.

Technical Problems

Technical problems involving image statistics, border definition, background subtraction, and motion analysis must be overcome for accurate assessment of ventricular performance. While these problems are clearly interrelated, they will be briefly discussed separately.

The Image Statistics

Imaging of the left ventricle presents certain statistical difficulties because the radionuclide bolus is injected into a peripheral vein, distant from the left side of the heart. During the first transit, the bolus lengthens and rapidly decreases in concentration. In addition, to resolve cardiac motion, count accumulation per frame is limited to 20 – 50 ms and the RAO view presents the maxi-

* Supported by grant of the Bundesinnenministerium, Federal Republic of Germany

Radiology Today 1. Ed. by M. W. Donner and F. H. W. Heuck

mum extension of the left ventricle so that relatively low count densities result over the left ventricle.
Nevertheless, dynamic imaging of the left ventricle can be successfully performed if the bolus input into the right side of the heart is compact, the scintillation camera has high count capabilities (short dead times), and several cardiac cycles during the transit of the bolus through the left ventricle are summed to form a representative cycle [4]. Introduction of a compact bolus into the right side of the heart is routinely accomplished by the injection of a highly concentrated radionuclide bolus (18 – 20 mCi ^{99m}Tc-pertechnetate dissolved in 0.5 ml saline) into a large antecubital fossa vein or the external jugular vein. The vein is then flushed with 15 ml saline at a flow rate of 6 – 8 ml/s.
The multicrystal scintillation camera records up to 400000 cps without saturation or the introduction of errors in the positioning of pulses, as it increasingly occurs with single crystal cameras at count rates over 80000. Incorrect positioning, however, can introduce a certain degree of distortion and a general loss of spatial resolution. The sensitivity of multicrystal cameras, expressed as cps observed per 1 mCi bolus, is 10000 – 16000 cps, in contrast to single-crystal cameras, which record only 4000 cps [5]. In fact, first-pass studies with multicrystal cameras, using the bolus injection method outlined above, have produced count rates exceeding 200000 cps in 360 consecutive examinations conducted in our laboratory (Fig. 1).
Six to nine cycles are summed to form a representative cycle of left ventricular function. With the aid of the electrocardiogram and visual control, the first frames of the selected beats are individually chosen; all corresponding frames are

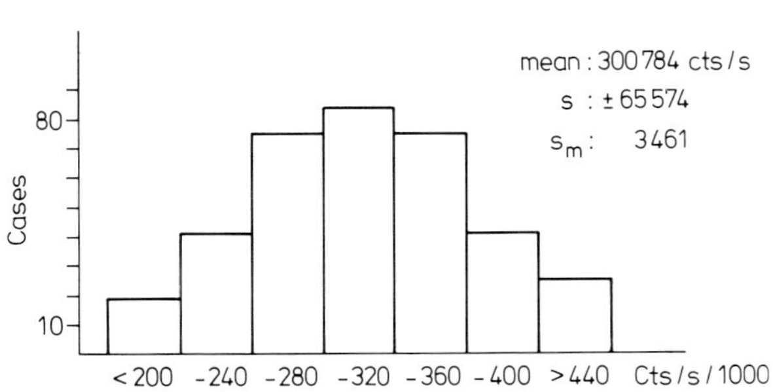

Fig. 1. During the first pass of the bolus through the heart, a maximum count rate of approximately 300000 can be obtained by using a multicrystal camera and a compact bolus of 18 – 20 mCi ^{99m}Tc-pertechnetate. Note that in 96% of the 360 cases, a count rate greater than 200000 cps was achieved [9]

subsequently added by a computer program. Precise determination of the initial frame of each cardiac phase avoids blurring of the information during the filling or emptying of cardiac chambers. Usually, only cycles on the washout side of left ventricular transit are added, guaranteeing adequate mixing and preventing the overlap of significant residual activity from the other chambers. The images of the representative cycle (RC) have higher count densities and, therefore, provide better statistical data. In addition, the resulting images of the representative cycle are linearly interpolated from a data matrix of 14 × 21 to one of 56 × 84 points.

Border Definition

Precise border definition on the representative cycle images is necessary for regional wall-motion analysis and for determination of LV size and volumes. Usually there is a gradual decrease in count density from the center of the heart chamber to the wall and the surrounding tissue or background. Therefore, detection of the heart border by simple visual control is frequently difficult, and assumption of a constant border background level is inaccurate, since the background varies from patient to patient and around the heart. Thus, the first step in assessment of ventricular function is to define the LV border and to eliminate from the image the background measured at that border [6].
Any border point has a statistical uncertainty corresponding to the square root of the count density at that point (Poisson statistics, standard deviation). Hence, the higher the count rate the relatively lower the percentage of statistical uncertainty. Definition of a border point is possible when the change to the contiguous point is larger than the corresponding statistical uncertainty. Thus, the steepness of change of count densities at the heart border becomes critical; in other words, a low background count and a high maximum count density over the heart chamber are of paramount importance [7]. Introduction of a compact tracer bolus into the right heart keeps the background count sufficiently low during LV transit and count densities over the left ventricle sufficiently high to facilitate an accurate border determination.
The border points are determined by taking the first derivative of the count density distribution in two perpendicular directions on the end-diastolic RC image. Both resulting first derivative images are squared and added to form the so-called spatial

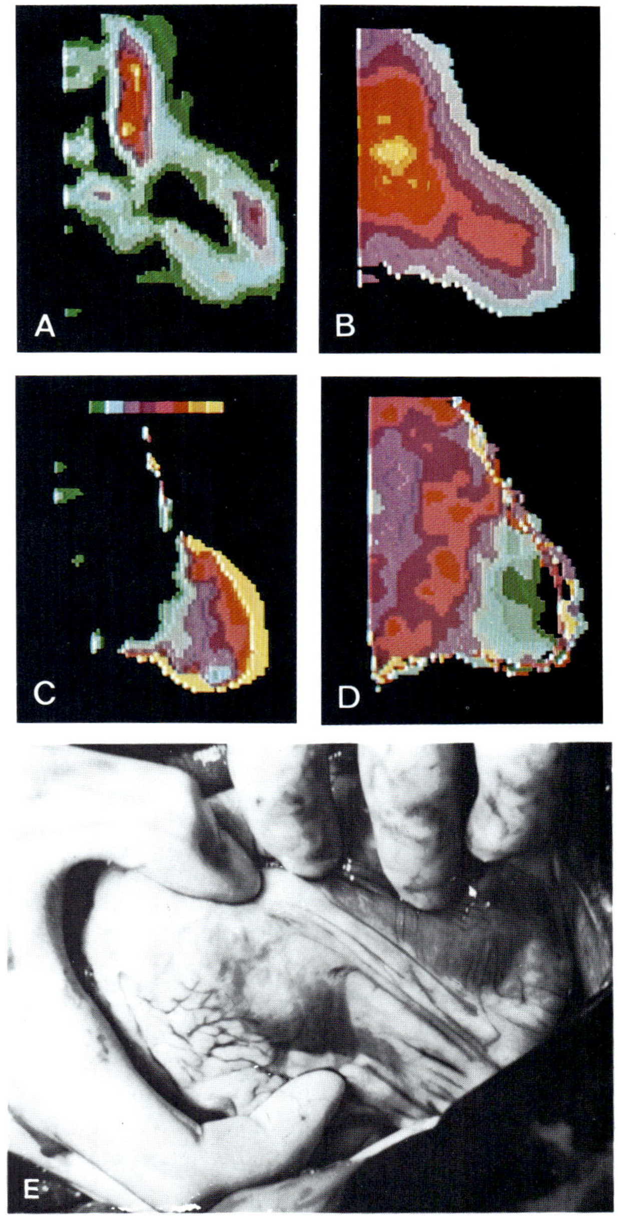

Fig. 2A – C. A 61-year-old patient with significant stenosis of the right coronary artery and first diagonal branch and 50% stenosis of the circumflex artery. **A** Spatial gradient image derived from the end-diastolic LV image of the representative cycle (right anterior oblique projection). Note the homogeneous increase in the gradient at the heart border. **B** End-diastolic frame after border definition. From each border point a different background is eliminated, corresponding to the points of increase of the gradients. **C** Regional EF image (10% incremental color scale). Hypokinesia is shown at the inferior wall (yellow band). Posterior to the apex, a small area of akinesia (shortening $<10\%$) and low regional EF (light blue and green) suggests a small aneurysm. **D** Systolic mean transit time image. In contrast to **A – C**, this is derived by subtraction of a constant background; the heart is foreshortened at the apex. The shortest mean transit time is shown at the anterior wall where contraction is best (black and dark green), while at the inferior wall the transit time is prolonged (light blue). The small purple dot behind the apex points to long systolic persistence of activity in that area and suggests a small retroapical aneurysm. **E** At coronary artery bypass surgery a small retroapical aneurysm of approximately fingertip size was found. (Photograph by courtesy of Professor Klinner.) [9]

gradient image. On these gradient images – for example, those processed for the end-diastolic and end-systolic images (Fig. 2) – the densities at the heart border are increased and the background levels decreased, thus enhancing the contrast between the heart and its background. In addition, the first derivative of the background around the heart is more uniform, so that by setting a constant cut-off level and by forming a mask, the background around the original image can be easily eliminated. The main advantage of these images, however, lies in their improved definition of the heart border. This technique makes possible the accurate subtraction of the contiguous background from each border point. Moreover, by the use of image brightness histograms, interobserver and intraobserver variations in defining the border levels can be reduced to a minimum [8, 9, 26]. Segmental wall motion of the left ventricle measured by this technique has shown a high correspondence with segmental wall motion visualized by cineangiocardiography for normokinesis and asynergy (see below).

This technique also allows magnification factors to be calculated by measuring the images of small, circular ^{99m}TC-pertechnetate-filled dishes or balloons of different diameters at various distances from the collimator. These magnification factors are needed for correction of actual volume measurements.

The Background Subtraction

Accurate estimation and subtraction of the background in front and behind the left ventricle from the RC image is the prerequisite for measurements of regional as well as global ejection parameters. One can presume that the background overlying the left ventricle spatially varies like that around the LV border (inhomogeneous background matrix). With first pass technique, the major part of the LV background derives from the lung, i.e., from the tail of the injected bolus. In fact, the background adjacent to the anterior wall of the LV is usually higher than that beneath the inferior wall, because the lingula segment overlaps the anterior wall. The degree of such an overlap varies from patient to patient according to the extension of the lingula toward the LV apex and inferior wall. Therefore, first an average lung image out of the sum of eight frames is prepared. Frames are chosen at the time interval when the ventricular time – activity curve presents a minimum between the first right ventricular and the second left ventricular part. At that time the major part of the bolus is in the lung periphery and pulmonary venous bed. By division with the heart mask previously obtained from the LV border definition, one produces the lung background matrix. This lung background, however, continues to wash-out until the time interval of the RC images, i.e., the washout phase of the left ventricle. Therefore, the lung background matrix has to be adjusted. For adjustement the background points adjacent to the LV border are used. The background border points on the lung image are linearly fitted (least square) to the corresponding points on the background image obtained after subtraction of the heart mask from the LV end-diastolic image (correlation coefficient $r = 0.95$ in 120 cases). Thus, the entire lung background matrix is lowered, so that the LV border background corresponds to the border background at the time of the LV images. Finally, the adjusted background matrix is subtracted from the images of the LV representative cycle [8, 9].

Motion and Ejection Analysis

The blurring effect of cardiac motion can be minimized by adapting the temporal resolution (frames per second) to the cardiac event and the information required. High temporal resolution, however, reduces count density, so that it may become difficult to reach statistically valid diagnostic conclusions, particularly on regional image analysis. Thus, frame rate is limited to the lowest acceptable level.

Generally, regional changes between two sequential images can be demonstrated by subtracting the two images of end-diastole and end-systole. Subtraction, however, increases regional statistical noise disproportionally because the statistical fluctuation derives from the sum of both images but relates to their difference. Hence within regions where changes are minimal, for example, where ventricular ejection is poor, statistical fluctuations are high on the subtraction image. Correspondingly, these regions are "noisy," poorly delineated, and difficult to separate from surrounding areas, and their function is not easily evaluated. However, it is precisely these regions that are the most important in regional diagnosis. Furthermore, by concentrating on only the two endpoints of the cardiac cycle one loses all information about what occurs throughout the

Fig. 3a – c. Normal functional images at rest (*left*) and at peak exercise (*right*). **a** Regional EF image (gray scale, 10%). Symmetric semianular EF bands, which decrease toward the outflow tract. Wall motion corresponds to 100% EF (dark band). At peak exercise wall motion increases and the high gray values advance to the outflow tract according to the increase in regional EF. Decrease of end-diastolic and particularly end-systolic ventricular size. Global EF at rest, 73%; at peak exercise, 81%. **b** Regional rates of ejection. Functional symmetry with maximum where the largest volume is completely displaced (*crescent-shaped zone*). With exercise this zone shifts to the outflow tract, since contraction of LV increases. **c** Regional mean transit time image. Low values lie at the ventricular periphery because of short persistence of activity in the region of wall motion. Increase in persistence and time values toward the outflow tract. Longest times immediately below the aortic valve and in the ascending aorta, where blood and activity remain at the end of systole. With exercise the bands corresponding to shorter times advance to the outflow tract due to stronger contraction [9]

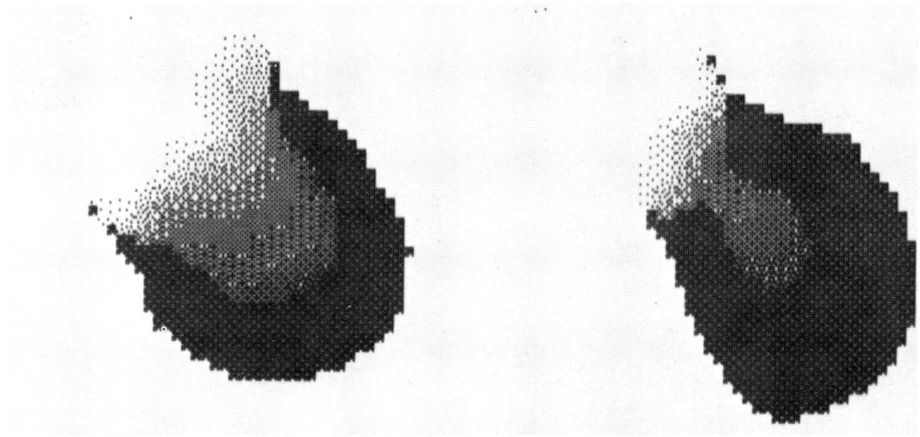

a

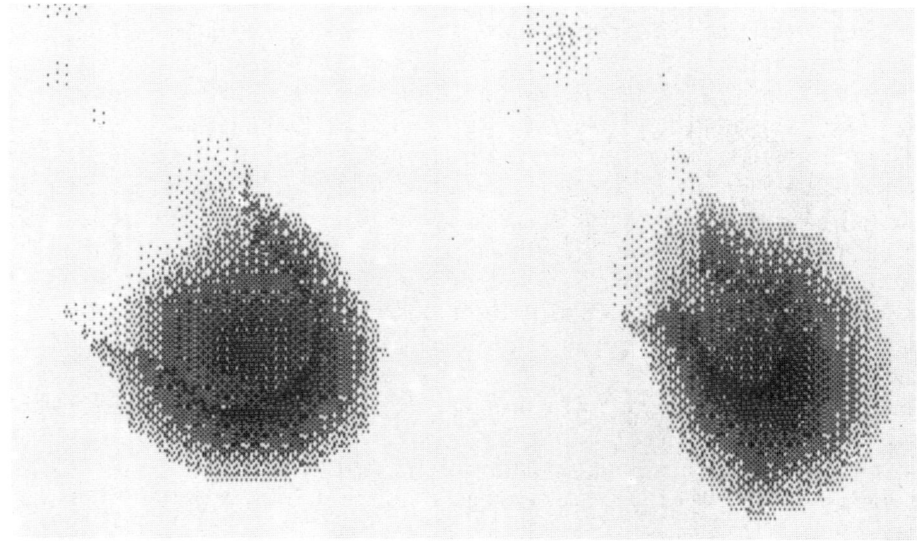

b

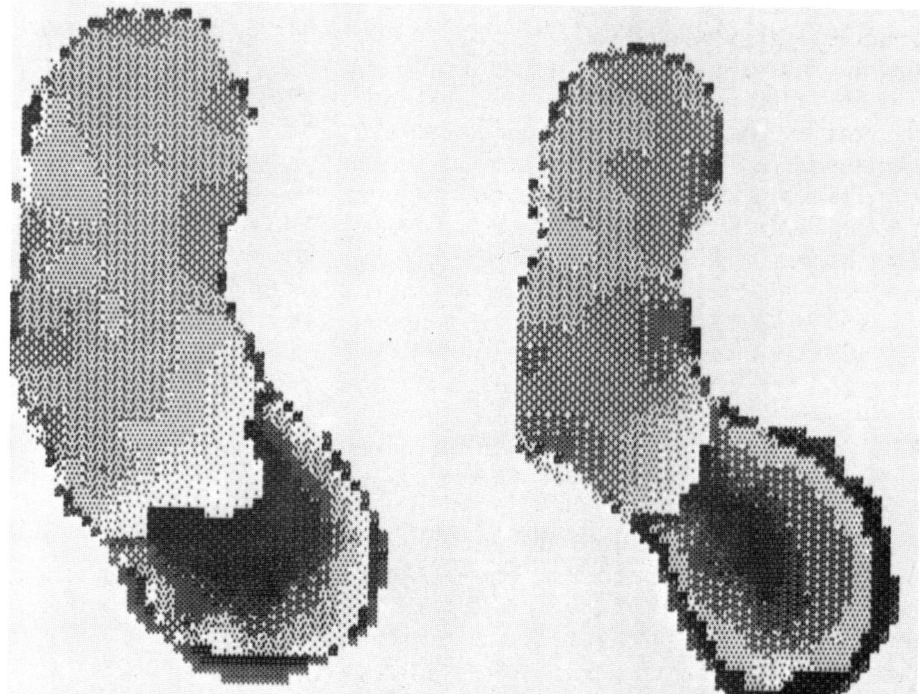

c

entire period of ventricular contraction or relaxation [10].

To overcome these drawbacks, all regional changes during a total cardiac phase or part of that phase can be fitted (via least squares) to a given mathematical function so that an automatic smoothing of the data occurs. Single "temporally smoothed" images (for example, end-diastolic and end-systolic images) can then be used to process subtraction images, which contain fewer random fluctuations than the subtraction images obtained from the original images (linear or cosine fit). The regional ejection fraction image thus processed (REFI image) presents the regional distribution of EFs for each pixel, i.e., cylinder measured through the heart (Fig. 3a). Normally, it shows semianular symmetric bands of equal range of values, which decrease from 100% EF corresponding to the wall motion where all blood is displaced to low EF in the subvalvular regions where residual volume remains at the end of systole. In regions with decreased ejection underneath wall motion disorders, these bands are interrupted or partly missing. Very low regional EF values point to extension of malfunction in depth. In this way regional ejection values provide some three-dimensional information.

Images that show the rate of linear decrease or increase in activity can also be processed [11]; these images collect all information during a selected cardiac phase and reflect the average trend of density change during that phase for all matrix points (regional "temporal" gradients). Normally, regional rates of ejection values again show symmetric bands of equal range of values (Fig. 3b). The maximum velocity band lies somewhat inside the ventricle where the largest volume is completely displaced during systole. Reduced regional ejection rate is characterized by interruption of high velocity bands and substitution by lower values. The regional mean transit time image practically represents the regional persistence of activity during systole, i.e., symmetric bands of long time value in the subvalvular region and band of short times at the periphery of the left ventricle (Fig. 3c). This image is of great value in the diagnosis of severe akinesias and aneurysms, which are characterized by low regional time values like in the aorta and immediate subvalvular area.

Noisy areas are automatically depressed by temporal smoothing, and the contrast between normal and abnormal regions is enhanced; areas with reduced or abnormal function are better delineated than on subtraction images, and the extent of malfunction becomes measurable. Therefore, trend images present a higher image quality and are diagnostically more reliable than subtraction images. Indeed, a high correlation has been found between areas of regional malfunction as shown on trend images and on cineangiocardiograms [10, 12],

For calculation of three territorial ejection fractions corresponding to the vascular territories supplied by the three major coronary arteries, the LV is subdivided into three zones according to the vascular distribution pattern seen on the coronary angiogram in the RAO view [8, 9]. Subdivision is performed on the end-diastolic and stroke volume images with the aid of the microprocessor computer system and a particular program. First, the percentage end-diastolic volume (ratio zonal counts to global counts) for each individual territory is computed. Whereas the end-diastolic volumes at rest and at exercise are usually different, it was assumed that the percentage end-diastolic volume remains approximately the same for the same territory during exercise. Therefore, fine adjustements of the two corresponding zones of the two studies are necessary to obtain percentage end-diastolic volumes not varying more than 2% from each other. Then, the territorial ejection fractions are separately calculated for the resting and exercise study and compared.

Clinical Applications

Global and regional information can be obtained at rest, after unloading the left ventricle by nitroglycerin administration, or while stressing it during exercise.

Information about global LV function is prognostically important and may influence the decision as to whether coronary artery bypass surgery or aneurysmectomy is indicated. Global assessments, however, include both regions with normal function and those with depressed function due to ischemia and/or scar formation. Hence, global parameters may to a certain degree mask regional disorders. Regional analysis, in addition, can be decisive in determining the treatment for patients with coronary artery disease.

Global Left Ventricular Function

Global information includes LVEF, end-diastolic volume, and derived measurements. Measurement of global LVEF by the first-pass technique correlates strongly ($r \sim 0.9$) with calculations from contrast angiocardiography [13–16]. It is a reliable parameter of performance that can be directly computed from a time-activity curve of the representative cycle. The measurement is independent of assumptions about ventricular geometry that are introduced in computations of volume by the standard angiographic formula. It also is not influenced by the projection used [13, 14, 17]. Furthermore, only small changes in ejection fraction were found on sequential measurements obtained over a 4-day period (4.4% ± 3.6%) [18], so that the radionuclide determination of EF also represents a reproducible global parameter of LV function. The same applies for the mean ejection rate determined from the same representative cycle (slope of a fit to a weighted least squares straight line).

End-diastolic volume can be computed by definition of the LV area on the end-diastolic image and the length of the major axis and by the use of the area – length method. Comparison between end-diastolic volumes determined by radionuclide techniques and by standard contrast biplane ventriculography showed a correlation coefficient of 0.89 in 33 patients [13]. In another study comparing ventriculography and radionuclide angiography, with both performed in the 30° right anterior oblique projection, the correlation coefficient of linear regression analysis was 0.93 [15]. From separate calculations of end-diastolic volume and ejection fraction, values can be derived for the end-systolic volume, stroke volume, cardiac output, and cardiac index. In 33 patients, comparison of cardiac output measured by an indocyanine green dye dilution curve and by radionuclide volumetric determination showed a correlation coefficient of 0.94 [19].

Regional Left Ventricular Function

Regional or segmental wall motion can be evaluated on first-pass radiocardiograms, particularly in the right anterior oblique projection. Analysis of the predictive value of the left and right anterior oblique projections in asynergy showed a higher sensitivity and specificity for the right anterior oblique view [20]. The right anterior oblique projection also showed a better correlation with contrast angiography than the left anterior oblique view in a grading of segmental involvement from 0 to 5+. Another study considering three regions revealed agreement with the radiographic angiograms in 69 to 78 regions [21].

Obviously, the prerequisite for accurate regional wall motion analysis, as for volume determination, is the precise definition of the LV border. By the use of spatial gradients for border detection (see above) and with measurements of wall motion in the right anterior oblique view, an average hemiaxis shortening for each of six segments per patient (210 segments in all) was computed in our laboratory on radionuclide and contrast angiograms of patients with coronary artery disease (Table 1). With normokinesis (hemiaxis shortening, 30%) there was a correlation of 91% (129/142) between radionuclide and contrast studies; with motion disorders the correlation was 90% (61/68). Thus, detection of segmental asynergy in the right anterior oblique view was achieved with a sensitivity of 90% and a specificity of 91% with the first-pass technique. A correlation of 88% (38/43) was found with hypokinetic segments (hemiaxis shortening between 10% and 30%). Similar results were obtained in a study of another group with evaluation of wall motion by two independent observers [14].

Table 1. Correlation between radionuclide and contrast angiocardiography in the evaluation of segmental wall abnormalities

	Correlation between studies	
	Number of segments[a]	Percentage
Normal motion	129/142	91
Asynergy	61/68	90
Hypokinesis	38/43	88

[a] Total number = 210 – measurements of hemiaxis shortening

Important additional information about regional ejection is contributed by the derived functional images, such as regional distribution of ejection fractions (Fig. 3), rate of regional systolic decrease and increase, and mean transit time images [4, 6, 10]. Akinesia and dyskinesia, in our experience, are best evaluated on the functional images which express the average function throughout all of systole because persistent akinesia or dyskinesia (of 300 – 400 ms) has greater clinical significance than does akinesia or dyskinesia that is limited to one or two images only (25 – 50 ms).

In our study of 210 segments, 13 of the 142 with normal motion – all of which were at the base of the heart – were found to be hypokinetic [15] or akinetic [1] on radionuclide investigation. Considering wall motion separately, these segments would represent false-positive radionuclide angiographic segments. With all 13 segments, however, the adjacent zone of the LV cavity showed depressed regional ejection on the functional images and a corresponding compromised vascular territory on the coronary angiogram. Therefore, the normokinetic contrast angiograms were considered falsely negative. The angiographic results can probably be explained as a consequence of the nitroglycerin the patients received during the procedure.

Seven of the 68 segments – all at the LV apex – that showed motion disorders on contrast angiocardiography were found to be normokinetic by radionuclide studies. These segments represent false-negative radionuclide angiographic findings; the corresponding vascular territory was found to be compromised on the coronary angiogram for all segments. The adjacent regions of the LV cavity, however, showed a depressed regional function on the functional images; in all cases, data from the functional images thus, in effect, corrected for the false-negative regional wall motion findings.

Thus, the information about regional wall motion and ejection obtained from first-pass radionuclide angiograms is both valuable and reliable. To increase the sensitivity and specificity, however, wall motion and ejection data from adjacent regions within the LV cavity should always be evaluated together.

Exercise Studies

First-pass radionuclide angiocardiography during exercise can be used in screening patients for coronary artery disease. During exercise, potentially jeopardized myocardium will contract abnormally in patients with relatively normal function at rest. Graded bicycle exercise is frequently used, with measurements made when cardiac performance is maximally stressed. Patients who can only be excercised until they exhibit angina and/or ischemic electrocardiographic changes or symptom-limiting fatigue are examined at that level. The direction and magnitude of the LV response is similar whether studies are performed with supine or upright exercise [16].

Global LV function changes under stress as follows: In normal individuals, end-systolic volume decreases significantly, end-diastolic volume decreases slightly, and global EF increases during exercise by at least 10 percentage points [13, 16, 22].

In a group of patients with significant one-vessel disease there was an equivalent increase in end-diastolic and stroke volume so that no change in EF resulted with exercise, whereas in a group of patients with multiple-vessel disease end-diastolic volume increased much more than stroke volume, so that the global ejection fraction decreased during stress (0.60 ± 0.14 to 0.53 ± 0.14) [13]. Most importantly, however, in both groups end-systolic volume increased, in contrast to a control group of normal individuals. Successful revascularization reversed the pathologic response pattern [13, 23]: the EF response to exercise returned to normal in patients who became asymptomatic. Although some residual cardiac dilatation occurred in the asymptomatic group during exercise, the end-diastolic and end-systolic volumes were less than before bypass surgery.

A decrease in global EF during exercise in patients with significant coronary artery disease has been seen by other investigators: (66% ± 2% to 57% ± 2%) [16] and (0.57 ± 4% to 0.45 ± 0.03) [22]. While a 12-lead exercise electrocardiogram yielded false-negative results in 36% of patients with coronar artery disease, the radionuclide EF results were diagnostically accurate in all but two patients with left anterior descending lesions of less than 70% and were also diagnostic in four patients with significant coronary artery disease on digoxin [24]. In patients in whom the EF does not change or decreases under stress, the resting EF is frequently normal, i.e., does not exclude significant coronary artery disease.

Regional LV function at rest may also be normal or may already show circumscribed motion and ejection disorders. Normally, segmental wall motion and regional ejection increase uniformly during exercise (Fig. 3). In areas supplied by stenosed coronary arteries, however, wall motion extent and regional ejection decrease. New or exaggerated regional wall motion abnormalities develop during exercise even in some patients in whom EF increases [16]. In patients with wall motion disorders at rest, EF can still rise significantly under exercise if the resting volume is low, i.e. between 35% and 55% [8, 9]. If only global information is considered, strong contraction in normal areas may mask depressed contractions in other areas, and no change or a slight increase in the EF may result. Therefore, regional wall motion and ejection analysis should always complement global evaluation. The exercise study usually enhances the regional contrast between the areas with normal and depressed function and is thus helpful in defining the location and extent of the compromised vascular territory and in determining whether disease of one or more vessels is present.

Exercise studies have been found particularly valuable in demonstrating the significance of a coronary stenosis and/or the adequacy of collateral perfusion [15]. Patients with coronary artery disease but insufficient collateralization were characterized by a significant decrease in EF and stroke volume in the presence of LV dilatation at peak effort. Frequently (in 16 of 19 patients), new areas of wall motion dysfunction appeared at peak exercise. Some of the patients (4/11) with visualized collaterals to all major coronary arteries also showed new areas of wall motion dysfunction and a decrease in EF at peak effort, suggesting functionally inadequate collateralization.

Exercise studies can also be helpful in the detection of latent heart failure before it becomes clinically manifest in patients with valvular heart disease (e.g., aortic insufficiency) [23]. Patients who had decreased EF with exercise before aortic and mitral valve replacement were found to represent a higher operative risk than patients who had an increased EF [23].

Nitroglycerin Administration

Screening for reversible as opposed to nonreversible depression of LV function has rested on two tests performed during invasive cardiac catheterization and contrast ventriculography: postextrasystolic potentiation and nitroglycerin potentiation. The latter, however, can be noninvasively performed using first-pass right anterior oblique radionuclide angiocardiography; global EF and regional wall motion and ejection can be examined before and after nitroglycerin administration. The examination allows one to determine whether function in severely hypokinetic or akinetic regions improves after nitroglycerin or remains unchanged, thereby suggesting extensive scar formation.

In 44 patients with documented myocardial infarction examined before and after sublingual nitroglycerin administration, we observed an average increase in global EF of 6%. In two other studies the increase was 6% [25] and 7% [15]. In the same patients the average resting EF rose from 40% to 46% with nitroglycerin, while after bypass surgery it rose from 32% to 40%. The preoperative EF after nitroglycerin and the postoperative EF after bypass surgery showed an acceptable correlation [15].

When EF, ejection velocity, and end-diastolic volumes at rest, after nitroglycerin, and postoperatively were compared [25], a significant difference was found between the resting and nitroglycerin data, but no significant difference between the nitroglycerin and postoperative data. Regional wall motion analysis on a total of 120 segments showed similar changes: no improvement of dyskinetic segments (8/120) after either nitroglycerin or bypass surgery and improvement of approximately half of hypokinetic and akinetic segments following nitroglycerin and surgery; only a small number (9/120) showed improvement after surgery that was not predicted by the results with nitroglycerin [17]. The studies showed a sensitivity of 81% and a specificity of 81% in predicting potential wall motion improvement after revascularization.

Regional wall motion was evaluated in our laboratory in 44 patients with documented myocardial infarctions [8]. After nitroglycerin administration, the number of segments with normal motion (25% shortening) increases by 51%, the number with hypokinesia (11 – 25% shortening) decreased by 22%, and the number with akinesia decreased by 60% (Table 2). All infarcted segments (44) showed motion disorders; 70% of the hypokinetic and 67% of the akinetic segments improved after nitroglycerin, but no response was observed in the four dyskinetic segments. Of 59 adjacent

Table 2. Regional wall motion before and after nitroglycerin administration

Wall motion	Number of segments		
	Before nitroglycerin	After nitroglycerin	Overall change (%)
Normokinetic	81	122 (+50.6%)	+18.6
Hypokinetic	102	80 (–21.6%)	–10.0
Akinetic	32	13 (–60.0%)	– 8.6
Dyskinetic	5	5	None

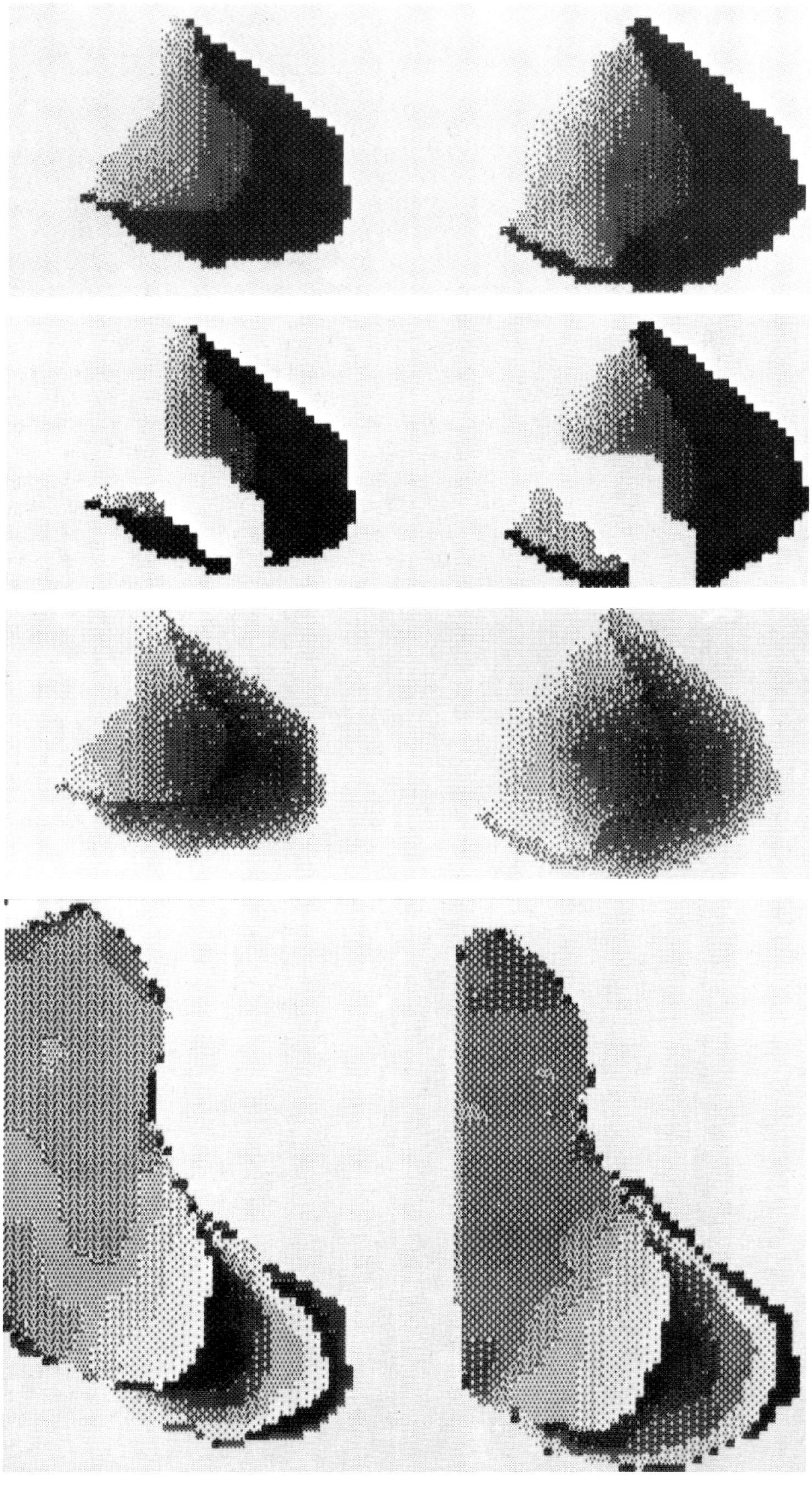

a

b

c

d

segments, 54% showed a motion disorder; three-fourths of these segments improved after nitroglycerin. No difference was observed in the response pattern of anterior and inferior infarcts.

Exercise Studies After Revascularization Surgery

Excercise functional images are particularly helpful for following patients after revascularization procedures since they can demonstrate the adequacy of bypass flow to the originally compromised territories. Segmental wall motion abnormalities that occur during exercise may disappear after successful bypass surgery, and a global LV decrease in wall excursion during exercise may markedly improve. However, to answer the two surgically relevant questions, i.e., whether the bypass graft remained open or provides no or inadequate flow, and whether revascularization was complete or incomplete leaving major stenosed branches not bypassed, regional analysis of function under stress is indispensable.

For 60 vascular territories (20 patients) regional territorial EFs have been calculated in our laboratory at rest and peak exercise. When revascularization was complete (n = 33), territorial EF rose from an average of 52% at rest to 58.4% (+12.5%) with exercise; when it was incomplete (n = 9, territorial EF fell from an average of 56.5% at rest to 48.7% with exercise (−13.8%). The difference between both groups was significant. In normal territories the increase with stress was from 50.6% to 58.4% (+15.4%). The increase in territorial EF with exercise in complete revascularized territories was similar to that of normal territories. In a distinct group of eight closed bypass grafts proven by coronary angiography, territorial EF fell from 53.1% to 48.5% (−8.7%). The difference versus the complete revascularized group was significant. The resting values of the three groups are quite similar; the exercise values only allow one to detect a closed bypass or an incomplete revascularized territory. A decrease in territorial EF is also seen in infarcted zones independent on whether revascularization was attempted or not.

◀ **Fig. 4a–d.** Regional functional images at rest (*left*) and at peak exercise (*right*). Two bypass grafts to the LAD and RC are open (proven by angiography performed by Dr. Deeg). Residual stenosis in the distribution of circumflex artery. Previous inferior infarction. **a** Regional EF image. With exercise severe hypokinesia at the inferior wall dorsally. The LV increases in size at end-diastole and end-systole, particularly in the area of the inferior wall. Global EF at rest, 69%; at peak exercise, 60%. **b** Territorial subdivision corresponding to three major vascular territories (cx territory light). One can appreciate the decrease of regional EF in the RC territory (previous infarct!) and the increase in the grafted LAD territory with exercise. Territorial EF values: RC, decrease from 75% to 49%; LAD, 75% at rest and exercise; cx, 56% at rest and 54% with exercise. In accordance with the open grafts and the previous inferior infarct three is no fall in the already high territorial EF in the LAD territory, but a significant decrease in the RC territory. **c** Regional rates of ejection. There is an appreciable reduction of velocities in the RC territory. **d** Regional mean transit time images. The longer times advance from the outflow tract to the inferior wall with exercise, pointing to a prolonged persistence in that region [9]

References

1. Ashbury WL, Schelbert HR, Verba JW (1978) Left ventricular ejection fraction – a review of several radionuclide angiographic approaches using the scintillation camera. In: Holman BL, Sonnenblick EH, Lesch M (eds) Principles of cardiovascular nuclear medicine. Grune & Stratton, New York, pp. 171 – 188
2. Pierson RN (1978) Application of ventricular function in the acute care environment: First transit and gated studies. Symposium on nuclear cardiology: Principles and applications, Milwaukee, October 1978
3. Strauss HW, Pitt B (1978) Gated cardiac blood-pool scan: Use in patients with coronary heart disease. In: Holman BL, Sonnenblick EH, Lesch M (eds) Principles of cardiovascular nuclear medicine. Grune & Stratton, New York, pp. 161 – 170
4. Schad N (1977) Nontraumatic assessment of left ventricular wall motion and regional stroke volume after myocardial infarction. J Nucl Med 18:333 – 341
5. MacIntyre WJ (1978) Imaging devices and computers in nuclear cardiology. Symposium on nuclear cardiology: Principles and applications, Milwaukee, October 1978
6. Nickel O, Schad N (1978) Image analysis of the heart action recorded with a high speed multicrystal gamma camera. Med Prog Technol 5:1 – 7
7. Budinger TF, Rollo FD (1978) Physics and instrumentation. In: Holman BL, Sonnenblick EH, Lesch M (eds) Principles of cardiovascular nuclear medicine. Grune & Stratton New York, pp. 17 – 51
8. Schad N, Nickel O (to be published) Assessment of left ventricular performance by functional images in cardiac imaging. In: Hipona FA (ed) Cardiac imaging. Grund & Stratton, New York
9. Schad N, Nickel O (1980) Nichtinvasive Beurteilung der regionalen Funktion des linken Ventrikels. Radiologe 20:56 – 69
10. Schad N, Nickel O (1978) Radionuclide angiography in coronary heart disease: Where do we stand? Cardiovasc Radiol 1:27 – 35
11. Noelpp UM, Schad N, Roesler H (1977) Trendszintigraphie. J Nucl Med 5:232
12. Ramos M, Rösler H, Noelpp U, Salzmann Ch, Fritschy P (1978) Trend scintigrams in the work-up of cardiac patients. 2nd international congress of nuclear medicine and biology, September 1978, p 4
13. Jones RH, Rerych SK, Newman GE et al. (1978) Noninvasive radionuclide procedures for diagnosis and management of myocardial ischemia. World J surg 2:811 – 828
14. Schmid DH (1978) First pass technique. Symposium on nuclear cardiology. Regensburg, September 1978
15. Tow DE, Parisi AF, Folland E et al. (1978) Quantitative radionuclide (RN) assessment of left ventricular function (LVF): Precision and correlation with contrast angiography. 2nd international congress of nuclear medicine and biology, September 1978, p 4
16. Marshall RC, Berger HJ, Reduto LR et al. (1978) Variability in sequential measures of left ventricular performance assessed with radionuclide angiocardiography. Am J Cardiol 42:531 – 536
17. Hellman CK (1978) Dynamic evaluation of ventricular function. Symposium on nuclear cardiology: Principles and applications, Milwaukee, October 1978
18. Rerych SK, Scholz PM, Newman GE et al. (1978) Cardiac function at rest and during exercise in normal and in patients with coronary heart disease: evaluation by radionuclide angiocardiography. Ann surg 187:7 – 22
19. Ally K, Patterson R, Horowith SF et al. (1978) Relative merit of RAO and LAO radionuclide angiocardiography in the detection of left ventricular regional wall motion abnormalities. 2nd international congress of nuclear medicine and biology, September 1978, p 139
20. Shields RA, Walton S, Wrigley C et al. (1978) Left-ventricular wall motion by first passage radionuclide angiocardiography. 2nd international congress of nuclear medicine and biology, September 1978, p 95
21. Suzuki Y, Kanemoto N (1978) Noninvasive measurement of right ventricular ejection fraction with radionuclide angiocardiography. 2nd international congress of nuclear medicine and biology, September 1978, p 52
22. Berger H, Reduto L, Johnstone D et al. (1978) Radionuclide assessment of global and regional left ventricular function during graded bicycle exercise in coronary artery disease. 2nd international congress of nuclear medicine and biology, September 1978, p 2
23. Jenge JA, Uszler JM, Freeman R et al. (1978) Upright exercise stress first pass radionuclide detection of coronary artery disease. 2nd international congress of nuclear medicine and biology, September 1978, p 95
24. Lumia F, Germon P, Maranhoe V et al. (1978) Comparison of radionuclide angiography with stress testing in the diagnosis of CAD. 2nd international congress of nuclear medicine and biology, September 1978, p 153
25. Kremers S, Kight J, Heck L (1978) Value of nitroglycerine radionuclide angiocardiography in preoperative evaluation of patients with coronary artery disease. 2nd international congress of nuclear medicine and biology, September 1978, p 23
26. Zita G, Zwick H, Kubicek F et al. (1978) Haemodynamic findings in pulmonary hypertension. 2nd international congress of nuclear medicine and biology, September 1978, p 53
27. Berger H, Zaret B (1978) Quantitative assessment of right ventricular performance by first-pass radionuclide angiocardiography: Clinical applications in cardiopulmonary disease. 2nd international congress

of nuclear medicine and biology, September 1978, p 53

28. Jones RH, Newman GE, Rerych SK et al. (1978) Restand exercise radionuclide angiocardiography in surgical patients. 2nd international congress of nuclear medicine and biology, September 1978, p 95

29. Schad N (1979) Assessment of ventricular function with first pass angiocardiography. Cardiovasc Radiol 2:149

30. Stewart DK, Dodge HT, Frimer M (1975) Quantitative analysis of regional myocardial performance in coronary artery disease. Cardiovascular imaging and image processing. Theory Pract 72

Coronary Arteries

U. Wegelius

The University Central Hospital of Turku, Department of Radiology, SF-20520 Turku 52

Summary

The past two years' literature concerning estimation of coronary artery stenosis and its sequelae, dynamic angiography, efforts in computerized digital coronary angiography, and percutaneous transluminal coronary angioplasty is reviewed.

A major question concerning the clinical evaluation of patients with coronary artery disease relates to the degree of coronary narrowing that constitutes functionally significant obstruction.

Although luminal diameter must substantially decrease before a pressure gradient or flow reduction is detected [25, 26, 38], there is no general agreement on the precise degree at which a narrowing can be considered significant. The American Heart Association Committee Report [1] accepts an 80% reduction of luminal diameter as significant, based on measurements which at operation demonstrated increased resting pressure gradients across narrowings of at least this magnitude [58]. Paulin [42] concludes in his report that the critical lumen diameter reduction probably lies somewhere between 50% and 95% stenosis and that it is impossible to define a sharp border between significant and nonsignificant narrowing for an individual situation. However, many investigators consider a 50% diameter reduction to be capable of producing ischemia [47, 7, 35, 12].

Thickness of the coronary artery wall will vary greatly due to genetic factors [44], age [25, 17], and state of diesease. The intimas of the large coronary arteries tend to be thicker than the intimas of muscular arteries of comparable size elsewhere in the body, and during middle-age the intimal thickness is several times that of the media [25, 17].

The media consists mainly of spirally oriented smooth muscle cells. Contraction of these cells causes active vasomotion of the vessel. Stress and strain, particularly in hypertension, lead to thickening of this layer. Until recently it has been a common supposition that significant atherosclerosis causes rigidity and prevents vasomotion, despite contradictory pathology studies by Leary half a century ago [35]. In reality the atherosclerotic involvement is often eccentric, leaving normal wall over part of the circumference [35, 18], and even concentric stenoses can change their diameter [40, 6, 10, 43, 12]. Studies of variant angina and the influence of different drugs indicate that stenotic segments usually are capable of active and dynamic vasomotion.

Angiographic studies have shown that vasodilators such as nitroglycerin can increase the luminal diameter of normal coronary arteries by 20% – 30% [19, 40, 32, 6] while constrictors such as ergonovine maleate cause a 20% – 30% decrease in luminal diameter [6, 31, 10]. These data suggest that major coronary arteries can, under physiologic conditions, approximately double their luminal diameter from their most constricted to their most dilated state.

MacAlpin [37] has calculated in a hypothetical model that the amount of smooth muscle contraction which is required to decrease the diameter of a normal artery by 39% will produce an 80% decrease of diameter if the arterial lumen is already affected by a 30% stenosis. Such a stenosis is usually not considered clinically significant (Fig. 1). A 50% stenosis will, according to the same calculations, lead to total occlusion of the arterial lumen. Undoubtedly, many atheromatous stenoses are calcified and rigid enough to be truly "fixed" stenoses. But it is just as certain that hemodynamically significant active vasomotion does occur at stenotic regions in some patients [40, 6, 10, 43, 12]. Therefore MacAlpin criticizes the use of the term spasm in cases where normal vasomotion in connection with arterial wall thickening causes obstruction and restricts the expression to cases where hypercontractility and therefore true spasm does exist.

Radiology Today 1. Ed. by M. W. Donner and F. H. W. Heuck

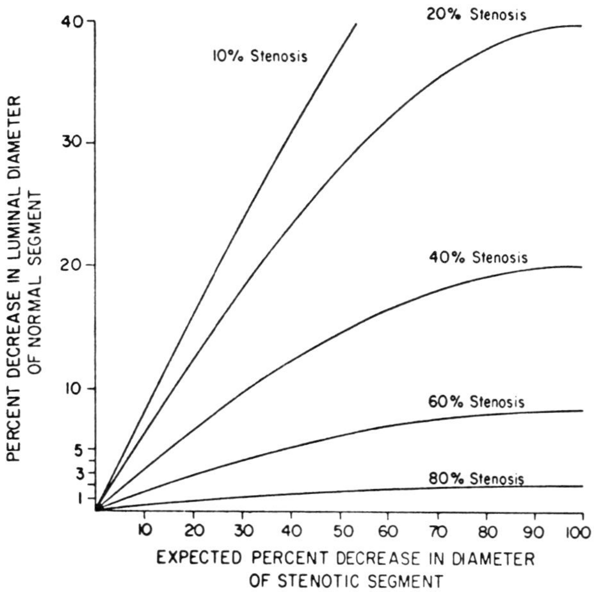

Fig. 1. Effect of luminal diameter decrease in hypothetical case of 10% – 80% diameter stenosis of coronary artery [37]

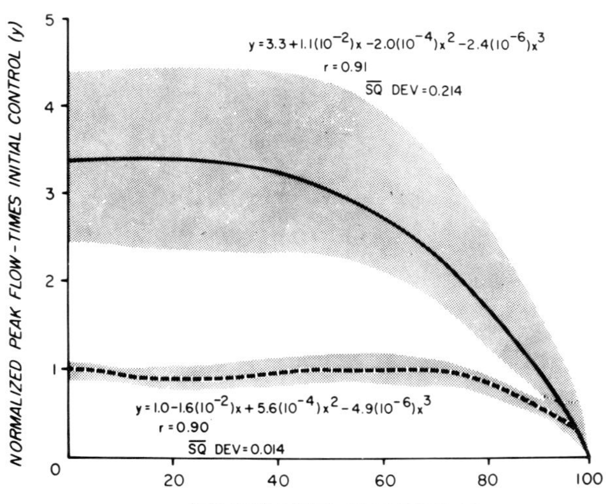

Fig. 2. The relation of circumflex arterial constriction by diameter to resting mean flow (– – –) and hyperemic response (———) after intracoronary injection of Hypaque in 12 dogs. Flows are expressed as ratios to control resting mean values at the beginning of each experiment. The *shaded area* indicates the limits of the relation plotted for individual dogs. *r*, correlation coefficient; *SQ DEV*, mean square of deviations [26]

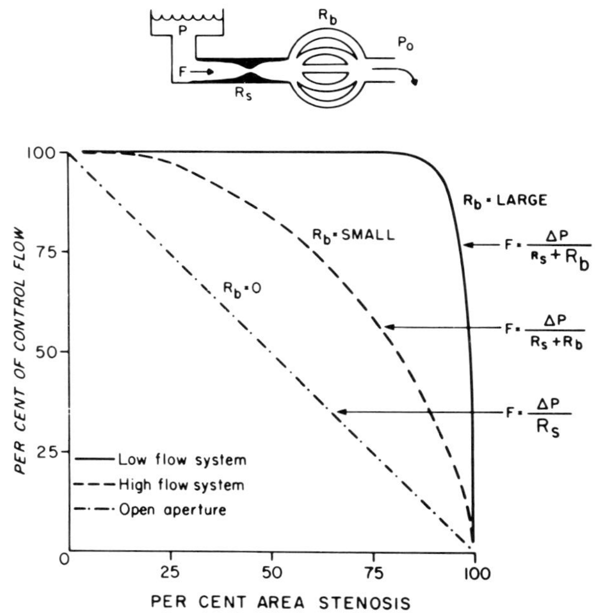

Fig. 3. Diagram representing the diseased coronary circulation as two resistances in series – the stenosis (R_s) and distal vascular bed (R_b). The effects of reducing R_b with vasodilators is shown by the *dashed line.* The equations on the right show the relation between resistance and flow (F). For a given total pressure gradient across the stenosis and distal vascular bed (ΔP), flow is determined primarily by R_b if R_b is large. P, arterial pressure; P_0, venous pressure. Increments in the value of stenotic resistance (R_s) have little effect until R_s approaches the value of R_b. When R_b is zero, R_s completely determines flow [23]

In their already classic animal experiment, Gould and co-workers [26] have shown the relationship of flow and stenosis (Fig. 2). By injecting the contrast agent Hypaque into the coronary artery, hyperemia was induced and the flow at rest increased by 3 – 4 times. A normal artery responds with maximal dilatation, which a stenosed artery is incapable of doing. The hyperemic response was decreased when there was a 30% – 45% decrease of the diameter, and it totally disappeared when the stenosis was 88% – 93%. On the other hand, under resting conditions the flow was not altered before stenosis was 85%.

In a diseased coronary bed the resistance is the sum of the resistance caused by stenosis (R_s) and the resistance of the arteriolar and capillary bed, called the bed resistance (R_b). Flow alterations are normally dominated by the bed resistance. In the case of a critical stenosis, the bed resistance still dominates in resting conditions. During stress the flow demand increases and the resistance due to stenosis starts to dominate and thus prevents the normal increase of flow (Fig. 3).

If active vasomotion can change the caliber of a stenotic segment of a coronary artery, the stenotic segment may not be rigid and might also passively change caliber in response to changes in intraluminal pressure. To show this Schwartz et al. [55] made noncircumferential stenoses on coronary arteries in animal experiments. A fall in perfusion pressure (PCBP) in the stenosed artery resulted in an increased resistance (R_s) to flow (F) across the stenosis.

$$\mathrm{PCBP}\downarrow \rightarrow \left(R_s = \frac{\Delta P}{F}\right)\uparrow \rightarrow F\downarrow .$$

According to Schwartz a passive narrowing of a stenotic segment explains the increased resistance. An increased coronary pressure, on the other hand, caused decreased resistance, presumably caused by passive distension of the narrowing.

$$\mathrm{PCBP}\uparrow \rightarrow \left(R_s = \frac{\Delta P}{F}\right)\downarrow \rightarrow F\uparrow .$$

Alterations in coronary pressure may therefore affect the severity of a coronary stenosis. Increased pressure causes dilatation of a narrowed segment; decreased pressure passively leads to a further narrowing of a nonfixed stenosis, which then may become a critical one. If, however, the stenosis is truly fixed, decreased pressure does not lead to increased but rather to decreased stenosis resistance. Therefore, the hemodynamics of a coronary stenosis depend importantly on the type and degree of stenosis present and whether it is capable of vasomotion, as has recently been pointed out by Schwartz and co-workers [56].

In an earlier paper [54] the same group as well as Walinsky et al. [59] showed that dilatation of the coronary bed distal to a critical stenosis (DVd) causes a decrease in distal coronary pressure (DCBP) and an increase in the resistance across the stenosis.

$$\mathrm{DVd} \rightarrow \mathrm{DCBP}\downarrow \rightarrow R_s\uparrow \rightarrow F\downarrow .$$

A further increase in the resistance across the stenosis occurs as the coronary pressure falls, providing an additional possible mechanism by which a fall in blood pressure may result in decreased myocardial blood flow.

In an open chest animal experiment Santamore and Walinsky [53] studied coronary flow response to vasoactive drugs prior to and after application of a critical arterial stenosis (Table 1). Controversially, isoproterenol and nitroglycerin, which dilated the distal coronary vasculature, increased the hemodynamic severity of the stenosis. This in-

Table 1. Coronary response to vasoactive drugs

	Normal artery			Stenosed artery			
	DCBP	F	R_b	DCBP	F	R_b	R_s
Methoxamine	↥	↓	↑	↑	↧	↑	↧
Vasopressin	↑	↓	↑	↑	↓	↑	↓
Isoproterenol	↧	↑	↓	↓	↧		↑
Nitroglycerin	–	↑tr.	↓tr.	↓tr.	–	↓tr.	↑tr.

↑ significant increase
↓ significant decrease
tr. transitory
↥ nonsignificant increase
↧ nonsignificant decrease

crease in stenosis resistance altered or even reversed the normal responses to vasodilators, namely a decrease in total coronary resistance and an increase in coronary blood flow. On the other hand, Doerner and co-workers [15] showed in a computer-based clinical angiographic analysis of normal and significantly stenotic (>50%) arterial segments that intravenous nitroprusside and sublingual nitroglycerin in clinical doses dilate both normal and diseased segments of large coronary arteries and decrease stenotic resistance. The discrepancy between clinical and experimental observations might at least in part depend on collateral circulation present in man but absent in the dog, as pointed out by Santamore and Walinsky [53].

Experimental animal studies have mainly dealt with short narrowings produced by a snare around the artery. In man, narrowings are often long. The hemodynamic importance of the length of a given obstruction has generally been disregarded. Feldman et al. [20] studied the influence of the length of a given coronary narrowing upon coronary hemodynamic responses in 14 dogs. Recordings were made as short fixed diameter reductions were progressively lengthened to 5, 10, and 15 mm by the addition of plastic occluders. Resting coronary blood flow decreased and pressure gradients developed across short (snare) narrowings greater than 80% (critical stenosis) (Fig. 4). Short 40%–60% narrowings had no significant resting hemodynamic influence; if their length was 10 or 15 mm, they consistently caused significant pressure gradients and flow reductions (Fig. 5). Feldman et al. tested the capability of the coronary artery to increase its flow by the temporary occlusion test. When a coronary artery is totally occluded for 10 s and then released, a reactive

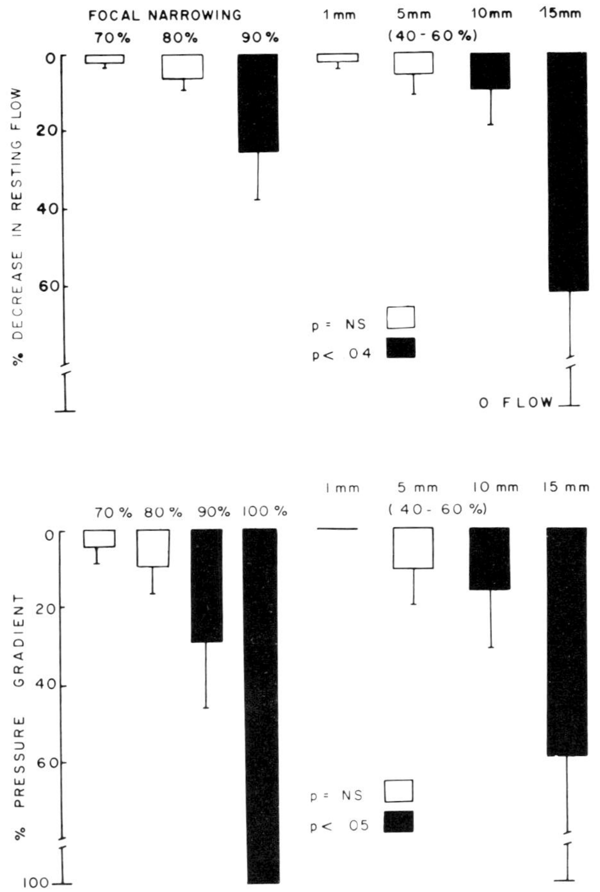

Figs. 4 and 5. Summary of resting data on coronary flow (Fig. 4) and pressure gradient (Fig. 5) for short and long narrowings [20]

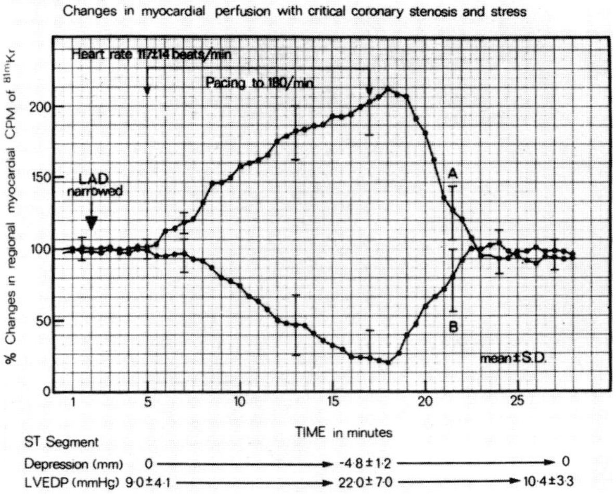

Fig. 6. This time-activity graph shows stable regional perfusion in regions of myocardium supplied by the circumflex (*A*) and the left anterior descending artery (*LAD*) (*B*) before and after *LAD* stenosis. Atrial pacing caused an abnormal redistribution of perfusion, which improved when pacing was stopped. The serial changes in the epicardial ECG and left ventricular end-diastolic pressure (*LVEDP*) are shown below. *CPM,* counts per minute [57]

hyperemia of short duration follows. In combination with a 60% focal narrowing, the reactive hyperemia peak flow was slightly decreased and delayed. Eighty percent focal narrowing decreased and prolonged reactive hyperemia markedly, while 90% obstruction almost completely abolished reactive hyperemia. If the length of a 60% narrowing is extended to 5 mm, reactive hyperemia is radically decreased and prolonged and a diastolic pressure gradient develops. A 10 mm long 60% narrowing causes a reaction similar to that of a 90% focal narrowing. A 15 mm long 60% narrowing almost completely stops flow and causes a pressure drop approximating total occlusion. The study showed significant influence of the length of a coronary artery narrowing on reactive hyperemic flow and the resting pressure gradient.

Selwyn et al. [57] studied the coronary angiogram under myocardial ischemia (Fig. 6). By atrial pacing or by ergonovine maleate-induced ischemia, regions transiently failed to opacify during angiography. Recording of myocardial perfusion under the same conditions produced redistribution with increases in perfusion (112 ± 14%) in nonischemic regions and decreases (78 ± 9%) in the affected ischemic segments. The effects of the ischemia produced by a combination of arterial constriction and atrial pacing or by injecting microspheres in an arterial branch and thus partially occluding the capillary bed were similar. This suggests that the reversible disappearance in angiography of a large coronary artery during an episode of myocardial ischemia may not necessarily be due to coronary spasm but rather a result of stenosis. It is suggested that stenosis prevents the normal flow increase in response to increased demand, thus secondarily producing ischemia, which decreases the myocardial flow and thereby decreases the flow in the feeding artery as well.

Estimation of absolute "normal" values for coronary luminal diameters during life has limited importance because of great anatomic and functional variations. In fact only a few estimations have been made. MacAlpin et al. [38] reported a study involving 26 normal patients; Rafflenbeul et al. [46] developed a method of quantitative analysis. Some of these results are listed in Table 2.

Table 2. Diameter values (mm) of coronary arteries of normal patients

		MacAlpin	Rafflenbeul
RCA	proximal	3.2 ± 0.6	3.55 ± 0.11
	middle		3.20 ± 0.11
	distal	2.7 ± 0.7	2.91 ± 0.11
RPD			2.10 ± 0.08
LCA	main	4.0 ± 0.7	4.24 ± 0.14
LAD	proximal	3.4 ± 0.5	3.45 ± 0.13
	distal	1.9 ± 0.7	1.94 ± 0.08
LCX	proximal	3.0 ± 0.7	3.03 ± 0.08
	middle		2.57 ± 0.1
LOM		2.4 ± 0.5	

Measurement of relative changes (percent stenosis) gives the best information if comparison of any artery in any patient has to be made. If, on the other hand, comparison of the effect of a chemical or physical intervention has to be made, measurements of absolute diameters are essential, as stressed by Gould [24].

Quantitative analysis of the coronary tree has been time consuming and limited especially by inter- and intraobserver error. Proper angiographic technique is available since multiangulated projections are used routinely. To overcome human error and obtain exact measurements of both normal and diseased coronary arteries, computerized analysis systems have been developed in recent years. In 1977 Brown et al. reported on a semiautomated computerized method for the analysis of biplane coronary angiograms [3, 5]. Sandor and Paulin have been very active in this field [50, 51, 52]. The most recent system is a semiautomated computer-based system developed by Sanders et al. [49]. Since 1978, Reiber and co-workers [47, 4] have been developing a system where a minimum of operator interaction is required. A selected cineframe of a coronary angiogram is converted into video format with a video-camera. The operator indicates with a writing tablet a number of positions of the center of the lumen of the

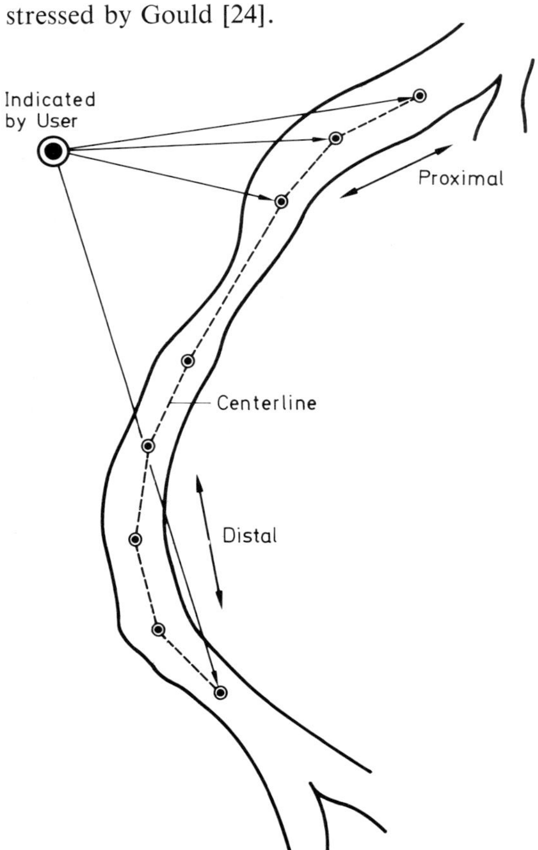

Fig. 7. To analyze a selected coronary artery lesion, the user indicates a number of center positions with the writing tablet. The interpolated straight lines function as tentative centerlines [47]

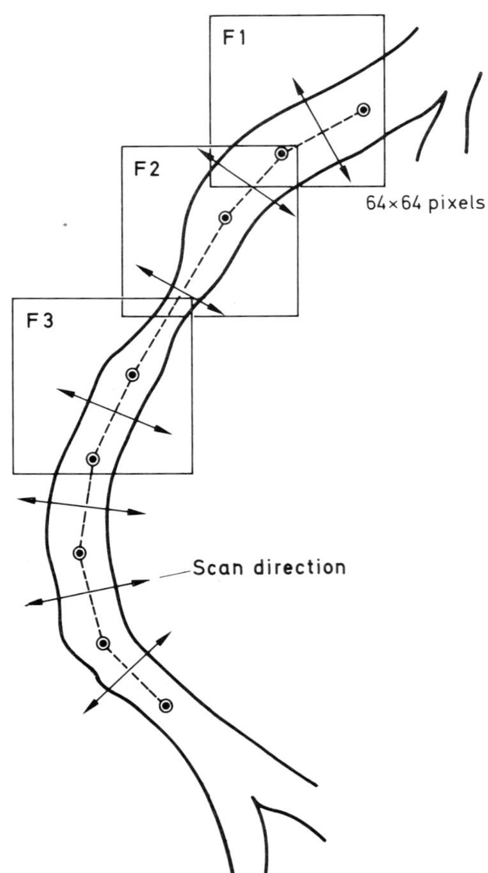

Fig. 8. For the schematic drawing of Fig. 7, the scan directions perpendicular to the corresponding centerline segments are given, as well as the positions of the 64 × 64 matrices to be digitized [47]

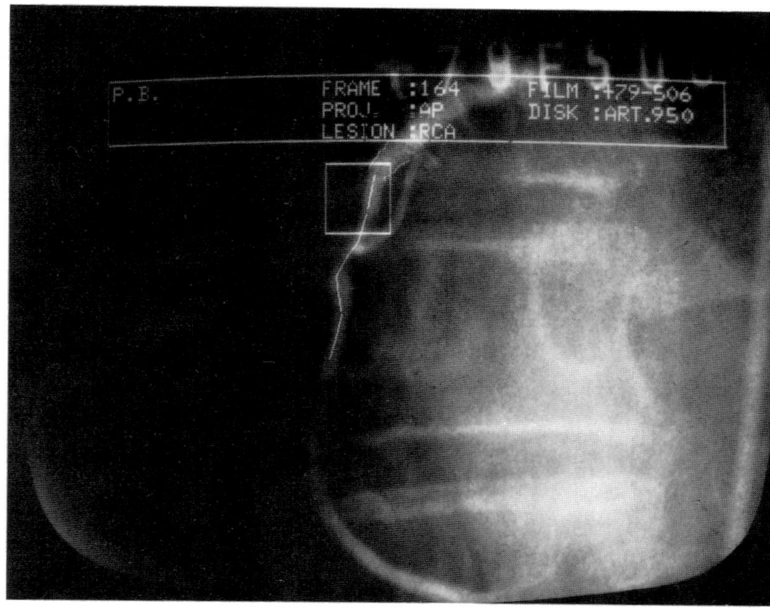

Fig. 9. Intermediate result. The edge points of the first 64 × 64 matrix, the boundaries of the second 64 × 64 region, and the tentative centerline are superimposed in the original video image [47]

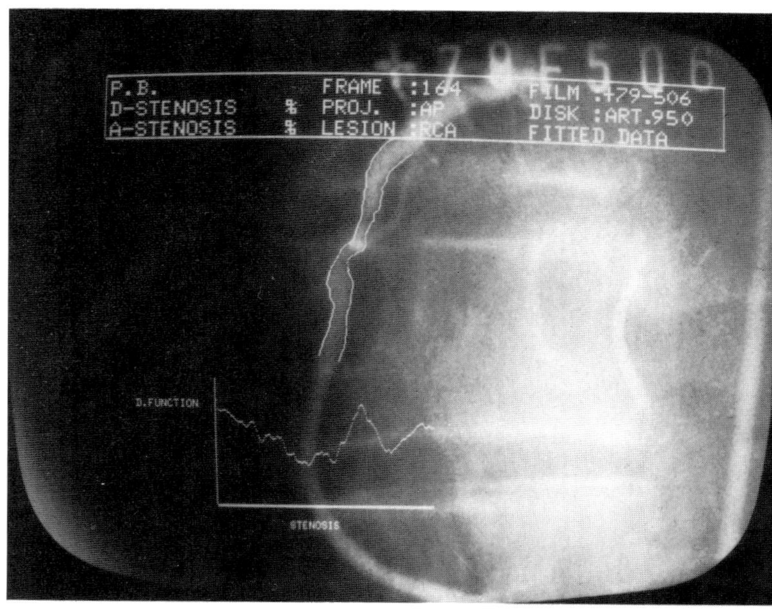

Fig. 10. The final detected contours. Diameter function (*D*) is calculated from these data. *D* function curve shown [47]

selected artery (Fig. 7). The interpolated lines define the region of interest that are to be digitized with the video A/D converter (Fig. 8); the image data are stored in the memory of a minicomputer. The contours of the artery are then established automatically. The detected contours are superimposed in the original video image for visual feedback (Figs. 9–11). The extent and degree of coronary obstructions are computed from the derived diameter function; the center position of the reference diameter region is indicated by the user. At present it takes approximately 1 min to analyze one lesion including the time required to define the centerline position manually.

The accuracy of the method validated in a phantom study gave highly significant results (r 0.99) with a low standard error of the estimate of 2.33%. In clinical studies, the average s.e. was 11.9% for the computerized system compared to an s.e. of 20.49% for visual interpretation with calipers.

So far the system has been used to calculate relative values only. Using the catheter tip as a reference, it is possible to calculate absolute measures.

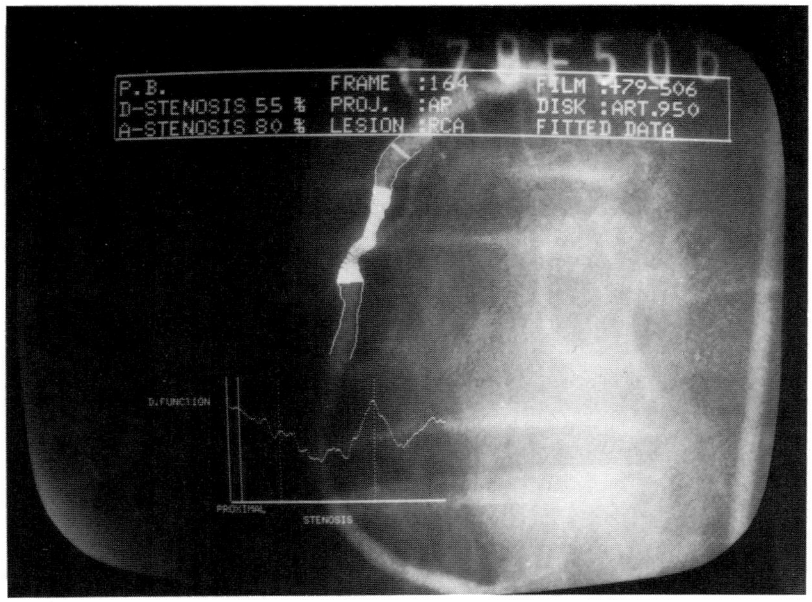

Fig. 11. Computer output of the lesion analyzed [47]

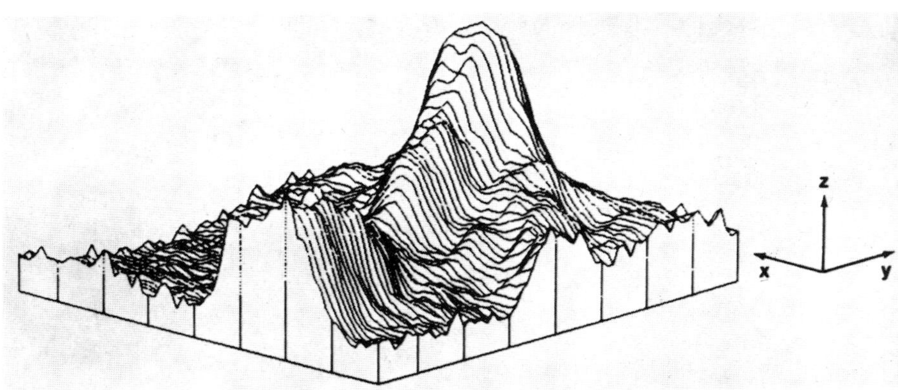

Fig. 12. Three-dimensional representation of the brightness function of one 64 × 64 matrix of Fig. 11, on compassing a coronary stenosis [47]

Three-dimensional reconstruction of arterial segments seems feasible using the information given by the brightness levels of the scanline pixels within the boundaries of the contrast-filled arteries (Fig. 12). Using the background subtraction successfully applied by Heintzen et al. [30] for left ventricular angiograms of children, automated delineation of the entire coronary tree is under development. Blood flow measurement through single coronary arteries by roentgen densitometry was done by Rutishauser et al. as long as 10 years ago [48]. Demski et al. [13] developed a computerized system based on densitometry and applied it in practice [14]. Unfortunately the method seems to have certain disadvantages mainly due to anatomic reasons. Theoretically the computerized quantitative analysis method of Reiber et al. promises better possibilities of segmental flow measurements in the coronary arteries. This will make quantitative functional studies of the coronary arteries a reality in routine radiology.

Since 1977 coronary angiography has not been a diagnostic procedure only. In that year Grüntzig [27, 28, 29] reported the first successful percutaneous dilatation of a coronary artery stenosis. With a specially designed inflatable balloon catheter the proximal noncalcified blockage was completely eliminated. Since then a cooperative study has been proceeding at centers in Zurich, Frankfurt, San Francisco, New York, Philadelphia, and Boston. It has been recommended that patients currently accepted for percutaneous transluminal coronary angioplasty (PTCA) must be younger than 60 years, have a history of angina of less than 1 year, have 70% or greater noncalcific proximal stenosis of one major coronary vessel with good distal runoff and preserved ventricular function, and have abnormal results of a stress test to ensure proper objective postdilation evaluation of improved myocardial perfusion [2].

By the end of 1979 some 400 patients had undergone the procedure. Experience is too limited to allow evaluation of randomized trials comparing PTCA with medical or surgical therapy. Probably not more than 5% of all patients referred for aortocoronary bypass are ideal candidates for this new and promising technique [39]. In experimental PTCA, Pasternak et al. [41] found loss of endothelium and platelet adhesion and thrombus formation at the site of damage. The immediate layering of platelets could be prevented by administration of low-molecular-weight dextran. In a postmortem study Lee et al. [36] found microanatomic changes in all wall layers, but no serious vascular tears. Dilatation beyond normal coronary diameter, however, caused rupture of the artery. For these authors, angioplasty was most successfully applied in proximal, discrete, noncalcified lesions of the RCA and LAD coronary arteries; calcified, tortuous, middle and distal lesions and the LCX coronary artery were entered with difficulty or were unapproachable. Dorros et al. [16] reported coronary artery intimal dissection to be an expected finding after PTCA and not a cause for alarm, since spontaneous healing and repair was seen in their patients. Mautner and Phillips [39] emphasize that experience with PTCA so far is limited and the results preliminary. With proper patient selection and improvement in technical skill, as well as in equipment, it is anticipated that the results will continually improve.

References

1. American Heart Association Committee Report (1975) A reporting system on patients evaluated for coronary artery disease. Circulation 51:7 – 34
2. Bentivoglio LG (1979) Bypassing the bypass with percutaneous transluminal coronary angioplasty. Am J Cardiol 43:866 – 867
3. Bolson EL, Brown BG, Dodge HT, Frimer M (1977) Computer analysis of coronary lesions. In: Proceedings of the Digital Equipment Computer Users Society, San Diego, Dec 1977, pp 453 – 458
4. Booman F, Reiber JHC, Gerbrands JJ, Slager CJ, Schuurbiers JCH, Meester GT (to be published) Quantitative analysis of coronary occlusions from coronary cine-angiograms. In: Proceedings Computers in Cardiology, Geneva 1979
5. Brown BG, Bolson E, Frimer M, Dodge HT (1977) Quantitative coronary arteriography. Estimation of dimensions, hemodynamic resistance and atheroma mass of coronary artery lesions using the arteriogram and digital computation. Circulation 55/2:329 – 337
6. Brown BG, Bolson E, Frimer M, Dodge HT (1978) Angiographic distinction between variant angina and nonvasospastic chest pain. Circulation 58 (Suppl II): II – 122
7. Burggraf GW, Parker JP (1975) Prognosis on coronary artery disease. Circulation 51:146 – 156
8. Caldwell JH, Ritchie JL, Hamilton GW (1979) Radioactive particle image of coronary blood flow distribution. In: Willerson JT (ed) Nuclear cardiology. Davis, Philadelphia, pp 213 – 223
9. Cannon PJ: Measurement of coronary blood flow using Xenon n-133. In: Willerson JT (ed) Nuclear cardiology. Davis, Philadelphia, pp 195 – 212
10. Cipriano PR, Guthamer DF, Orlick AE, Ricci DR, Wexler L, Silverman JE (1977) Effects of ergonovine maleate on coronary arterial size. Circulation 56 (Suppl III): III – 83
11. Cole JS, Trost RF, Wright KE et al. (1973) Who should have coronary arteriography? Geriatrics 28:125 – 129
12. Curry RC, Pepine CJ, Varnell JH, Sabom MB, Conti CR (1978) Clinical usefulness and safety of the ergonovine test in patients with chest pain. Am J Cardiol 41:369
13. Dembski JC, Decker D, Epple E, Heuck F, Zeitler E (1976) Koronare Flußmessungen mit der Cinedensitometrie I. ROEFO 124:59 – 67
14. Dembski JC, Decker D, Epple E, Heuck F, Scharf-Bornhofer E, Zeitler E (1978) Koronare Flußmessung mit der Cinedensitometrie II. ROEFO 128: 391 – 396
15. Doerner TC, Brown BG, Bolson E, Frimer M, Dodge HT (1979) Vasodilatory effects of Nitroglycerin and Nitroprusside in coronary arteries – a comparative analysis. Am J Cardiol 43:416
16. Dorros G, Spring DA (1980) Healing of coronary artery intimal dissection after percutaneous transluminal angioplasty. Am J Cardiol 45:423
17. Ehrich W, de la Chapelle C, Cohn AE (1931) Anatomic ontogeny. B. Man 1. A study of the coronary arteries. Am J Anat 49:241
18. Eliot RS, Edwards JS (1974) Pathology of coronary atherosclerosis and its complications. In: Hurst JW (ed) The heart, arteries and veins, 3rd edn. McGraw-Hill, New York, pp 1003 – 1016
19. Feldman RL, Pepine CJ, Curry RE, Conti CR (1978) Coronary artery responses to graded doses of nitroglycerin. Circulation 58 (Suppl II):II – 25
20. Feldman RL, Nichols WW, Pepine CJ, Conti CR (1978) Hemodynamic significance of the length of a

coronary arterial narrowing. Am J Cardiol 41: 865 – 871
21. Fisher HW, Thomson KR (1978) Contrast media in coronary arteriography: A review. Invest Radiol 13/5:450 – 459
22. Gensini GG (1975) Coronary arteriography. Futura, Mount Cisco New York, pp 241 – 320
23. Gould KL (1978) Assessment of coronary stenoses with myocardial perfusion imaging during pharmacologic coronary vasodilatation. Am J Cardiol 42:761 – 768
24. Gould KL (1980) Dynamic coronary stenosis. Am J Cardiol 45:286 – 292
25. Gould SE, Joannides G (1968) Diseases of the coronary vessels. In: Gould SE (ed) Pathology of the heart and blood vessels, 3rd edn., Thomas, Springfield, pp 545 – 600
26. Gould KL, Lipscomb K, Hamilton GW (1974) Physiologic basis for assessing critical coronary stenosis. Instantaneous flow responce and regional distribution during coronary hyperemia as measures of coronary flow reserve. Am J Cardiol 33:87 – 94
27. Grüntzig AR (1976) Perkutane Dilatation von Coronarstenosen – Beschreibung eines neuen Kathetersystems. Klin Wochenschr 54:543 – 545
28. Grüntzig AR (1978) Transluminal dilatation of coronary-artery stenosis. Lancet 1:263
29. Grüntzig AR, Senning A, Siegenthaler WE (1979) Nonoperative dilatation of coronary-artery stenosis. Percutaneous transluminal coronary angioplasty. N Engl J Med 301:61 – 68
30. Heintzen PH (1978) Review on the research and some aspects upon the modern development of densitometry, particularly roentgen-videocomputer techniques. Ann Radiol (Paris) 21:343 – 348
31. Heupler FA, Proudfit WL, Razavi M, Shirey EK, Greenstreet R, Sheldon WC (1978) Ergonovine maleate provocative test for coronary artery spasm. Am J Cardiol 41:631
32. Hood WP, Amende J, Rüdiger S, Lichtlen P (1978) Effects of intracoronary nitroglycerin on global and regional ventricular function. Circulation 58 (Suppl II):II – 27
33. Humphries J, Juller L, Ross RS et al. (1974) Natural history of ischemic heart disease in relation to arteriographic findings: a twelve year study of 224 patients. Circulation 49:489 – 497
34. Lawrie DJ, Levinsky RA, Lewis RM et al. (1975) A mathematical model describing the effects of coronary artery stenosis on coronary blood flow in resting and stressed dogs. Cardiovasc Res Cent Bull 13:52 – 60
35. Leary T (1935) Coronary spasm as a possible factor in producing sudden death. Am J Heart J 10:338
36. Lee G, Ikeda RM, Joye JA, Bogren HG, DeMaria AN, Mason DT (1980) Evaluation of transluminal angioplasty of chronic coronary artery stenosis. Value and limitations assessed in fresh human cadaver hearts. Circulation 61:77 – 83
37. MacAlpin RN (1980) Contribution of dynamic vascular wall thickening to luminal narrowing during coronary arterial constriction. Circulation 60: 296 – 301
38. MacAlpin RN, Abbasi AS, Grollman JH, Eber L (1973) Human coronary artery size during life. Radiology 108:567 – 576
39. Mautner RK, Phillips JH (1979) Percutaneous transluminal coronary angioplasty. JAMA 242: 1625 – 1626
40. Oravetz R, Lee F, Baker L, Titus P, Joye JA, Kaku R, Bogren H, Mason DT (1978) Prominent dilatation of stenotic coronary artery lesions following sublingual nitroglycerin by quantitative arteriography. Circulation 58 (Suppl II):II – 25
41. Pasternak RC, Baughman KL, Fallon JT, Block PC (1980) Scanning electron microscopy after coronary transluminal angioplasty of normal canine coronary arteries. Am J Cardiol 54:591 – 598
42. Paulin S (1979) Grading and measuring coronary artery stenoses. Cathet Cardiovasc Diagn 5:213 – 218
43. Pepine CJ, Feldman RL, Nichols WW, Conti CR (1977) Coronary angiography: potentially serious sources of error interpretation. Cardiovasc Med 2:747
44. Pesonen E, Norio R, Sarna S (1975) Thickenings in the coronary arteries in infancy as an indication of genetic factors in coronary heart disease. Circulation 51:218
45. Proudfit WL, Shirley EK, Sones FM (1966) Selective cine-coronary arteriography: correlation with clinical findings in 1000 patients. Circulation 33:901 – 910
46. Rafflenbeul W, Heim R, Dzuiba M, Henkel B, Lichtlen P (1976) Morphometric analysis of coronary arteries. In: Lichtlen PR (ed) Coronary angiography and angina pectoris. Thieme, Stuttgart, pp 255 – 265
47. Reiber JHC, Booman F, Tan HS, Gerbrands JJ, Slager EJ, Schuurbiers JCH, Meester GT (to be published) Computer processing of coronary occlusions from X-ray arteriograms. Proceedings of the International Conference on Information Processing in Medical Imaging, Paris, July 2 – 6, 1979
48. Rutishauser W, Stucky J, Schad N, Wirtz P (1966) Kreislaufsmessungen mittels Röntgen-Cinedensitometrie. Verh Dtsch Ges Kreislaufforsch 32:252 – 256
49. Sanders WJ, Alderman EL, Harrison DC (1979) Coronary artery quantitation using digital image processing techniques. Comp. in Card., Geneva, Sept 1979. pp 26 – 28
50. Sandor T, Paulin S (1977) Computer-aided evaluation of coronary cine-angiograms. In: Proceedings of the Digital Computer Users Society, Boston, Massachusetts, May 1977. pp 1249 – 1251
51. Sandor T, Paulin S (1977) Cine-densitometric analysis of coronary arteriograms. In: Proceedings of the Vth International Conference on Information Processing in Medical Imaging, Nashville, 1977. pp 1 – 12
52. Sandor T, Als AV, Paulin S (1979) Cine-densitometric measurement of coronary arterial stenoses. Cathet Cardiovasc Diagn 5:229 – 245

53. Santamore WP, Walinsky P (1980) Altered coronary flow responses to vasoactive drugs in the presence of coronary arterial stenosis in the dog. Am J Cardiol 45:276–285
54. Schwartz JS, Carlyle PF, Cohn JN (1979) Effect of dilation of the distal coronary bed on flow and resistance in severely stenotic coronary arteries in the dog. Am J Cardiol 43:219
55. Schwartz JS, Carlyle PF, Cohn JN (1980) Effect of coronary arterial pressure on coronary stenosis resistance. Circulation 61:70–76
56. Schwartz JS, Carlyle PF, Cohn JN (1980) Fixed vs. non-fixed coronary stenosis: The response to a fall in coronary pressure. Am J Cardiol 45:390
57. Selwyn AP, Fox K, Clay T (1979) The effect of acute regional myocardial ischemia on the angiographic anatomy of coronary arteries. Circulation 60:1335–1342
58. Smith SG, Gorlin R, Herman MV et al. (1972) Myocardial blood flow in man: effects of coronary collateral circulation and coronary artery bypass surgery. J Clin Invest 51:2556–2565
59. Walinsky P, Santamore WP, Wiener L, Brest AN (1979) Dynamic changes in the hemodynamic severity of coronary artery stenosis in a canine model. Cardiovasc Rese 13:113–118

Frequency Analysis and Filtering in Cardiac Nuclear Medicine

J.-A. Feser

c/o C.H.F. Müller, Unternehmensbereich der Philips GmbH, Abteilung Nuklearmedizin, Alexanderstrasse 1, D-2000 Hamburg 1

Examination of ventricular function with high temporal and local precision is an important problem in cardiac nuclear medicine. Ejection fraction and contractility in global size and regional distribution can be assessed in a non-invasive way: A gamma camera with a processing and display system offers such a diagnostic possibility. However, the acquired data have a strong noise overlay, resulting from statistical noise and background activity.

Reduction of background activity is difficult, for only the blood with its possible high activity concentration can be used as a carrier for radionuclides to investigate the relatively quick movements of the heart. As yet, the usable measurement time is too short for emission tomographic methods.

The sensitivity of the gamma camera cannot be improved without loss of spatial resolution. Moreover, the trend in gamma camera development is to improve resolution at the cost of sensitivity. Enhancement of applied activity is limited by the tolerable dose load of the patient.

Measurement time can indeed be multiplied by ECG-triggered cyclic superposition of single heartbeat acquisition, but this method is limited by patients with an unstable heart frequency. Even equipment for elimination of atopic heartbeats is only of help within the durable acquisition time for patient and personnel.

Single smoothing algorithms give a good cosmetic effect, but have the disadvantage of quenching the extrema overlaid to the first bolus passage. This leads to an underestimation of ejection fraction. Smoothing of ECG-gated images may smear over the diagnostically important edges of the ventricles. It also neglects the temporal correlation between successive frames given by the motion of the organ.

In this situation frequency analysis offers a good possibility of filtering the measured information by consideration of the organ-inherent motion and the given resolution of the gamma camera in such a way that the diagnostically relevant parameters may be assessed with great accuracy and exact repetition.

Fourier Analysis of First Bolus Passage

Each function f(t) may be superimposed within a given time interval T by harmonic waves.

$$f(t) = A_0 + \sum_{k=1}^{n} A_k \sin(k\Omega t + \varphi_k) \quad \text{with } \Omega = \frac{2\pi}{T}.$$

Fourier analysis solves this problem by calculating the amplitudes A_k and the phases φ_k of the harmonics k. The accuracy of this fit is dependent upon the number of harmonics considered.

The passage of a 20 mCi Tc-99m pertechnetate bolus is superimposed by the activity changes during the single heartbeats. Ejection fraction is assessed by the difference of the local extrema of the curve. Due to the small count number per image at a frame rate of about 20 images per second, the statistical noise within the produced bolus curve is considerable. Complete frequency analysis of the bolus curve gives a frequency spectrum with prominent amplitude levels at the frequency of the bolus passage and at the frequency of the heart beats. Frequencies higher than the heart frequency are associated with noise and cut off at back-transformation. The transformed curve then fits noise free into the measured curve with specified phase and under special consideration of the heart frequency. For transformation of the background curve even the heart frequency is cut off. The result is a noise-free "center-line of gravity." For calculation of ejection fraction three representative heartbeats of the net left ventricular curve are averaged at the peak of the bolus passage.

Radiology Today 1. Ed. by M. W. Donner and F. H. W. Heuck

Fourier Analysis of Gated Bloodpool Studies

ECG-gated bloodpool studies show a representative heartbeat composed of about 30 single frames with an acquisition time of about 20 ms. For each pixel of the frame matrix one may calculate the corresponding time-activity curves along all frames of the heart cycle (a 64 × 64 matrix gives 4096 curves) and analyze it by the Fourier method. For the motion of the heart is nearly harmonic, frequencies higher than the second harmonic may

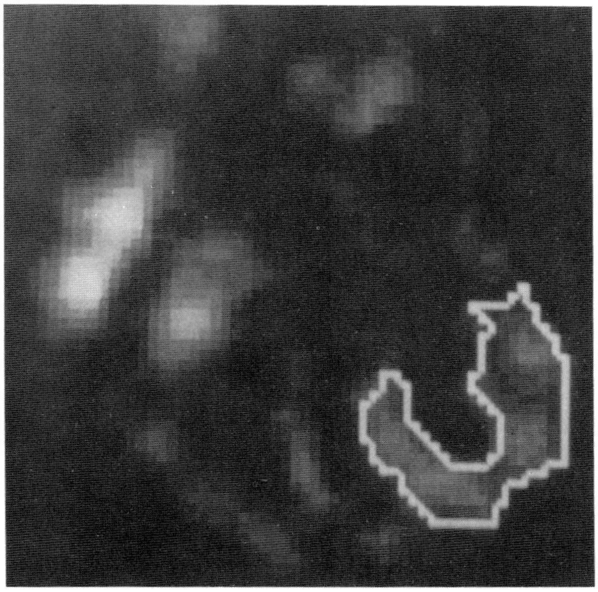

Fig. 1. Functional image of first Fourier amplitude. Gated bloodpool study in left-anterior-oblique position. The region of interest (ROI) shows an area with high amplitudes within the left ventricle. It corresponds to the wall motion between endsystole and end-diastole

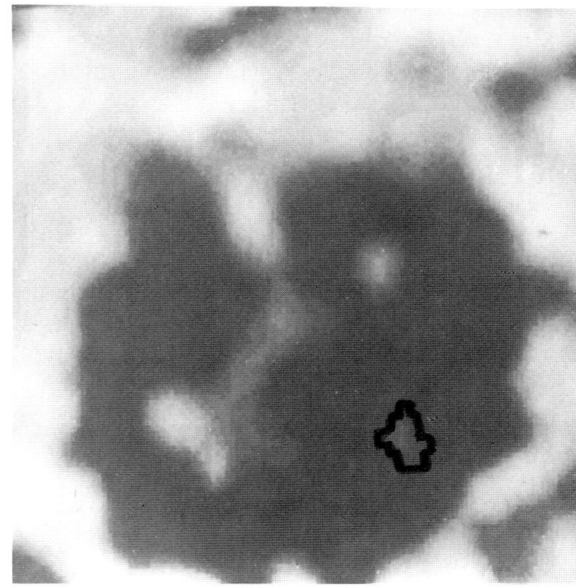

Fig. 3. Functional image of first Fourier phase. ROI marks a phase shift area within left ventricle

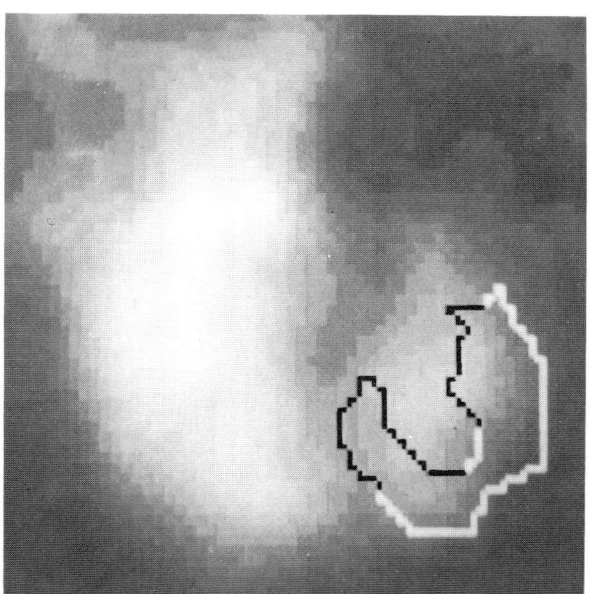

Fig. 2. End-diastolic scintigram overlaid with wall motion. ROI from Fig. 1

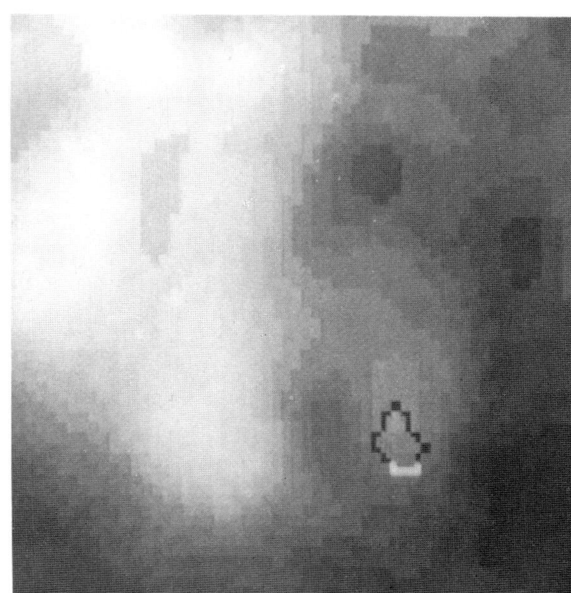

Fig. 4. End-systolic scintigram overlaid with phase shift ROI from Fig. 3. Indication for dyskinesia in lower part of ventricle

be considered as noise and cut off at back-transformation. The production of a new frame cycle out of the transformed curves gives a coherent motion of corresponding parts of the organ. This "temporal smoothing" can be seen very impressively at playback in cinemode. It also effects a noise-free left ventricular curve.

The first harmonic corresponds with the blood flow in the atria, ventricles, and coronary arteries. The normal heart shows synchronous contraction over the area of both ventricles and a similar contraction over both atria, but with a big phase shift. Ventrical areas with akinesia or hypokinesia are detected in the functional image of the first amplitude; dyskinetic regions can be found in the first phase image.

The second harmonic may correspond with the motion of the valves, but may also show areas of organ motion different from pure sinusoidal form.

Left Ventricular Edge Detection

Assessment of ejection fraction from gated bloodpool studies requires a very exact fixation of LV edges during the motion of the heart cycle. Differentiating the normal scintigrams was very unsatisfactory because of the local statistical noise. Using the Hawman filter one obtains a noise-free image without smearing over the edges by ordinary smoothing. This filter is based upon the idea that the spatial resolution of the gamma camera fixes the upper limit for the spatial frequency of the modulation transfer function (MTF). Therefore higher frequencies are due to statistical noise and can be cut off. Hence the MTF can be approximated by a modified cosine-function. The deconvolution of a scintigram by this MTF results in a filtered noise-free image whose differentiation leads to satisfactory determination of the edge of the left ventricle. Marking the septum with the help of the first amplitude functional image and defining the border to the atrium with the help of the first-phase functional image may reduce drastically the number of iterations.

Execution of this edge-detection procedure for every frame of a gated bloodpool study leads to a *region of interest* gliding with the ventricle motion, whose count numbers result in an LV volume curve representing best the dynamics of the ventricle.

References

1. Adam WE et al. (1979) Equilibrium (gated) radionuclide ventriculography. In: Cardiac nuclear medicine. Springer, Berlin Heidelberg New York, pp 21 – 33
2. Pretschner DP et al. (1979) Quantitative Auswertung von Myocardszintigrammen. Der Nuklearmediziner [Suppl]:48 – 58
3. Pretschner DP (1980) Prinzipien parametrischer Darstellung in der Nuklearmedizin. Der Nuklearmediziner 2:91 – 106
4. Jaszczak RJ, Chang LT, Stein NA, Moore FE (1979): Whole-body single-photon emission computed tomography using dual, large-field-of-view scintillation cameras. J Phys Med Bio 24:1127

Oblique Views in Angiographic Visualisation of Cardiovascular Morphology

B. Schmidt-Redemann, H. O. Fürste, and K. Haap

Universitäts-Kinderklinik, Abteilung pädiatrische Kardiologie,
Mathildenstrasse 1, D-7800 Freiburg

Progress in cardiovascular surgery has made it possible to correct even complicated cardiovascular malformations, and the differentiated representation of pathological cardiovascular structures has become essential for the exact indication of the type of operation.

Conventional angiocardiographic methods of diagnosis are restricted to contrast representation in posterior-anterior and vertical views. Since Bargeron and co-workers introduced axial-angled views into cine-angiocardiographic investigation in 1977 [1], the diagnostic implications of these methods have been significantly extended due to the fact that structural superimpositions could largely be eliminated. The methods hitherto adapted for conducting these angled views utilised the possibility of rotating and elevating the patient within the beam of a fixed image intensifier [3]. A further development was the employment of a U-shaped parallelogram which could be adjusted around the patient's horizontal and vertical axes [2, 4].

The biplane C-arm combination allowing iso-centering at all projection levels in the direction of the heart finally met the need for an unrestricted viewing technique. A broad table makes possible free rotation of the image intensifier, which is fixed to the two C-arms by synchronisation. The investigator stands in the middle of the rotating unit and is able to manipulate the catheter freely. A zoom-magnifier with direct indication of the magnification factor ensures that the position of the catheter in the desired cardiovascular structures is represented biplanely in the image inten-

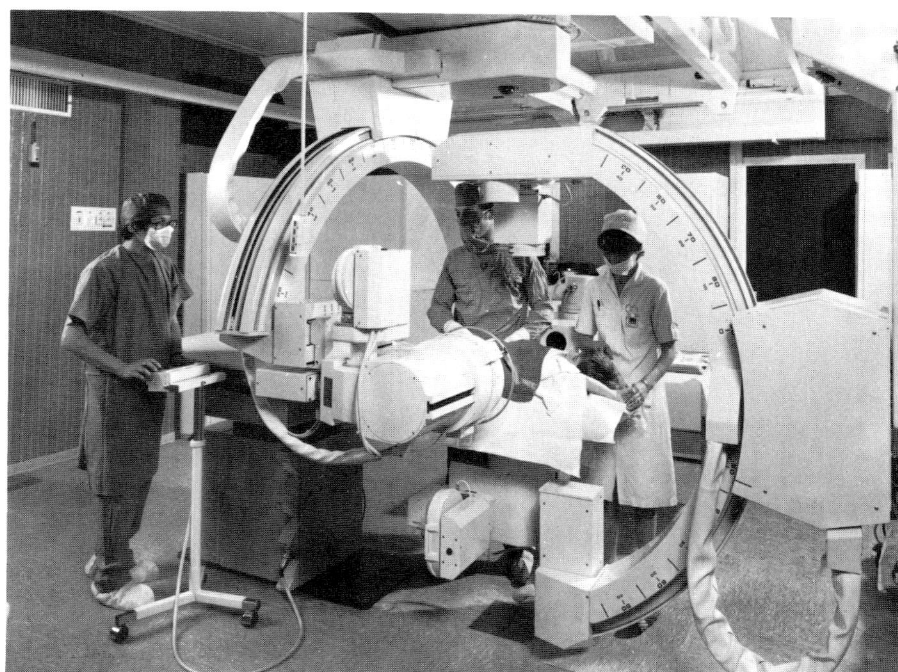

Fig. 1. Automated programme for cine procedure

Radiology Today 1. Ed. by M. W. Donner and F. H. W. Heuck

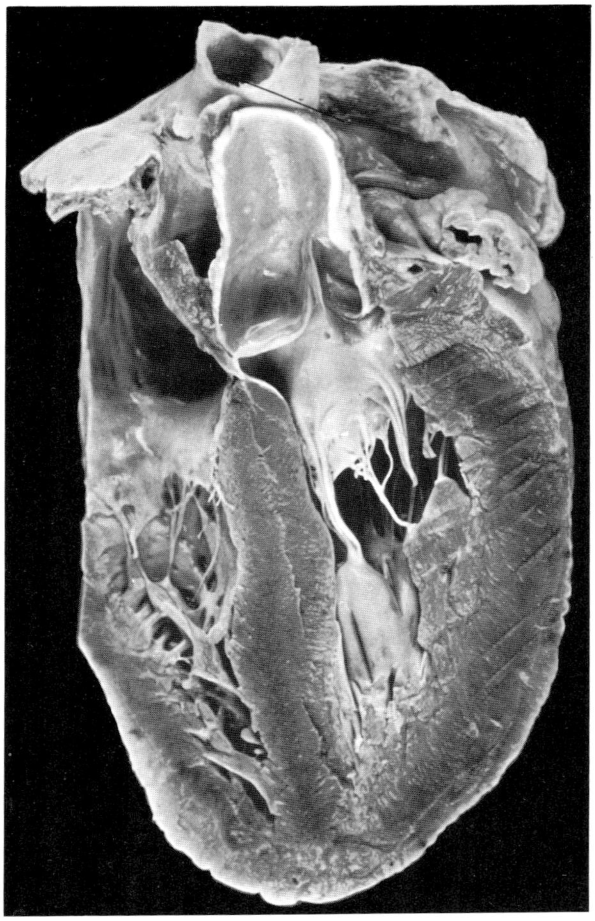

Fig. 2. Biplane C-arm equipment for synchronised cine-angiography

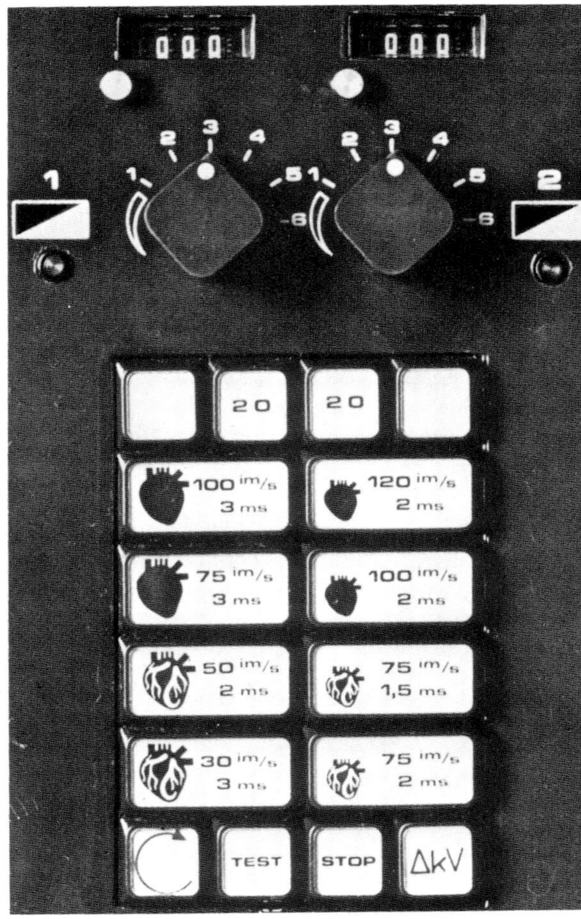

Fig. 3. Post-mortem specimen of the heart (four chamber view)

sifier-television equipment. The two intensifiers are synchronised in such a way that fixed coupling in certain angle positions, for example at 90° to each other, is possible. By this method direct observation and profile representation of the cardiovascular morphology is obtained (Fig. 1).

For the sake of better didactic understanding of these angled views, hearts were cut at the levels suitable for viewing. These cross-section samples offer a very concrete picture of the cardiovascular structures thus represented at certain levels of incision (Fig. 2).

The X-ray generator must be adapted to the latest evolution of the C-arms by liberating the user from complicated adjustments. This generator is characterized by:

1. Stepless kV adjustment from 50 to 150.
2. Stepless mA adjustment from 50 to 3000.
3. Stepless time adjustment from 0.0003 to 1 s.
4. Rapid sequence up to 200 fps.
5. Visualisation of tube load percentage and number of exposures permitted.

This generator provides a cine module including eight present programs covering all the cine parameters. Each pushbutton (see Fig. 3) preselects the frame rate, focal spot, mA, and exposure time. Before initiating the first cine sequence the "test" pushbutton will predetermine the starting kV value for the cine run. This value is placed in memory store during the examination. When a cine run is initiated the basic kV will be corrected during the first three frames of each run, and by this method maximum contrast is provided during the various phases of the coronary examination for example.

The angle views listed below correspond to experience made in the past years and are an extension and supplementation of current literature on the subject [8, 10].

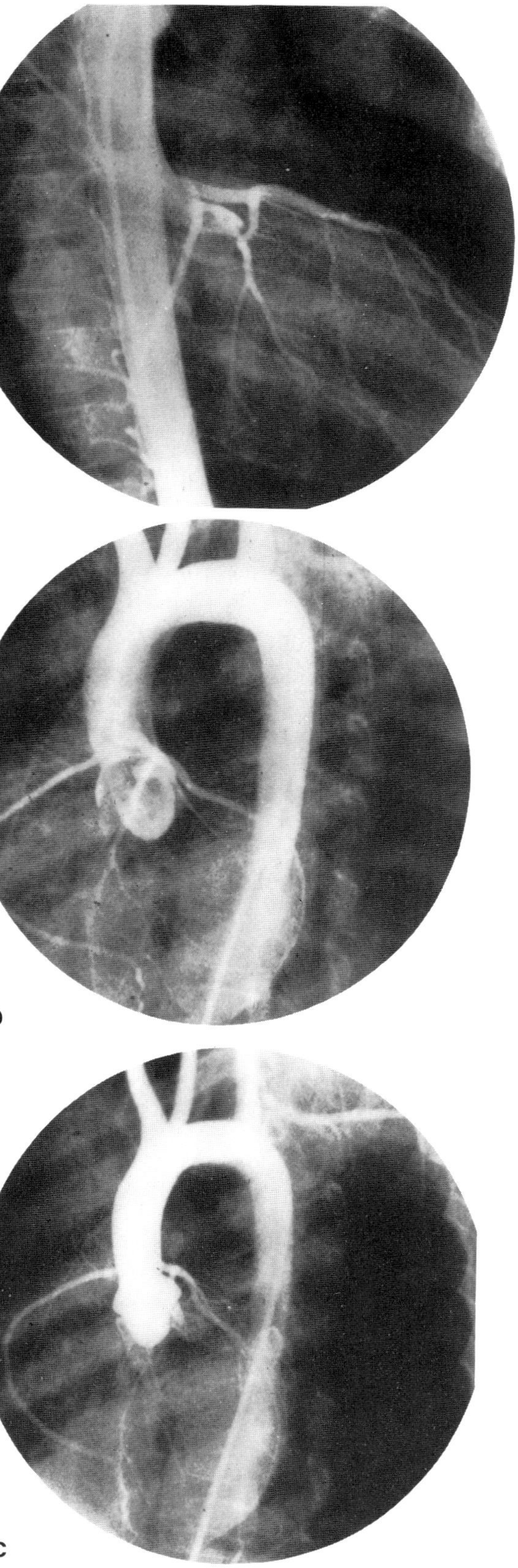

a

b

c

Fig. 4a – c. Non-selective angiography of an abnormal origin of the right coronary artery. Left-anterior-oblique view

Cranial 25° – 35°, Left Oblique 70° – 80° (Four Chamber View)

The anatomical guideline for this view is the connection between the anterior and posterior mitral valve as well as the connecting structure of the free wall of the left ventricle with the posterior part of the ventricular septum. The localisation of the catheter in the apex of the left ventricle likewise assists the sensitive focussing for rotation around the patient's vertical axis. If necessary a test injection makes determination of the exact angle possible. This method helps to localise the anatomical vertical axis of the heart, which varies considerably between individuals. The second C-arm allows the profile representation of the heart structures visible from this view. The septal curvature of the free wall of the left ventricle during the systolic phase in the area of its connection with the mitral valve, which is recognisable by a fibrous edge, assists the exact regulation of the C-arm in this vertical position [6, 7].

Particularly for making a differentiated diagnosis of the various forms of endocardial cushion defects, this viewing method, corresponding as it does to a four chamber view, is far superior to conventional views, since these do not take into consideration a structural superimposition in the area of the left ventricular outflow tract and the mitral valve (Fig. 4).

Cranial 15° – 25°, Right Oblique 25° – 35° (Long Axis View)

The relationship between mitral valve and left ventricular outflow tract, for example in the case of asymmetrical hypertrophy of the septum or prolapse of the anterior cusp of the mitral valve, can be precisely diagnosed in this view, both as regards extent and functional course. The vertical C-arm, here at an angle of 90°, represents the atrioventricular septum in the right-posterior-oblique view and in profile and assists the differentiation of the position, function and number of the AV valves, for example in the case of univentricular heart. By right ventricular injection the trabeculation of the septum marginalis can be particularly well represented.

In contrast to the vertical view of the left-anterior-oblique C-arm, the position of 20° – 30° inclines more sharply left-anterior-oblique.

Table 1. Angled views in angiocardiography

Cranial	45° – 55°
Left oblique	10° – 20°
Indications:	Tetralogy of Fallot Pulmonary artery stenosis (peripheral) Pulmonary artery (anomalous origin) Pulmonary atresia (postop. prosthetic reconstruction) Pulmonary arterial banding
Cranial	35° – 45°
Left oblique	20° – 30°
Indications:	Fontan conduit Atrioventricular canal (left ventricular – right atrial shunt)
Cranial	15° – 25°
Left oblique	20° – 30°
Indication:	Haemodynamic corrective operation of transposition of the great arteries (TGA) (Mustard or Senning)
Cranial	25° – 35° (four chamber view)
Left oblique	70° – 80°
Indications:	Atrial septal defect Left ventricular outflow tract obstruction in TGA Aortic stenosis (subvalvular) Ventricular septal defect, membranous, septal, multiple Anomalies of the coronary arteries (in tetralogy of Fallot and TGA) Atrioventricular canal Common AV valve Endocardial cushion defects Single ventricle
Vertical projection	(90° against four chamber view)
Indications:	*Right ventricle:* Muscular portion of the ventricular septum right to left shunt Connection between ventricular septum and tricuspid valve Dynamic of left ventricle outflow tract in TGA
Cranial	15° – 25°
Right oblique	25° – 35° (long axis view)
Indications:	*Left ventricle:* Mitral valve Portion of the anterior ventricular septum Posterior papillary muscle of the mitral valve Relationship of the anterior mitral cusp to the left ventricular outflow tract in IHSS Bicuspid aotric valve *Right ventricle:* Ostium of the infundibular chamber Sinus and inflow tract of right ventricle Ebstein's anomaly of the tricuspid valve Abnormal muscle bundle in the right ventricular outflow tract (Waterston shunt)
Vertical projection	(90° against long axis view)
Indications:	*Left ventricle:* Representation of the anterior mitral cusp in profile Valvular and subvalvular pulmonary stenosis in TGA Perimembranous ventricular septal defect

Cranial 45° – 55°, Left Oblique 10° – 20°

This so-called "sitting up position" as described by Kattan in 1970 serves above all to represent the area of the pulmonary arteries and to make possible a more precise identification of the pulmonary arteries in the case of genuine or pseudo-truncus arteriosus communis persistence. The outflow tract of the right ventricle reconstructed by means of Hancock's prosthesis can be particularly well observed in this view; peripheral pulmonary stenoses, not infrequently met with in the area of the right pulmonary artery in Fallot's tetralogy, are also visible in detail.
In our experience it is also possible to draw conclusions about the function of arteriovenous anastomoses by examining the density of the contrast medium.

Cranial 35° – 45°, Left Oblique 20° – 30°

This view serves to represent a left ventricular-right atrial shunt, something which was not at all easy to represent hitherto by conventional methods. Two-dimensional echocardiography with the injection of contrast medium into the left ventricle makes equivalent diagnosis possible in this area. A Fontan conduit can be controlled in its function and position after correcting tricuspid atresia (Figs. 5 and 6).

Cranial 15° – 25°, Left Oblique 20° – 30°

The haemodynamic total corrective operation according to Mustard and Senning requires angiocardiographic functional control, provided non-invasive methods of investigation do not suggest dysfunction of the interatrial buffle or leakage of the newly created atrial septum [11].

Future Developments

As a perspective for the future we have conceived the following projects for the standardisation of angled views:

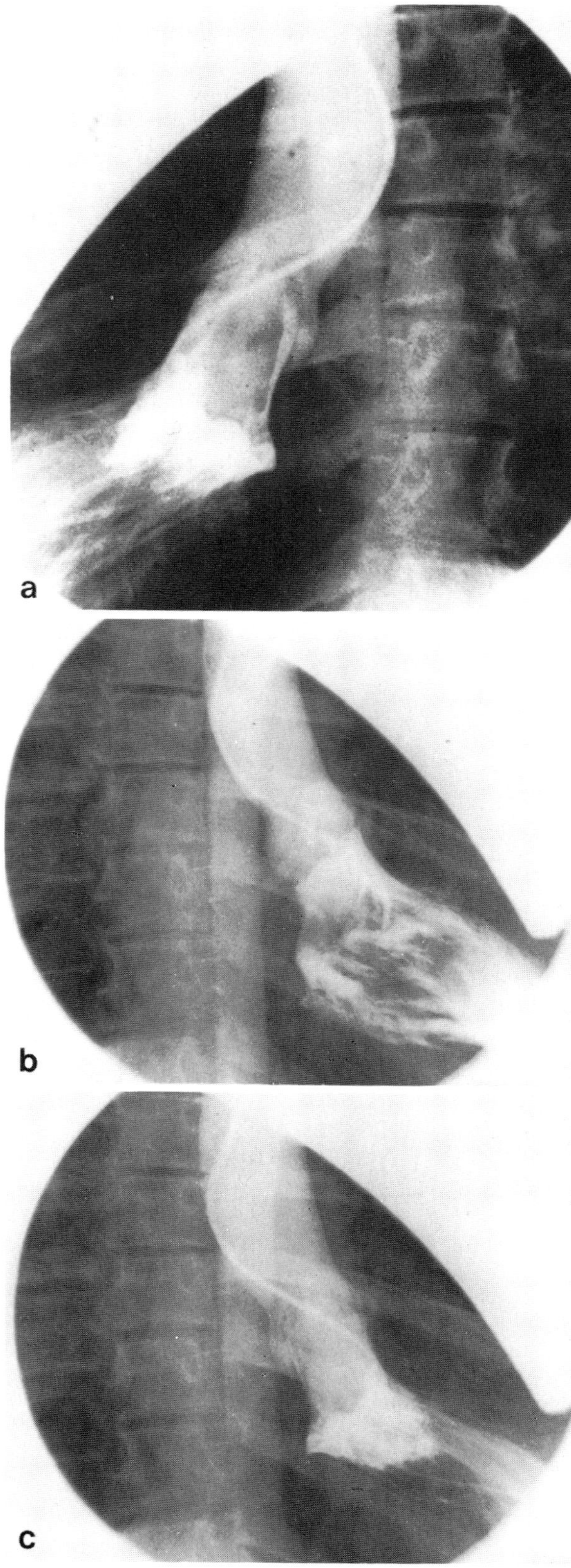

Fig. 5a – c. Selective angiography of a stenosis of the aortic valve. Right-anterior-oblique view

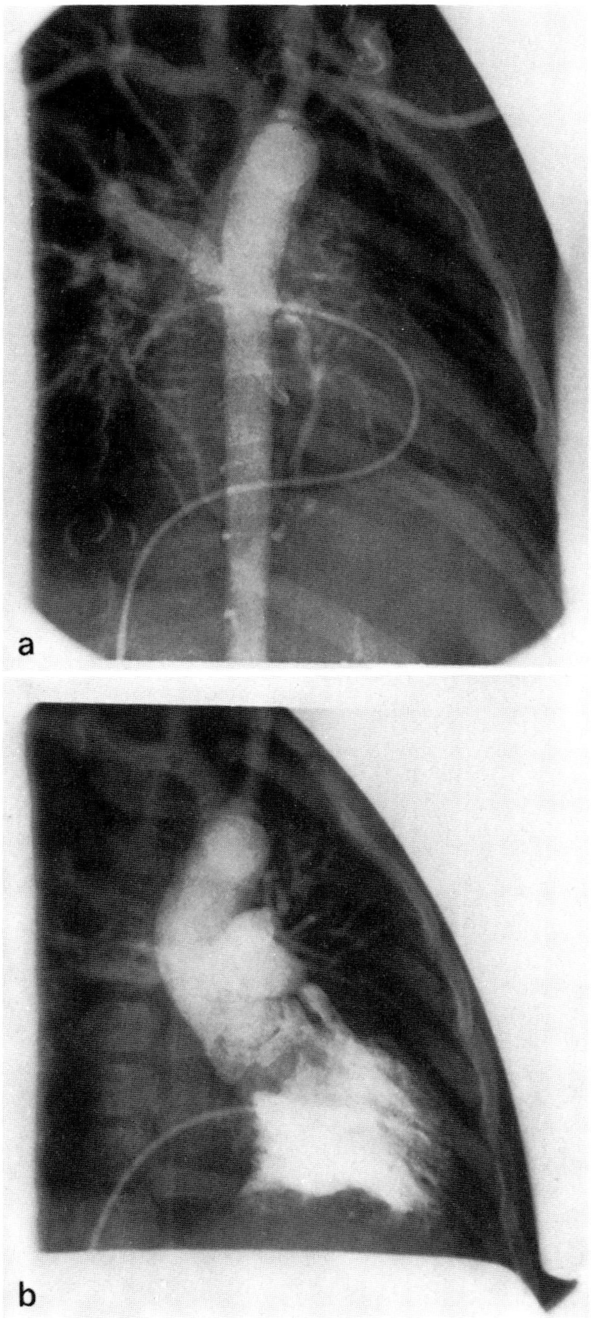

Fig. 6. a Selective angiography. Bronchial arteries in tetralogy of Fallot. **b** Same patient as in **a.** Selective angiography by injection of contrast medium into the right ventricle. Right-anterior-oblique view

The post-mortem specimen of a young child with a topographically exact copy of the cardiovascular system will be cine-angiocardiographed at the best possible angle view after marking the individual structures with a contrast material. The angle data thus obtained, which correspond to normal values, will serve as guidelines for the angle views to be established in the horizontal and vertical planes [9].

In accordance with the experiments conducted by Köhler and Schneider, it is further planned to employ Cardan suspension of hearts in a Plexiglass cylinder to demonstrate pathological-anatomical alterations after marking them with a contrast material. They will then be filmed from the corresponding angles with the biplane C-arm device described above. This method guarantees the transmission of the intravital axis position of the heart. It will thereby be possible to compare angled views for the representation of pathological structures in their deviation from the norm and at the same time make known these experimentally obtained angle data for general application.

References

1. Bargeron LM, Elliott LP, Soto B, Bream PR, Curry CG (1977) Axial cineangiography in congenital heart disease. I. Concept, technical and anatomical considerations. Circulation 56:1075
2. DenBoer JA (1976) Distribution of scattered radiation around the cardio diagnost. Medicamundi 21:121
3. Elliott LP, Bargeron LM Jr, Bream PR, Soto B, Curry CG (1977) Axial cineangiography in congenital heart disease. II. Specific lesions. Circulation 56:1086
4. Fellows KE, Keane JF, Freed MD (1977) Angled views in cineangiocardiography of congenital heart disease. Circulation 56:485
5. Freedom RM, Olley PM (1976) Pulmonary arteriography in congenital heart disease. Cathet Cardiovasc Diag 2:309
6. Kattan KR (1970) Angled view in pulmonary angiography. A new roentgen approach. Radiology 94:79
7. Sansa M, Tonkin IL, Bargeron LM Jr, Elliott LP (1979) Left ventricular outflow tract obstruction in transposition of the great arteries. An angiographic study of 75 cases. Am J Cardiol 44:88
8. Schmidt-Redemann B, Böhm N, Piechaud P, Tibert M, Schaupeter W, Fürste HO (to be published) Neue Projektionsmethoden zur cineangiocardiographischen Darstellung angeborener Herzfehler. Z Kardiol
9. Soto B, Bargeron LM Jr, Elliott LP, Barnes G, Bream PR, Curry CG (to be published) Special projections for angiographic study of congenital heart malformations. Exibit, 49th Scientific sessions, Am Heart Assoc. Miami Beach, Tl. Oct. 1976
10. Tonkin JL, Sasa M, Bargeron LM Jr, Elliott LP (1978) The radiographic recognition of developing left ventricular outflow tract obstruction in complete transposition. Circulation 58/II:69

Preliminary Evaluation of New Nonionic Contrast Media

U. Speck, G. Mannesmann, W. Mützel, and G. Schröder

Schering AG, Pharma-Forschung, Abteilung Biodynamik, Müllerstrasse 170–178, D-1000 Berlin 65

A number of physical and chemical properties of currently used ionic contrast agents were suspected to be responsible for the general toxicity as well as for the cardiovascular side effects of these products. The properties discussed in this regard are shown in Table 1.

The tolerance of former urographic and angiographic agents such a acetrizoate was severely limited by their lipophilic properties. The same is true for the cholegraphic contrast media. Considering the well-tolerated triiodinated compounds such as diatrizoates, iothalamates, and the other very similar products, three important factors limiting cardiovascular tolerance have been identified during the past 20 years: hypertonicity, the choice and concentration of cations, and the calcium ion binding of stabilizing agents like sodium EDTA.

Hypertonicity is believed to be the most important factor with regard to local tolerance during angiographic examinations. In 1969 Almen [1] proposed several principles to reduce osmotic pressure of contrast media from which polymerization and elimination of electrical charge leading to nonionic molecules were realized during the past 10 years. Problems occurred concerning solubility, stability, production cost, and toxicity of individual compounds or certain chemical classes of products. These problems led to compromises with regard to the pharmaceutical formulation of the new contrast agents, their cost per gram iodine, and their tolerance with regard to side effects caused by properties other than osmotic pressure, e.g., allergylike reactions.

Nevertheless, decreasing hypertonicity and eliminating the cations have been shown to be the most promising ways to improve cardiovascular tolerance of contrast media. New nonionic agents synthetized and developed with this object in mind in our laboratories or together with Nyegaard & Co., Oslo, were compared to ionic contrast media with high and with reduced osmotic pressure. Some of the results obtained with the new products are presented in this paper.

The compounds tested and their osmotic pressures are shown in Fig. 1. Osmolality of blood is about 290 mosmol. Currently used ionic contrast agents are strongly hypertonic. The first nonionic contrast agent with reduced osmotic pressure was metrizamide, a well tolerated but rather expensive product delivered as freeze-dried powder due to its limited stability. By dimerization Guerbet was able to produce an ionic contrast medium with significantly reduced osmotic pressure at lower cost and with better stability. New nonionic products combine the stability of ionic agents with the better tolerance of nonionic compounds. Dimerization of nonionic molecules led to blood-isotonic contrast media with high iodine content [12].

Table 1. Properties of X-ray contrast agents influencing their tolerance

Property	Significance for cardiovascular tolerance	References
Lipophilicity	Vasodilatation	[4]
Hypertonicity	Vasodilatation, cardiodepression (?), bradycardia	[7, 9, 13]
Electrical charge of ions		
Type and proportion of cations	Arrhythmia, ventricular fibrillation	[3, 8, 10]
Ca-binding (e.g. EDTA)	Decreased contractility	[9, 14]
Viscosity	Impaired microcirculation	[1]
Structure specific factors	Various	[11]

Radiology Today 1. Ed. by M. W. Donner and F. H. W. Heuck

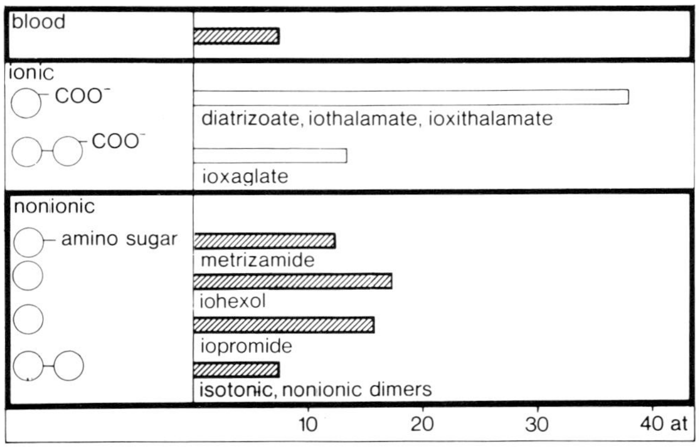

Fig. 1. Osmotic pressure of blood in comparison with contrast media for angiography (contrast medium, 300 mg iodine/ml)

General toxicity of contrast agents is known to be related to their lipophilicity [11]. Lipophilicity of various contrast agents as measured as partition coefficient between butanol and water is presented in Table 2. One has to realize that the electrical charge of ionic contrast agents contributes to a high degree to their hydrophilic properties and good tolerance. On the other hand, for technical reasons it is easier to measure the lipophilicity of acids in their undissociated state at low pH. Since these problems do not occur with nonionic molecules it is not appropiate to compare the figures given in Table 2 for ionic and nonionic compounds.

Nevertheless, the higher lipophilicity of ioxaglate compared with the well-tolerated ionic contrast agent ioglicate indicates that ioxaglate should be more chemotoxic than ioglicate. The lack of electrical charge on the second triiodobenzene is the reason why ioxaglate is more lipophilic than the known ionic contrast media.

Nonionic contrast agents are very hydrophilic due to a great number of hydroxy groups attached to the molecules.

A correlation similar to that between lipophilicity and toxicity exists between protein binding and toxicity. As one example of an interaction of contrast agents with proteins, the inhibition of human serum complement-mediated hemolysis [11] is presented in Table 3. Ioxaglate proved to be the most active agent in this test system, nonionic contrast media influencing the complement system only to a lesser extent.

In agreement with these results, the LD_{50} of nonionic contrast agents after IV injection in rats is distinctly higher than that of ionic contrast media (Table 4). The best intravenous tolerance was found for a nonionic dimer, probably because of its low osmotic and molar load for the animals

Table 2. Lipophilicity of various contrast agents (partition coefficient butanol/buffer pH 1)

Contrast agent	Partition coefficient
Meglumine ioglicate	0.62[a]
Meglumine ioxaglate	0.89[a]
Metrizamide	0.27
Iohexol	0.061
Iopromide	0.069
Nonionic dimer	0.090

[a] Undissociated acid

Table 3. Inhibition of complement mediated hemolysis, concentration necessary to inhibit 50% of activity

Contrast agent	I_{50}
Meglumine ioglicate	5.3
Meglumine ioxaglate	3.5
Metrizamide	11.5
Iohexol	13
Iopromide	15
Nonionic dimer	11.5

Table 4. LD_{50} of various ionic and nonionic contrast agents in the rat after intravenous injection; 95% confidence limits in parentheses

Contrast agent	LD_{50} (g iodine/kg body weight)
Meglumine-sodium ioglicate	8.72 (8.04 – 9.27)
Meglumine-sodium ioxaglate	8.41 (7.70 – 9.13)
Metrizamide	12.97 (11.99 – 14.03)
Iohexol	~ 13
Iopromide	12.92 (11.70 – 14.22)
Nonionic dimer	16.05 (14.24 – 18.37)

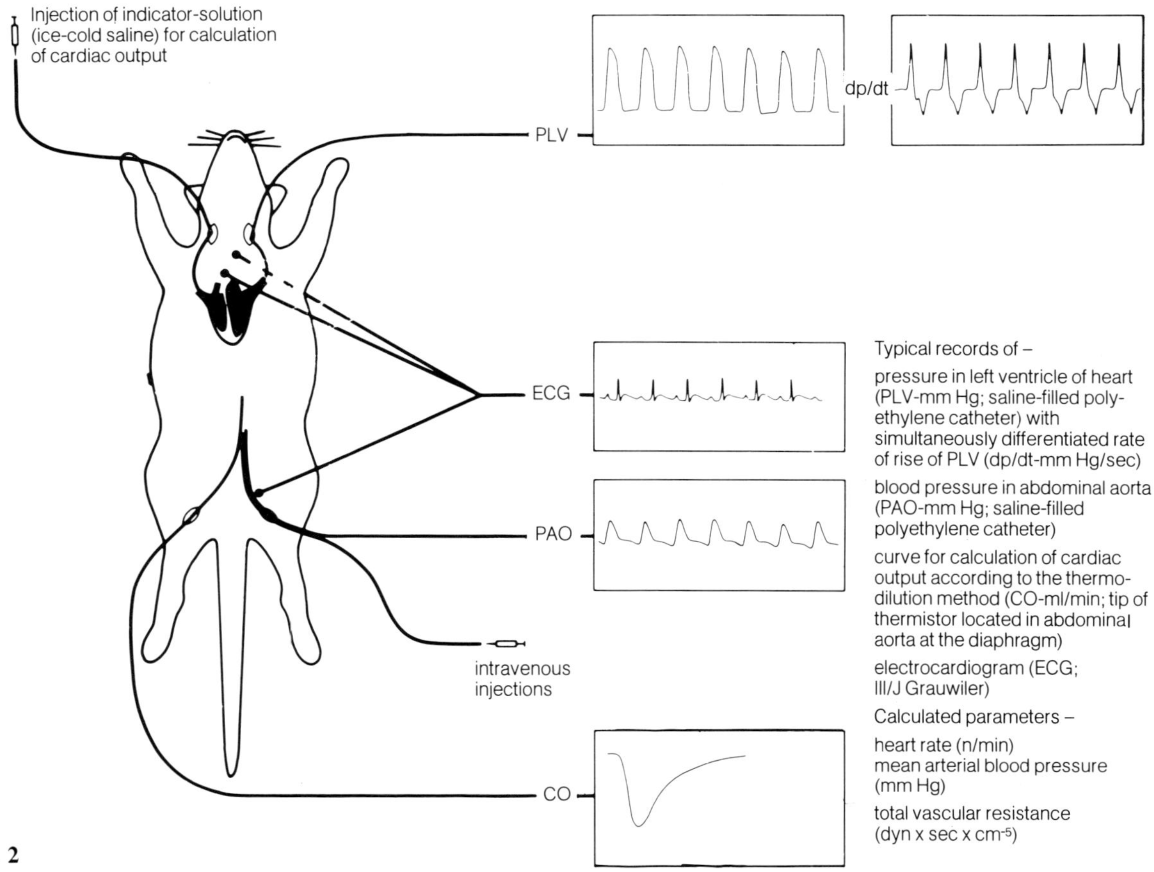

Fig. 2

at the same iodine dosage. Ioxaglate was not better tolerated than hypertonic ionic contrast media in spite of its lower osmotic pressure.

Of course, only a few comparative clinical data are available on the cardiovascular tolerance of new contrast media. For the comparison of new agents with well-known contrast media we have to refer to animal experiments. According to our experience with regard to cardiovascular tolerance, even experiments in the rat give a good prediction of the side-effects of X-ray contrast media in humans [6] (Fig. 2).

To get a first impression a bolus IV injection of 3 ml contrast medium/kg body weight or a volume control was given within 10 s to ten animals each. We compared contrast agents from four chemical classes:

a) Meglumine ioglicate, a well-tolerated but hypertonic triiodinated ionic contrast medium.
b) Meglumine-sodium ioxaglate, a monocarboxy-dimer with reduced osmotic pressure.
c) Metrizamide, iohexol, iopromide, nonionic triiodinated contrast media, slightly hypertonic.
d) A nonionic dimer, blood isotonic due to the addition of salts.

In a first series meglumine ioglicate (300 mg iodine/ml, Rayvist) was compared to meglumine-sodium ioxaglate (320 mg iodine/ml, Hexabrix), metrizamide (320 mg iodine/ml, Amipaque), and saline as volume control (Fig. 3).

Under the experimental conditions even the saline solution produced an increase in blood pressure and cardiac contractility as a consequence of the large injection volume. Meglumine ioglicate caused the known effects of hypertonic contrast agents: a short-lasting hypotension due to depression of contractility of the heart and vasodilatation followed by a compensatory increase in contractility and blood pressure. With metrizamide no pronounced reactions were observed. In contrast to ioglicate and similar to the volume control immediately after injection of metrizamide a slight increase of blood pressure and contractile force occurred.

The injection of ioxaglate was followed by a distinct increase of blood pressure. Contractility changes resemble metrizamide more than ioglicate. Ioxaglate is the only contrast agent which led to an early and marked increase in vascular resistance. The occurrence and significance of this new type of

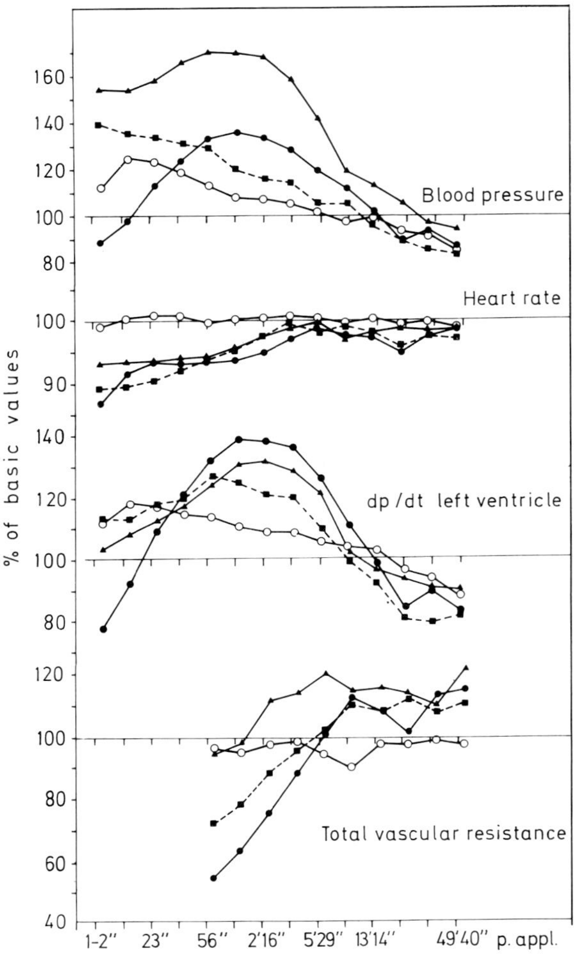

Fig. 3. Cardiovascular effects of contrast media in rats; first series. ○, control; ●, meglumine ioglicate; ■, metrizamide; ▲, meglumine-sodium ioxaglate

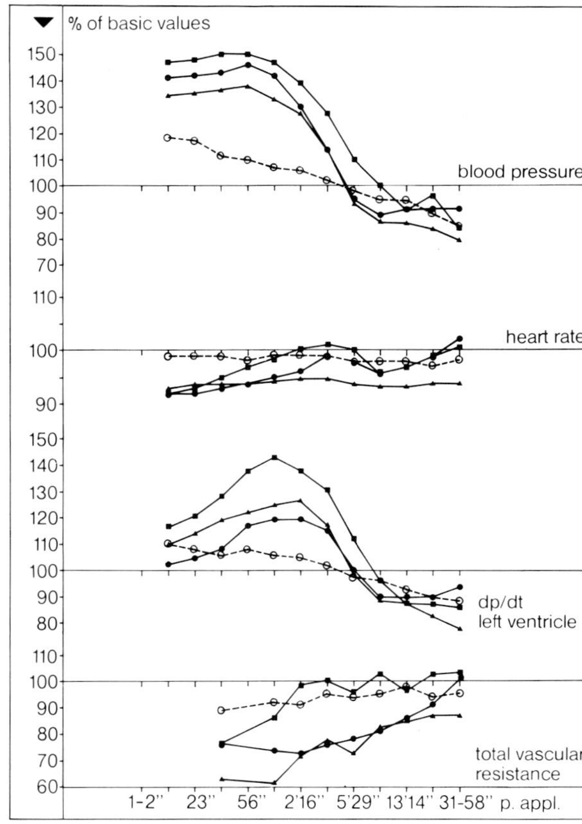

Fig. 4. Cardiovascular effects of contrast media in rats; second series. ○, control; ■, metrizamide; ●, iopromide; ▲, iohexol

side effect should be investigated under clinical conditions.

In a second series the new monomeric nonionic contrast media iohexol and iopromide were compared to metrizamide (Fig. 4). In spite of the high dosage and fast injection rate the effects were only moderate and shortlasting (logarithmic time axis in figures). All three contrast media caused no decrease but rather an increase in blood pressure. The influence on heart rate was negligible. Contractility was increased to 140% of preinjection values by metrizamide but only slightly influenced by iopromide. A small positive inotropic effect was reported by Higgins [5] after intracoronary administration of two other nonionic contrast media in dogs. Decrease of vascular resistance was very small with metrizamide and somewhat more pronounced with iopromide and iohexol, which is in accordance with the increasing osmotic pressure of these agents.

In a third experiment the cardiovascular tolerance of an isotonic nonionic dimer (300 mg iodine/ml) was compared to metrizamide and the hypertonic contrast medium meglumine ioglicate. Blood pressure and cardiac contractility showed a shortlasting increase over control values. Influence of the nonionic dimer on peripheral vascular resistance was less pronounced than with all other agents tested (Fig. 5).

Conclusion

During the last 10 years new types of contrast agents have been synthesized and tested for their tolerance. They differ from the known triiodinated ionic hypertonic contrast media with respect to several physicochemical properties which are believed to be responsible for toxicity as well as for cardiovascular side effects. Monoacid dimers are more lipophilic than conventional ionic contrast media, thus bearing a greater risk of general

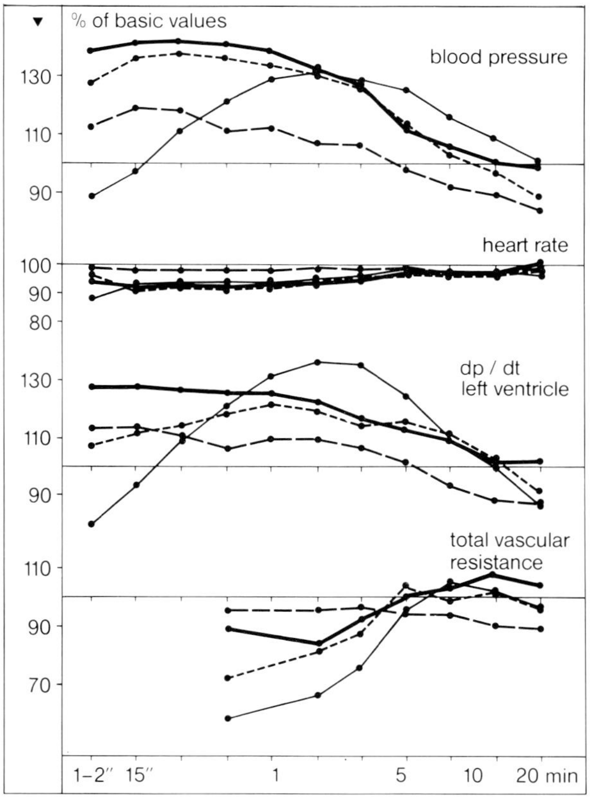

Fig. 5. Cardiovascular effects of contrast media in rats; third series. - — -, control; ——, meglumine ioglicate; - - - - -, metrizamide; ▬▬, nonionic dimer

toxicity. The toxicity of nonionic agents is not dependent upon electrical charge, the effects of cations, and hypertonicity, since these factors are absent or at least reduced. The known cardiovascular side effects of hypertonic contrast media such as vasodilatation, cardiodepression, and hypotension occur only to a minor extent. However, new types of reactions were observed in the animal experiments, e.g., hypertension and increase in cardiac contractility leading to a higher oxygen demand of the myocardium. The clinical significance of the positive inotropic effect of contrast media has been discussed in the literature as possibly being deleterious under ischemic conditions [2, 8].

References

1. Almen T (1969) Contrast Agent design. Some aspects on the synthesis of water soluble contrast agents of low osmolality. J Theor Biol 24:216
2. Als AV, LaRala JR, Miner NC, Paulin S (1978) Differential effects of sodium meglumine calcium metrizoate on the inotropic state of normal and ischemic myocardium. Radiology 128:499
3. Carter AM, Olin T (1976) Ionic composition and cardiotoxicity of dimeric contrast media at injection into the coronary arteries of rabbits. Acta Radiol [Diagn] (Stockh) 17:433
4. Coel MN, Lasser EC (1971) A pharmacologic basis for peripheral vascular resistance changes with contrast media injections. AJR 111:802
5. Higgins CB, Sovak M, Schmidt WS, Kelley MJ, Newell JD (1980) Direct myocardial effects of intracoronary administration of new contrast materials with low osmolality. Invest Radiol 15:39
6. Mannesmann G, Müller B, Goedecke H, Maaß B (1979) Cardio- and hemodynamic characterization of X-ray contrast media after intravascular administration. Pharmacol Ther [B] 5:115
7. Paulin S (to be published) Radiographic contrast experiments in the isolated canine heart and in the isolated rat papillary muscle. Contrast Material Symposium, Colorado Springs, 1979, Invest Radiol
8. Paulin S, Adams DF (1971) Increased ventricular fibrillation during coronary arteriography with a new contrast medium preparation. Radiology 101:45
9. Popio KA, Ross AM, Oravec JM, Ingram JT (1978) Identification and description of separate mechanism for two components of renografin cardiotoxicity. Circulation 58:520
10. Snyder CF, Formanek A, Frech RS, Amplatz K (1971) The role of sodium in promoting ventricular arrhythmia during selective coronary arteriography. AJR 113:567
11. Sovak M, Ranganathan R, Lang JH, Lasser EC (1978) Concepts in design of improved intravascular contrast agents. Ann Radiol (Paris) 21:283
12. Speck U, Mützel W, Mannesmann G, Pfeiffer H, Siefert HM (to be published) Pharmacology of nonionic dimers. Contrast Material Symposium, Colorado Springs, 1979. Invest Radiol
13. White CW, Eckberg DL, Inasaka T, Abboud FM (1976) Effects of angiographic contrast media on sinoatrial nodal function. Cardiovasc Res 10:214
14. Zipfel J (1979) Kardiale Nebenwirkungen der Koronarangiographie mit und ohne Ca^{++}-Zusatz. Z Kardiol 68:282

Interventional Radiology: Overview

R. I. White, Jr.

Johns Hopkins Medical Institutions, Department of Radiology and Radiological Science, 601 N. Broadway, Baltimore, MD 21205 (USA)

Introduction

An outgrowth of diagnostic angiography was the realization that an intravascular catheter could be used for much more than delineating arterial and venous anatomy. Viewed in simplest terms, interventional radiology is considered to comprise any catheter technique for selectively opening up or closing down a circulation. In the latter category, techniques for infusing vasopressin to control gastrointestinal hemorrhage or chemotherapeutic agents for selectively perfusing metastatic tumors are considered in addition to therapeutic embolization techniques.

Use of specialized angiographic catheters and wire guides have also led to successful interventional procedures in the biliary and urinary tracts.

Percutaneous Transluminal Angioplasty

Barely 16 years ago, in 1964, Dotter and Judkins described the technique employing telescoping catheters to recanalize femoral arteries [1]. The technique was nurtured and further developed by the pioneering efforts of Porstmann, Van Andel, and Zeitler [2, 3, 4]. Andreas Grüntzig conceived a major technical breakthrough with his development of the double lumen balloon sheath catheter in 1974. He was able to demonstrate that compression of soft atheromatous plaque was associated with an enlarged lumen and healing at the site of dilatation. Angioplasty was extended to the renal and visceral arteries and, in 1977, to the coronary arteries [5, 6, 7, 8].

In 1978, American cardiovascular radiologists took up the technique in earnest [7, 8, 9]. Intermediate and long-term results are now being documented on both sides of the Atlantic. In his contribution to this symposium, Professor Zeitler details techniques and results of angioplasty in a variety of circulations. The following observations only highlight some of the more recent work in this field:

Iliac and Femoral Artery Angioplasty

In the United States, angioplasty of the deep femoral artery is being performed with greater frequency. In general, many of the techniques as practiced are used in combination with distal surgical approaches. For example, upstream dilatation of ipsilateral iliac stenoses are performed before femoral-femoral and femoral-popliteal surgical bypasses.

Great effort is made to obtain thorough preangioplasty hemodynamics at the time of the diagnostic study [10, 11]. In addition to oblique angiography, pressures are measured on either side of the stenosis, and peak systolic gradients at rest and after priscoline-induced reactive hyperemia are calculated (Fig. 1).

Several important questions remain to be answered. Chief among these are the type and duration of antiplatelet drugs and anticoagulation prescribed after angioplasty.

Renal Angioplasty

Best results have followed dilatation of fibromuscular hyperplasia, followed by atherosclerotic and renal transplant stenoses [12]. The guiding catheter and dilatation balloon developed by Grüntzig for renal angioplasty have been largely replaced by coaxial techniques using superselective angiography with small catheters, flexible guidewires, and ultimately balloon catheters.

Radiology Today 1. Ed. by M. W. Donner and F. H. W. Heuck

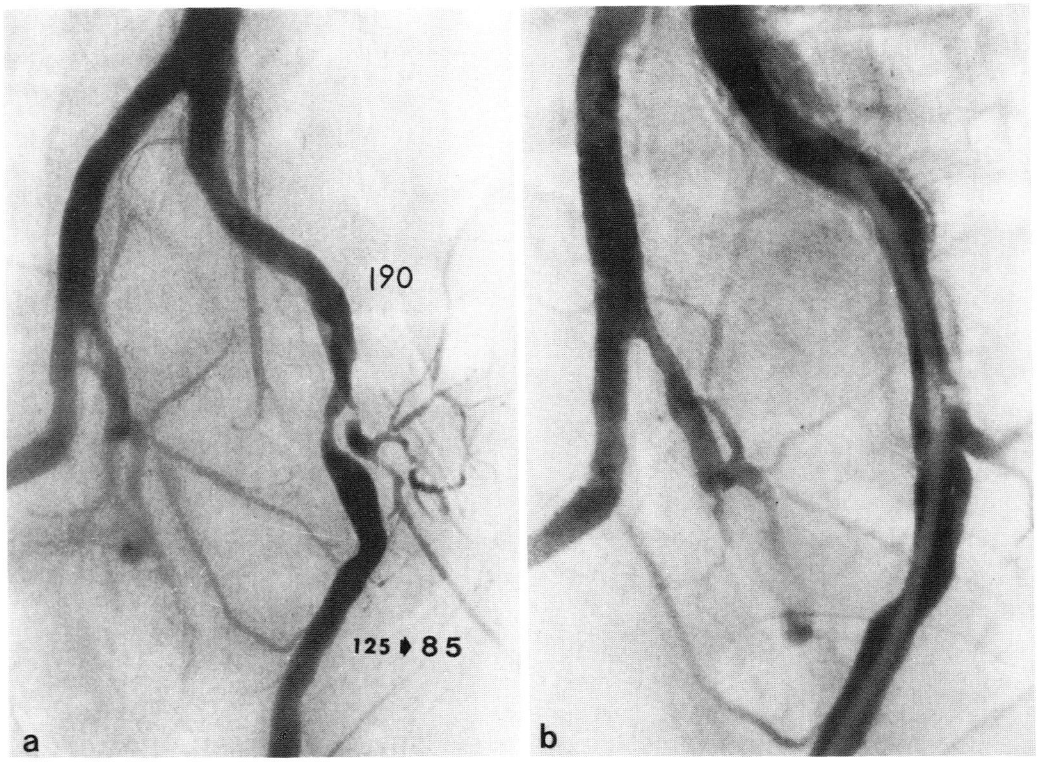

Fig. 1. a Iliac stenosis with peak systolic gradient of 65 mm at rest rising to 105 mm after priscoline. **b** After angioplasty, gradient was obliterated and symptoms were relieved

Coronary Artery Angioplasty

Coronary artery angioplasty has been limited to 5% – 10% of proximal right and left coronary artery lesions. With the best technique, emergency coronary bypass is required in 10% of patients undergoing the procedure. Now that Grüntzig and his colleagues have demonstrated the feasibility of this technique, it is anticipated that additional technical breakthroughs in catheter design will permit more access to distal lesions and more safety in performing the procedure.

Gastrointestinal Hemorrhage

After the demonstration by Baum, Rösch, and others of the feasibility of diagnosing acute upper and lower gastrointestinal bleeding sites by angiography, selective infusion of vasopressin was begun to control hemorrhage [13, 14, 15]. The experience has been duplicated in many centers, and it is now possible to stop most forms of small vessel bleeding from gastritis and stress erosions by selective vasopressin infusions. It was further demonstrated that continuous low dose intravenous vasopressin reduced portal pressure and caused vasoconstriction of esophageal varies to the same degree as selective infusions in the superior mesenteric artery [16]. In clinical studies, low dose intravenous vasopressin appeared to have the same efficacy as mesenteric arterial infusions for controlling hemorrhage from esophageal varices.

For large vessel bleeding from duodenal and gastric ulcers and some Mallory-Weiss hemorrhages, vasopressin did not appear to control most patients and therapeutic embolization of the left gastric and/or gastroduodenal artery was developed with particulate materials like Gelfoam [17]. Results have been quite acceptable with 75% of patients expected to stop by these techniques [18, 19]. Of course, controlling hemorrhage is only part of the therapy and patients must be vigorously managed with antiacids and in some instances surgery.

In most affected patients, arterial bleeding stops of its own accord after a period of stabilization and angiographic techniques are not employed until the patient has continued evidence of bleeding. This is true for all forms of gastrointestinal bleeding

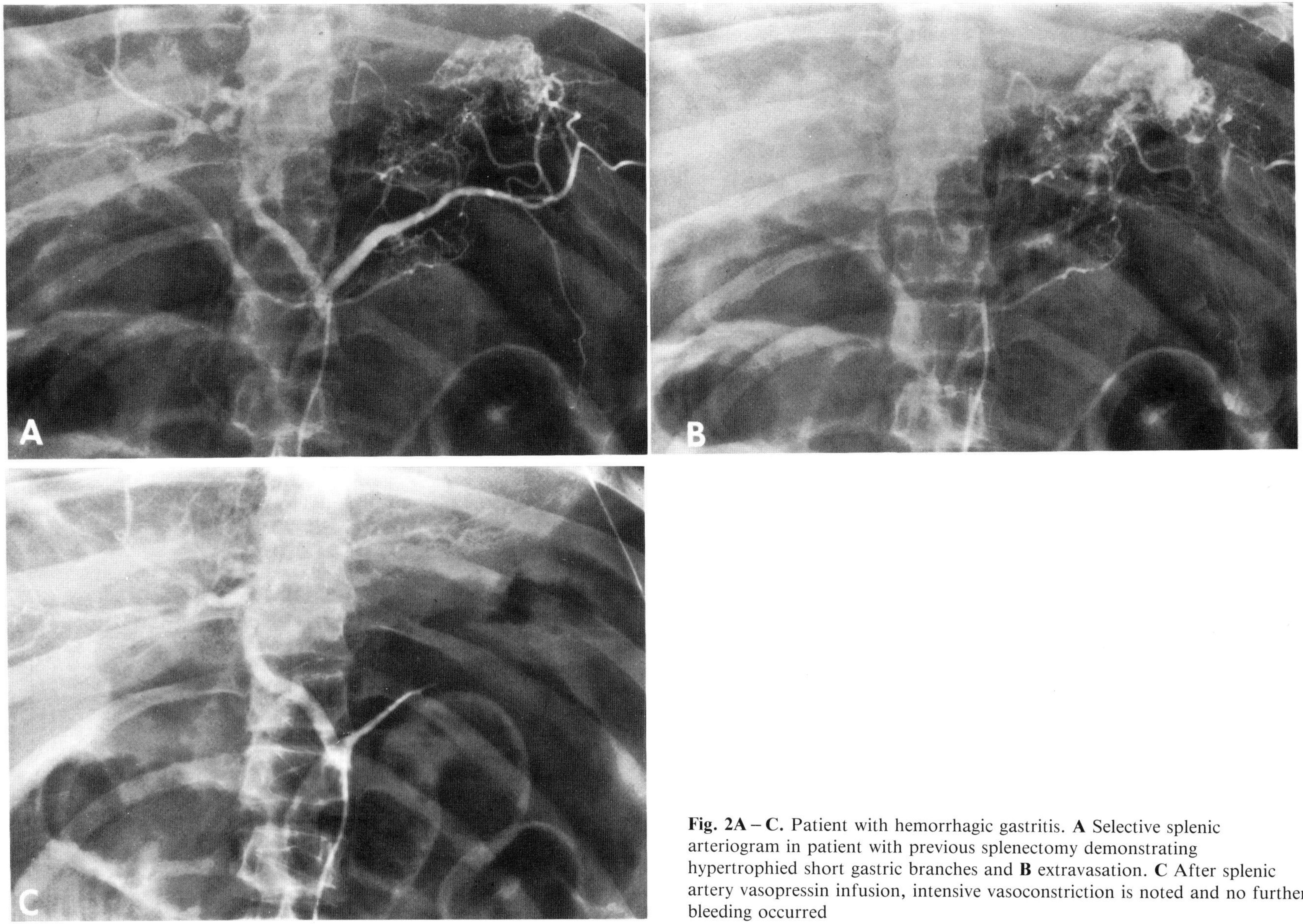

Fig. 2A – C. Patient with hemorrhagic gastritis. **A** Selective splenic arteriogram in patient with previous splenectomy demonstrating hypertrophied short gastric branches and **B** extravasation. **C** After splenic artery vasopressin infusion, intensive vasoconstriction is noted and no further bleeding occurred

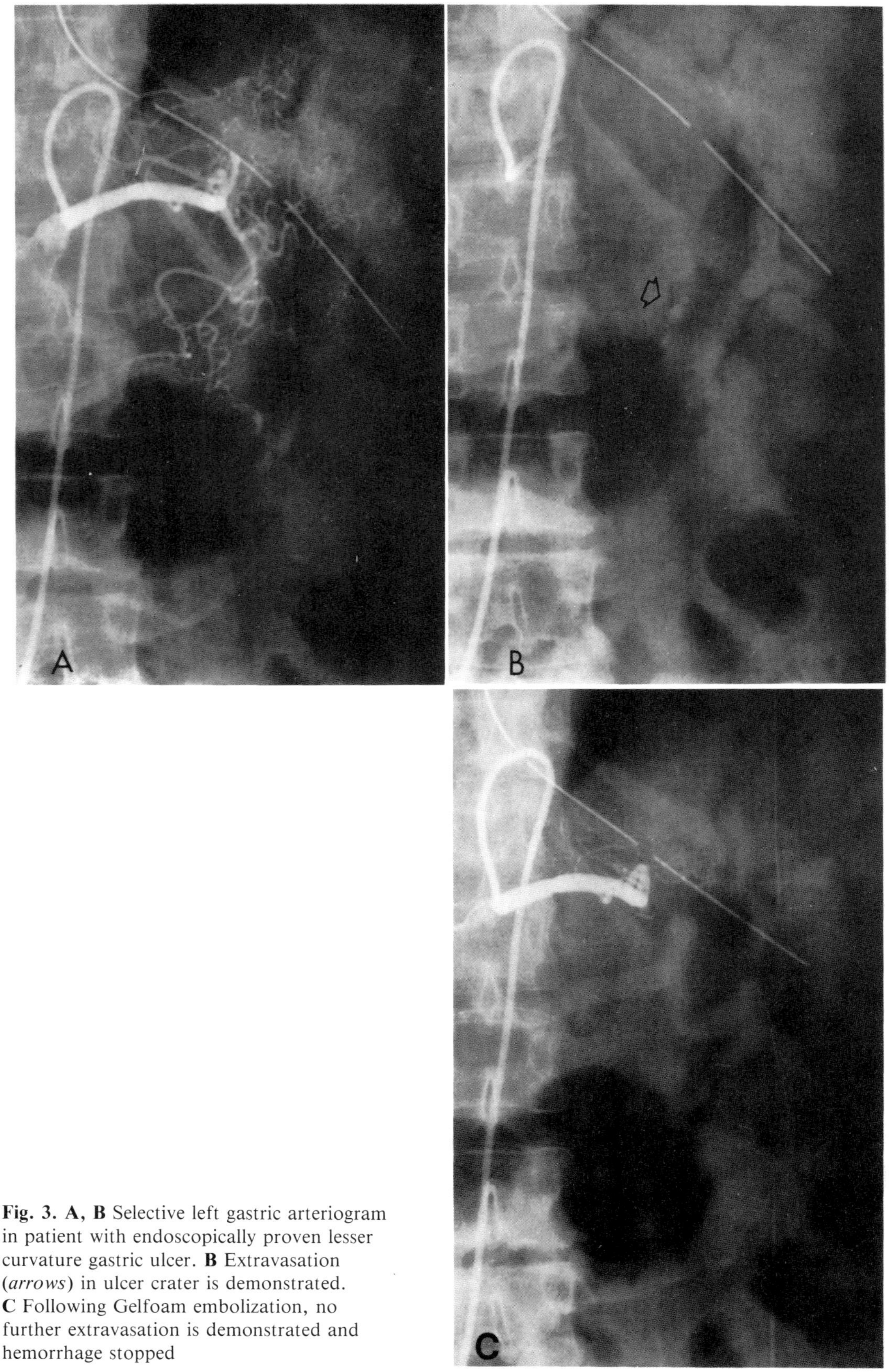

Fig. 3. A, B Selective left gastric arteriogram in patient with endoscopically proven lesser curvature gastric ulcer. **B** Extravasation (*arrows*) in ulcer crater is demonstrated. **C** Following Gelfoam embolization, no further extravasation is demonstrated and hemorrhage stopped

except in patients with hemorrhage from esophageal varices, where the incidence of rebleeding and ultimate death are so high. In this selected group of patients, if vasopressin infusions are not successful, then transhepatic coronary vein occlusion techniques are tried in lieu of emergency portal-systemic shunts [20, 21]. As yet, final evidence has not been obtained as to the efficacy of coronary vein occlusion techniques in altering long-term patient survival.

Experience has demonstrated that the success of the technique is largely dependent on the cooperation of the medical, surgical, and radiologic staffs. All patients are infused in an Intensive Care Unit under close monitoring, and for best results decisions are arrived at jointly by all physicians participating in the care of that patient (Figs. 2 and 3).

Selective Perfusion with Chemotherapy for Metastatic Tumors

In the past 2 decades, enthusiasm for selective infusion techniques has waxed and waned. Recently, with a whole new group of chemotherapeutic agents on the horizon, selective infusion techniques are being used with greater frequency [22, 23]. Best results seem to occur with metastatic liver and pelvic neoplasms. Goals of therapy are to produce a high concentration of drug in the target organ and to minimize systemic side effects.

Therapeutic Embolization

The literature in this area has expanded greatly in the past decade and, in particular in the past 5 years, largely as a result of the great many diseases that can be approached by these techniques and the large number of materials available for embolization [24, 25, 26]. Before treating a patient with these techniques, the radiologist must have a thorough background in embolic materials, the types of circulations to be embolized, and a knowledge of the natural history of the disease. Questions including length of action of the embolic material and associated inflammatory or possible carcinogenic effects should be considered.

The enthusiasm for embolization techniques has been dampened in part by lack of a material which produces long-lasting occlusion and also techniques that permit reversible occlusion up to a certain point in the procedure. Additionally, superselective catheterization may be difficult but absolutely necessary for embolization with particulate materials or tissue adhesives. Finally, risk of inadvertent embolization of neighboring organs is always present when using particulate materials (Figs. 4 and 5).

Duration of occlusion and inflammatory responses to the materials are often considered together. Short-lived materials (<48 h) include autologous clot, either natural or modified with aminocaproic acid. Intermediate length materials (>48 h – 30

Table 1. The properties and uses of materials employed in embolization techniques

Material	Inflammation	Size of particle	Application
Autologous clot	Minimal	Variable	Historical
Gelfoam	Moderate-self limited	Large particles (1 – 3 mm)	Hemorrhage, preoperative neoplasms
Oxycel	Moderate-self limited	Variable	Difficult to use consistently
Avitene	Moderate-self limited	Variable	Devascularization of head and neck neoplasms – contraindicated in AVM[a]
Ivalon	Minimal	Variable – slurry to 1 – 3 mm particles	Particles helpful for distal devascularization of AVM
Coils	Wool – moderate Dacron and Ivalon – minimal	Variable – pediatric to large	Preoperative neoplasms, hemorrhage, AVMs
Balloons	Minimal	1 – 8 mm silicone 1 – 12 mm latex	Preoperative devascularization of neoplasms, hemorrhage, post-traumatic fistula, pulmonary arteriovenous malformations
Isobutyl cyanoacrylate	Mild-to-moderate	Liquid	Preoperative devascularization of neoplasms, control of hemorrhage, AVMs
Liquid silicone	Minimal	Liquid	Preoperative devascularization of neoplasms or AVMs or devascularization of organs

[a] Arteriovenous malformations

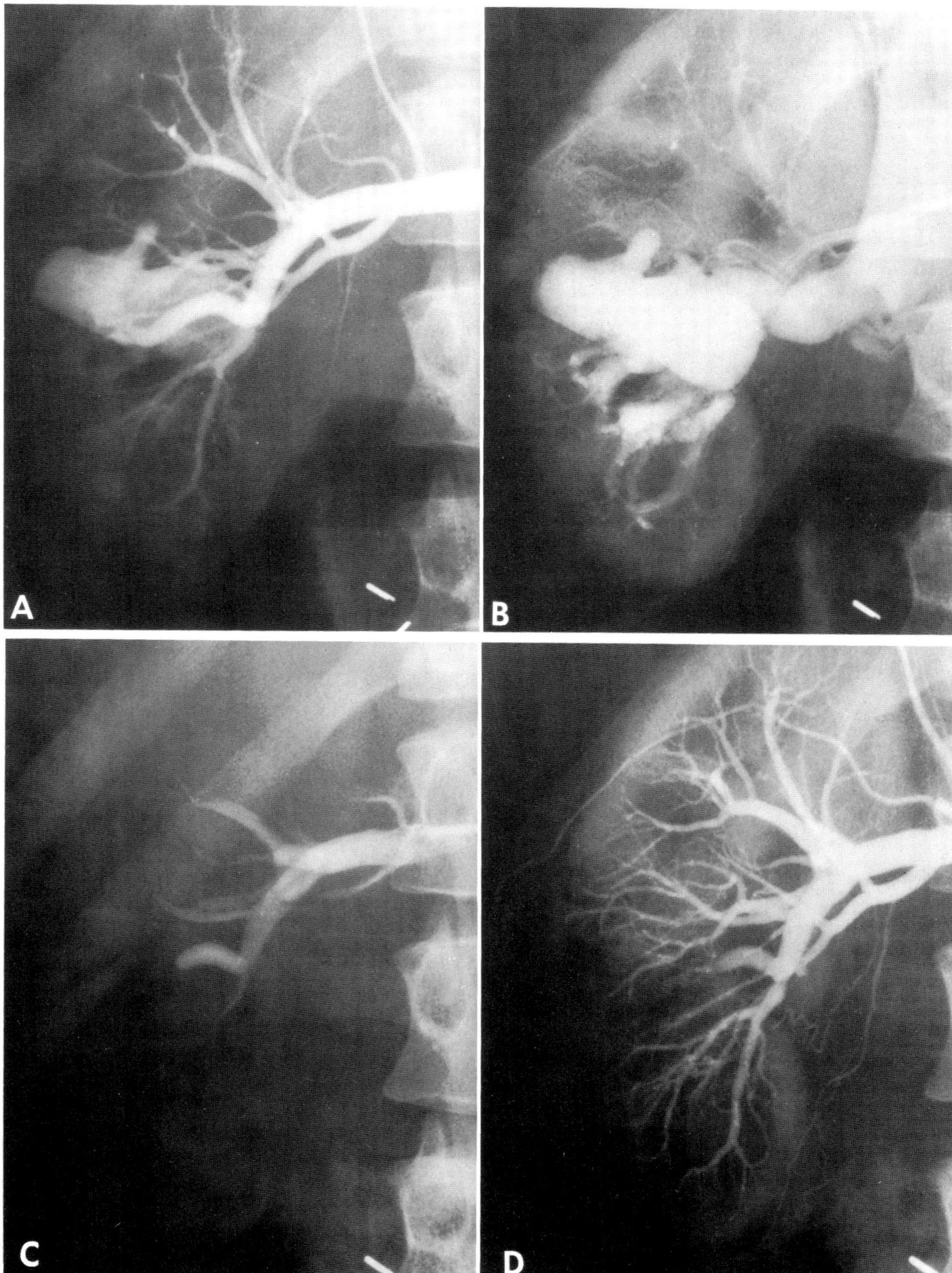

Fig. 4A – E. Renal angiograms demonstrating traumatic arteriovenous fistula formation following a stab wound of the right lower pole. **B** Early renal venous and inferior vena caval opacification. **C** Following balloon occlusion, the lower pole artery is blocked, with **D** preservation of the rest of the renal circulation and minimal distal infarction. Hematuria was immediately controlled, and 20 days later the balloon was identified on a follow-up radiograph [25]

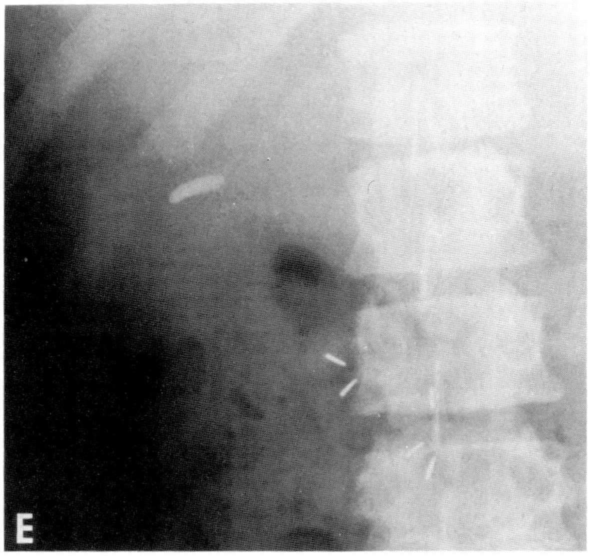

Fig. 4E. Legend see p. 55

days) include Gelfoam, oxidized cellulose, and microfibrillar collagen. Long-acting materials (>30 days) include detachable balloon, coils, polyvinyl alcohol (Ivalon), isobutyl cyanoacrylate (IBC), and silicone. The latter two agents are liquid and harden after injection; they appear to have the most promise for obliterating the interstices of congenital arteriovenous malformations. Table 1 lists some of the properties of these materials and the diseases they are used for.

Percutaneous Biliary Bypass

An outgrowth of the resurgence and interest in skinny needle transhepatic cholangiography was the realization that the biliary tract was readily

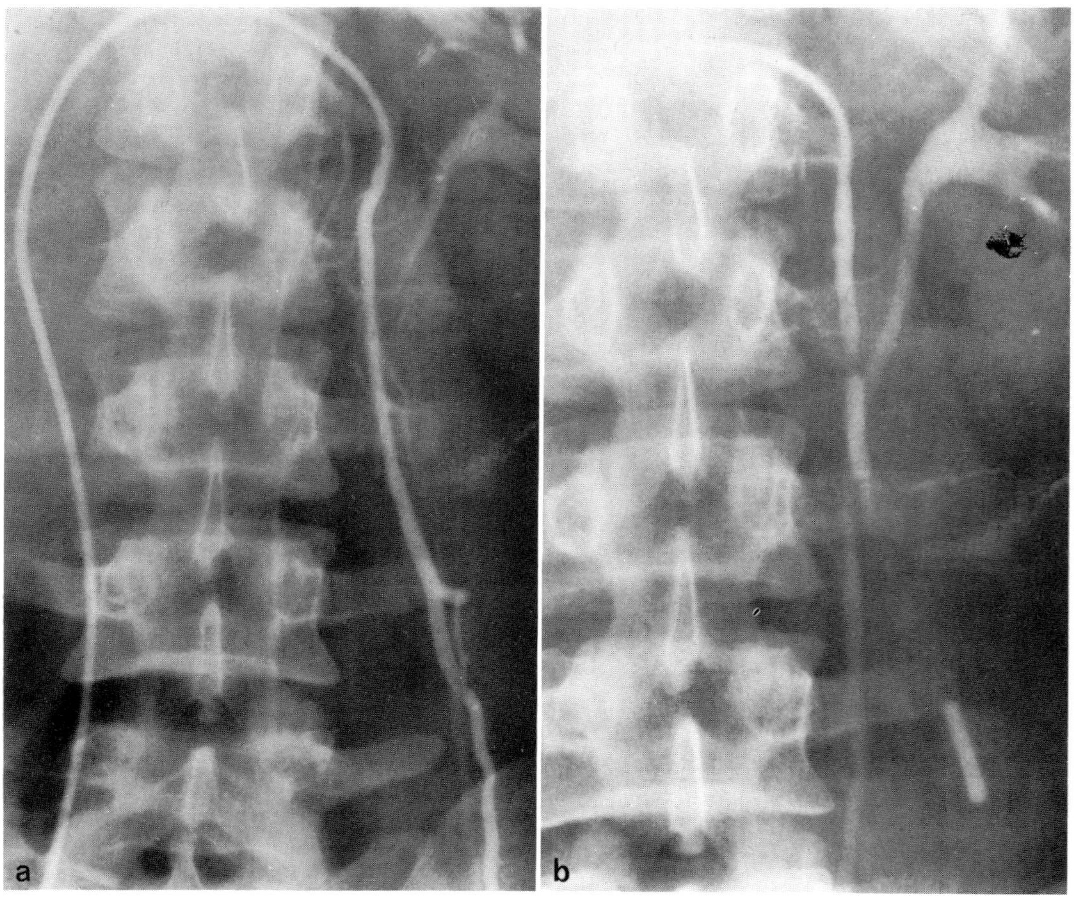

Fig. 5a, b. Testicular venogram before and after occlusion with large detachable silicone balloons. Balloons are precisely placed above any potential collaterals which could produce recurrent varicocele

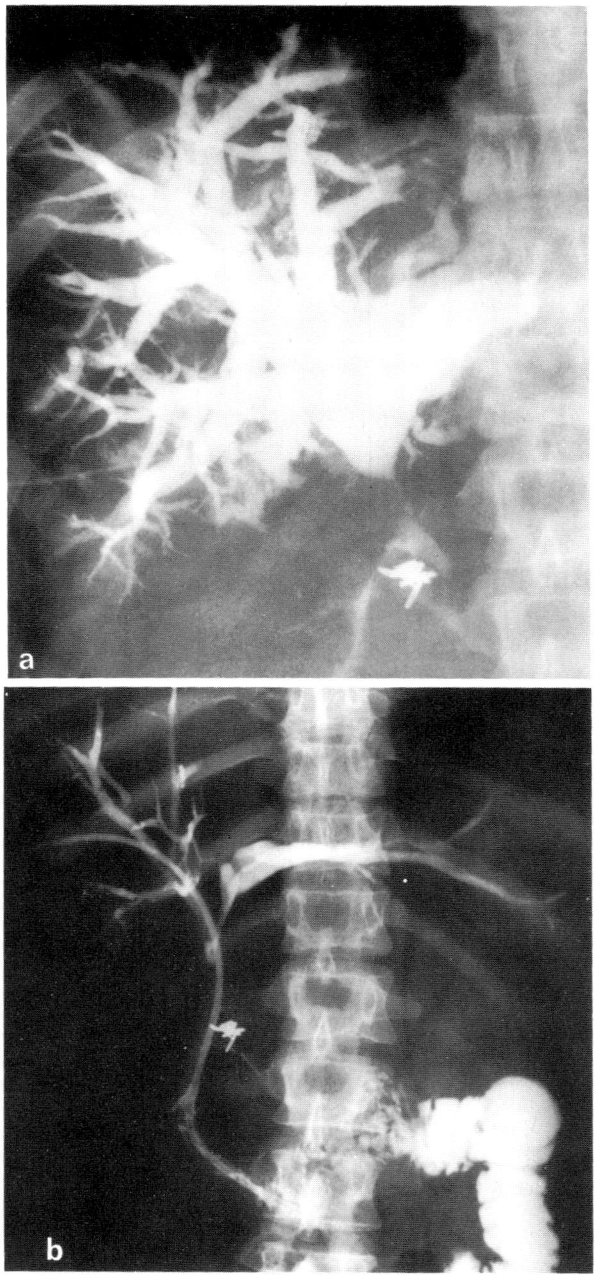

Fig. 6. a Stenosis of choledochojejunostomy with recurrent jaundice treated by percutaneous transhepatic biliary decompression. **b** Stent with multiple sideholes is placed across stenotic anastomosis and left in duodenum

accessible with modern guidewires and catheters for both external and internal drainage procedures [27, 28, 29]. It is now possible to palliate successfully malignant jaundice by transbiliary catheter stenting. Relief of jaundice permits the patient to receive intravenous hyperalimentation and thus be a stronger candidate for surgery or, in some instances, surgery can be avoided and the patient maintained by catheter drainage when the natural course of the disease is guarded. Additionally, patients with acute biliary obstruction and infection, who are poor surgical candidates, can be drained nonsurgically while receiving systemic antibiotics. After the patient has recovered, the offending lesion causing obstruction can be removed with less surgical risk to the patient (Fig. 6). These same procedures can be applied to obstruction in the urinary tract and also for draining retroperitoneal abscesses.

Concluding Remarks

These techniques have accounted for a marked change in the cardiovascular radiologist's practice. The actual performance of the interventional radiology procedure requires first, good repoire with the patient; second, close consultation with the referring physician prior to the procedure; and third, close follow-up of the patient after the procedure [30, 31]. Whenever indwelling catheters are left in the biliary tract or the vascular system, they must be monitored closely by the attending radiologist on a daily basis or more frequently as necessary. The results of these therapies have been most gratifying, and they will continue to provide us with a challenge for improving upon them and, in so doing, delivering better care to our patients.

References

1. Dotter CT, Judkins MP (1964) Transluminal treatment of arteriosclerotic obstruction. Description of a new technic and a preliminary report of its application. Circulation 30:654–670
2. Porstmann W (1973) Ein neuer Korsett-Ballonkatheter zur transluminalen Rekanalisation nach Dotter unter besonderer Berücksichtigung von Obliterationen an den Beckenarterien. Radiol Diagn (Berl) 14: 239
3. Van Andel GJ (1976) Percutaneous transluminal angioplasty: The dotter procedure. VanGorcum, Assen
4. Zeitler E, Gruntzig A, Schoop W (1978) Percutaneous vascular recanalization: Technique application clinical results. Springer, Berlin Heidelberg New York

5. Gruntzig AR, Senning A, Siegenthaler WE (1979) Nonoperative dilatation of coronary-artery stenosis. N Engl J Med 301:61 – 68
6. Gruntzig A, Kuhlmann U, Vetter W, Lutolf U, Meier B, Siegenthaler W (1978) Treatment of renovascular hypertension with percutaneous transluminal dilatation of a renal-artery stenosis. Lancet 1:801 – 802
7. Millan VG, Madias NE (1979) Percutaneous transluminal angioplasty for severe renovascular hypertension due to renal-artery medical fibroplasia. Lancet 1:1993 – 1935
8. Katzen BT, Chang J, Kukowsky GH, Abramson EG (1979) Percutaneous transluminal angioplasty for treatment of renovascular hypertension. Radiology 131:53 – 58
9. Yune HY, Schwarten DE, Klatte EC, Grim CE, Weinberger MH (to be published) Clinical experience in percutaneous transluminal angioplasty of stenotic renal arteries. Radiology
10. Udoff EJ, Barth KH, Harrington DP, Kaufman SL, White RI Jr (1979) Hemodynamic significance of iliac artery stenosis: Pressure measurements during angiography. Radiology 132:289 – 293
11. Kaufman SL, Fara JW, Udoff EF, Harrington DP, White RI Jr (1979) Hemodynamic effects of vasodilators across iliac stenoses in dogs. Invest Radiol 14/6:471 – 475
12. Sniderman KW, Sos TA, Sprayregen S, Saddekni S, Cheigh JS, Tapla L, Tellis V, Veith FJ (1980) Percutaneous transluminal angioplasty in renal transplant arterial stenosis for relief of hypertension. Radiology 135/1:23 – 26
13. Baum S, Nusbaum M (1971) The control of gastrointestinal hemorrhage by selective mesenteric arterial infusion of vasopressin. Radiology 98:497 – 505
14. Rosch J, Dotter CT, Rose RW (1971) Selective arterial infusions of vasoconstrictors in acute gastrointestinal bleeding. Radiology 99:27 – 36
15. Athanasoulis CA, Waltman AC, Novelline RA, Kurdy AG, Sniderman KW (1976) Angiography: Its contribution to the emergency management of gastrointestinal hemorrhage. Radiol Clin North Am 14:265 – 280
16. Kaufman SL, Maddrey WC, Harrington DP, White RI Jr (1977) Hemodynamic effects of superior mesenteric arterial and intravenous vasopressin infusions in patients with portal hypertension. Invest Radiol 12/3:210 – 214
17. Bookstein JJ, Chlosta EM, Foley D, Walter JF (1975) Transcatheter hemostasis of gastrointestinal bleeding using modified autogenous clot. Radiology 113:277 – 285
18. Eisenberg H, Steer ML (1976) The nonoperative treatment of massive pyloroduodenal hemorrhage by retracted autologous clot embolization. Surgery 79:414 – 420
19. Reuter SR (1979) Embolization of gastrointestinal hemorrhage. AJR 133:557 – 558
20. Lunderquist A, Vang J (1974) Transhepatic catheterization and obliteration of the coronary vein in patients with portal hypertension and esophageal varices. N Engl J Med 291:646 – 649
21. Widrich WC, Johnson WC, Robbins AH, Nabseth DC (1978) Esophagogastric variceal hemorrhage: Its treatment by percutaneous transhepatic coronary vein occlusion. Arch Surg 113:1331 – 1338
22. Wirtanen GW: Percutaneous transbrachial artery infusion catheter techniques. AJR 117:696 – 700
23. Clouse ME, Ahmed R, Ryan RB, Oberfield RA, McCaffrey JA (1977) Complications of long term transbrachial hepatic arterial infusion chemotherapy. AJR 129:799 – 803
24. Athanasoulis CA (1980) Therapeutic applications of angiography. (First of Two Parts). N Engl J Med 302/20:1117 – 1125
25. White RI Jr, Kaufman SL, Barth KH, DeCaprio V, Strandberg JD (1979) Embolotherapy with detachable silicone balloons. Technique and clinical results. Radiology 131/3:619 – 627
26. Terry PB, Barth KH, Kaufman SL, White RI Jr (1980) Balloon embolization for treatment of pulmonary arteriovenous fistulas. New Engl J Med 302/21:1189 – 1190
27. Molnar W, Stockum AE (1978) Transhepatic dilatation of choledochenterostomy strictures. Radiology 129:59 – 64
28. Ring EJ, Oleaga JA, Freiman DB, Husted JW, Lunderquist A (1978) Therapeutic applications of catheter cholangiography. Radiology 128:333 – 338
29. Hansson JA, Hoevels J, Simert G, Tylen U, Vang J (1979) Clinical aspects of nonsurgical percutaneous transhepatic bile drainage in obstructive lesions of the extrahepatic bile ducts. Ann Surg 189:58 – 61
30. White RI Jr (1980) Interventional radiology in the 1980s (editorial). AJR 134/4:859 – 860
31. Baum S (1980) The radiologist intervenes (editorial). N Engl J Med 302/20:1141 – 1142

Transluminal Dilatation: Overview

E. Zeitler

Klinikum Nürnberg, Radiologisches Zentrum, Flurstrasse 17, D-8500 Nürnberg

Thanks to the technical improvement of the original Dotter [3, 4] catheter, the knowledge of the important role that platelet inhibitors play [20], and the close supervision of the patient during the first 48 h after treatment, this technique can now be successfully applied in the treatment of occlusive arterial disease [1, 2, 5, 6, 7, 12, 15, 18, 19, 20]. Between 1968 and the present, we have utilized it 1217 times in 1071 patients.

Nowadays, we use the following catheter types: (a) teflon step catheters [1] (Zeitler) [19, 20]; (b) teflon dilating catheters [2] (Van Andel) [2] in different sizes; and (c) double-lumen catheters [3] (Grüntzig) [6], but not the "coaxial dilating set" (Dotter) [3, 4]. Experiences with the Dotter technique have been made in the Aggertalklinik in 820 patients with 922 recanalizations.

Results

From 1217 cases, follow-up checks were made in 81 extremities of 79 patients with stage II superficial femoral arterial occlusion (Fig. 1) over a period of more than 5 years, this being a well-defined patient group treated between December 1968 and November 1971.

Twenty-one legs were successfully recanalized using 8-French Teflon catheters – today called bypassing catheters – and 60 cases were treated with the coaxial dilating set developed by Dotter. During the follow-up period, 20 patients died and three legs had to be amputated (3.7% in 7 years) because of rethrombosis and resulting gangrene. During the first 2 years the rethrombosis rate appeared to increase (to 40%), but it then slowed down until the 5th year.

1, 2 Cook Europe ApS, DK-2860 Söborg
3 Schneider Medintag, CH-8053 Zürich

Additionally, a cooperative study from 12 clinics [21] is now available covering 1184 cases treated up to March 1977. A third of these cases had gangrene. The primary success rate was 74%; the early reocclusion rate within 2 weeks was 11%.

Our long-term follow-up study manifested that of the arteries treated, 26% were still patent after 5 years, and 20% after $6\frac{1}{2}$ years.

Previous follow-up examinations of different obliterations dilated with the Grüntzig balloon catheter manifested a higher patency rate after 1 and 3 years (Tables 1 and 2). However, maintenance of an anticoagulation therapy or treatment with aggregation inhibitors has considerable influence on the results. We observed that about 80% of the

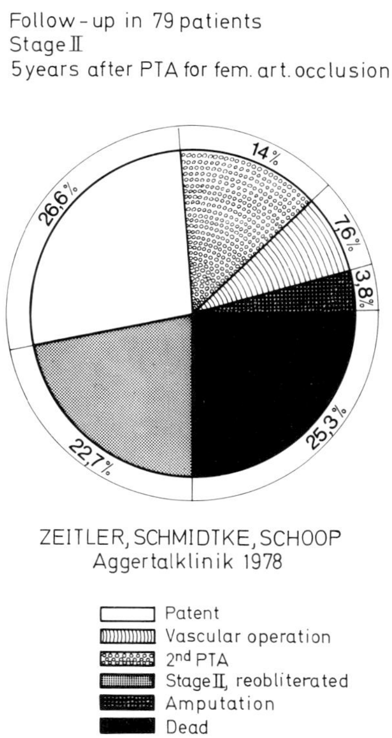

Fig. 1. Follow-up control after PTA in patients with superficial femoral occlusion and claudication

Radiology Today 1. Ed. by M. W. Donner and F. H. W. Heuck

Table 1. Results of PTA with different types of catheters

Artery	*n*	+[a]	1-year patency rate	Author
Iliac artery stenosis	262	79%	77%	Zeitler (A)[b]
	56	92%	79%	Mathias[c]
	45	84%		Zeitler (Nbg.)[d]
Femoral artery stenosis	131	84%	78%	Zeitler (A)[b]
	108	98%	74%	Mathias[c]
	75	95%	84%	Zeitler (Nbg.)[d]
Femoral artery occlusions (smaller than 10 cm)	304	81%	80%	Zeitler (A)[b]
	159	90%	69%	Mathias[c]
	107	79%	82%	Zeitler (Nbg.)[d]
(larger than 10 cm)	133	54%	52%	Zeitler (A)[b]
Popliteal artery stenoses	51	75%		Zeitler (A)[b]
+ popliteal artery occlusions	53	92%	67%	Mathias[c]
Tibial artery obstructions	73	90%	73%	Mathias[c]

[a] + good angiographic and clinical result in the first 10 days
[b] Zeitler (A) = Aggertalklinik: original Dotter catheter,
single Teflon catheter,
Fogarty balloon catheter,
caged balloon catheter,
Grüntzig balloon catheter
[c] Mathias, Freiburg, (personal information): Grüntzig balloon catheter
[d] Zeitler, Nbg.: single Teflon catheter
Teflon step catheter
Grüntzig balloon catheter

Table 2. PTA in leg arteries

Clinic		Patients	*n*	+[a]	Patency rate	Complications[b]
Aggertalklinik						
1968–1976	Zeitler et al.	820	922	72.0%		2.2%
1976–1980	Roth et al.		901	78.0%	3 years	0.2%
Kantonspital Zürich		Iliac artery stenosis	115		83.4%	
Grüntzig, Schneider (personal information)		Femoro-popliteal obliterations	356		71.0%	1.5%
Uni-Klinik Freiburg Mathias (personal information)		353	375	93.5% 422 segments		2.5%
Uni-Klinik Munich Ingrisch (personal information)		129	129	84.0%		1.1%
Klinikum Nürnberg 1976–1980		251	295	St. II: 91.0% St. IV: 70.0%		2.2% 1.4%
			3093	81.0%	80.0%	1.6%

[a] + good angiographic and clinical results in the first 10 days
[b] Complications, which need vascular surgery

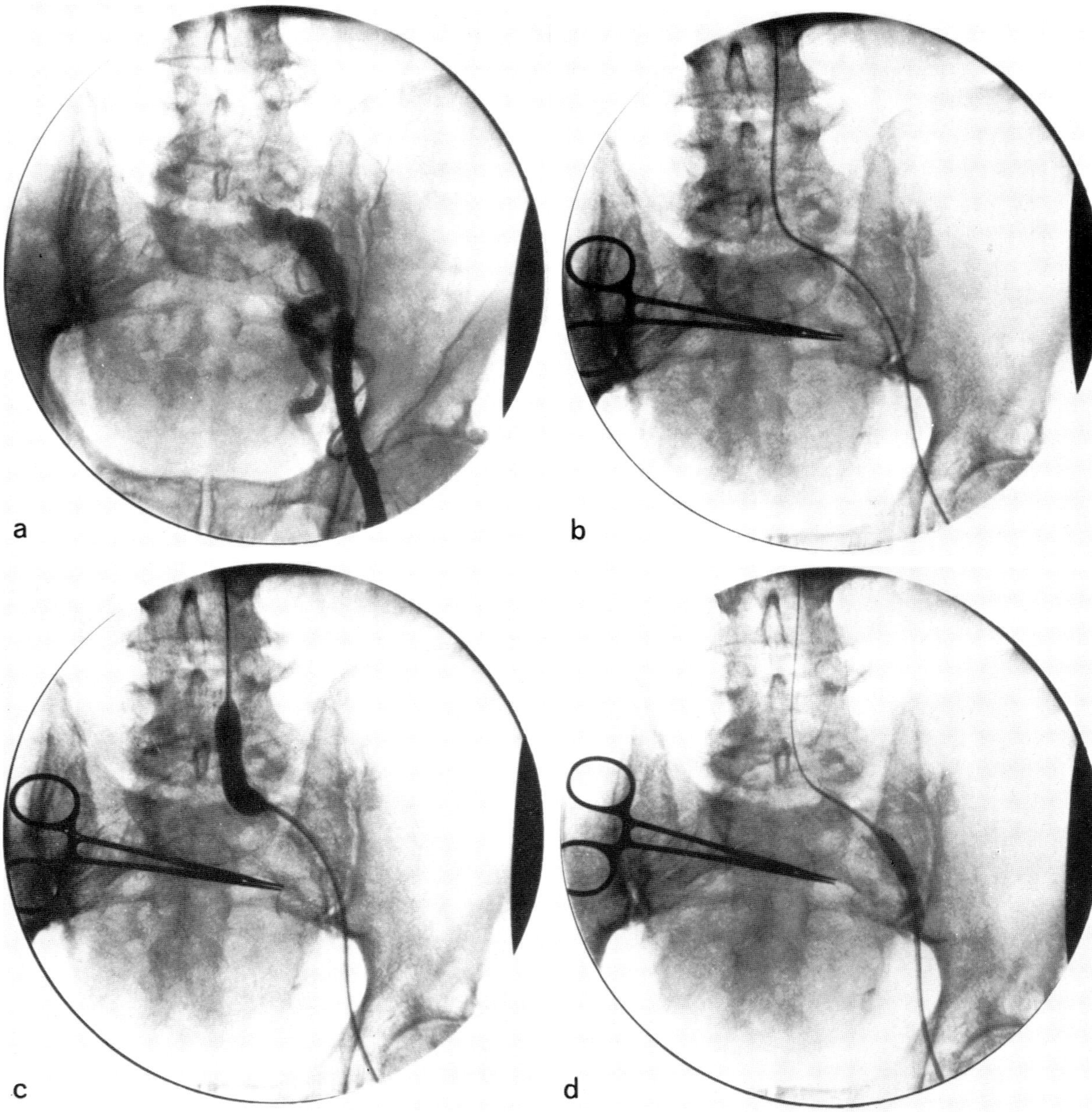

Fig. 2a–d. Technique of PTA in iliac artery stenosis. **a** Angiography from the groin; **b** bypassing the stenosis with a guide wire and location of the stenosis; **c** inflation of the balloon in the proximal part of the iliac artery; **d** inflation in situ of the stenosis

cases in the group with anticoagulation therapy remained patent for up to 30 months, whereas the reobliteration rate was 40% in patients without such therapy. As during the subsequent observation period no more than five patients had continued anticoagulation treatment, assessment of this therapy was impossible. In only one out of these 5 cases was the femoral artery reobliterated, one patient had a stenosis (but not an occlusion) 3 years after treatment, he and 3 others were still patent five years later.

Today, follow-up treatment is preferably performed with aggregation inhibitors. At present, the reobliteration rate is less than 15% in the 1st year.

In the Aggertalklinik, percutaneous transluminal dilatation of iliac artery stenoses (Fig. 2) was carried out in 262 iliac arteries (single, 220;

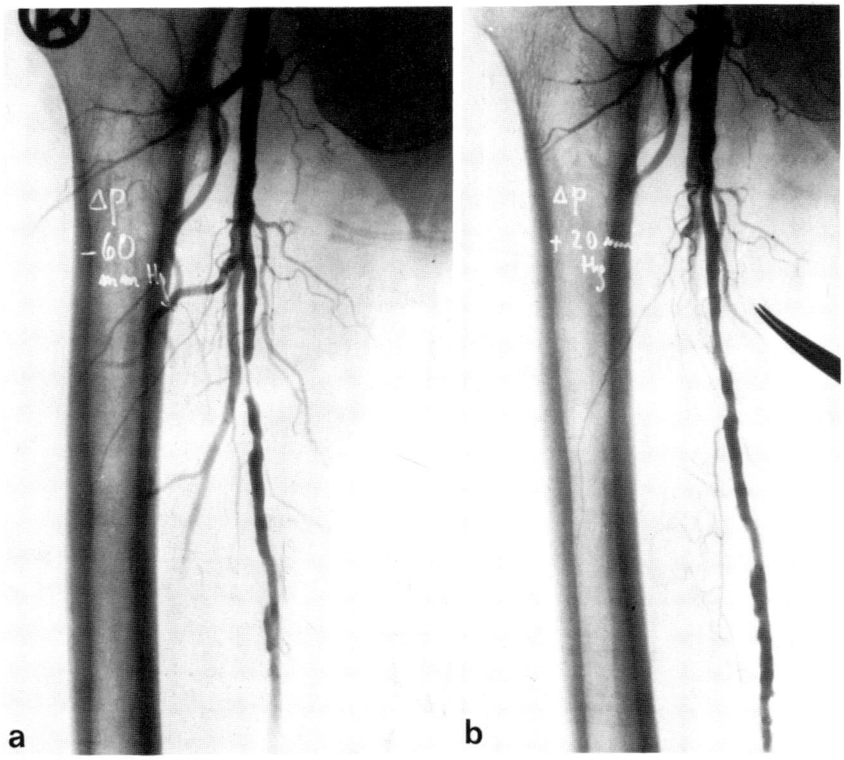

Fig. 3a, b. Stenosis in the proximal superficial femoral artery with blood pressure gradient between arm and ankle. **a** Before, and **b** after dilatation

multiple, 42). In 78%, the hemodynamic and clinical state was clearly improved. The joint study in 12 clinics with 206 additional patients in whom the Grüntzig [7] balloon catheter was used showed a primary success rate of 92%.

Table 3. Angioplasty of the inguinal arteries (Roth, Aggertalklinik)

Location	n	+	−	+ %	− %
Distal external iliac artery	14	13	1	93	7
Common femoral artery	20	10	10	50	50
	11 Stenoses	7	4	64	36
	9 Occlusions	3	6	33	67
Proximal superficial femoral artery	12	10	2	83	17
Deep femoral artery	22	16	6	73	27
	18 Stenoses	14	5	74	26
	3 Occlusions	2	1	67	33
Total	68	49	19	72	28

Whereas in the early years of the technique, stenoses and short obstructions in the distal superficial femoral artery and stenoses in iliac arteries were the most important indications for percutaneous transluminal angioplasty (PTA), today stenoses in the proximal superficial femoral artery (Fig. 3), in the deep femoral artery, and in the common femoral artery (Table 3) are also good indications. The material from Roth [15] in the Aggertalklinik demonstrates the results which it is possible to obtain in these locations with the balloon catheter dilating technique.

It is also possible to dilate long-distance stenoses of the superficial femoral artery (Fig. 4) in patients with Bürger-Winiwarter syndrome. In the 31-year-old male shown in Fig. 4, we passed the stenosis with a very thin guide wire and a 5-Fr Teflon catheter. Over the guide wire we changed the Teflon catheter against the Grüntzig balloon catheter 6 cm in length and 4 mm in diameter. After a stepwise dilatation control angiography demonstrated a patent lumen of the superficial femoral artery. Doppler ultrasound controls 3 days, 1 month, and 4 months later revealed a good hemodynamic result. The pressure gradient between brachial and posterior tibial artery changed from −70 to +10 mmHg.

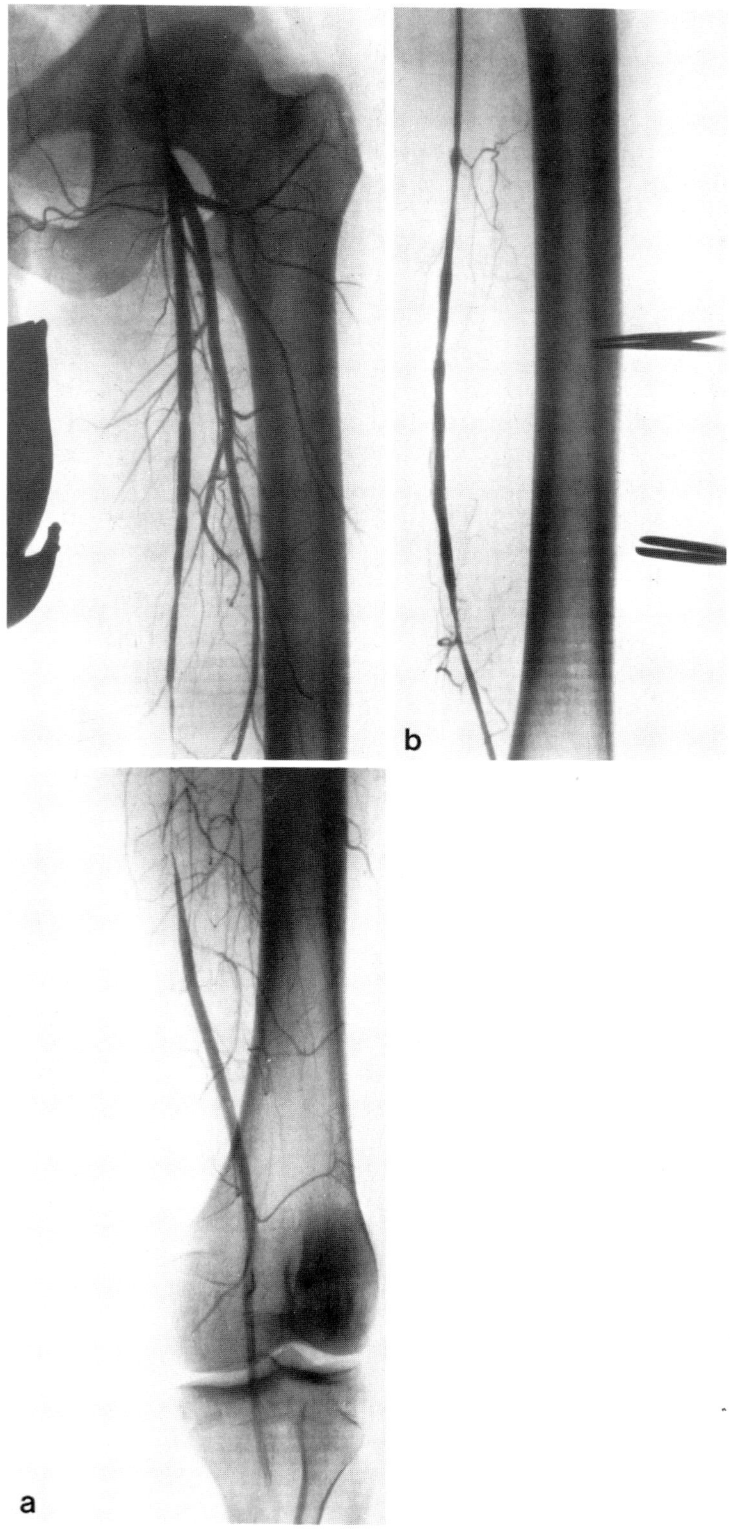

Fig. 4a, b. Long-distance stenosis in a patient with thrombangiitis obliterans. **a** Angiography before PTA; **b** control angiography

Follow-up studies were made in 88 successfully treated patients (19 November 1968 – 31 December 1973) with iliac artery stenoses in whom treatment had been performed more than 34 months previously. Sixteen of them had died in the meantime. In 57% of all treated patients or 69% of the remaining patients the good primary result still persisted 3 years later, and in 61% even 5 years later.

Hemodynamic Results

1. As early as 1971 we reported on the reduction of the blood pressure difference between brachial artery and posterior tibial artery from 79 to 38 mmHg (52% of the initial value) in 26 patients [19].
2. In 1974, Grüntzig et al. reported that the systolic pressure difference between brachial and posterior tibial artery was reduced by 78% after surgical reconstruction of femoral artery occlusions, and by 55% after percutaneous angioplasty [7].
3. The blood pressure was controlled in each case before and after dilatation of iliac artery stenoses (Fig. 5). Only dilatations with remarkable reduction of the blood pressure gradient were considered to positive.
4. The systolic pressure difference (Δp) between brachial and posterior tibial artery – measured with the ultrasound Doppler device – reveals a reduction of the pressure difference by 55% in successfully recanalized patients, and of 45% in all of those cases in which treatment of the obliterations was not successful.
5. In 1978, Bollinger [2a] showed in a comparative study that after reconstructive surgery ($n = 67$) the pressure difference (Δp) sank from 60 to 7 mmHg, and 12 months later it was about 19 mmHg. After percutaneous recanalization ($n = 50$) Δp sank from 60 to 19 mmHg, and 12 months later it was nearly equal to the medium pressure difference of 20 mmHg in operated patients. Simultaneously, Bollinger referred to the significant differences in the patient material, i.e., operated patients and those who underwent percutaneous treatment.

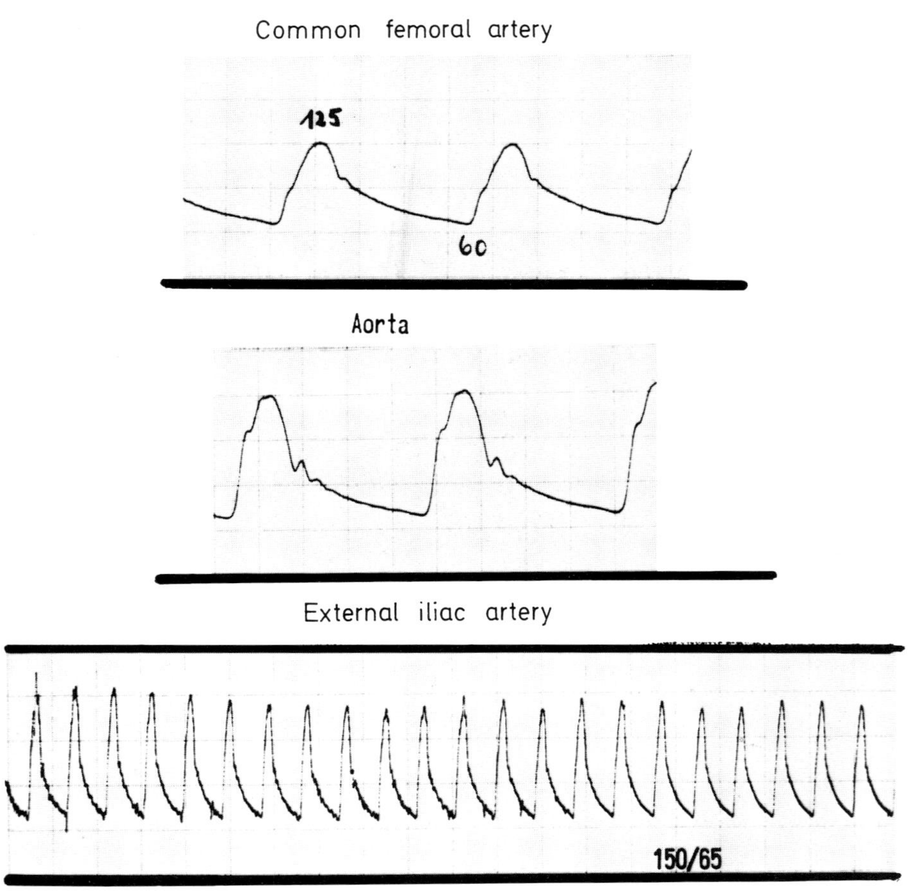

Fig. 5. Blood pressure control before and after dilatation of the iliac artery stenosis in the same case as in Fig. 2

Follow-up examinations 2 and 3 years later confirmed these primary hemodynamic improvements. Complete removal of the pressure difference, however, can be expected only in cases without concomitant obliterations in the lower leg arteries or in cases in which such obliterations can be successfully removed.

Patients with Gangrene

In addition to these previous and long-term results with the treatment of peripheral vascular disease in patients mostly with claudication, we can also report on angioplasty in patients with gangrene, rest pain, and claudication carried out in the Klinikum in Nürnberg (Tables 4–6).

The conspicuous factor in the 143 patients with rest pain and gangrene was the greater number of female patients and the mean age of 61 years, the oldest patient being an 87-year-old female. In 60% of patients, clinical diabetes was evident. In none of these cases were all lower leg arteries patent, and in 50% only 1 tibial artery was patent. In 100 cases (70%) we noted a primary success. Complications occurred in two cases, necessitating surgical intervention.

Depending on the length of the obliterated segment and the outflow, we used either a Teflon bypassing catheter (9 Charrière) or, additionally, one of the Andel's Teflon catheters (9, 10, or 12 Charrière) or a Grüntzig balloon catheter. In cases with poor peripheral outflow it is necessary to work very quickly to avoid prolonged ischemia. Femoro-

Table 4. Percutaneous catheter treatment, lower extremities (Nürnberg, 1 July 1976–23 April 1980)

No. of patients	251	Treatments	295
Mean age (31–87):	61 years	Sex: Male	167 (66.5%)
		Female	84 (33.5%)
		Multiple PTA in the same patient:	
1. Only puncture of deep femoral art. or unsuitable oblit.	13 (4.5%)	Left and right:	21 patients (8.2%)
		Iliac and sup. fem. art.:	6 patients (2.5%)
		Same location 2nd time:	12 patients (5.6%)
2. Stage II	159 (47.0%)		
3. Stage III/IV	143 (48.5%)		

Table 5. Percutaneous catheter treatment of the lower extremities in patients with claudication (stage II) (Nürnberg, 1 July 1976–23 April 1980)

Obliteration/result	+[a]	(+)	−[b]	N	(+ in %)
Aortic stenosis	1	–	–	1	91
Iliac art. stenosis	29	–	3	32	
Iliac art. occlusion	1	–	1	2	
Femoropopl. art. stenos.	42	2	1	45	93
Deep femoral art. stenos	1	–	–	1	
Femoropopl. occlusion					
<10 cm	41	–	5	46	89
>10 cm	8	–	4	12	67
Lower leg art. oblit.	4	–	5	–	
	127	2	19	139	91

Recidivism (2 weeks): 3 (2.2%)
Complications (op.): 3 (2.2%)
[a,b] See Table 6

Table 6. Percutaneous catheter treatment of the legs; patients with rest pain (stage III) and gangrene (stage IV) (Nürnberg, 1 July 1976–23 April 1980)

Obliteration/result	+[a]	(+)	−[b]	*n*	(+ in %)
Iliac art. stenoses	9	2	2	13	69
Femoropopl. art. stenos.	25	1	–	26	96
Deep femoral art. stenos.	3	–	–	3	
Femoropopl. occlusion					
<10 cm	43	8	10	61	70.5
>10 cm	14	2	13	29	48
Lower leg art. oblit.	6	1	4	11	54.5
	100	14	29	143	70

Recidivism (2 weeks): 9 (6.3%)
Complications (op.): 2 (1.4%)

[a] + good angiographic and clinical result within 2 days
[b] – without clinical improvement

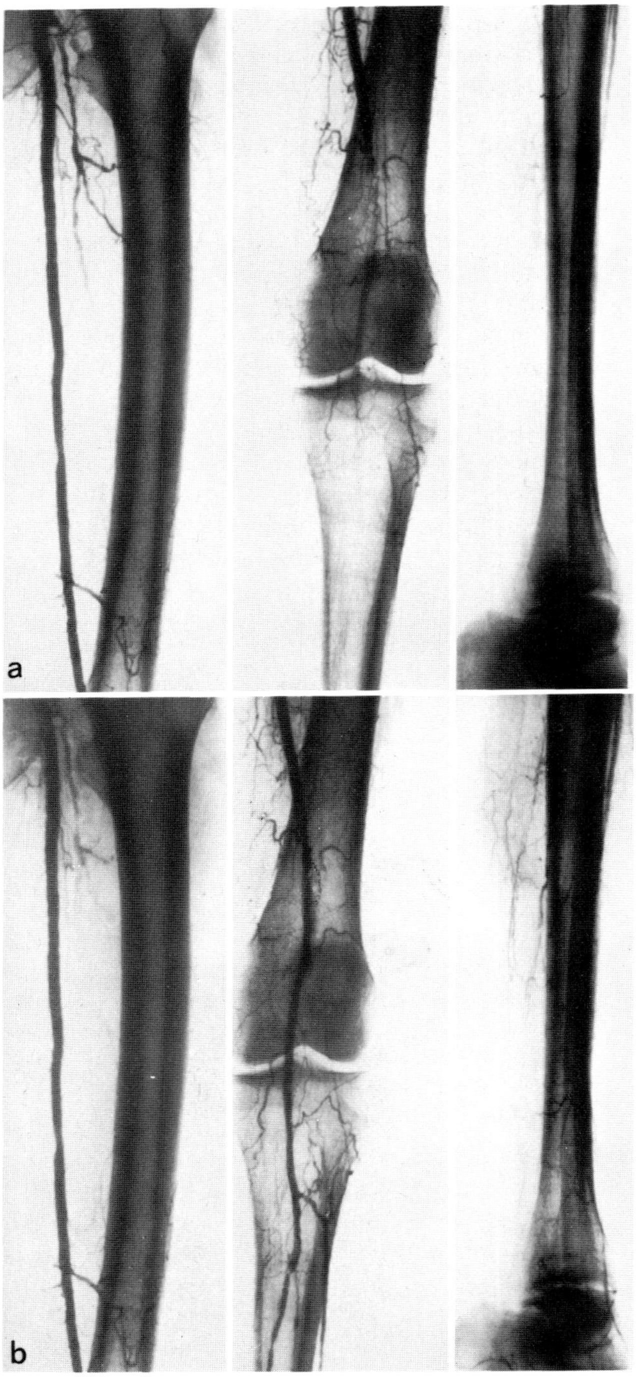

Fig. 6a, b. 87-year-old diabetic female with gangrene in the right foot, and with a distal femoral and distal popliteal artery occlusion plus obliteration of tibial arteries. **a** Before PTA; **b** after effective recanalization

popliteal stenoses were dilated with the Grüntzig catheter after successful passage with the guide and the Teflon catheter.

Seventy percent of cases with occlusion less than 10 cm in length and 96% of those with femoropopliteal stenoses (Fig. 6) were successfully treated. Only in 8% of all cases in which angioplasty was initially successful did amputation prove unavoidable.

Complications

In a joint study [20] with 1401 patients from four clinics, 35 complications (2.5%) occurred after angioplasty, requiring surgical intervention. Thrombotic occlusion, small emboly, and hemorrhage at the puncture site were the most frequent incidents. This is the reason why experience plays such an important role.

Table 7. Risks of percutaneous catheter treatment in leg arteries [20]

Risk	Rate of occurrence
1. Lethality	0% – 0.1%
n, 2800	
3rd – 7th postop. day	Cardiac failure, twice Pulmonary embolism, once
2. Emergency operations:	2.5%
n, 1401	(0 – 8.7%)
3. Amputation rate:	
After PTA Stage II:	3.7% (8 years)
Stage III:	5.0%
Stage IV:	40.0% (1 – 2 years)

During the combined treatment of obliterations by radiologist and surgeon and during therapy of possible complications cooperation is very important. The risks of PTA in leg arteries are summarized in Table 7.

Pharmaceutical Regimen

Following various randomized studies, the majority of interventional radiologists today use standardized accessory pharmaceutical treatment (Table 8). However, in older patients and in patients with hypertension, gastric ulcers, carcinoma, and after brain infarction, Coumarins are contraindicated. In such cases, aggregation inhibitors are probably of value for long-term regulation

Renal Artery Dilatation

Following successful percutaneous transluminal dilatation of renal arteries [8, 9, 10, 13, 14] with a modified Grüntzig coaxial balloon catheter, a large number of dilatations were performed in the past 2 years (Table 9). We know the primary success rate in 362 renal arteries. It is important that proximal and peripheral stenoses in the renal arteries can be successfully dilated in cases of arteriosclerotic and fibromuscular lesions. Also, renal artery stenoses in transplanted kidneys [11, 16] (nine patients up to now) could effectively be dilated with good angiographic and clinical results.

Measurement of blood pressure in the aorta and behind the stenosis (Fig. 7) is important as an indication for dilatation. Only in cases with a systolic blood pressure gradient of more than 20 mmHg is dilatation indicated. Moreover, blood pressure control after dilatation furnishes important information about the result.

It is possible to dilate stenoses in both renal arteries (Fig. 8) in the same procedure. Today, the coaxial balloon catheter system but also simple balloon catheters for iliac and femoral arteries are in use. In most cases the transfemoral route is effective, and very seldom does the axillary route prove necessary. In many cases a Sidewinder catheter II is very helpful to enter and bypass the renal artery stenosis. Above a guide wire in place, the balloon catheter can be shifted along the stenosis and dila-

Table 8. Accessory pharmaceutical treatment

Timing	*Treatment*
2 days before	Acetosal (ASA) 3 × 0.5 g
After puncture	Intraart. heparin 5000 I.U.
After PTD/PTR[a]	ASA for 6 – 10 days
Long term regulation	Coumarins, starting 2nd or 3rd day after PTD/PTR

[a] Percutaneous transluminal recanalization

Table 9. Percutaneous dilatation of renal artery stenoses

Author/team	*n*	+	Complications
Casarello	12	11	
Chang	4	4	
Cope	2	2	
Derier	5	5	
Freiman	2	2	
Grüntzig	24	23	
Ingrisch	14	11	
Jassovic	20	16	1 (+)
Katzen	7	7	
Lohmann	1	1	
Löhr	32	25	1
Mahler	14	11	
Mathias	5	4	1
Millen	5	5	
Passariello	2	2	
Pereiras	5	5	
Porstmann	6	5	
Puylaert	54	46	4
Roth	28	25	
Schwarten	70	65 (93%)	3
Sörensen	7	4	
White	15	13	1
Zeitler	17	14	
	362	314 (87.0%)	11 (3.0%)

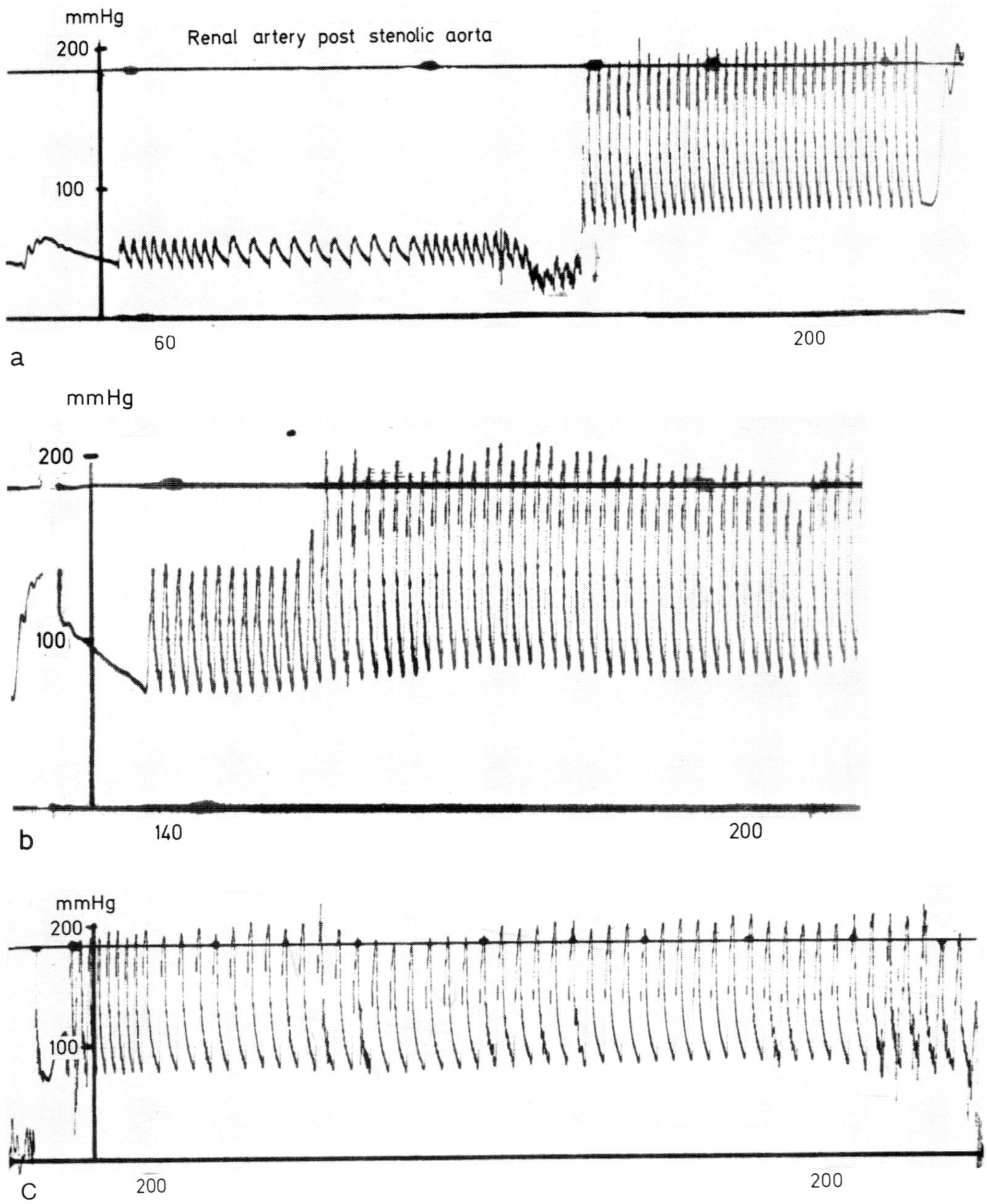

Fig. 7a – c. Blood pressure control in a patient with a renal artery stenosis on the left side. **a** Pressure gradient before dilatation; **b** pressure gradient after the first dilatation procedure; **c** after effective dilatation

tation is possible. Inflation of the balloon for the dilatation of renal artery stenoses in most cases needs between 2 and 4 atm.

Today, follow-up controls are carried out only in small patient groups [9, 10, 14]. Recidivism is mostly seen in patients without anticoagulation therapy. We have dilated three stenoses in a second session between 3 and 9 months after PTA.

Periarterial hematomas around the renal artery have also been seen in some cases. These patients must be kept under continuous supervision for 2 days. Immediate surgical intervention, however, is not necessary. Only if a subintimal dissection occurs during the dilatation procedure must vascular surgery be performed within the next 24 h. In future, more experience must be gained in this field. However, it seems that the therapy for renovascular hypertension is changing totally.

Following the good results with PTA in leg, coronary (Table 10), and renal arteries, some seldom special indications have also been reported (Table 11).

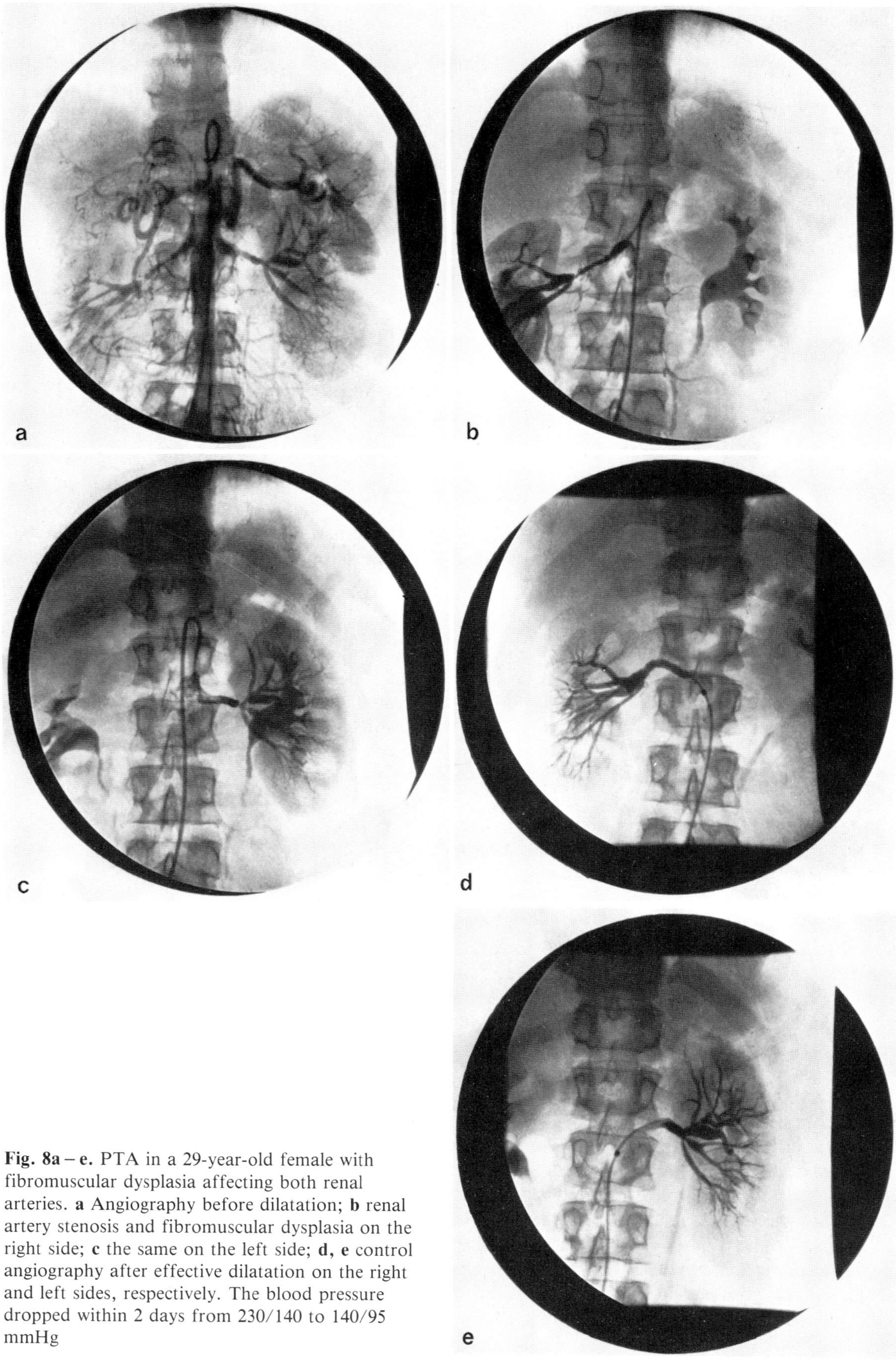

Fig. 8a – e. PTA in a 29-year-old female with fibromuscular dysplasia affecting both renal arteries. **a** Angiography before dilatation; **b** renal artery stenosis and fibromuscular dysplasia on the right side; **c** the same on the left side; **d, e** control angiography after effective dilatation on the right and left sides, respectively. The blood pressure dropped within 2 days from 230/140 to 140/95 mmHg

Table 10. PTA in coronary arteries (Grüntzig, Zurich) (*n*, 145)

Result	Percentage
Passage possible	86
Patency rate 1 year	93
2nd dilatation	11
Acute heart surgery within 24 h	8
Myocardial infarction (Q-wave)	3

Table 11. Special indications for PTA, new experiences

Indication	Author
Fibromuscular dysplasia: renal a.	
carotid a.	Mathias, 1980
Postoperative strictures	Martin, 1980
Venous stenoses in AV fistulas	Zeitler, 1978; Martin, 1980
Common femoral a.	Roth, 1979
Superior mesenteric a.	Grüntzig, 1980
Aortic stenoses	Velasquez, 1980; Zorn-Bopp, 1980; Zeitler
Vein graft stenosis	Alpert, 1979

Discussion

Early and late results in PTA with the new improved technique using the Grüntzig balloon catheter system and single Teflon catheters demonstrate that in centers with skilled cardiovascular radiologists not only good angiographic findings but also clinically impressive improvements are possible. In cases with successful PTA measurable increases of the peripheral systolic blood pressure in the ankle and of the systemic blood pressure after renal artery dilatation or the absence of angina pectoris could be noted after effective balloon catheter dilatation. The number of severe complications can be kept low.

The great advantage of this method is that general anesthesia and operation risk can be avoided. Treatment is always carried out under local anesthesia and the patient's stay in hospital varies between only 3 and 6 days. If reobliteration occurs, angioplasty can be repeated and the chances for a by-pass operation remain unchanged. A thrombendarterectomy after PTA, however, has only a slight chance of success.

In the interest of the patient an increasing partnership with the surgeons must be aimed at. In those patients, however, with localized obliterations in coronary, renal, iliac, and femoropopliteal regions, where the obstruction cannot be passed, the surgical risk after PTA is not higher than before.

Summary

Follow-up studies over more than 5 years in patients with superficial femoral arterial occlusions and iliac artery stenoses manifested the efficacy and the good results which can be obtained with the Dotter procedure.

The special balloon catheters developed by Grüntzig, a standardized accessory pharmaceutical regimen, and an increasing number of clear indications are the basis for very good long-term results, with patency rates approaching 70% after 3 years. Clinical follow-up controls with the Doppler technique demonstrate the hemodynamic effectivity.

More and more new indications such as coronary [6, 17] and renal artery stenoses have manifested that PTA is a useful procedure for most arterial lesions, assuming special care and skill of the performer.

References

1. Alpert JR, Ring EJ, Berkowitz HD, Freiman DB, Oleago JA, Gordon R, Roberts B (1979) Treatment of vein graft stenosis by balloon catheter dilatation. JAMA 242:2769–2771
2. van Andel GJ (1976) Percutaneous transluminal angioplasty. Excerpta Medica, Amsterdam

2a. Bollinger A (1978) Appraisal of the therapy. In: Zeitler E, Grüntzig A, Schoop W (eds) Percutaneous vascular recanalization: Technique, applications, clinical results. Springer, Berlin Heidelberg New York, pp 194–195

3. Dotter CT, Judkins MP (1964) Transluminal treatment of arteriosclerotic obstruction. Description of a technique and a preliminary report of its application. Circulation 30:654
4. Dotter CT, Rösch J, Anderson JM, Antonovic R (1974) Transluminal iliac artery dilatation. Nonsurgical catheter treatment of atheromatous narrowing. JAMA 230:117

5. Freiman DB, Ring EJ, Oleago JA, Berkowitz HD, Roberts B (1979) Transluminal angioplasty of the iliac, femoral and popliteal arteries. Radiology 132:285 – 288
6. Grüntzig A (1977) Die perkutane transluminale Rekanalisation chronischer Arterienverschlüsse mit einer neuen Dilatationstechnik. Gerhard Witzstrock, Baden-Baden Köln New York
7. Katzen BT, Chang J, Lukowsky G, Abramson E (1979) Percutaneous transluminal angioplasty for treatment of renovascular hypertension. Radiology 132:53 – 58
8. Kuhlmann U, Grüntzig A, Vetter W, Lütolf U, Siegenthaler W (1978) Percutaneous transluminal dilatation: A new treatment of renovascular hypertension. Klin Wochenschr 56:703 – 707
9. Lux E, Seybold D, Grosse-Vorholt R, Zeitler E, Gessler U (1980) Perkutane transluminale Katheterdilatation von Nierenarterien-Stenosen bei Patienten mit renovaskulärer Hypertonie. Fortschr Med 98/15: 563 – 568
10. Mahler F, Krneta A, Haertel M (1979) Treatment of renovascular hypertension by transluminal renal artery dilatation. Ann Intern Med 90:56 – 57
11. Mathias K, Rau W, Kauffmann G (1979) Katheterdilatation einer Arterienstenose nach Nierentransplantation. Dtsch Med Wochenschr 104:437 – 438
12. Mathias K, Spillner G, Staiger J, Ahmadi A, Werner JP (1979) Perkutane transluminale Revascularisation von Unterschenkelarterien. Chirurg 50:158 – 163
13. Puylaert C (1979) Renal artery stenosis dilatation in hypertension. Combined Meeting European College of Angiography and the American Society of Cardiovascular Radiology, Dublin, June 1979
14. Richter E-I, Grüntzig A, Ingrisch H, Mahler F, Mathias K, Roth FJ, Sörensen A, Zeitler E (1980) Percutaneous dilatation of renal artery stenosis. Ann Radiol (Paris) 4:275 – 278
15. Roth FJ, Cappius G (1980) Angioplastie der Leistenarterien. German Radiol Society Meeting, Cologne 1980
16. Snidermann KW, Sos TA, Strayregen S, Saddekni S, Cheigh JS, Tapia L, Tellis V, Veith FJ (1980) Percutaneous transluminal angioplasty in renal transplant arterial stenosis for relief of hypertension. Radiology 135:23 – 25
17. Spodick DH (1979) Percutaneous transluminal coronary angioplasty: Opportunity fleeting. JAMA 242:1658 – 1659
18. Velasquez G, Castaneda-Zuniga W, Formanek A, Zollikofer Ch, Barreto A, Nicoloff D, Amplatz K, Sullivan A (1980) Nonsurgical aortoplasty in leriche syndrome. Radiology 134:359 – 360
19. Zeitler E, Schoop W, Zahnow W (1971) The treatment of the occlusive arterial disease by transluminal catheter angioplasty. Radiology 99:19
20. Zeitler E, Grüntzig A, Schoop W (1978) Percutaneous vascular recanalization: Technique, application, clinical results. Springer, Berlin Heidelberg New York

Therapeutic Technology

L. Ekelund

University Hospital, Department of Diagnostic Radiology, S-22185 Lund

With the advent of abdominal sonography and computed tomography, angiography became less important as a primary diagnostic tool, especially in tumor diagnosis. However, the experience gained from angiography has formed the basis for a new therapeutic technology developed during the 1970s. Specialized radiologic experience and equipment are thus being used to treat a variety of disorders. The aim of this presentation is to summarize the present concepts of intravascular embolic therapy with special reference to renal and hepatic neoplasms, to briefly discuss the technology of transluminal dilatation of renal artery stenosis, and finally to consider techniques and indications for percutaneous nephrostomy.

Transcatheter Occlusion of the Renal Artery

Indications include gross hematuria secondary to trauma, arteriovenous fistula, aneurysm, or tumor. Furthermore, preoperative embolization may be employed to decrease the blood loss at nephrectomy. In renal carcinoma intractable pain and inoperability have also been reasons for embolization. End-stage renal disease in poor surgical candidates requiring nephrectomy may be another indication.

Several embolic materials have been tried clinically as well as experimentally. These include autologous clot, muscle tissue, Gelfoam, cyanoacrylate, stainless steel coils, and detachable balloons [1 – 10]. Experimental long-term follow-up of embolization with autologous clot, Oxycel, and Gelfoam in swine has shown that these agents are not suitable for permanent vascular occlusion because of recanalization [11]. We have had the same experience with Spongostan (99% gelatine, similar to Gelfoam) in clinical embolization of renal tumors as well as in experiments in rats [12, 13]. These types of embolic material are thus not suited for long-term occlusive therapy in patients with inoperable neoplasms. Being particulate materials, there is also a risk of secondary spread of emboli due to reflux [14]. This may be avoided, however, if embolization is performed via a balloon catheter [15].

Isobutyl-2-cyanoacrylate is a monomer which is said to produce permanent vascular occlusion in the renal artery [6, 7, 16]. Experiments in rats and rabbits indicate its usefulness in providing long-term occlusion [6, 16]. We have used this agent in six patients with renal carcinoma [12]. In one patient partial recanalization was demonstrated by 1-month follow-up angiography. In this connection it is of interest to compare the results of Lunderquist et al., who used cyanoacrylate for obliteration of the gastric coronary vein and bleeding esophageal varices [17]. Follow-up PTP (percutaneous transhepatic portography) in eight patients demonstrated recanalization in six. Consequently, cyanoacrylate does not cause a permanent vascular occlusion in all instances. This agent is also difficult to handle and furthermore there is a risk of reflux of embolic material as demonstrated in experiments with rabbits [6].

Wallace et al. developed a stainless steel coil with wool strands (provided in the Gianturco arterial occluder set, Cook Inc., United States) for permanent vascular occlusion [8]. We have used this technique in ten patients with inoperable renal carcinoma (Fig. 1) and so far we have had no complications nor seen any evidence of recanalization in follow-up arteriograms. However, the risk of peripheral embolization remains [18], and there is also one case report of recanalization and pseudoaneurysm formation as demonstrated by 1-month follow-up angiography [19]. The effect of cyanoacrylate and steel coils on embolized tissues has been studied in experiments with pigs [20].

Promising results with detachable silicone balloons have recently been reported. These can be used for

Radiology Today 1. Ed. by M. W. Donner and F. H. W. Heuck

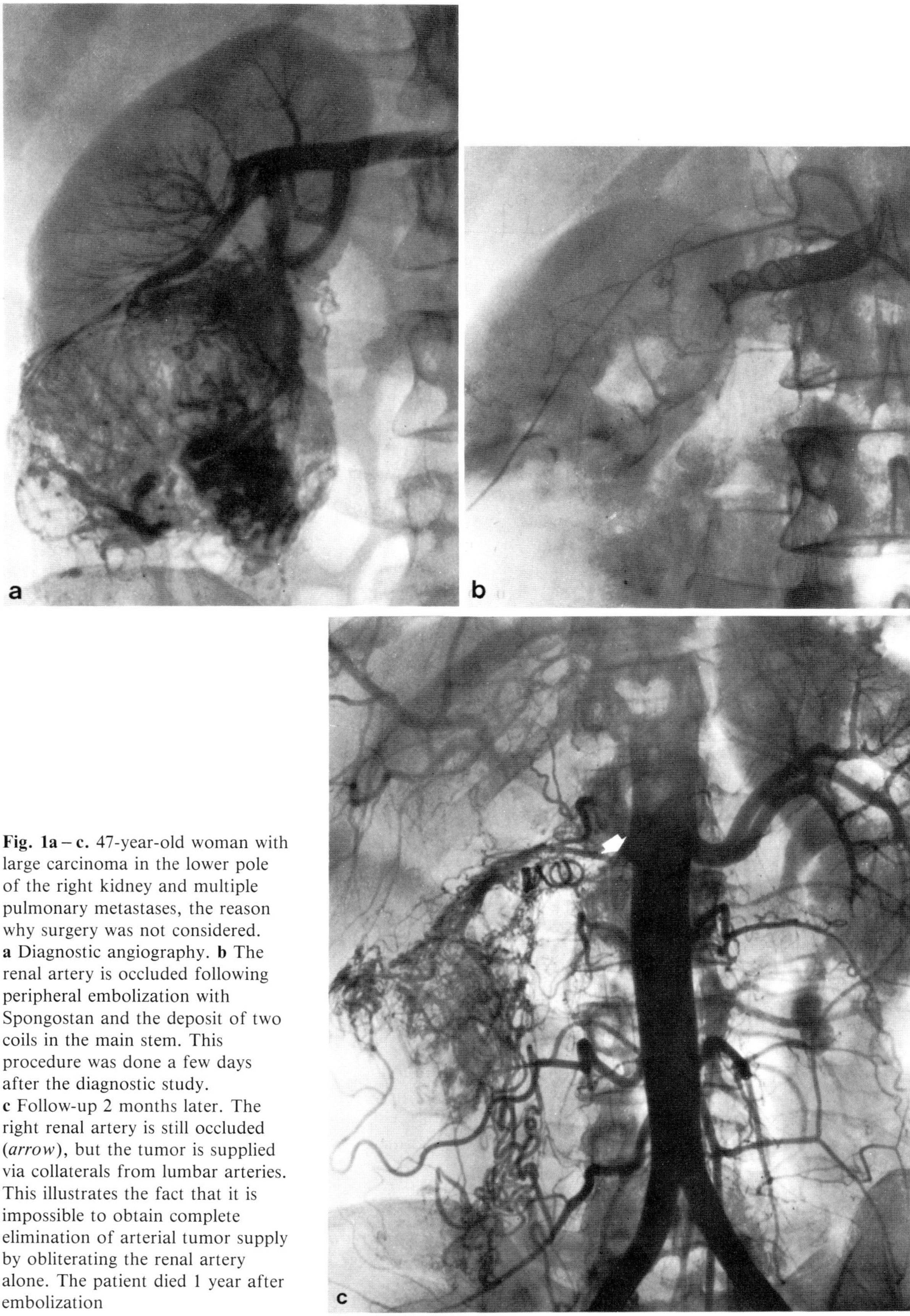

Fig. 1a–c. 47-year-old woman with large carcinoma in the lower pole of the right kidney and multiple pulmonary metastases, the reason why surgery was not considered. **a** Diagnostic angiography. **b** The renal artery is occluded following peripheral embolization with Spongostan and the deposit of two coils in the main stem. This procedure was done a few days after the diagnostic study. **c** Follow-up 2 months later. The right renal artery is still occluded (*arrow*), but the tumor is supplied via collaterals from lumbar arteries. This illustrates the fact that it is impossible to obtain complete elimination of arterial tumor supply by obliterating the renal artery alone. The patient died 1 year after embolization

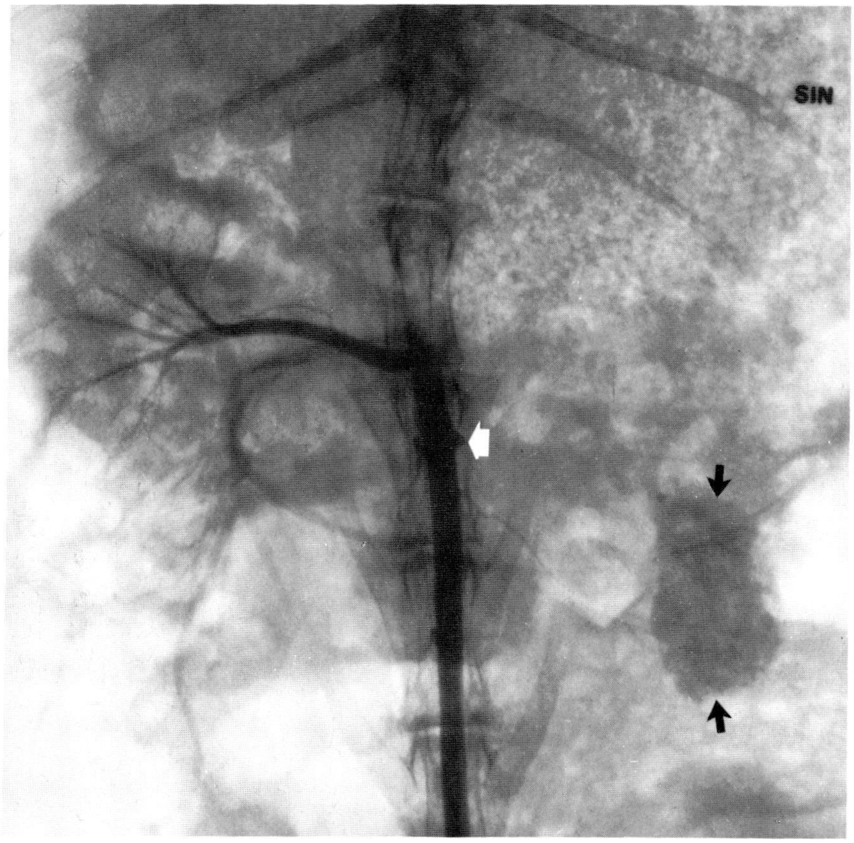

Fig. 2. Abdominal aortogram in a rabbit 7 weeks following the injection of 1 ml 95% ethanol into the left renal artery. This artery is occluded (*white arrow*) and the left kidney calcified and shrunken (*black arrows*). The findings were verified at microscopy

preoperative as well as for permanent vascular occlusion [10].

Preoperative occlusion with a balloon catheter seems to be the preferred method fo facilitate nephrectomy [21]. The balloon is placed in the renal artery and inflated before surgery. Using this technique, the risks that can be expected with embolization are avoided.

In the search for a safer, more permanent, and technically easier method of producing renal artery occlusion we investigated the sclerosing effect of 95% ethanol in animal experiments [22]. Longstanding occlusion of the renal artery with ensuing infarction of the kidney could be produced by a small and tolerable dose (Fig. 2). Several of the inherent drawbacks of currently used embolic agents may be eliminated in this way. Preliminary reports showing similar promising results with absolute ethanol in dog experiments have recently been published [23].

Transcatheter electrocoagulation has also been used for vessel occlusion [24]. We have tried a similar technique with electrolysis in an experimental pig model and have been able to initiate occlusion of the renal artery using fairly low currents (Fig. 3).

It has been suggested that an immunologic response may be associated with the induction of tumor necrosis. Whether or not the survival time can be improved, it is evident that local tumor symptoms may be palliated in patients with renal carcinoma who are not considered for surgery. We have even seen temporary remission of pulmonary nodules regarded as metastases in two patients following palliative embolization of arterial renal tumor supply.

Transcatheter Occlusion of the Hepatic Artery

Experience with hepatic embolization is limited [4, 25]. The fact that the liver has a dual blood supply and that primary as well as secondary hepatic neoplasms receive their main blood supply from the hepatic artery provides an interesting theoretical background for transcatheter arterial occlusion of

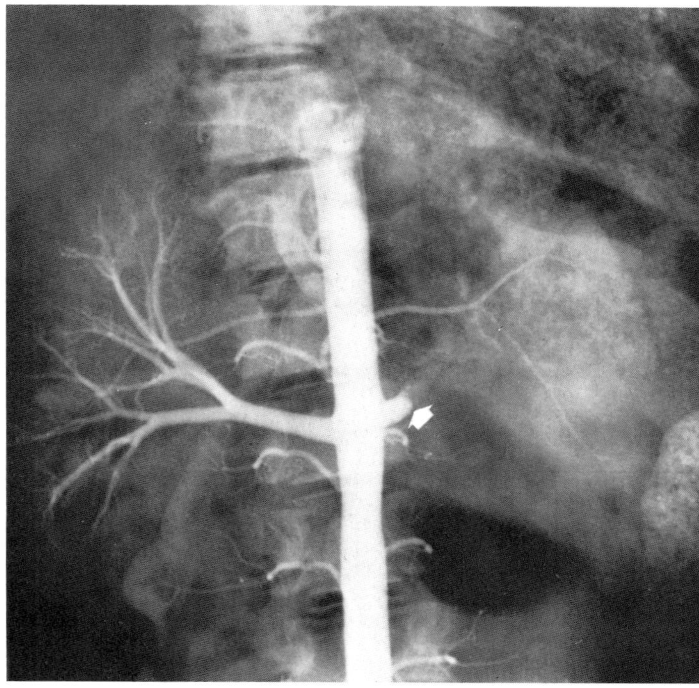

Fig. 3. Abdominal aortogram in a pig following electrocoagulation of the left renal artery, which is occluded (*arrow*)

liver tumors. After arterial Gelfoam or Spongostan embolization liver metastases may decrease in size [8, 26]. Additional obliteration may be obtained by use of steel coils. However, extensive embolization of the hepatic artery may result in liver failure, intrahepatic abscesses, and death [27]. These authors also investigated the difference between proximal and peripheral hepatic artery obstruction in monkeys. Gelfoam obstructed proximally, arterial collaterals developed rapidly, and liver function remained normal. Peripheral hepatic artery embolization with silicone was more effective in preventing the development of collateral circulation, but involved a significant risk of hepatic failure or abscess. We have studied the angiographic and microscopic findings in rats with experimental hepatic tumors that were subjected to transcatheter arterial embolization with Spongostan [13, 28]. Partial recanalization of the hepatic artery could already be seen after a few days. Reduced vascularization of tumors could be demonstrated, and in some animals even a decrease in tumor size (Fig. 4). However, necrosis of normal liver tissue could also be demonstrated by microscopy, and the risk of inducing necrosis of preserved tissue in tumor-infiltrated livers should be borne in mind when embolization is considered. Contraindications for hepatic embolization are hepatic insufficiency, portal hypertension, and portal vein thrombosis.

Transluminal Dilatation of Renal Artery Stenosis

In 1978 a preliminary report on balloon catheter dilatation of experimental renal artery stenosis in the dog appeared, and the authors discussed the possible clinical implications of this technique [29]. In the same year Grüntzig et al. reported on a successful percutaneous transluminal dilatation of a renal artery stenosis in a hypertensive patient [30]. Since then this technique of balloon catheter dilatation of stenotic renal arteries has been used with increasing frequency, and the preliminary results are very encouraging [31 – 34]. The procedure may be used to dilate both arteriosclerotic and fibromuscular stenoses. Short fibrotic stenoses are probably best suited for this kind of therapy. A breakthrough in this connection was the recent development of a new type of balloon with a distensible segment of polyvinyl chloride, which is placed on a double-lumen catheter [35]. The balloon can resist high pressure and is far superior to other types of balloon catheters made of latex. We have used this catheter for the dilatation of experimentally produced renal artery stenoses in the pig with overall good long-term results (Fig. 5). The angiographic results were correlated with the histologic findings, and the main effect of dilatation seems to be a disrupture of the internal elastic lamina (Ekelund L., Jonsson N., Stridbeck H., un-

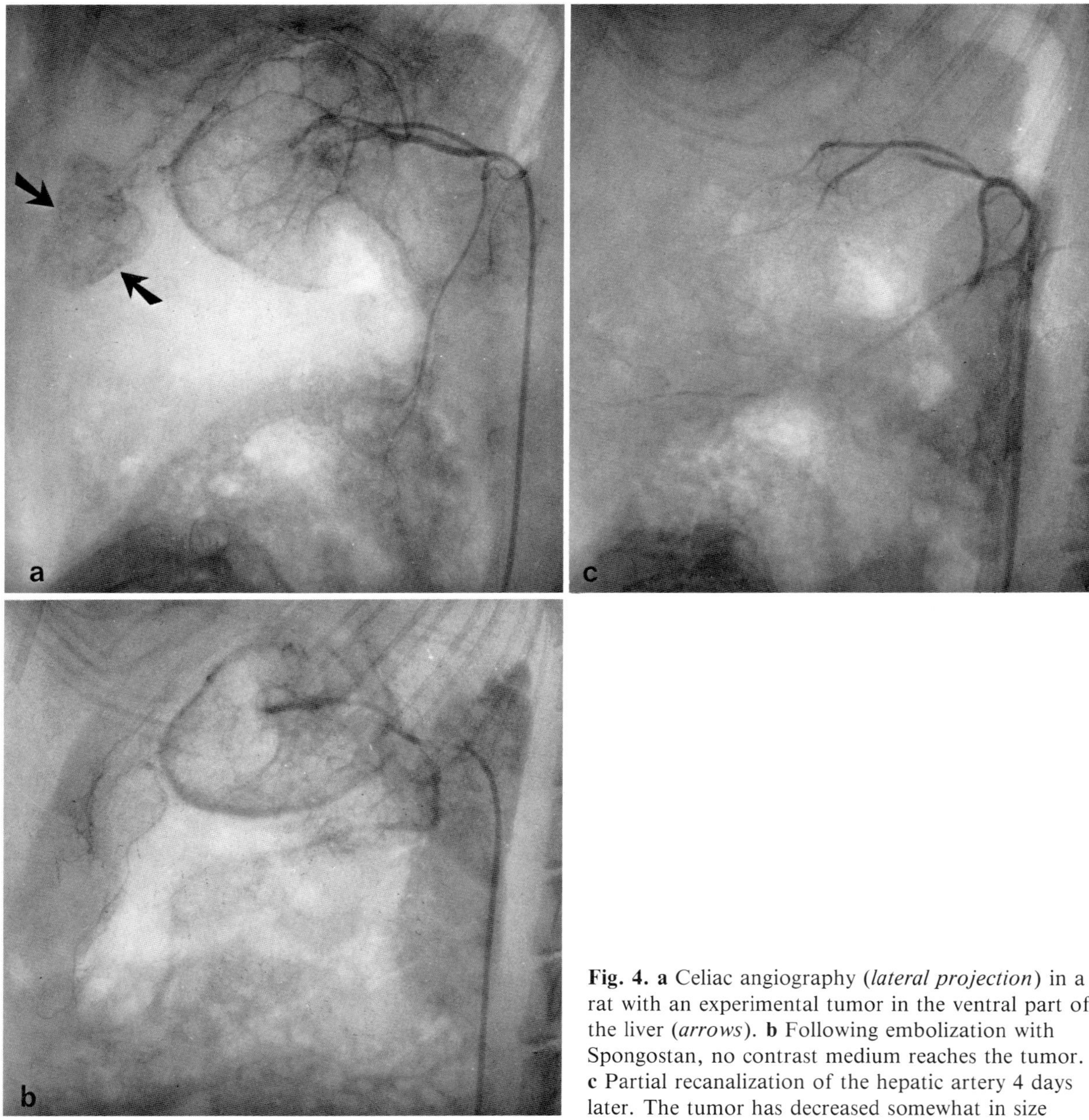

Fig. 4. **a** Celiac angiography (*lateral projection*) in a rat with an experimental tumor in the ventral part of the liver (*arrows*). **b** Following embolization with Spongostan, no contrast medium reaches the tumor. **c** Partial recanalization of the hepatic artery 4 days later. The tumor has decreased somewhat in size

published data). However, a word of caution is warranted, as we have seen rupture of the dilated segment with poststenotic pseudoaneurysm formation and subsequent exsanguination of the experimental animal.

Percutaneous Nephrostomy

Percutaneous nephrostomy for temporary urinary drainage has been used increasingly during the past decade, and it is therefore important to discuss variation in techniques, catheters, and especially the incidence of complications. The procedure may be performed with the patient prone [36] or supine – oblique, which is more comfortable for the patient [37 – 39]. If the kidney is still functioning, contrast medium is injected intravenously to localize the renal pelvis. Biplane fluoroscopy is helpful in patients with only mild dilatation of the renal pelvis. A puncture site in the posterior axillary line below the 12th rib is selected. The same catheter – needle combination as for percutaneous cholangiography is used. After the metallic needle has been withdrawn and urine sample been taken for

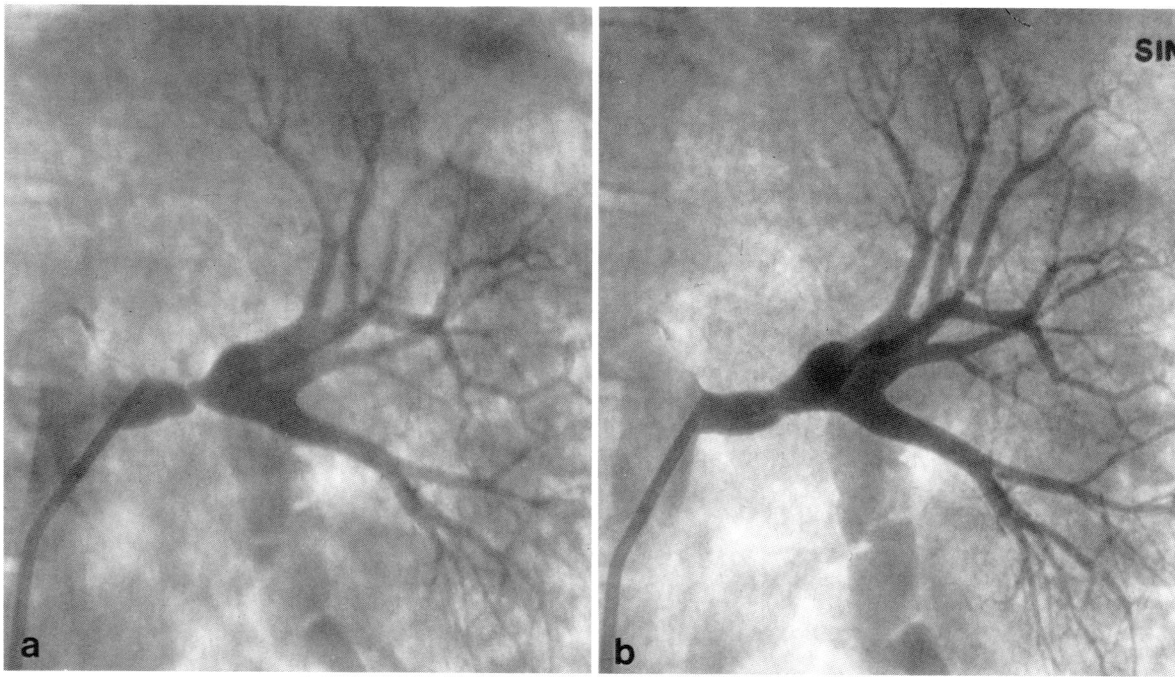

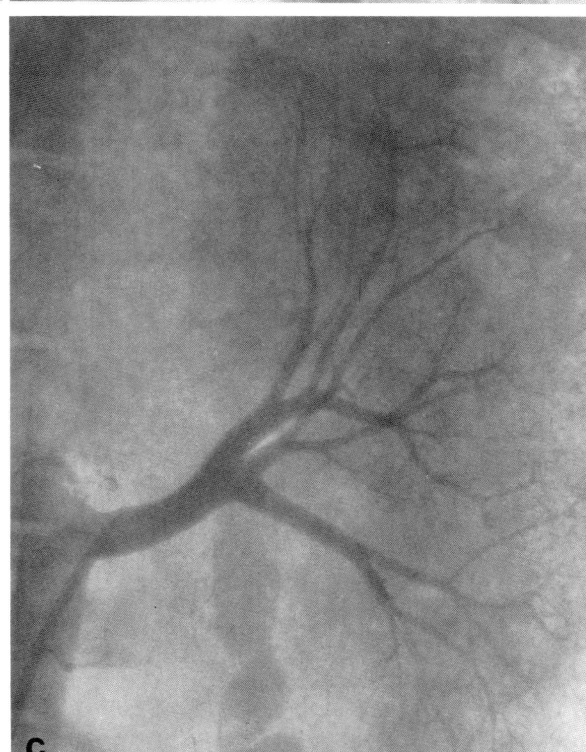

Fig. 5. a Selective angiography of the left kidney in a pig 6 weeks following the creation of a renal artery stenosis showing marked poststenotic dilatation. **b** Immediately after balloon catheter dilatation; **c** 8 weeks later no evidence of stenosis remains

culture, a guide-wire is introduced followed by an angiographic catheter with multiple side holes, which is placed either in a loop in the renal pelvis or, if possible, in the proximal part of the ureter. Sometimes, when difficulties of inserting the catheter over the guide-wire arise, the use of a recently developed guide-wire for percutaneous transhepatic cholangiography may be extremely helpful [40]. Careful fixation of the catheter to the skin is very important. In cases with nonvisualized collecting systems, ultrasound or CT guidance may be very helpful [41, 42].

Depending on the indications, a nephrostomy tube may be kept in place for varying lengths of time. Which type of catheter to use is a debated matter. We have been generally satisfied with the angiography catheter for up to 12 months and see no need for routine exchange unless obstruction or dislodgment occurs. For permanent drainage, a Foley-type catheter may be installed by widening the tract using larger tubes over a period of days or weeks [37]. However, repeated changes with dilatations of the canal are often unpleasant and painful.

Percutaneous nephrostomy does not carry the hight mortality of open surgical nephrostomy [43]. Transient hematuria is commonly seen following the procedure and should not really be regarded as a complication. Small perinephric hematomas are found at 8% of subsequent operations or autopsies [44]. The incidence of major complications was 4% in a recent series of 53 percutaneous nephrostomies, the most frequent being symptomatic infection [36].

It is generally agreed that percutaneous nephrostomy is of great value for temporary urinary diversion in benign conditions as an alternative to open surgical nephrostomy and to emergency correction of ureteral obstruction. In patients with obstruction from malignant disease the situation is far more complex and an expectant attitude has been advocated in order not to prolong a desolate and often painful life with incurable cancer. The procedure should not be recommended for the patient with incapacitating end-stage malignant disease, for which no further adequate antitumor therapy is left.

References

1. Chuang VP, Reuter SR, Walter J, Foley WD, Bookstein JJ (1975) Control of renal hemorrhage by selective arterial embolization. AJR 125:300–306
2. Cho KJ, Stanley JC (1978) Non-neoplastic congenital and acquired renal arteriovenous malformations and fistulas. Radiology 129:333–343
3. Almgård LE, Slezak P (1977) Treatment of renal adenocarcinoma by embolization. A follow-up of 38 cases. Eur Urol 3:279–281
4. Goldstein HM, Wallace S, Anderson JH, Bree RL, Gianturco C (1976) Transcatheter occlusion of abdominal tumors. Radiology 120:539–545
5. Chang J, Katzen BT, Sullivan KP (1978) Transcatheter gelfoam embolization of posttraumatic bleeding pseudoaneurysms. AJR 131:645–650
6. Günther R, Schubert U, Bohl L, Georgi M, Marberger M (1978) Transcatheter embolization of the kidney with butyl-2-cyanoacrylate. Experimental and clinical results. Cardiovasc Radiol 1:101–108
7. Freeny PC, Bush WH Jr, Kidd R (1979) Transcatheter occlusive therapy of genitourinary abnormalities using isobutyl-2-cyanoacrylate (bucrylate). AJR 133:647–656
8. Wallace S, Gianturco C, Anderson JH, Goldstein HM, Davis CJ, Bree RL (1976) Therapeutic vascular occlusion utilizing steel coil technique. Clinical applications. AJR 127:381–387
9. Riedl P, Flamm J (1979) Kontrollangiographische Befunde nach palliativer Nierenarterienokklusion mit der GAW-Spirale. ROEFO 130:398–403
10. White RJ, Kaufman SL, Barth KH, De Caprio V, Strandberg JD (1979) Therapeutic embolization with detachable silicone balloons. JAMA 241:1257–1260
11. Barth KH, Strandberg JD, White RJ (1977) Long term follow-up of transcatheter embolization with autologous clot, oxycel and gelfoam in domestic swine. Invest Radiol 12:273–280
12. Ekelund L, Månsson W, Olsson AM, Stigsson L (1979) Palliative embolization of arterial renal tumor supply. Acta Radiol [Diagn] (Stockh) 20:323–336
13. Ekelund L, Stigsson L, Jonsson N, Sjögren HO (1977) Transcatheter arterial embolization of normal livers and experimental hepatic tumours in the rat. Acta Radiol [Diagn] (Stockh) 18:641–651
14. Gang DL, Dole KB, Adelman LS (1977) Spinal cord infarction following renal artery embolization. JAMA 237:2841–2842
15. Greenfield AJ, Athanasoulis CA, Waltman AC, Le Moure ER (1978) Transcatheter embolization; prevention of embolic reflux using balloon catheters. AJR 131:651–655
16. Giuliani L, Carmignani G, Belgrano E, Puppo P (1977) Embolization of renal carcinomas with isobutyl-2-cyanoacrylate. Experimental study and first clinical applications. Urology 10:197–202
17. Lunderquist A, Börjesson B, Owman T, Bengmark S (1978) Isobutyl-2-cyanoacrylate (bucrylate) in obliteration of gastric coronary vein and esophageal varices. AJR 130:1–6
18. Tisnado J, Beachley MC, Cho SR, Amendola M (1979) Peripheral embolization of a stainless steel coil. AJR 133:324–326
19. Jhaveri HS, Gerlock AJ, Ekelund L (1978) Failure of steel coil occlusion in a case of hypernephroma. AJR 130:556–557
20. White RJ, Strandberg JV, Gross GS, Barth KH (1977) Therapeutic embolization with long-term occluding agents and their effects on embolized tissues. Radiology 125:677–687
21. Marberger M, Georgi M (1975) Balloon occlusion of the renal artery in tumor nephrectomy. J Urol 114:360–363
22. Ekelund L, Jonsson N, Treugut H (to be published) Transcatheter obliteration of the renal artery by ethanol injection. Experimental results. Cardiovasc Radiol

23. Ellman B, Green C, Eigenbrodt E, Curry T, Peters P (1979) Total renal infarction employing absolute ethanol. Invest Radiol 14:388
24. Thompson WM, Johnsrude IS, Jackson DC, Mc Alister S, Miller MD, Pizzo SV (1979) Vessel occlusion with transcatheter electrocoagulation: Initial clinical experience. Radiology 133:335 – 340
25. Doyon D, Mouzon A, Jourde AM, Regensberg C, Frileux C (1974) L'embolisation artérielle hepatique dans les tumeurs malignes du foie. Ann Radiol (Paris) 17:593 – 603
26. Pueyo I, Jimenez JR, Hernández J, Burgarolas A, Garcia-Moran M, Garcia-Muniz JL, Arroyo F (1978) Carcinoid syndrome treated by hepatic embolization. AJR 131:511 – 514
27. Doppman JL, Girton M, Kahn ER (1978) Proximal versus peripheral hepatic artery embolization: Experimental study in monkeys. Radiology 128:577 – 588
28. Stigsson L, Ekelund L, Jonsson N, Sjögren HO (1979) Transcatheter arterial embolization of experimental hepatic tumours in the rat. Acta Radiol [Diagn] (Stockh) 20:422 – 432
29. Ekelund L, Gerlock J Jr, Goncharenko V, Novak G (1978) Balloon catheter dilatation of renal artery stenosis in the dog. A preliminary report. Eur Urol 4:298 – 302
30. Grüntzig A, Vetter W, Meier B, Kuhlmann U, Lütolf U, Siegenthaler W (1978) Treatment of renovascular hypertension with percutaneous transluminal dilatation of a renal artery stenosis. Lancet 1:801 – 802
31. Sörensen R, Grüntzig A, Apitzsch DE, Oelkers W, Pellnitz W (1979) Transluminale Angioplastie von Nierenarterienstenosen zur Behandlung des renalen Hochdrucks. ROEFO 131:575 – 580
32. Katzen BT, Chang JC, Lukowsky GH, Abramson EG (1979) Percutaneous transluminal angioplasty for treatment of renovascular hypertension. Radiology 131:53 – 58
33. Schwarten DE, Yune HY, Klatte EC, Grim CE, Weinberger MH (1979) Clinical experience in percutaneous transluminal angioplasty of stenotic renal arteries. Radiology 135:601 – 604
34. Tegtmeyer CJ, Dver R, Teates CD, Avers CR, Carey RM, Wellons HA, Stanton LW (1980) Percutaneous transluminal dilatation of the renal arteries: Techniques and results. Radiology 135:589 – 599
35. Grüntzig A (1977) Die perkutane transluminale Rekanalisation chronischer Arterienverschlüsse mit einer neuen Dilatationstechnik. Witzstrock, Baden-Baden
36. Stables DP, Ginsberg NJ, Johnson ML (1978) Percutaneous nephrostomy: A series and review of the literature. AJR 130:75 – 82
37. Fernström I, Andersson L (1977) Percutaneous puncture nephrostomy. Springer, Berlin Heidelberg New York (Encyclopedia of urology, suppl V/1)
38. Barbaric ZL, Wood BP (1977) Emergency percutaneous nephropyelostomy: Experience with 34 patients and review of the literature. AJR 128:453 – 458
39. Ekelund L, Karp W, Klefsgård Ö, Lindstedt E, Lundquist SB (1980) Percutaneous nephrostomy – Indicational and technical considerations. Urol Radiol 1:227 – 231
40. Lunderquist A, Lunderquist M, Owman T (1979) Guide wire for percutaneous transhepatic cholangiography. Radiology 132:228
41. Pederson JF, Cowan DF, Kristensen JK, Holm HH, Hancke S, Jensen F (1976) Ultrasonically-guided percutaneous nephrostomy. Radiology 119:429 – 431
42. Haaga JR, Zelch MG, Alfidi RJ, Stewart BH, Dougherty JD (1977) CT-guided antegrade pyelography and percutaneous nephrostomy. AJR 128:621 – 624
43. Holden S, McPhee M, Grabstald H (1979) The rationale of urinary diversion in cancer patients. J Urol 121:19 – 21
44. Fowler JE Jr, Meares EM Jr, Goldin AR (1975) Percutaneous nephrostomy: Techniques, indications and results. Urology 6:428 – 434

Main Points Concerning New X-ray Contrast Media for Angiography: Their Advantages, Disadvantages, and Special Indications

W. Clauss

Schering AG, Fachbereich Medizin, Department Radiologie, Müllerstrasse 170 – 178, D-1000 Berlin 65

There can be no doubt that the synthesis of metrizamide (Amipaque) enabled Nyegaard to make a decisive advance in the field of developing contrast media (CM). Amipaque has set new standards for the use of CM in myelography as well as in several subareas of angiography.
The toxic effect of CM for angio- and urography can be traced mainly to chemotoxicity (e.g., lipophilia, protein binding), osmotic pressure (e.g., pain, thrombogenic effects, volume stress), and electrical charge (e.g., epileptogenicity). These factors will more or less influence the tolerance of all conventional CM with high osmotic pressure, e.g., Angiografin and Conray, but in Amipaque there remains only the influence of chemotoxicity (Fig. 1).
The essential advantages but also some disadvantages of Amipaque that are caused by the complicated synthesis and the insufficient stability of its solutions are demonstrated in Table 1.
All firms working on research into CM have recognized the great importance of decreasing the osmotic pressure, especially for reducing pain during peripheral angiography. Now, which possibilities are available for lowering the osmotic

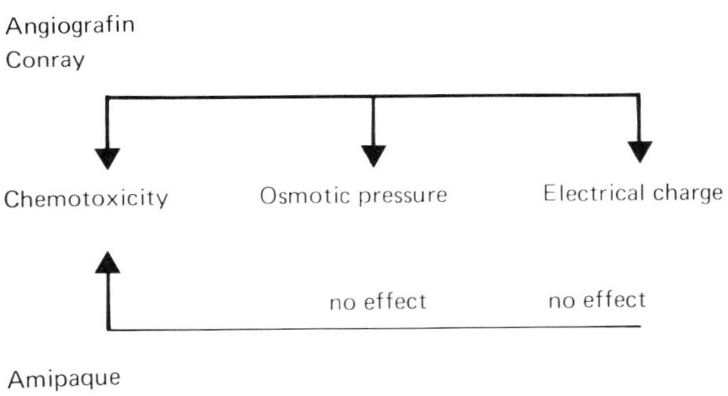

Fig. 1. Reasons for the toxicity of contrast media

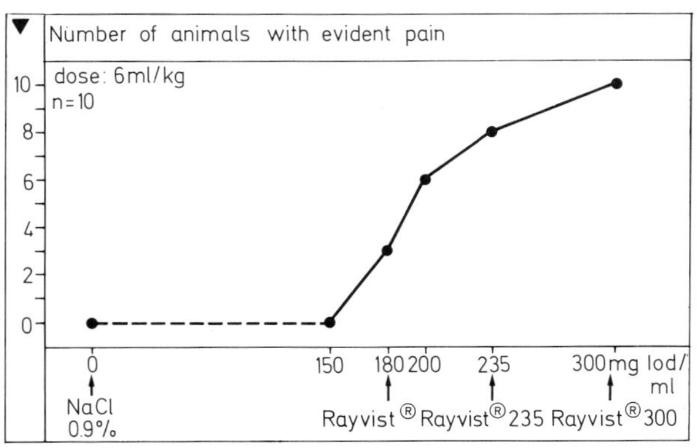

Fig. 2. Vascular pain after injection of meglumine ioglicinate at various concentrations into the femoral artery of rats

Table 1. Amipaque: Essentials on chemistry and pharmacology

Chemistry:
- new type of contrast medium
- production costs are very high
- stable only as dry powder

Physicochemistry:
- lower osmotic pressure and
- nonionic character

are responsible for better tolerance of Amipaque

Pharmacology:
- neural tolerance
- – low epileptogenicity
  – no arachnitis
- good general tolerance
  – lower toxicity
  – better cardiovascular tolerance
- local tolerance in blood vessels
  – no pain
  – less endothelium injury
  – no thrombosis
  – less blood-brain barrier damage
- lower diuresis

Pharmacokinetics:
- very similar to diatrizoate

Radiology Today 1. Ed. by M. W. Donner and F. H. W. Heuck

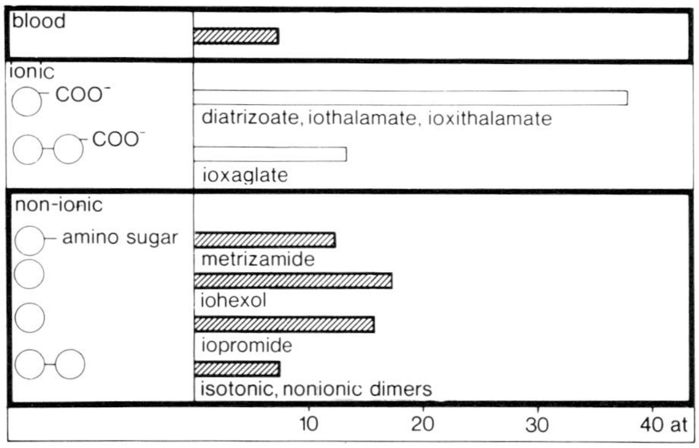

Fig. 3. Osmotic pressure of blood in comparison with contrast media for angiography (contrast medium, 300 mg iodine/ml)

ZK 35 760 (Schering AG)

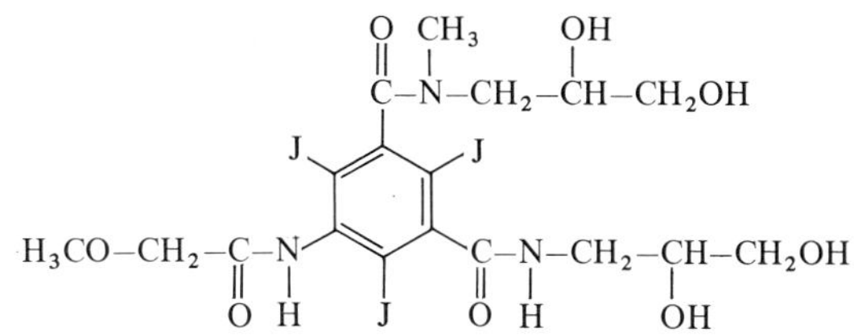

5–methoxyacetylamino–2,4,6–triiodisophthalic acid–[(2,3–dihydroxy–N–methylpropyl)–(R,S)–2,3–dihydroxy– propyl)] diamide

(IUPAC)

Fig. 4. Nonionic substance newly developed by Schering

IOHEXOL (Nyegaard)

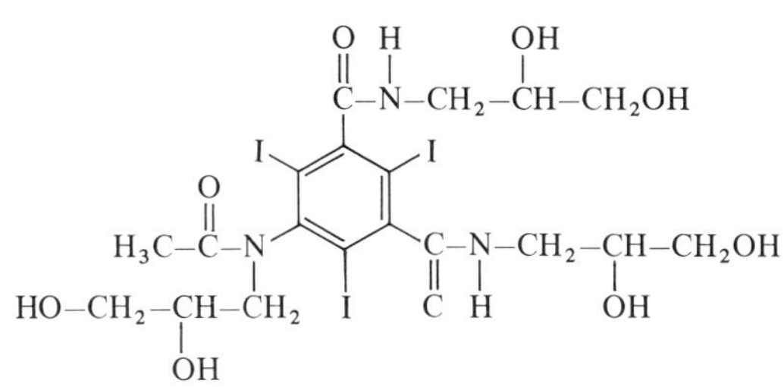

5–[N–(2,3–Dihydroxypropyl)–acetamido]–2,4,6–triiodisophthalacid–bis (2,3–dihydroxypropyl) diamid

(IUPAC)

Fig. 5. Iohexol

pressure and approximating it as closely to the blood pressure as possible? The simplest method is to be found in diluting the well-known ionic contrast media (Fig. 2). However, as the concentration grows weaker the iodine content also sinks rapidly, so that after reaching the goal of a painless concentration one has to take an impairment of the diagnostics into account. A lowering of the osmotic pressure can be better achieved, however, by synthesizing new compounds, which also allows a sufficiently high iodine concentration to be maintained. Figure 3 demonstrates the osmotic pressure of ionic and nonionic CM in comparison with that of blood.

Contrast media of nonionic origin (e.g., Amipaque) do not dissociate in aqueous solutions. This results in a low osmotic pressure and the lack of electric charge. In the case of the ionic dimeric compound ioxaglate (Hexabrix) it has been possible to lessen the number of particles in the solution and so to lower the osmotic pressure. An electric charge, however, remains, and in our opinion must be considered as one of the reasons why the use of this compound is contraindicated in myelography because of its high epileptogenicity. There are also some other disadvantages to observe in general tolerance of Hexabrix that underline the necessity of developing new compounds of nonionic origin for angio- and urography.

At present in the Federal Republic of Germany and Berlin there are three nonionic substances in the early phase of clinical testing: one from Bracco (Iopamidol), one from Nyegaard (Iohexol, developed together with Schering), and one from Schering (Figs. 4 and 5). All these CM are offered as stable solutions ready for use. Today it is too early to discuss the first result in patient treatment, but they all are looking to become real successors to Amipaque. As is the case with several well-known ionic X-ray contrast media, these compounds are aminoisophthalic acid derivatives.

Instead of one carboxyl group (e.g., Conray; Rayvist), however, both carboxyl groups were replaced in the nonionic compounds by hydrophilic residues. This allowed the acid character of the compounds known to us to be avoided, and it needs no base for giving rise to a water-soluble salt.

In concluding I would like to ask: For what indications will the CM of the nonionic (Amipaque) and ionic dimeric (Hexabrix) types be used and for what indications will the conventional CM of ionic type also be used in the future due to the costs and the lacking or insufficiently documented advantages of the new generation of preparations? The initial answers to these questions are to be seen in Table 2.

Table 2. Indications for the use of various contrast media

	Nonionic	Ionicdimer	Ionicmonomer
Indication	Amipaque	Hexabrix	Angiografin Rayvist 300 Telebrix 300
Myelography	+	–	–
Computer tomography	–	–	+
Cerebral arteriography	+	(+)	(+)
Arteriography (painful)	+	+	(+)
Arteriography (painless)	(+)	(+)	+
Coronarography	+	(+)	– Urografin 76: (+)
Phlebography	+	(+)	(+)
Urography	–	–	+

+, indicated
(+), indicated with reservations
–, not indicated

New Contrast Media for Angiography: Their Benefits, Drawbacks, and Specific Indications

E. Schmiedel

Byk Gulden Lomberg, Chemische Fabrik GmbH, Byk-Gulden-Strasse 2, D-7750 Konstanz

An outstanding characteristic of the "new" contrast media for angiography – also called the "new generation" of contrast media – is their low osmolality and consequent low osmotic pressure. Compared with conventional agents, the incidence of osmotic side effects is lower. Benefits are expected in the form of improved tolerance and reduced examination risk, especially in angiography when visualization of the arterial system calls for injection of large doses at high flow.

Table 1 gives osmolalities for the conventional, classic hyperosmolar contrast agents as opposed to the low-osmolar contrast agents in terms of iodine content. A comparison of osmolalities and iodine content is relevant in that osmolality in a contrast agent depends among other things on the concentration of iodine. Iodine content, besides dose, flow, injection site, and vascular province, constitutes an essential determinant of radiopacity in angiography.

At nearly comparable iodine content, the new contrast agents metrizamide, ioxaglic acid, and Jopamidol excel in terms of their osmolality, which is considerably lower than that of the conventional agents, without being isotonic with the blood; osmolality of the blood varies between 290 and 300 mosmol/kg. The preparation of an isotonic solution with one of these three agents would necessarily be at the expense of iodine, the content of which would then be less than 200 mg/ml. A contrast agent of this type is, however, inconceivable, at least in arteriography.

Another aspect of practical value in a contrast medium is its availability in a form ready for injection, a requirement currently met by all agents except metrizamide.

Table 1 also indicates whether the solution of contrast medium is ionic or nonionic. Occasionally, the quality of being non-dissociated or nonionic is erroneously considered an indispensable prerequisite for low-osmolar contrast agents. Yet, when it comes to osmotic side effects, the essential question is not whether the contrast agent is ionic or nonionic, but whether its osmolality is low. How osmolality is reduced, by which chemostructural principle, is of secondary importance in this connection.

By contrast, the clinical benefits derived from a reduction of osmolality and the indications that result for application of the new contrast agents in angiography are of truly practical importance.

Contrast agents of low osmolality are known to cause less subjective side effects, such as *pain* and *heat sensations,* both in intensity and incidence, when intraarterially injected. The better tolerance of low-osmolar contrast agents has been confirmed by ample clinicoradiologic experience and sufficiently documented in several studies. Thus, Tillmann et al. [6] compared Hexabrix with Telebrix 300 in a double-blind intraindividual study with pelvis – leg arteriography. The incidence of subjective side effects, such as pain, was significantly lower when Hexabrix was injected. Under the same indication and following the same methodologic principle, Holm et al. [1] compared Hexabrix with Urografin 60%. Again, the difference between the two contrast media was significant.

On the basis of these clinical findings, it appears appropriate to propose the following indications for use: selective coronarography, angiocardiography, and angiography involving large doses in patients with unstable hemodynamics, especially when preangiographic readings indicate that bradycardia is to be expected.

The rapid injection of large doses of hyperosmolar contrast media causes a rise in serum osmolality by as much as 35 mosmol/kg immediately after injection. With multiple injections at short intervals, the *initial hyperosmolar phase* persists, a phenomenon evidenced by Mann et al. [2]. To produce isotonicity, fluid from the perivascular space is transported to the blood stream, resulting in transient hypervolemia. Osmotic hemodilution of

Radiology Today 1. Ed. by M. W. Donner and F. H. W. Heuck

Table 1. Contrast media for angiography

	Agents of high osmolality	Agents of low osmolality		
	Classic products	Metrizamide[a]	Ioxaglic Acid[b]	Jopamidol[c]
Osmolality (mosmol/kg)	1500 – 2000	480	580	616
Iodine content (mg/ml)	280 – 380	300	320	300
Ready-for-injection	+	–	+	+
Ionic	+		+	
Nonionic		+		+

[a] Amipaque: Nyegaard & Co A/S, Oslo; Schering AG, Berlin/Bergkamen
[b] Hexabrix: Laboratoire Guerbet, Paris; Byk Gulden Pharmazeutika, Konstanz
[c] Jopamidol: Bracco Industria Chimica S.p.A. Milano; Byk Gulden Pharmazeutika, Konstanz

this type – detectable in hematocrit decline – is less pronounced when low-osmolar agents are employed. Taking this temporary osmotic hypervolemia into account, angiography in hypertensive patients, especially if requiring visualization of several vessels and administration of large overall doses, appears to be another indication for low-osmolar contrast agents.

Another osmotic phenomenon which has been observed for years with hyperosmolar contrast media is *erythrocyte deformation* resulting from dehydration. This deformation causes a reduction in erythrocyte flexibility or increased rigidity and consequent deterioration of the flow characteristics of the blood and leads to a reduction in capillary perfusion. Aspelin and Schmid-Schönbein [9] were particularly concerned with these rheological aspects, showing that injection of hyperosmolar contrast agents into the right ventricle causes a temporary rise in pulmonary arterial pressure. This rise is much less pronounced when contrast agents of low osmolality are used. Considering the lower osmotic activity, the number of indications for low-osmolar contrast agents may be reasonably extended to include dextrocardiography, pulmonary angiography, and mediastinal phlebography, the latter implying rapid bilateral injection of large doses and high concentrations of contrast medium in the pulmonary artery.

Another typical osmotic activity in hyperosmolar contrast agents is *diuresis,* especially following administration of large doses, which may lead to intermittent electrolyte imbalance and thus contribute to the precipitation of adverse effects in pediatric patients. With low-osmolar contrast agents, the increase in urine output is only small, since less fluid is required for elimination and tubular reabsorption is more substantial than after administration of hyperosmolar agents. Thus, in angiography requiring large doses, such as in dehydrated patients and children, the employment of low-osmolar contrast agents suggests itself.

Occasionally, the addition of a local anesthetic to the contrast medium is believed to create the same beneficial effect as when using a contrast medium of low osmolality. This belief was not confirmed by Schmitt et al. [4], who conducted an intraindividual comparative study using Hexabrix and Angiografin plus Lidocain.

Significant differences were found in the incidence of pain, heat sensations, and mimical reactions between the two agents, despite the addition of a local anesthetic to the hyperosmolar contrast agent, in this case Lidocain.

As can be seen from Table 1, the osmolality of metrizamide is slightly lower than that of Hexabrix at identical iodine content: the osmolality of Hexabrix is 580 mosmol/kg, that of metrizamide, 490 mosmol/kg, the iodine content being 320 mg/ml for both agents. The question as to whether the difference of 90 mosmol/kg has any clinical relevance was investigated by Zachrisson et al. [8] in a double-blind intraindividual comparative study. No significant difference was found in the provocation of pain and heat sensations between the two contrast agents.

Considering their better tolerance, low-osmolar contrast agents appear preferable for certain types of examination: peripheral arteriography, visualization of the external carotid artery, retrograde brachial overpressure angiography, and levocardiography, especially in pediatric patients.

What other benefits exist besides the lower incidence of subjective side effects? Are there further reasons for using the low-osmolar contrast agents in angiography?

Contrast media of high osmolality, injected intra-arterially in large doses, cause a temporary *fall in blood pressure,* especially after intracoronary or left ventricular application. The fall in blood pressure is brought about by an initial cardio-depressive effect which is followed by vasodilation caused by the high osmolality of the contrast agents. Such agents also have a bradycardiac effect which is particularly prominent in selective coronarography. Blood pressure fall and *bradycardia* may contribute to elicit adverse effects in coronarography and levocardiography, causing a deficit in myocardial perfusion which prolongs the presence of contrast agent in the coronary system. Conversely, injection into the right ventricle or pulmonary artery causes a *rise in blood pressure* in the lesser circulatory system owing to the presumed decrease in erythrocyte flexibility from osmotic activity which, in turn, reduces capillary flow in the lung.

There is sufficient clinical evidence confirming that this influence on blood pressure and heart rate depends on the osmolality of the solution of contrast medium injected. In their above study, Holm et al. [1] observe that the fall in blood pressure after Hexabrix is significantly less than after Urografin 60%. The finding was confirmed by Weikl [7] in an intraindividual comparative study with selective coronarography involving Hexabrix and Urografin 76%. When Hexabrix was used, the fall in blood pressure was less pronounced and bradycardia was less severe, the effect being significant in both cases.

The lower *neurotoxic effect* constitutes another advantage of the new contrast media. It is particularly evident in metrizamide, which is employed in myelography, and Jopamidol, which is currently in the clinical trial stage amongst others for myelographic application. Simon [5] studied Hexabrix and Conray in two separate patient groups for their influence on the EEG in cerebral angiography. Following injection of the hyperosmolar Conray 60 into the carotid artery, temporary changes in the EEG were recorded in every fourth patient, while no pathologic changes appeared in the EEG of any one patient when Hexabrix was used. Owing to their low neurotoxicity, low-osmolar contrast agents are recommended for cerebral angiography and spinal arteriography as well as for angiography in predisposed patients or patients with preangiographic neurologic symptoms.

Finally, attention should be drawn to the fact that *endothelial alterations* are less severe with low-osmolar contrast agents. Osmotic alterations of the endothelium are likely to favor the appearance of postphlebographic thromboses and thrombophlebitides. To demonstrate this, Mellmann et al. [3] compared endothelial lesions caused by Hexabrix with those induced by Telebrix 300 in an intraindividual study involving peripheral phlebography after administration of labeled fibrinogen and gamma-camera scintigraphy. When Telebrix 300 was used, a circumscribed activity uptake was detectable in 32% of the cases, compared with only 6% after administration of Hexabrix. The number of indications for contrast media of low osmolality may thus be further increased to include peripheral phlebography.

References

1. Holm M, Praestholm J (1979) Ioxaglate, a new low osmolar contrast medium used in femoral angiography. Br J Radiol 52:169
2. Mann S, Zeitler E (1975) Verhalten der Serumosmolarität bei hohen Kontrastmitteldosen im Rahmen der Angiographie. ROEFO 122/2:135
3. Mellmann J, Bornemann H (1979) Phlebographie als Ursache tiefer Beinvenenthrombosen? Röntgenologische und nuklearmedizinische Befunde bei Verwendung unterschiedlicher Kontrastmittel. Symposion Zukunft der Angiographie-Schmerzfreiheit?, 7. Juli 1979, Frankfurt/Main. Byk Gulden Pharmazeutika, Constance
4. Schmitt HE, da Silva A (1979) Zum Schmerzproblem bei der peripheren Arteriographie. VASA 8:295
5. Simon R (1979) Interindividuelle randomisierte Studie mit AG 6227 und Conray 60 in der zerebralen Angiographie. Symposion Zukunft der Angiographie-Schmerzfreiheit?, 7. Juli 1979, Frankfurt/Main. Byk Gulden Pharmazeutika, Constance
6. Tillmann U (1979) Pain in peripheral arteriography – a comparison of a low osmolality contrast medium with a conventional compound. Br J Radiol 52:102
7. Weikl A (1979) Kardiale Nebenwirkungen von Hexabrix bei der Koronarangiographie – ein klinischer Vergleich zu einem Standardkontrastmittel. Symposion Zukunft der Angiographie-Schmerzfreiheit?, 7. Juli 1979, Frankfurt/Main. Byk Gulden Pharmazeutika, Constance
8. Zachrisson B-F et al. (1980) Two new contrast media in peripheral arteriography. A double blind study in patients with arterial insufficiency in the legs. ROEFO 132/2:208
9. Almén T, Aspelin P, Levin B (1975) Effect of ionic and non-ionic contrast medium on aortic and pulmonary arterial pressure. Invest Radiol 10:519

Pulmonary Radiology

Chest Radiology Today: Overview

R. G. Fraser

The University of Alabama in Birmingham, School of Medicine, Department of Diagnostic Radiology, 619 South 19th Street, Birmingham, AL 35233 (USA)

The purpose of this contribution is to review the current status of chest radiology in the world today, and to indicate new developments that have taken place during the past couple of years. I wish also to address briefly the question "where are we going?" The first of these tasks – an update of current knowledge – has proven relatively easy. I have reviewed the radiologic literature, chiefly American, of the past 2 or 3 years and have selected those contributions which I have felt have been most significant. I must emphasize the fact that I have only casually surveyed contributions made to chest radiology in the physiologic, pathologic, medical, and surgical journals. This is perhaps a serious omission since it is probable that the explosion of knowledge that has occurred in the field of chest disease over the past few years has been more physiologic and clinical than radiologic. With the exception of computerized tomography, I must conclude that major advances in the radiologic diagnosis of chest disease have been less than auspicious.

Methods and Techniques

First, a basic consideration: Which radiographic technique provides the optimal chest roentgenogram? To answer that question, at least in part, I would like to review some of the deliberations of a symposium entitled *The Optimization of Chest Radiography* held in Madison, Wisconsin in the spring of 1979 at which many experts in the field discussed the multiple factors involved in obtaining and interpreting the optimal chest roentgenogram. Abstracts from this symposium were published recently [1].

As one might imagine, opinions on certain matters were divided, sometimes widely. For example, although it was generally agreed that the large X-ray absorption differences in various areas of the chest make it most difficult to obtain a chest radiograph with ideal exposure and diagnostic quality in all areas, there was some dissension as to what constitutes the ideal kilovoltage. One group of observers [2] stated that a high kVp technique reduces the dominance of bone and provides a better match to film latitude, resulting in better visibility of vasculature, nodular lesions, air tissue boundaries, and diffuse low-contrast soft tissue features. Steiner and his group [3], in a comparative study of 350 and 120 kVp techniques, found that neither was superior in all categories but rather that each played a complementary role in image perception in the thorax. Further, Tuddenham [4] suggested that the perception of diagnostically critical shadows in a chest radiograph is more often limited by subjective factors than by the technical characteristics of the recording. He argued that the characteristics of the various structures in the chest are so dissimilar that "ideal" imaging of all structures in a single recording is simply not possible. He concluded that the radiologist must either adopt a technique that selectively optimizes the recording of the type of structure of greatest diagnostic interest in a particular clinical situation, recognizing that the recording of other structures may be inferior, or must accept a compromise recording in which all structures are reasonably well but none ideally imaged. My own attitude, if I may be allowed a personal bias, is that a kVp of about 150 provides that reasonable compromise. This symposium also discussed a number of aspects of observer performance, including ROC curves, conspicuity, the influence of structured background on visual search, the effects of scattered radiation on radiographic quality, and the use of new techniques such as slit radiography in reducing scatter and improving quality.

One further word on technique. During the past several years, the world has experienced a gradual but significant depletion in its silver supply. Added

Radiology Today 1. Ed. by M. W. Donner and F. H. W. Heuck

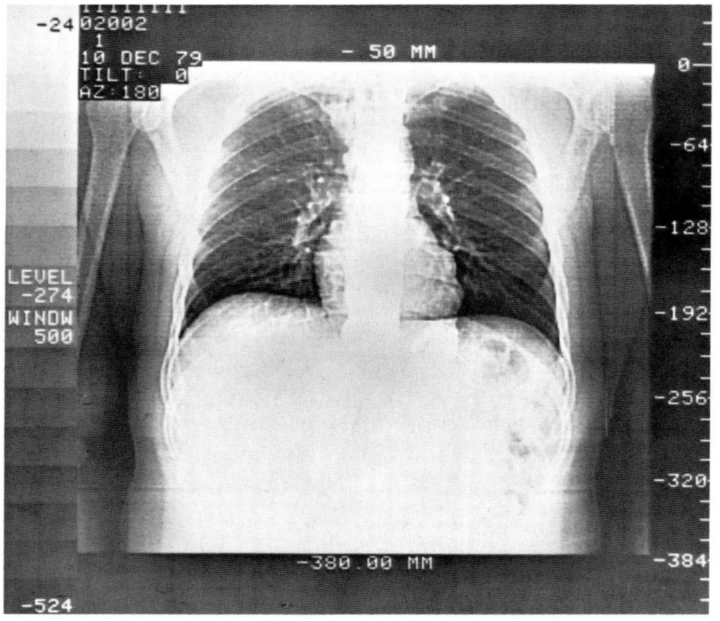

Fig. 1. Digital radiography. A computerized radiograph (scout view image) of the chest obtained on a G. E. 8800 CT scanner

to this in recent months has been the sharply escalating cost of this metal, and it is clear that something will have to be done in future years to provide an imaging system that will reduce the requirement for silver. Work is already progressing on several fronts to produce alternative methods of imaging that would accomplish this aim, including digital radiography with computer contrast correction and image evaluation [5], nuclear magnetic resonance and microwave systems, and improvements in film systems such as dry processed, nonhalide film. Although images of the chest produced by techniques such as digital radiography are as yet imperfect (Fig. 1), the provision of electronic subtraction of images following intravenous injection of contrast media may revolutionize the diagnosis of a variety of vascular disorders, including pulmonary embolism.

It would be inappropriate in an overview not to mention computerized tomography and the astonishing impact it has had on diagnosis over the past few years. While CT appears to be considerably less applicable in the thorax than in the abdomen or head, it has almost revolutionized our knowledge of mediastinal anatomy, both normal and pathologic, and has been employed to great advantage in several other applications dealt with in other contributions to this symposium.

While still in the area of basic knowledge, I would like to mention the superb studies that have been carried out by Dr. Tony Proto of Cincinnati, Ohio, in analyzing normal anatomic structures visible on lateral roentgenograms of the thorax [6]. He has visually dissected the complex of shadows visible in lateral projection and has described in exquisite detail the anatomy of structures which to the best of my knowledge have not before been properly recognized or described. I commend this reference for perusal and study.

Advances in the Diagnosis of Chest Disease

Infections

In the field of infectious disease, we have seen few significant advances. In some diseases, such as tuberculosis, a decreased frequency reflects improved public health measures and therapeutic innovations; in others, such as the nosocomial infections acquired by patients whose host defenses have been compromised as a result of organ transplantation and immunosuppressive therapeutic regimens, we have made little or no progress in our ability to recognize and separate the various causes with the possible exception of *Pneumocystis carinii*. Whether we will ever be able to accomplish this is a moot question, but the observation underlines the fact that, for the present at least, our capabilities go little further than to recognize that disease is present and to perform percutaneous needle biopsy when indicated [7].

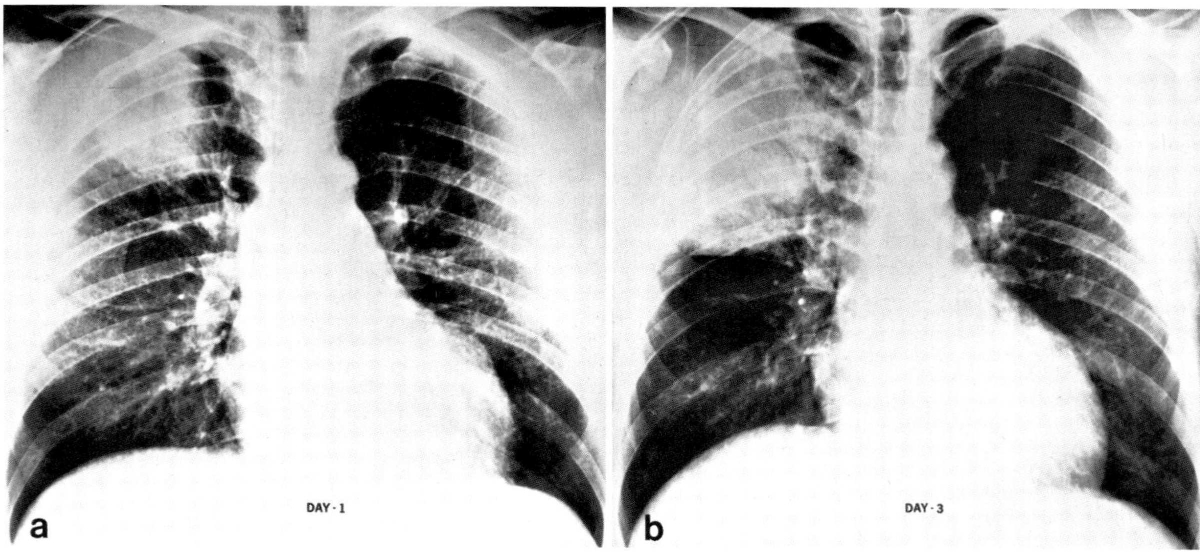

Fig. 2a, b. Acute Legionnaire's pneumonia. This 29-year-old white male was admitted to hospital with high fever, chills, drenching sweats, and extreme fatigue. **a** His admission chest roentgenogram revealed homogeneous consolidation in the right upper lobe consistent with acute air-space pneumonia. **b** Two days later, the consolidation had extended to involve most of the upper lobe and exhibited a prominent air bronchogram. This progression of disease is a common feature of acute Legionnaire's pneumonia. Uneventful recovery. (Courtesy of Dr. Fred Valdmanis, Hastings, Michigan)

Although new diseases are not recognized very often these days, during the past few years North America has experienced a spate of epidemics of a brand new infection, Legionnaire's disease. Presenting as a fulminant, often fatal pneumonia, it was first recognized among a group of American legionnaires holding a convention in Philadelphia [8]. The epidemic caused near hysteria and ultimately the demise of the great old hotel in which the meeting was being held. Eventually, the organism was successfully isolated at the National Communicable Disease Center in Atlanta as a pleomorphic, weekly gram-negative bacillus which requires special staining techniques for its demonstration [9]. It tends to occur in previously normal patients although immunosuppressed patients are at greater risk [10]. The roentgenographic presentation is of an acute air space pneumonia (Fig. 2), bilateral in 50% of patients [11, 12]. Therapeutic response to erythromycin or tetracycline tends to be prompt.

Drug-Induced Disease

Of increasing interest and importance in recent years has been iatrogenic lung disease, specifically that associated with drugs. Drug-induced pulmonary reactions vary widely in their roentgenographic manifestations in the chest, including such changes as simple overinflation as in asthma, a diffuse bubbly pattern characteristic of bronchopulmonary dysplasia caused by a complex group of influences including oxygen toxicity and high inflation pressures, and widespread interstitial and air space disease caused notably by a variety of cytotoxic agents. In January 1979, Seltzer and Herman [13] reviewed this subject in great detail, producing an exhaustive list of drugs capable of causing pulmonary reactions. For example, 21 drugs were deemed capable of producing tracheobronchial hypersensitivity (asthma), aspirin leading the list; seven drugs as causing eosinophilic lung disease; ten as being responsible for interstitial and alveolar disease, either alone or in combination; 14 as causing vasculitis; and 21 as being potential causes of systemic lupus erythematosus. I think that some radiologists, among whom I am numbered, have a tendency to forget drug-induced disease when considering the differential diagnosis of abnormal roentgen patterns, and since the incidence of these reactions is likely to increase rather than diminish, it is clear that we must be constantly aware of their possibility and thoroughly familiar with their various manifestations.

Neoplasms

In the field of lung cancer, it is clear that we have made very little progress during the past 2 or 3 years. The overall 5 year survival for lung cancer remains a dismal 10% or less [14]. Despite the fact that the great majority of cases are related to cigarette smoking and that the disease is thus a largely preventable one, efforts to reduce smoking unfortunately have not been very successful except among physicians. There is now little doubt that in unselected populations annual chest radiography in mass screening programs for lung cancer detection is useless and in fact counterproductive [15]. Although the value of semiannual radiography has been more controversial, a 1972 report from the Philadelphia Pulmonary Neoplasm Research Project [16] concluded that semiannual screening contributes little toward solving the lung cancer problem: of 6136 male volunteers who had semiannual chest roentgenograms for the detection of bronchogenic carcinoma, 121 (2%) developed cancer, but only 10 (8%) of these survived 5 years.

However, there does seem to be a small ray of light at the end of this abysmal tunnel of darkness. Some 10 years ago, the National Cancer Institute of the United States formed a "Cooperative Early Lung Cancer Group" consisting of three centers of higher learning, the Mayo Clinic, the Johns Hopkins University, and the Memorial-Sloan Kettering Cancer Center in New York. Although the protocols of these three centers were not identical, they were designed to generate data that would be complementary and supportive [17]. The Mayo Clinic has published preliminary results of its studies [18], and I would like to review some of these briefly. This program was designed to detect curable lung cancer in a "high-risk" population of men, 45 or more years of age and all heavy cigarette smokers. These men were screened initially by means of chest radiographs, sputum cytology tests, and questionnaires. The men were randomly assigned either to a close surveillance study group, rescreened every 4 months, or to a comparison group advised to undergo yearly rescreening. Results as of 1978 indicated that the initial and 4-monthly screenings made possible the detection and localization of lung cancers at a time when the majority were either occult or localized and resectable for cure. Survival appeared better for those men whose lung cancers were detected by the initial screening than for those in a similar nonscreened population. *Despite this,* however, the lung cancer death rates in the two populations were similar. It is clear that further observation is essential before any definite conclusions can be reached regarding the value of 4-monthly rescreening, even in such a high-risk population.

While the diagnosis of lung cancer has not been facilitated to any extent by gallium-67 scanning, selenium methionine-75 seems to hold considerable promise: in one study [19], uptake of this isotope was positive in *all* 42 cases of cancer of all types and negative in all eight cases of infectious disease.

The solitary pulmonary nodule controversy remains topical. The four possible courses of action following identification of a solitary nodule – watchful waiting, fiberoptic bronchoscopy, needle aspiration biopsy, and thoracotomy – each has its strong proponents, and it is apparent that we still have further to go in establishing an investigational protocol that will fit every situation. The studies by Stanley Siegelman in the investigation of solitary nodules by CT look very promising indeed and are discussed elsewhere in this symposium.

While still on the subject of cancer, it now appears clear that any controversy that may have existed regarding diagnostic persistence in working up a patient with metastatic cancer to the lung and an unknown primary site has finally been put to rest. In a retrospective analysis of 255 patients with metastases of unknown origin, Steckel and Kagan [20] found that 231 patients (over 90%) had since died. Of 34 patients with autopsy information, no primary lesion was found in 20. In the remaining 14 cases, prior knowledge of the primary site would not have influenced either therapy or prognosis. These authors make a plea for judicious restraint in the use of diagnostic imaging procedures to search exhaustively for a primary cancer site, a position with which I feel sure most radiologists would be in complete and enthusiastic agreement.

One further potentially exciting development in the field of lung cancer that has appeared on the horizon during the past 2 or 3 years is the pioneering work being performed by Björn Nordenström of Sweden on bioelectric potentials in the vicinity of lung neoplasms and on the possible applications of electrotherapy [21]. This work has not yet been published, but I understand that we can look forward to learning of its capabilities from a book to be published sometime during the next several months.

Pulmonary Thromboembolism

I suspect that all would agree that progress in methods of investigation and management of patients with suspected thromboembolism has been rather limited. One large retrospective study [22] offered assurances that a negative angiogram in patients with suspected pulmonary embolism positively excludes that diagnosis. Although in some countries, notably the United States, pulmonary arteriography is still regarded as the single most definitive technique for investigating suspected pulmonary thromboembolic disease [23, 24], such a position is not held universally in all institutions, even in the United States, and many physicians still rely heavily on ventilation/perfusion scanning to make a reasonably confident diagnosis without recourse to angiography. The improvement in ventilation scanning brought about by the use of krypton-81m [25] rather than low-energy xenon-133 is such that a negative $\dot{V}/\dot{Q}$ scan now virtually excludes the diagnosis of embolism.

Inhalational Diseases

In the field of occupational lung disease, the ILO, at a meeting in Geneva in August 1979, saw fit to modify its 1971 *International Classification of Radiographs of the Pneumoconioses* and has now published a draft of its new 1979 classification. What they have done in essence – and I say this without necessarily being critical – is to increase the complexity of the recording of the shape and size of small opacities by requiring that two descriptive letters be recorded. Thus, if the reader considers that all or virtually all opacities are of one size and shape, then this should be noted by recording the symbol twice, separated by an oblique stroke (e.g., q/q). If, however, another shape or size is seen, then this should be recorded as the second letter (for example, q/t). By a little simple arithmetic, it can be established that there are 36 possible combinations of small opacities which the reader must recognize and record, clearly a monumental task of visual acuity. If one adds to this the twelve point scale of profusion, the astonishing number of 432 combinations of abnormalities are possible. While there is no doubt that the ILO has put much thought and wisdom into this decision and that the classification may indeed work well for the epidemiologist, the complexity of interpretation from the chest radiologist's viewpoint boggles the mind!

While still in the field of the pneumoconioses, it is now safe to say that any doubt that may have existed about the astonishing incidence of lung cancer among asbestos workers who smoke has now been put to rest. As pointed out by Selikoff and Hammond in a recent editorial [26], the brunt of the asbestos lung cancer burden is borne by asbestos workers who smoke. These investigators reported on a 10-year follow-up study of 8220 asbestos insulation workers who had volunteered their smoking histories at the outset of the study in 1967; 6841 had a history of cigarette smoking, 1379 did not. For comparison, a group of 73763 men in the American Cancer Society's prospective cancer prevention study was analyzed as controls; these men had the same distribution of smoking habits and were alike in most other respects except that they had not been exposed to asbestos. Death rates for lung cancer (per 100000 man-years, standardized for age) were as follows: 11.3 for men who neither worked with asbestos nor smoked cigarettes; 58.4 for men who worked with asbestos but did not smoke; 122.6 for cigarette smokers who had not worked with asbestos; and 601.6 for men who had been exposed to both cigarettes and asbestos. The latter finding is ominous indeed: among asbestos workers who smoke, one in every five deaths is due to lung cancer.

Interventional Radiology

It does not appear as if major advances have been made in the commonest form of interventional radiology, percutaneous biopsy of parenchymal and mediastinal disease. New needles have been described [27, 28] but there still remains a disturbing 15% incidence of false negative results in many people's hands.

However, a contribution of major clinical application was the report by Remy and associates [29] on the treatment of hemoptysis by bronchial artery embolization. In 49 actively bleeding patients, hemorrhage was arrested in 41, permanently in 35. Another 55 patients were treated prophylactically.

Adult Respiratory Distress Syndrome

Finally, a word about that most devastating of pulmonary injuries, the adult respiratory distress syndrome (ARDS). The appellation ARDS was coined by Petty and Ashbaugh in 1971 [30] to describe a clinical picture of severe, unexpected, and life-threatening acute respiratory distress occurring after a widely diverse group of clinical insults. Despite intensive investigations that have been performed on many fronts to clarify its pathogenesis, it does not look as if we are much further ahead in understanding this complex condition. The radiologic manifestations are usually easily recognized: the acute phase is characterized by massive pulmonary edema, followed on sequential examinations by one of three courses – complete clearing, diffuse pulmonary fibrosis, or death. On the basis of superb ultrastructural studies, Ewald Weibel [13] has demonstrated the exceptional vulnerability of the delicate tissue of the alveolar septa and its limited capacity to repair damage. He concluded that the lungs' limited capacity to repair follows a most specific reaction pattern that essentially determines the course of ARDS.

By contrast to the rather limited state of our knowledge of ARDS, we have made considerable progress in the field of intensive care radiology, discussed in this symposium by Dr. Pokieser.

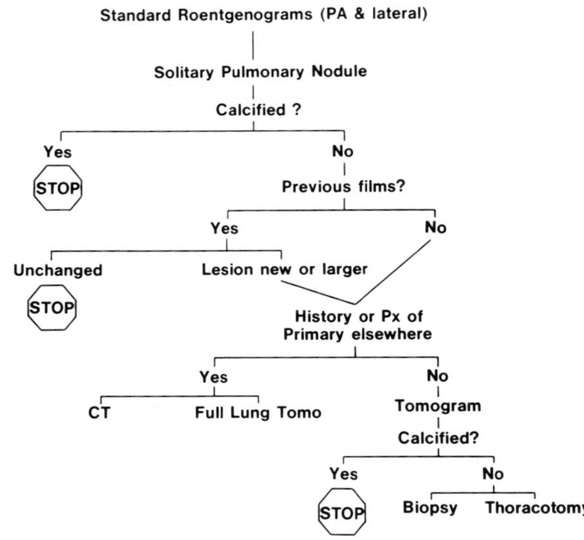

Fig. 3. A possible investigative algorithm for a solitary pulmonary nodule

Chest Radiology in the 1980s

I would like to devote the rest of this contribution to a consideration of the responsibility of the radiologist in the practice of chest radiology during the 1980s and perhaps beyond. What I am about to say is to some extent philosophical, but nevertheless is sufficiently practical to be appropriate to an overview such as this. I am going to ask, and hopefully answer, three important questions concerning our responsibilities as I see them.

Let us start with the premise that an abnormality has been discovered on standard PA and lateral roentgenograms of the chest. At this stage, the first important question to ask is: *Which imaging procedure or sequence of procedures should be carried out next to provide the maximum amount of useful information? In the course of the investigation, at what point should we call stop?*

In answer to this question, I think there would be some agreement among older radiologists that at one time a patient admitted to hospital for investigation of, for example, a solitary pulmonary nodule, was more or less automatically given the shotgun approach and put through a series of investigations including excretory urography, barium examination of the upper GI tract and colon, an oral cholecystogram, and even a skeletal survey, all searching for a possible primary site for a solitary metastasis. It is to be hoped that such useless expenditure of time, effort, and money has largely been abandoned for, as mentioned earlier, it must have rated somewhere near zero on the cost effectiveness scale. Nowadays our approach to the solitary pulmonary nodule has become somewhat more logical as a result of rather extensive experience gained over the years. Accepting that each institution must evolve its own approach based upon experience with available equipment and the expertise of the radiologist, a common investigative algorithm might be as illustrated in Fig. 3.

I believe it essential that we develop algorithms to fit every group of radiographic abnormalities that we recognize. Although admittedly, many algorithms exist fairly firmly in our minds – for example, the sequence of procedures to be carried out in a patient with suspected pulmonary embolism – it is important that we commit them to paper, not to be stuck away in a drawer somewhere but to be constantly visible for the education and guidance of our clinical colleagues.

Another example of a fairly common algorithm is that associated with segmental homogeneous consolidation (Figs. 4, 5). I feel that far too often in this type of radiographic presentation there exists a strong tendency to proceed directly from the plain roentgenograms to tomography or even bronchography. The important question arises as to why carry out tomography or more particularly bronchography at this stage of the investigation? The physician faced with a patient with suspected lung cancer seeks the optimum pathway (1) to establish a definitive diagnosis and (2) to assess the measurable extent of the disease. Once the presence or absence of neoplasm has been established, only then is it reasonable to move along the appropriate investigative pathways, progressing initially from

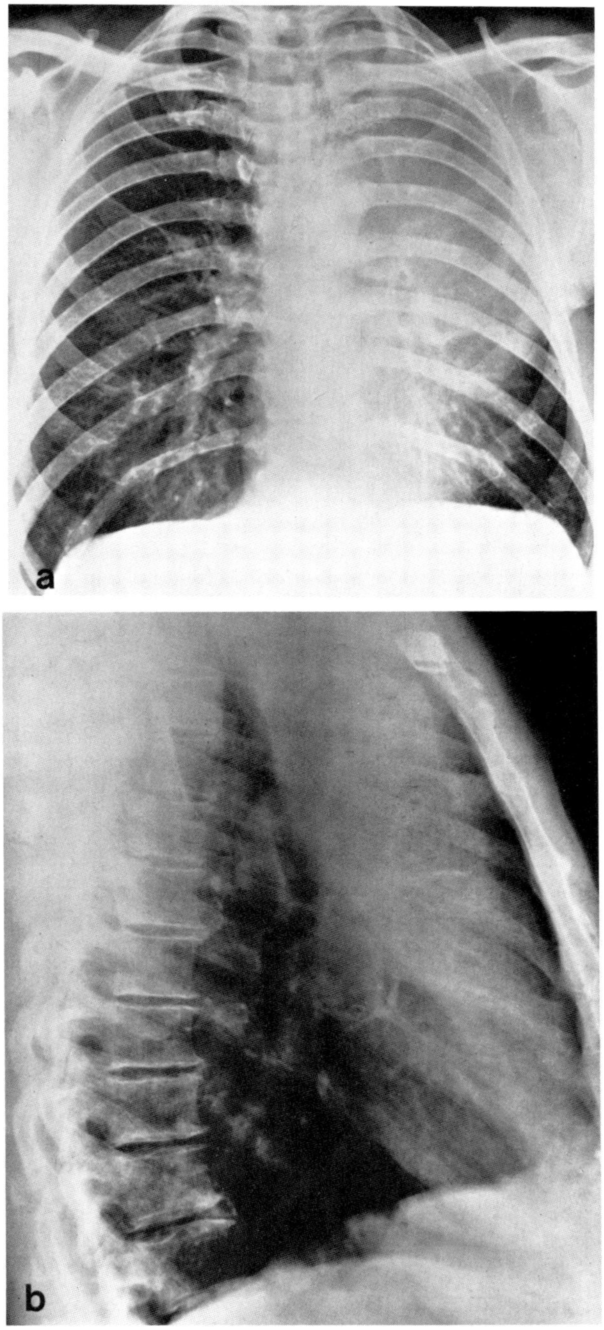

Fig. 4a, b. Obstructive pneumonitis, left upper lobe. **a** Posteroanterior and **b** lateral roentgenograms reveal a homogeneous opacity occupying the whole of the left upper lobe associated with moderate loss of volume. There is no air bronchogram. This appearance is almost pathognomonic of an obstructing endobronchial lesion. Proven squamous cell carcinoma, left upper lobe bronchus

procedures carrying the least cost and risk to the patient to those involving substantial hazard.

The second question we must ask is *to what extent should the radiologist be responsible for structuring the diagnostic workup?* I think we all agree that excessive diagnostic procedures are being performed nowadays, and one solution to decreasing the demand for X-ray services is to relieve the referring physician of his traditional responsibility for structuring the radiologic workup of a patient. Historically, either the referring physician or his house staff officer has determined which diagnostic studies should be performed on his patient, and there is no doubt that we have all been greatly concerned about the inefficiency of this approach. Expensive and often hazardous studies are being performed essentially at the whim of the referring physician, and I submit that the only way in which we are going to control this wasteful overutilization is for the radiologist to have more say in deciding which examinations to perform and when, obviously with input from the referring physician. Although on the surface this situation might be regarded as an intrusion into what the referring physician perceives as a basic right, his concern will be considerably assuaged if he has been previously exposed to the protocol governing that specific situation and if he recognizes the considerable saving in hospital time and money that will accrue from such prompt attention.

Accepting that the performance of examinations according to established algorithms ensures that a diagnosis is made as economically and with as much speed as possible, a further method of saving time is for additional examinations to be performed on the spot. Let me give you an example. Roentgenograms of the chest have been made on a 40-year-old asymptomatic man and the films viewed immediately at the end of the automatic processor. A solitary pulmonary nodule is visualized. The patient denies having had previous roentgenographic studies of his chest and is sent immediately (or as soon as feasibly consistent with room scheduling) to a radiographic room for tomography. Calcium is identified within the lesion. Voila! The matter is settled. There is no 24- or 48-h delay in the report reaching the referring physician to comply with your recommendation for tomographic examination. There is no needless extension of the patient's hospitalization for a lesion that was proven within a matter of minutes to be inconsequential. We call this "progressive investigative radiology," PIR or πR for short.

I think we would all agree that the best system of all in facilitating proper patient assessment is daily

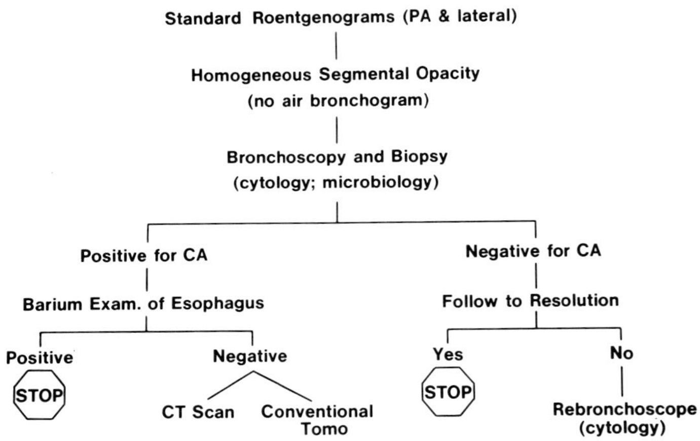

Fig. 5. A possible investigative algorithm for the type of lesion illustrated in Fig. 4

consultation between referring physician and radiologist on a personal basis. Such meetings provide a continuing dialogue which permits prompt evaluation of a patient's progress and enables a decision to be made as to the most fruitful investigations to be performed to clarify a problem.

Now for the third important question: *In what ways can the radiologist play a useful role in controlling or reducing burgeoning health costs?* It has been estimated that anywhere from 35% to 50% of the work load of departments of radiology in the United States relates to the thorax, and we are thus potentially in a position to reduce overutilization of X-ray services to a greater extent in the chest area than in any other section of the body. There are four areas that require brief consideration in this regard.

1. So-called *administrative X-rays* on asymptomatic patients, including routine checkups and preoperative or admission chest roentgenograms. The studies of Stuart Sagel and his colleagues at the Mallinckrodt Institute in St. Louis [32] have provided useful information concerning the potential yield of routine screening chest examinations obtained solely because of hospital admission regulations or scheduled surgery. From an analysis of over 10000 chest roentgenograms of a hospital-based population, they concluded that routine screening examinations were not warranted at all in patients under the age of 20 years, and that the lateral projection could be safely eliminated from routine examinations in patients from 20 to 39 years of age but should be included whenever chest disease was suspected and in screening examinations of patients 40 years of age or older. Now that the high costs of medical care are being critically examined, the radiologist should give due consideration to observations such as these.
2. *"Defensive" medicine,* which seeks to protect the physician from legal problems or possible malpractice litigation. This factor has obviously resulted in dramatic overutilization of certain radiologic services, but generally speaking is not an important issue in the thorax.
3. The subject that I addressed earlier in this paper – the requirement for a set of *algorithms* that would set down in precise fashion the order in which radiologic examinations should be performed in order to yield the greatest amount of information at lowest cost.
4. Finally, the item on which I would like to end my paper, our tendency to overutilize certain expensive procedures whose diagnostic yield tends to be rather low.

The first of these are the multiple ancillary techniques that can be employed to supplement standard PA and lateral chest roentgenograms. I refer specifically to oblique roentgenography, fluoroscopy, apical lordotic views, stereoscopy, and expiratory roentgenography. Although I expect howls of protest, I personally find that these procedures add little to information gained from good quality PA and lateral roentgenograms. There are, as always, certain exceptions: for example, oblique roentgenograms may be of considerable value in identifying pleural plaques in patients with asbestosis; fluoroscopy sometimes can be of use in evaluating diaphragmatic excursion and in establishing the anatomic location of an intrathoracic lesion; expiratory roentgenography reveals air trapping and as such can be useful in confirming the presence of airway obstruction. But generally speaking, how often are these procedures truly cost-effective? I submit not very often.

Tomography. I would like to make an earnest plea for restraint in the use of this technique. All too often, tomographic examinations are requested to provide better visualization of a lesion that is clearly identifiable on standard roentgenograms. What additional information do we gain? Seldom if ever will tomography establish a pathologic diagnosis even though the anatomic nature of the lesion may be somewhat better appreciated. A more direct approach such as bronchoscopic or percutaneous needle biopsy is obviously preferable. There are a number of exceptions to these statements such as the identification of cavitation not clearly visible on plain roentgenograms, the identification of calcium within a solitary peripheral nodule, or the better visualization of confusing shadows that make up the hila.

Bronchography. There is little if any doubt in my mind that this procedure has largely outlived its usefulness. Supporters of the procedure speak enthusiastically of its ability to distinguish infectious and neoplastic pulmonary lesions by revealing characteristic deformity of the airways. But the important question remains, if efficacious treatment depends on the identification of the offending microorganisms or neoplastic cells, why employ bronchography to make a general distinction between the two processes in the first place? With few exceptions, the diagnosis of pulmonary disease depends on microbiologic or morphological examination, and the many recently developed procedures to obtain adequate material for study in most cases permit precise diagnosis without recourse to bronchography. To my mind, there is only one indication for bronchography nowadays – the investigation of the presence and extent of bronchiectasis in a patient in whom surgical resection of diseased lung would be feasible.

Finally, let me make a plea for the independence of consultants in the practice of medicine. When examinations are requested that we know will have little positive yield and that we feel will have little beneficial impact on the course of the patient's illness, let us resist tenaciously. In my experience, when such a situation is discussed with the referring physician, seldom will he or she feel offended that we are unwilling to go along with his request. The radiologist who is not willing to take the risk of incurring a physician's anger by refusing to perform unproductive examinations not only fails to act in the best interests of the patient but also damages our position as consultants in the whole medical care system.

References

1. The optimization of chest radiography. AJR 134:199
2. Charbonnier F, Barbour J (1980) The physical basis for high voltage chest radiography. AJR 134:200
3. Steiner RM, Tuddenham W, McArdle G, Gorson R (1980) High kilovoltage chest radiography: a comparison of 350 and 120 kVp techniques. AJR 134:200
4. Tuddenham WJ (1980) Rationale for high kVp chest radiography. AJR 134:200
5. Foley WD, Lawson TL, Scanlon GT, Heenschen RC, DiBianca F (1979) Digital radiography of the chest using a computed tomography instrument. Radiology 133:231
6. Proto AV, Speckman JM (1979) The left lateral radiograph of the chest. Part I. Med Radiogr Photogr 55:30
7. Castellino RA, Blank N (1979) Etiologic diagnosis of focal pulmonary infection in immunocompromised patients by fluoroscopically guided percutaneous needle aspiration. Radiology 132:563
8. Fraser DW, Tsai TR, Orenstein W, et al. (1977) Legionnaires' disease: description of an epidemic of pneumonia. N Engl J Med 297:1189
9. McDade JE, Shepard CC, Fraser DW, Tsai TR, Redus MA, Dowdle WR (1977) Legionnaires' disease: isolation of a bacterium and demonstration of its role in other respiratory disease. N Engl J Med 297:1197
10. Bock BV, Kirby B, Eddstein PH, et al. (1978) Legionnaires' disease in renal transplant recipients. Lancet 1:410
11. Dietrich PA, Johnson RD, Fairbank JT, Walke JS (1978) The chest radiograph in Legionnaires' disease. Radiology 127:577
12. Reed JC, McLelland R, Nelson P (1978) Legionnaires disease. AJR 131:892
13. Seltzer SE, Herman PG (1979) Drug-induced pulmonary reactions associated with abnormal chest radiograph. J Cont Ed Radiol 1:25
14. Cancer patient survival report, no 5 (1977) U.S. Department of Health, Education and Welfare, Public Health Service. National Institutes of Health DHEW Publication, no (NIH) 77-992
15. Gilbertsen VA (1964) X-ray examination of the chest: an unsatisfactory method of detection of early lung cancer in asymptomatic individuals. JAMA 188:1082
16. Boucot KR, Weiss W (1973) Is curable lung cancer detected by semiannual screening? JAMA 224:1361

17. Manual of procedures (1978) Cooperative Early Lung Cancer Group, National Cancer Institute, Bethesda
18. Fontana RS, Taylor WF (1978) Screening for lung cancer: the Mayo lung project. Ann R Coll Phys Surg Can 11:309
19. Lilker ES, Gregorovicz V, Bayley A, Bibey R, Spratt E (1977) Detection of lung carcinoma by ^{75}Selenium selena methionine (^{75}Se) lung scans. Am Rev Respir Dis 115 [Suppl]:136
20. Steckel RJ, Kagan AR (1980) Diagnostic persistence in working up metastatic cancer with an unknown primary site. Radiology 134:367
21. Nordenström B (1979) Biokinetic considerations in the radiographic manifestations of pulmonary masses. Fleischner Symposium on Chest Disease, Stockholm June 1979
22. Novelline RA, Baltarowich OH, Athanasoulis CA, Waltman AC, Greenfield AJ, Mc Kusick KA (1978) The clinical course of patients with suspected pulmonary embolism and a negative pulmonary arteriogram. Radiology 126:561
23. Weidner W, Swanson L, Wilson G (1967) Roentgen techniques in the diagnosis of pulmonary thromboembolism. AJR 100:397
24. Sagel SS, Greenspan RH (1977) Nonuniform pulmonary arterial perfusion: pulmonary embolism? Radiology 99:541
25. Goris ML, Daspit SG, Walter JP, McRae J, Lamb J (1977) Applications of ventilation lung imaging with ^{81m}Krypton. Radiology 122:399
26. Selikoff IJ, Hammond EC (1979) Asbestos and smoking (editorial). JAMA 242:458
27. Ballard GL, Boyd WR (1978) A specially designed cutting aspiration needle for lung biopsy. AJR 130:899
28. Rosenberger A, Adler O (1978) Fine needle aspiration biopsy in the diagnosis of mediastinal lesions. AJR 131:239
29. Remy J, Arnaud A, Fardou H, Giraud R, Voisin C (1977) Treatment of hemoptysis of embolization of bronchial arteries. Radiology 122:33
30. Petty TL, Ashbaugh DG (1971) The adult respiratory distress syndrome. Clinical features, factors influencing prognosis and principles of management. Chest 60:233
31. Weibel ER (1979) Looking into the lung: What can it tell us? Fleischner lecture, 1979. AJR 133:1021
32. Sagel SS, Evens RG, Forrest JV, Bramson RT (1974) Efficacy of routine screening and lateral chest radiographs in a hospital-based population. N Engl J Med 291:1001

CT Densitometry of the Lung

W. Döhring, G. Linke, and H.-S. Stender

Medizinische Hochschule Hannover, Institut für Klinische Radiologie, Karl-Wiechert-Allee 9, D-3000 Hannover 61

In computed tomography (CT), a distinction must be made between the pictorial visualization of a body cross-section and the quantitative analysis of an organ. In the following, we report on the quantitative ventilation analysis of the lungs using computed tomography. First, the theoretical basics are explained and subsequently characteristic examples are demonstrated.

The Method of Quantitative CT Ventilation Analysis of the Lung

Methodical discussion starts from the matrix of the attenuation values measured and deals with two problems: the isolation of the respiratory lung parenchyma in a thoracic computer tomogram and the conversion of the pulmonary attenuation values into suitable ventilation parameters. In order to solve these problems, a new FORTRAN IV program system was developed for the Siemens computer tomographs [1, 2].

Computerized Isolation of the Respiratory Lung Parenchyma

In addition to the respiratory lung parenchyma, a computer tomogram of the thorax contains extrathoracic image portions (i.e., positioning material of the patient and ambient air), extrapulmonary thorax portions (i.e., chest wall and mediastinum) as well as larger vessels and bronchi inside the lung. These image portions, which do not belong to the respiratory lung parenchyma, adversely affect CT measurements of the pulmonary ventilation (e.g., when the mean value or the relative frequency distribution of the gas content in a larger measurement area or even a total lung cross-section are to be determined). The disturbing structures can be eliminated by means of a digital masking technique. The basic principle of this technique is shown in Fig. 1; its standard performance can be subdivided into four individual steps.

During the first step the entire matrix of the original image is scanned line by line from left to right and column by column from top to bottom until a set threshold value is reached. This threshold value must, on the one hand, be higher than the attenuation values of all extrathoracic image elements, on the other hand, it must not exceed the maximum attenuation values of the chest wall which still form a continuous external contour. The sum of the scans up to the preset threshold value give a so-called external mask. If the matrix of the original image is covered with this external mask, the masked extrathoracic image portions (here a mat, a blanket, and the ambient air) are eliminated and only the thoracic picture points remain.

In a second step those picture elements of the isolated thorax cross-section can be separated with the aid of a so-called interval mask whose attenuation values lie outside of a preset attenuation value interval. If we take the value 0 for the lower interval limit and for the upper interval limit an attenuation value which lies between the attenuation values of the lung on one hand and the attenuation values of the chest wall and the mediastinum on the other hand, then only the lung remains with the prevailing portion of its larger vessels.

The still existing medium-sized and larger pulmonary vessels with their marginal zones and the remaining transition zones of the lung towards the chest wall and the mediastinum are eliminated in a third step by means of a so-called difference mask. This mask embraces all picture points of the isolated lung which follow in some line or in some column an upward jump of the attenuation values of a preset magnitude or precede such a downward jump of the values.

Radiology Today 1. Ed. by M. W. Donner and F. H. W. Heuck

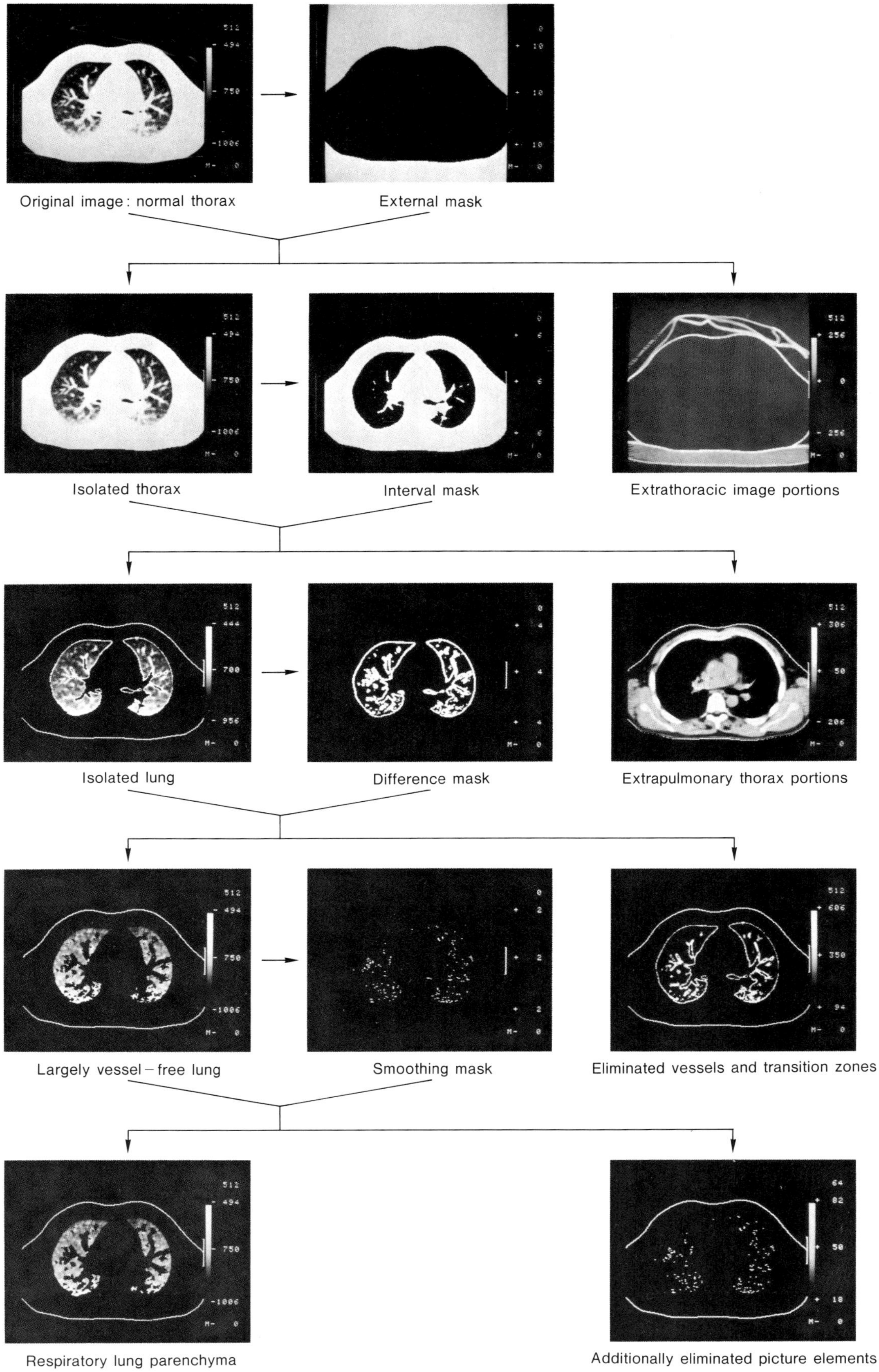

Fig. 1. Isolation of the respiratory lung parenchyma from a computer tomogram by means of a digital masking technique

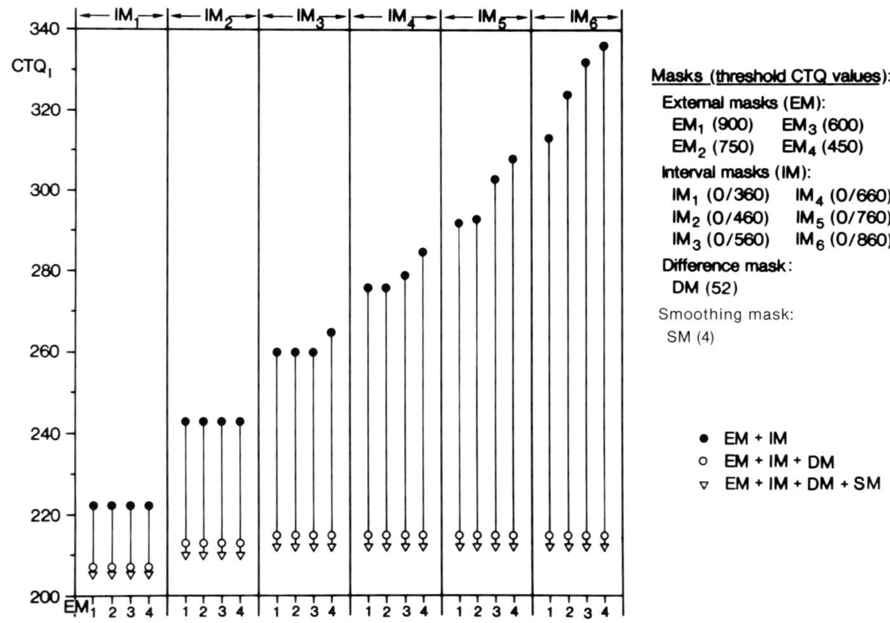

Fig. 2. Determination of mean pulmonary CT quotients (CTQ_I; cf. Table 1) in the application of various external masks (EM_1 up to EM_4) of various interval masks (IM_1 up to IM_6), a difference mask (DM) and a smoothing mask (SM). The difference mask compensates completely for the effect of differences in the threshold values of the external masks and the interval masks

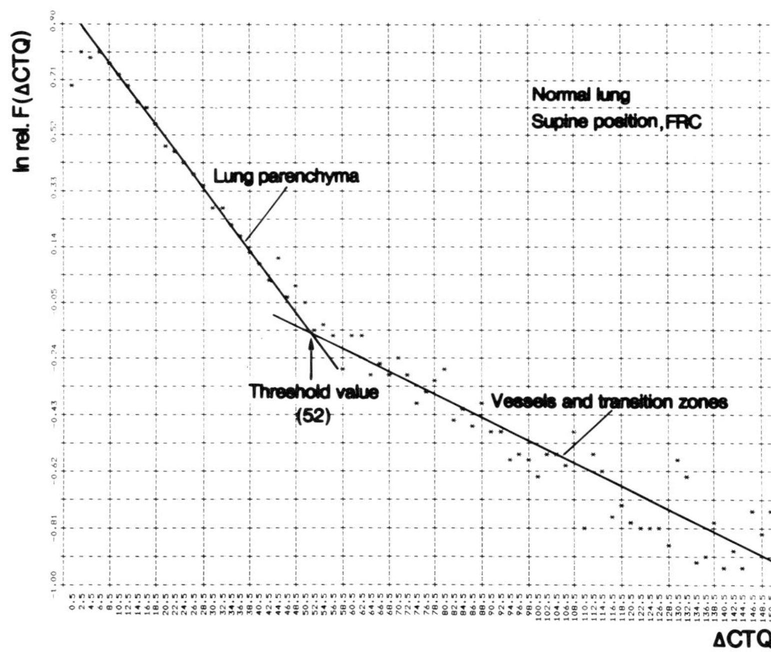

Fig. 3. Logarithmically represented frequency distribution of the differences in the CT values of an isolated vascular lung for the determination of the threshold value for the difference mask

Here as a rule, some individual picture points still remain amidst the larger vessels. These can be eliminated in a fourth step with so-called smoothing mask. This eliminates all picture elements which after application of the preceding masks were no longer left with a preset number of directly neighbouring picture points.

The threshold values for the external mask and the interval mask can be determined on the basis of the original image. In view of the isolation of the respiratory lung parenchyma their selection is completely uncritical because the difference mask is capable of compensating for the effects of considerable differences in the threshold values for the external mask and the interval mask (Fig. 2). The selection of a suitable threshold value for the difference mask also proved to be unproblematic: If the logarithm of the absolute or the relative frequency of the attenuation value differences in the picture of the isolated vascular lung is

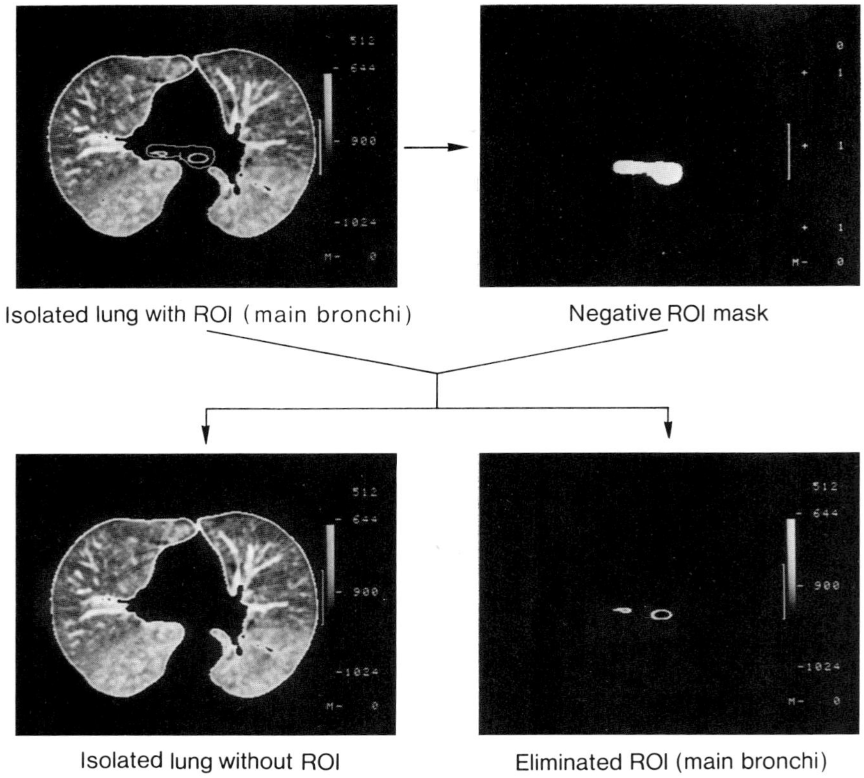

Fig. 4. Elimination of the main bronchi with a ROI mask

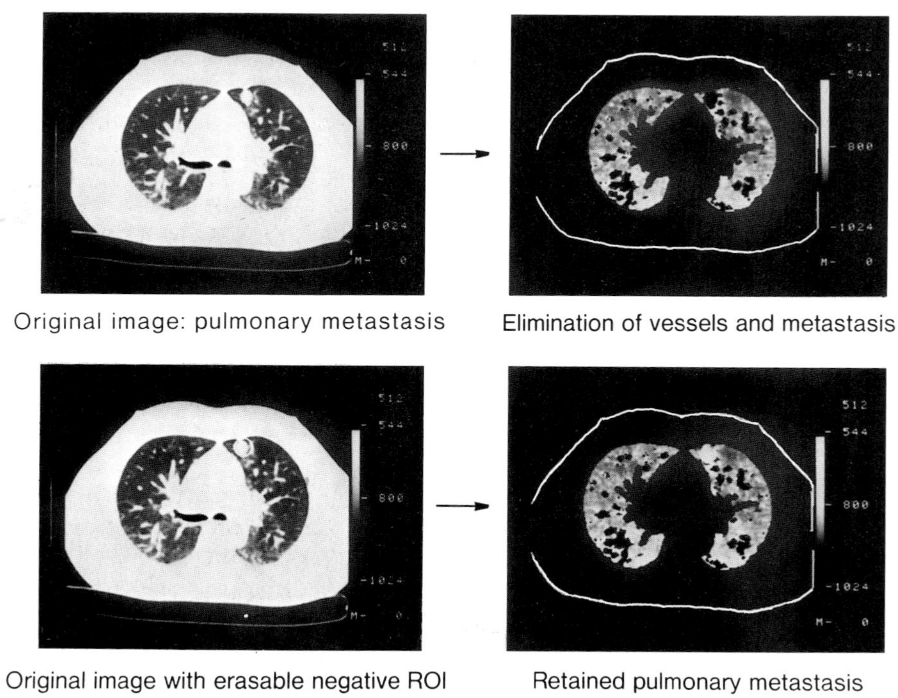

Fig. 5. Pulmonary metastasis eliminated with an interval mask, a difference mask and a smoothing mask (*upper panel*) and retained with an erasable ROI mask (*lower panel*)

represented as a function of these attenuation value differences, then even under pathological conditions an initial straight line with a steep gradient corresponding to the respiratory lung parenchyma and a flat terminal straight line corresponding to the pulmonary vessels and the transition zones can be distinguished. The value of the abscissa corresponding to the intersection of the two straight lines indicates the suitable threshold value of the difference mask with adequate accuracy (Fig. 3). This value can also be determined by the computer itself, so that in most cases the entire isolation of the respiratory lung parenchyma can also be obtained by computer control in the form of a batch string without any additional intervention. So far the application of the smoothing mask has shown that the demand for four neighbours for each picture element of the respiratory lung parenchyma is reasonable.

There are special cases in which the respiratory lung parenchyma cannot yet be adequately identified with the four standard masks described; for these special cases the programming system has been expanded. The expansion is demonstrated by two examples (Figs. 4, 5):

It is not always possible to eliminate the main bronchi, as indicated in Fig. 1, with the interval mask, the difference mask and possibly the smoothing mask. However, reliable separation of these structures is possible with a so-called region of interest (ROI) mask (Fig. 4). Here, an ROI containing the main bronchi is marked on the matrix of the original image with the aid of the Evaluskop (independent evaluation unit of the Siemens computer tomographs); subsequently a mask according to the ROI is formed and the original image is covered up with this mask, so that the entire ROI with the bronchi disappears from the original image.

With the customary application of the interval mask, the difference mask and the smoothing mask, frequently denser lung structures (e.g. nodules and atelectases) whose separation is undesirable are eliminated. These structures can be retained with a so-called erasable ROI mask (see Fig. 5). In this case a marked ROI which contains the lung area to be retained is protected from the influence of other masking procedures.

Conversion of Pulmonary Attenuation Values Into Suitable Ventilation Parameters

Having demonstrated that the respiratory lung parenchyma can be identified in a thoracic computer tomogram, the next step is to show that it is possible to convert the pulmonary attenuation values into suitable ventilation parameters understandable for lung specialists.

In CT derived quantities are employed instead of the measured linear attenuation coefficient μ (see Table 1); at present the CT value (or Hounsfield unit) defined as the relative deviation of the linear attenuation coefficient from the corresponding value for water in ‰ is most frequently used. Measurements of such attenuation values for ventilation analyses in selected lung areas or total thoracic cross-sections were performed by Rosenblum, Mauceri, Wellenstein, Bassano, Cohen and Heitzman [6] and by Wegener, Koeppe and Oeser [7, 8]. In the case of quantitative examinations it has frequently proved expedient to use the so-called CT quotient (CTQ) [1] instead of the generally used CT value; here the relative deviation $\frac{\mu - \mu_{H_2O}}{\mu_{H_2O}}$ of the CT value is replaced by the corresponding ratio $\frac{\mu}{\mu_{H_2O}}$. The dimensionless CT value is often falsely described as "density". The density, however, can be determined from a CT value or CT quotient only if the relationship of the total mass attenuation coefficient $\left(\frac{\mu}{\varrho}\right)$ to the corresponding water value $\left(\frac{\mu}{\varrho}\right)_{H_2O}$ is known. In lung measurements, using the radiation energies of commercially available computer tomographs (60 – 80 keV), this relationship can be taken to be equal to 1, the error being less than 0.5%. In this case, the absolute lung density in mg/cm^3 quantitatively agrees with the pulmonary CT quotient CTQ_l and the corresponding CT value CT_l increased by 1000.

The density ϱ_l of a lung region is made up of a proportion of density ϱ_t of the air-free tissue and the density ϱ_g of the respiratory air. For ventilation analyses, the density of the air-free lung tissue can be assumed to be 1.06 g/cm^3 with sufficient accuracy even under pathological conditions. Moreover, the mass of the respiratory air can be neglected with respect to the mass of the air-free lung tissue. From this a relationship existing between the absolute lung density on the one hand and the portion of the air-free tissue T as well as the air content G on the other hand can derived (see Fig. 6).

From the lung densities ascertained by CT, a number of further ventilation parameters can be computed in addition to the regional portion T_r of

Table 1. Measured quantities in CT

I. *Directly measured quantity:*

Linear attenuation coefficient $\mu = \mu(Z, \varrho, E)$

Z = atomic number
ϱ = density
E = energy

II. *Derived quantities:*

1. CT value [4]

$$CT = \frac{\mu - \mu_{H_2O}}{\mu} \cdot a \text{ with } a = \begin{cases} 500 \text{ EMI unit} \\ 1000 \text{ Hounsfield unit (HU)} \end{cases}$$

2. (Scaled) CT quotient [1]

$$CTQ = \frac{\mu}{\mu_{H_2O}} \cdot a, \quad \text{e.g. with} \quad a = 1000$$

3. Absolute density, if $\left(\frac{\mu}{\varrho}\right) \Big/ \left(\frac{\mu}{\varrho}\right)_{H_2O}$ known

$$\varrho = \frac{\left(\frac{\mu}{\varrho}\right)_{H_2O}}{\left(\frac{\mu}{\varrho}\right)} \cdot \frac{\varrho_{H_2O}}{a} \cdot \underbrace{(CT + a)}_{= CTQ}$$

In lung (l) measurements with usual radiation energies (E = 60 to 80 keV):

$$\left(\frac{\mu}{\varrho}\right)_l \approx \left(\frac{\mu}{\varrho}\right)_{H_2O} \rightarrow \varrho_l = \frac{\varrho_{H_2O}}{a} \cdot (CT_l + a)$$

i.e. $\boxed{(CT_l + a) \text{ or } CTQ_l \text{ with } a = 1000 \triangleq \varrho_l \text{ in mg/cm}^3}$

the air-free tissue and the regional air content G_r (see Table 2): namely the ratio $\left(\frac{V'_g}{V_g}\right)_r$ and the relative difference or the relative change $\left(\frac{\Delta V_g}{V_g}\right)_r$ of regional air volumes as well as absolute and relative ventilation distribution functions (e.g. ϕ_r = absolute gas volume distribution and RGD = relative gas content distribution). The absolute gas volume distribution formally corresponds to the air volume of a fictitious lung section with the air content G_r of the regional measuring area r and the tissue volume V_{tR} of a generally larger reference area R. The relative gas content distribution indicates the magnitude by which the regional air content G_r of a measuring region r deviates from the mean gas content G_R of a reference region R. Because the measuring plane is fixed in CT, comparison of regional lung volumes in different respiratory phases is allowed only if the examined lung region is ventilated homogeneously.

Practical Application of Quantitative Ventilation Analysis of the Lung by CT

In the following some examples of the quantitative ventilation analysis for normal and diseased lungs are presented. For this purpose, the mask techniques demonstrated in Figs. 1 and 4a are used and only the gas content G and the relative gas content distribution RGD are taken from the ventilation parameters enumerated in Table 2.

Figure 7 shows the chest cross-sections and the isolated respiratory lung parenchyma of a normal test person which were taken at the end of maximum inspiration (TLC, total lung capacity) as well as at the end of an expiration of normal depth and of extreme depth (FRC, functional residual capacity; RV, residual volume). The gas content (G) was calculated along the right pulmonary columns marked with the Evaluskop and traced by a printer (decwriter II, Digital Equipment). The

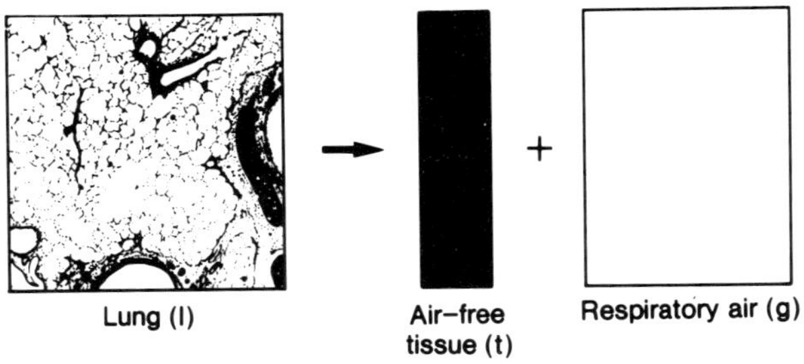

$$\varrho_l = T \cdot \varrho_t + G \cdot \varrho_g$$

$$T = \frac{V_t}{V_t + V_g}, \quad G = \frac{V_g}{V_t + V_g}$$

$$\varrho_t = 1{,}06\ \mathrm{g/cm^3} \quad \text{(const.!)}$$

$$G \cdot \varrho_g \ll T \cdot \varrho_t$$

$$\rightarrow \boxed{\varrho_l = T \cdot \varrho_t \quad \text{and} \quad \varrho_l = (1 - G) \cdot \varrho_t}$$

ϱ = density
V = volume
T = portion of air-free tissue
G = gas content

Fig. 6. Relationship between the absolute density, the portion of air-free tissue and the gas content in the lung

ordinates indicate the air content from 0 to 1000‰ and the abscissae indicate the row index of the picture matrix. The curves describe quantitatively how the pulmonary gas content decreases with increasing expiration and how a gravity-dependent gradient develops at the same time. Such measurements have shown that the in vivo density of normal lungs is lower than is frequently assumed; this finding is supported by the pathological anatomical investigations carried out by Joachim, Riede and Mittermayer (1978).
In Fig. 8 comparison is made of the differences in the regional gas content which were present in a female patient affected by lung fibrosis and in a male patient with a pronounced emphysema in the respiratory rest position (FRC) along comparable columns. The fibrosed lung shows a clearly reduced air content as compared with a normal lung; a ventrodorsal gradient of the gas content distribution is clearly identified. Compared with this the emphysematous lung reveals a clearly increased air content so that owing to larger emphysematous bullae partially a regional gas content of 100% exists; the ventrodorsal gas distribution is irregular in this case.
Figures 9 and 10 show distributions of the relative (!) frequency of the gas content in transverse sections through a normal lung and through a lung affected by alveolar proteinosis which were taken in different respiratory phases (TLC, FRC and RV). In the case of alveolar proteinosis, the inspiratory and expiratory gas content was substantially lower than that of a normal lung. On expiration the gas content fell off markedly in both persons tested. The normal lung showed at total lung capacity a uniform ventilation distribution; during expiration its increasing gravity-dependent density gradient caused the curve rise to level off. In the lung affected by alveolar proteinosis the gas content was inhomogeneously distributed also at maximum inspiration; on expiration the inhomogeneity decreased in the regions with a lower gas content.
Figure 11 demonstrates in the case of alveolar proteinosis that analogously to CT values the computed regional gas content (G) and the relative difference between the regional gas content and the gas content of the total examined pulmonary cross-section (RGD) can be displayed in grey shades or colours and measured by means of a joystick. With the aid of a so-called attenuation value transformation [3] the gas conent can also be imaged in freely selectable intervals (ΔG).

Final Remarks

When comparing CT with the conventional methods of ventilation analysis for circumscribed pulmonary regions (Table 3), the following can be stated: The undisputed merit of bronchospirometry over the radiological and nuclear medical measuring methods is to be seen in the fact that the measuring volume is well-defined irrespective of respiratory motion. But it has the disadvantage of being invasive for the patient and this was the reason why it was largely replaced by emission methods. The usual emission methods of measurement, just like the transmission methods, entail the disadvantage that they do not permit any differentiation regarding the measuring depth; moreover, the relative measuring parameters, the so-cal-

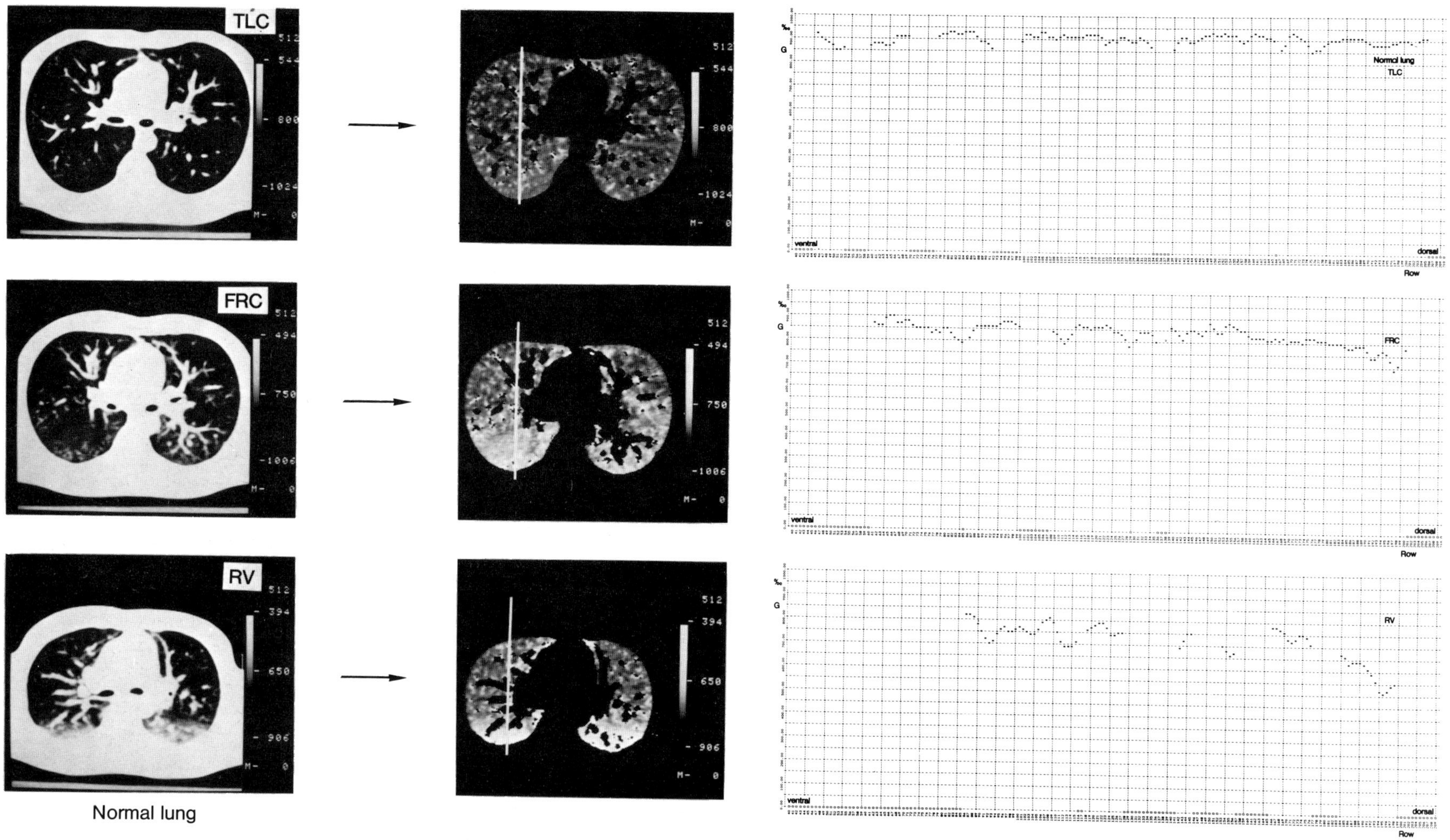

Fig. 7. Thoracic computer tomograms and isolated respiratory lung parenchyma of a supine healthy test person taken at the end of maximum inspiration (*TLC*) and with expiration of normal depth (*FRC*) and maximum depth (*RV*). The graphs represent the distribution of the gas content along the marked right pulmonary columns (*ordinates:* gas content G, *abscissa:* row index of the picture matrix)

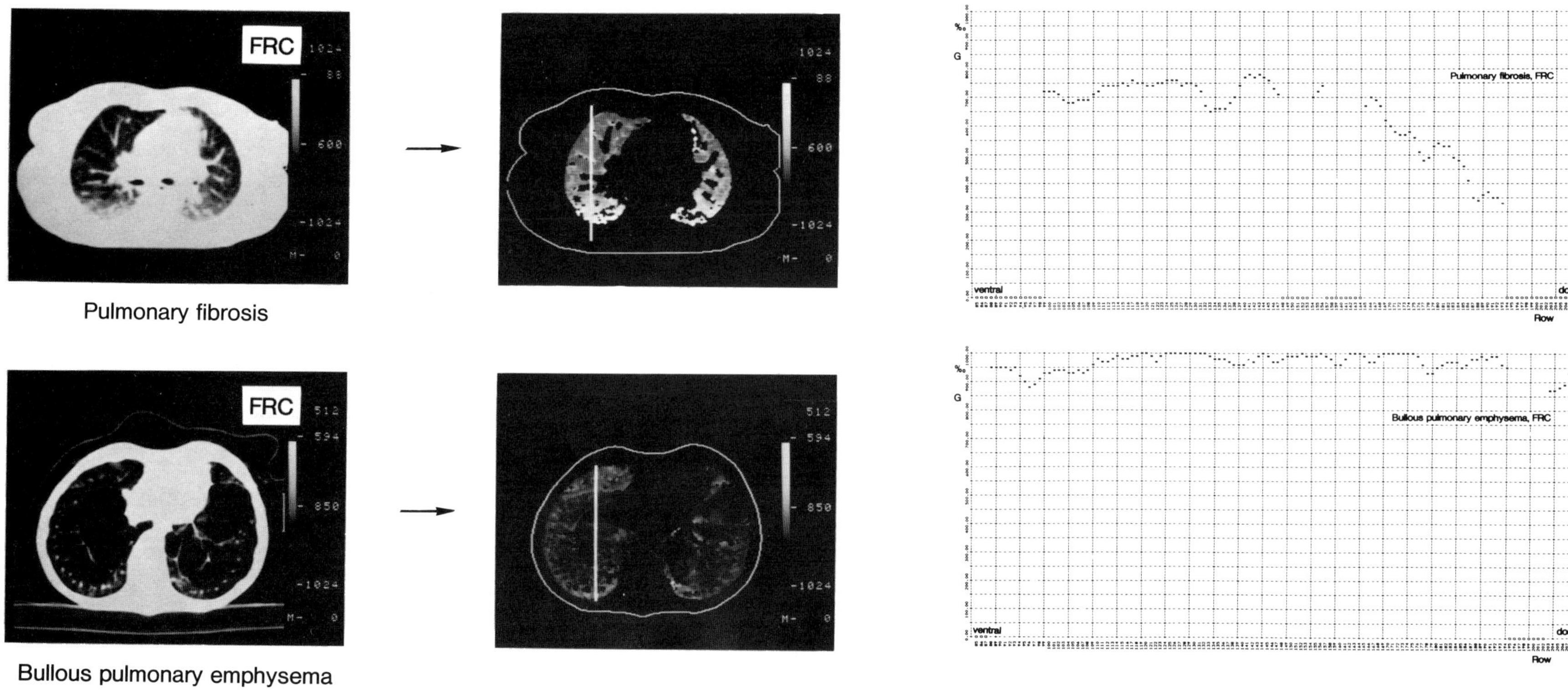

Fig. 8. Thoracic computer tomograms and isolated respiratory lung parenchyma of supine patients with lung fibrosis and lung emphysema taken at the endexpiratory resting position (*FRC,* functional residual capacity). The graphs represent the distribution of the gas content along the marked right pulmonary columns

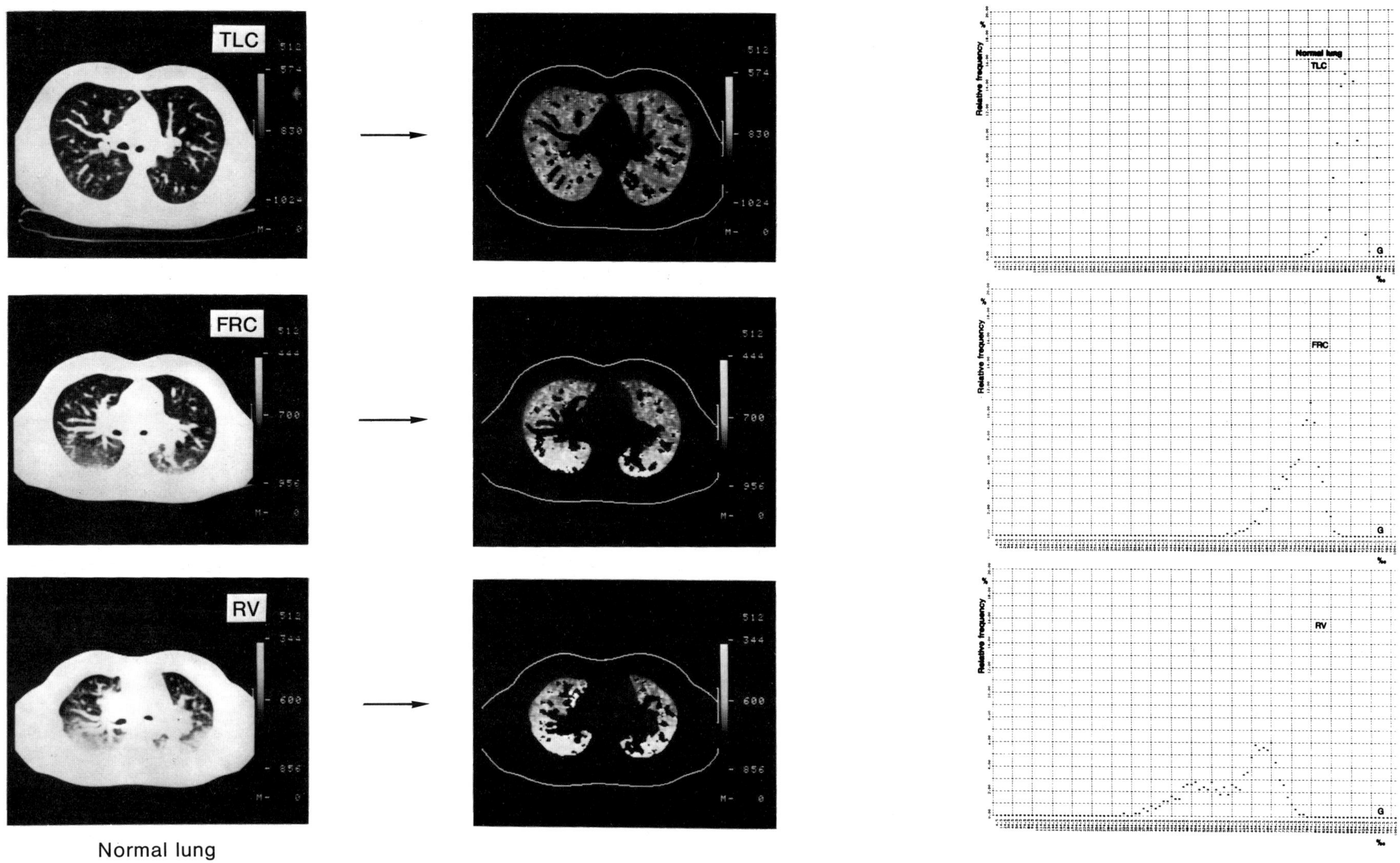

Fig. 9. Thoracic computer tomograms and isolated respiratory lung parenchyma of a supine test person with a normal lung taken at different respiratory phases. The graphs represent the relative frequency distribution of the gas content in the isolated lung sections

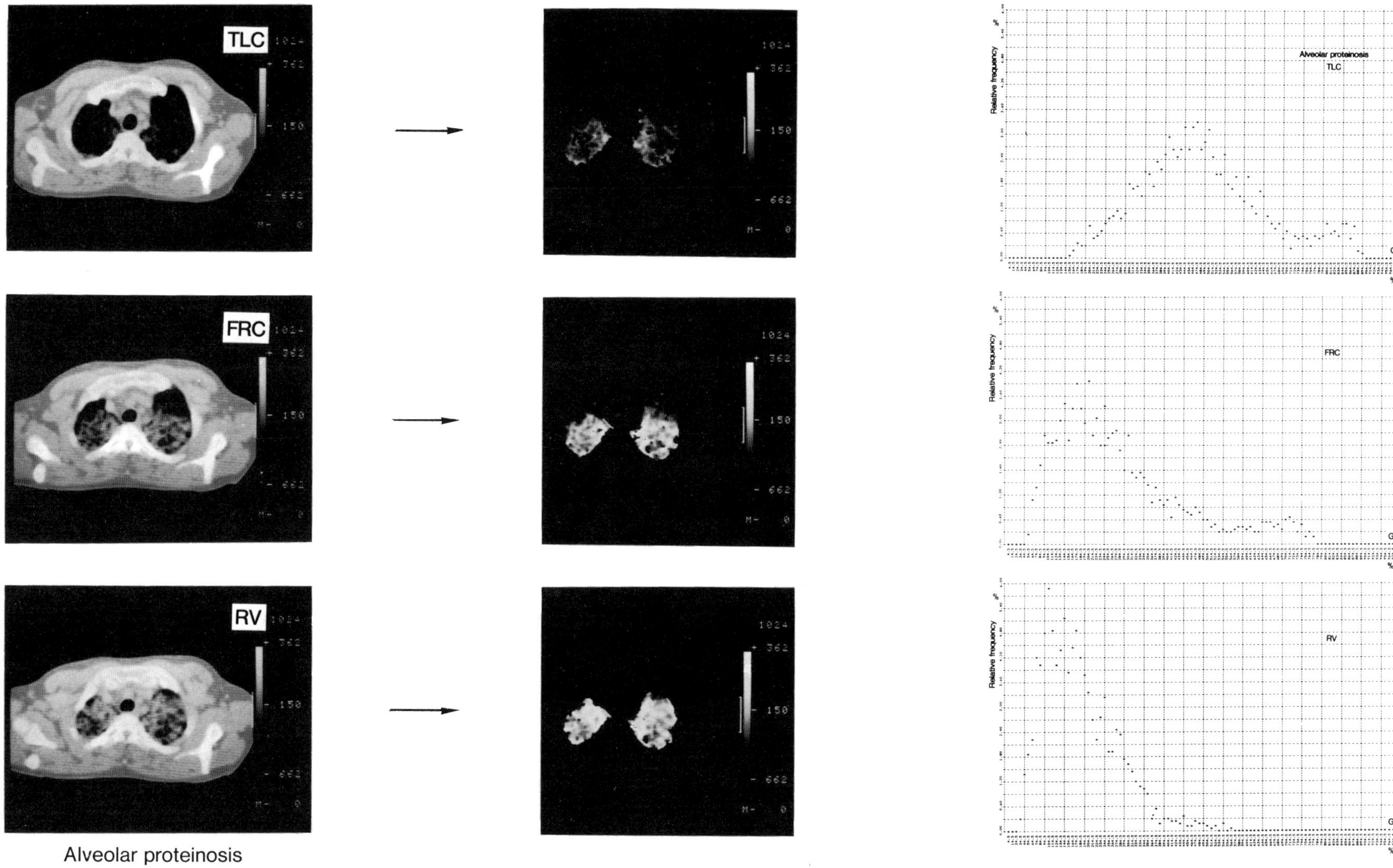

Fig. 10. Thoracic computer tomograms and isolated respiratory lung parenchyma of a supine patient with alveolar proteinosis taken at different respiratory phases. The graphs represent the relative frequency distribution of the gas content in the isolated lung sections

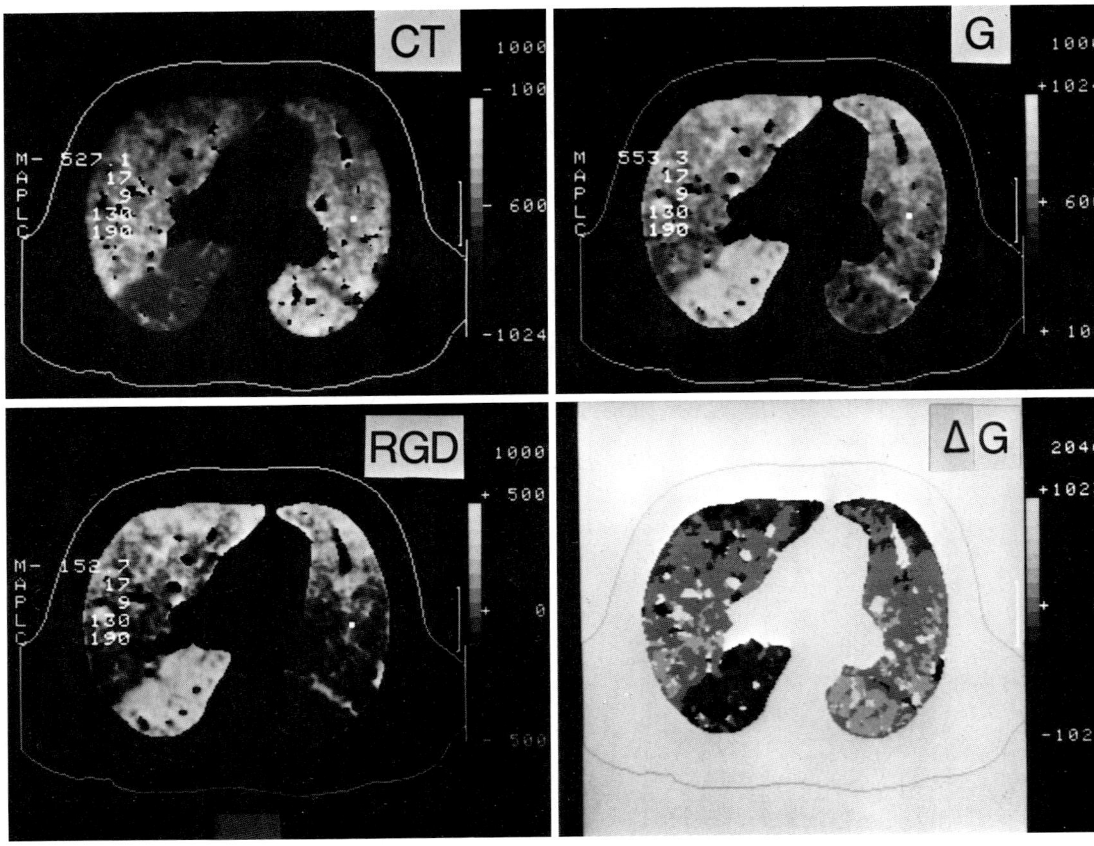

Fig. 11. Pictorial representation and joystick measurements of the *CT* value, the gas content (*G*) and the relative differences between the regional gas content and the gas content of the total lung section (*RGD*). Imaging of selected intervals of the gas content (ΔG); the increasingly darker grey shades represent ranges between 1% and 50%, 51% and 70%, 71% and 80%, and 81% and 100%

led regional lung volumes, furnish only limited information, especially under pathological conditions. A basic advantage of CT densitometry, similar to Compton densitometry which equipmentwise has not yet reached perfection, is that it allows determination of absolute parameters (e.g. density and gas content). A disadvantage is that both densitometric procedures do not permit distinction between alveolar air and inspiratory air.

It seems possible that the distribution of the pulmonary perfusion also can be estimated by CT when intravenous bolus injections of iodine-containing contrast media are given.

Furthermore, the described mask technique and evaluation programs which were originally designed for lungs exclusively, with supplemented software can also be applied to other organs, e.g. for the isolation and quantitative investigation of the brain, the vertebrae, the kidneys and regions of the liver [2].

Summary

Computed tomography permits quantitative analysis of pulmonary ventilation. Those evaluations are adversely affected by extrapulmonary image portions and larger pulmonary vessels. However, these disturbing structures can be eliminated with the aid of a digital mask technique. So-called CT quotients can be derived from the CT values of the isolated respiratory lung parenchyma. Regionally determined attenuation values allow the calculation of the absolute density, the air-free tissue portion and the gas content of circumscribed pulmonary regions; in addition, they allow the computation of ratios and relative differences in regional air volumes and they can be used to derive absolute and relative ventilation distribution functions. When a lung region examined during various respiratory phases is ventilated homogeneously, it

Table 2. Pulmonary ventilation parameters, regionally measurable by means of CT

1. *Portion of air-free tissue:*

$$T_r = \frac{\varrho_{lr}}{\varrho_t}$$

2. *Gas content:*

$$G_r = 1 - \frac{\varrho_{lr}}{\varrho_t}$$

3. *Ratios and relative differences (or relative changes) of regional gas volumes:*

a. $(V_t + V_g)_r = \text{const.}$

$$\left(\frac{V'_g}{V_g}\right)_r = \frac{\varrho_t - \varrho'_{lr}}{\varrho_t - \varrho_{lr}} \quad \text{and} \quad \left(\frac{\Delta V_g}{V_g}\right)_r = \frac{(\varrho_l - \varrho'_l)_r}{\varrho_t - \varrho_{lr}}$$

b. $V_{tr} = \text{const.}$

$$\left(\frac{V'_g}{V_g}\right)_r = \frac{(\varrho_t - \varrho'_{lr}) \cdot \varrho_{lr}}{(\varrho_t - \varrho_{lr}) \cdot \varrho'_{lr}} \quad \text{and} \quad \left(\frac{\Delta V_g}{V_g}\right)_r = \frac{(\varrho_l - \varrho'_l)_r \cdot \varrho_t}{(\varrho_t - \varrho_{lr}) \cdot \varrho'_{lr}}$$

4. *Absolute ventilation distribution functions:*

e.g. Absolute gas volume distribution at varying degrees of lung inflation $\left(\leftarrow G_r = \frac{\phi_r}{V_{tR} + \phi_r}\right)$

a. R = total lung

$$\phi_r = \frac{(\varrho_t - \varrho_{lr}) \cdot \varrho_{lR}}{(\varrho_t - \varrho_{lR}) \cdot \varrho_{lr}} \cdot V_{gR} \quad \text{with} \quad V_{gR} = \left(1 - \frac{\varrho_{lR}}{\varrho_t}\right) \cdot (V_t + V_g)_R$$

b. R = lung area

$$\phi_r \cdot \left(\frac{V_{t0}}{V_t}\right)_R = \frac{(\varrho_t - \varrho_{lr}) \cdot \varrho_{lR}^2}{(\varrho_t - \varrho_{lR}) \cdot \varrho_{lR_0} \cdot \varrho_{lr}} \cdot V_{gR}$$

5. *Relative ventilation distribution functions:*

e.g. Relative gas content distribution at constant lung volume

$$RGD = \frac{(\varrho_{lR} - \varrho_{lr})}{(\varrho_t - \varrho_{lR})}$$

Table 3. Procedures for quantitative analyses of regional pulmonary ventilation

1. Bronchospirometry
2. Radiological and nuclear medical transmission measuring techniques
3. Emission measuring procedures via inhalation or injection of inert gases
4. Densitometry by means of
   a) Compton scattering
   b) Computed tomography

is also possible to determine the changes of its air volume. The use of the digital mask technique is illustrated by examples of normal and diseased lungs; the examples also show determinations of the gas content and of a relative gas distribution function; in this context profile sections, recordings of relative frequency distributions and CT image transformations are demonstrated.

References

1. Döhring W, Linke G (1979) Die Grundlagen der quantitativen pulmonalen Computertomographie. ROEFO 130:133 – 143

2. Döhring W, Linke G (1980) Isolation of organs using a digital masking technique in quantitative investigations by CT. 5th CARVAT: International Meeting on Body CT, Rome 1980
3. Döhring W, Linke G (to be published) Modifizierte CT-Bildwiedergabe durch Schwächungswertetransformationen. ROEFO
4. Hounsfield GN (1973) Computerized transverse axial scanning (tomography): Part I. Description of system. Br J Radiol 46:1016–1022
5. Joachim H, Riede UN, Mittermayer Ch (1978) The weight of human lungs as a diagnostic criterium (Distinction of normal lungs from shock lungs by histologic, morphometric and biochemical investigations). Pathol Res Pract 162:24–40
6. Rosenblum LJ, Mauceri RA, Wellenstein DE, Bassano DA, Cohen WN, Heitzman ER (1978) Computed tomography of the lung. Radiology 129:521–524
7. Wegener OH, Koeppe P, Oeser H (1978) Measurement of lung density by computed tomography. J Comput Assist Tomogr 2:263–273
8. Wegener OH, Koeppe P, Oeser H (1979) Lung density measurements by computed tomography. In: Gerhardt P, van Kaick G (eds) Total body computerized tomography. Thieme, Stuttgart, pp 32–39

CT of the Solitary Pulmonary Nodule

S. S. Siegelman, E. A. Zerhouni, F. P. Leo, E. L. Nickoloff, N. F. Khouri, and F. P. Stitik

Johns Hopkins Medical Institutions, Department of Radiology and Radiological Sciences, 601 N. Broadway, Baltimore, MD 21205 (USA)

Introduction

The management of a patient over the age of 40 years with a solitary pulmonary nodule (SPN) detected by plain chest roentgenography has been a source of concern for more than 3 decades [1 – 6]. Excision of an SPN, including resection of the involved lobe, became a feasible technique in the early 1950s. As data on such cases accumulated it became apparent that a significant percentage of innocent-appearing peripheral pulmonary nodular lesions actually represented lung cancers [1]. The prevailing philosophy regarding such lesions is that tissue diagnosis (occasionally by needle biopsy but more frequently by thoracotomy) is mandatory in order to exclude the possibility of a malignant lesion. We summarized the results of the five largest reported series of thoracotomies for SPNs and noted that most resected lesions were actually benign [1 – 6]. In almost every case in which thoracotomy was carried out for a benign lesion, the operation would have been unnecessary if the nature of the lesion could have been determined by noninvasive methods. The need for surgery was indeed a reflection of the inadequacy of diagnosis techniques.

Are there any reliable noninvasive methods of determining that an SPN is benign? Two criteria exist: The absence of growth and the detection of significant calcification. The absence of growth over a 2-year period of observation is an excellent criterion for establishing that a pulmonary nodule is benign [1]. The information has no pertinent application, however, to the patient with a newly discovered lesion. Most authorities would deem it imprudent to use a policy of watchful waiting in a patient with a possible lung malignancy [7].

The presence of calcification within a lesion is generally a reliable sign that the lesion is benign. When pulmonary nodules are shown to contain definite calcium deposits by plain chest roentgenography or standard tomography it is assumed that the lesions are benign. Support for this approach is as follows:

1. Holin et al. [8] and McClure et al. [9] each followed up over 200 patients with calcified nodules for over 5 years. No single lesion was found to be malignant.
2. At the Mayo Clinic between 1940 and 1954, 48 calcified SPNs were excised and all proved to be granulomas or hamartomas [3, 10].

Although calcification is a reliable guide to benign lesions, the detection of significant calcium content within the lesion by conventional radiographic means is not always a simple matter. Calcium is easier to recognize when the calcium deposits create a distinctive pattern. As noted in Fig. 1, calcium may be deposited as a central nidus, concentric rings, or in a popcorn pattern. The contrast between the denser, calcified portions of the lesion and the adjacent, less dense, noncalcified areas facilitates recognition of the calcium. However, when the calcium is diffusely distributed throughout the lesion in a regular homogeneous fashion, it becomes more difficult to recognize. Bloch performed several simple experiments with calcium solutions to underscore the difficulty of detecting diffuse calcification within a lesion [11]. The determination of calcium content in a lesion which appears homogeneous on a standard tomographic examination is often subjective, difficult, and arbitrary. It occurred to us that computed tomography (CT) should be an important, objective, ancillary method of assessing the nature of an SPN. Calcium, with its high atomic number relative to other tissue structures, should attenuate X-rays and produce a higher CT number for any tissue with appreciable calcium content. Using a 120 kV, 20 mA, and 5 mm slice thickness scans, we measured the CT number of a series of solutions of calcium chloride and found a linear relationship between calcium content and CT number (Fig. 2). It was our hypothesis that CT might be capable of

Radiology Today 1. Ed. by M. W. Donner and F. H. W. Heuck

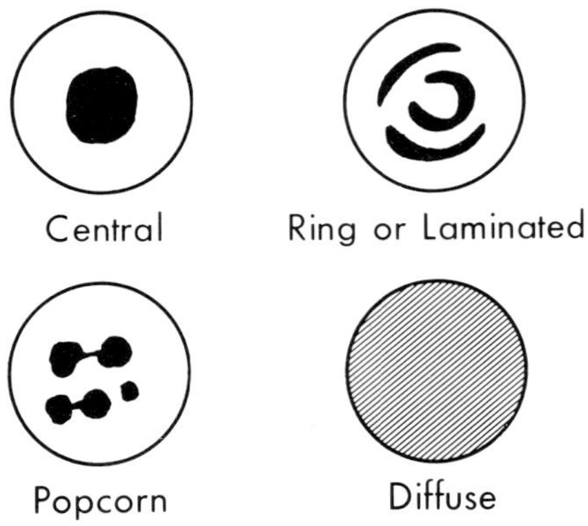

Fig. 1. Patterns of calcification in benign lesions. The diffusely calcified lesion is most difficult to recognize

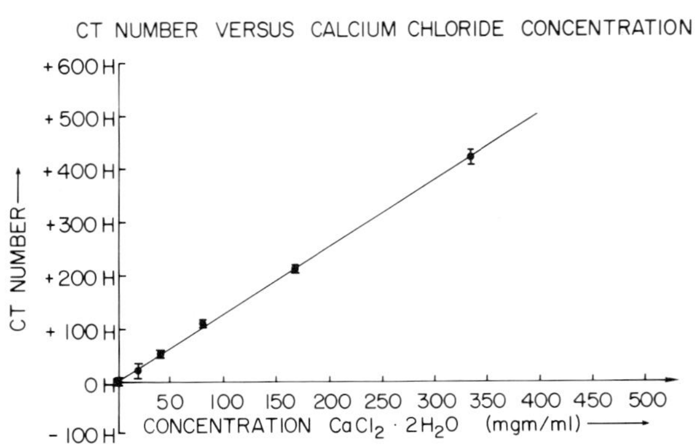

Fig. 2. The relationship between calcium content and CT number. To register a CT # greater than 164 HU, a solution must contain more than 150 mg $CaCl_2$ per milliliter

detecting calcium deposits in lesions which could not be certified as calcified by standard chest roentgenography or standard lung tomography.

A formal study of CT of the SPN was undertaken and completed. The results of this investigation were published in the American Journal of Roentgenology [12]. The reader is directed to the published manuscript for details of technique, results, and discussion of the findings. The purposes of this current communication are: (1) to summarize briefly the results of the initial investigation, (2) to emphasize the technical factors necessary for successful duplication of the method of examination, (3) to illustrate several additional cases of benign and malignant SPNs studied by CT, (4) to provide additional discussion based upon experiences with the method of examination.

The Published Study

Only SPNs which were deemed noncalcified by standard tomography were examined. Thin sections (always less than half the diameter of a nodule) were obtained as close as possible to the center of the lesion. The study was done with the Pfizer (Model 500) Scanner using a 6 in. radius of reconstruction and a 512 × 512 matrix. A computer printout of the scan with the highest CT numbers was used for analysis. A representative CT number based on the 32 highest contiguous voxels was calculated. Among 45 primary lung malignancies, the mean representative CT number was 92 HU with a standard deviation of 18 HU. Nodules with a representative CT number above 164 HU were all found to be benign. Among the 58 malignant lesions (45 primary malignancies and 13 metastases) no lesion had a representative CT number above 150 HU. Two typical primary lung malignancies are illustrated in Figs. 3 and 4. Two typical benign lesisons are shown in Figs. 5 and 6. The features of a benign lesion were:

1. Representative CT number above 164 HU.
2. Highest CT numbers within the center of the nodule.
3. Centrally located cluster of voxels with CT numbers greater than 175 H.

The results of the first 100 nodules examined are as follows:

100 nodules → benign by CT, 24
100 nodules → indeterminate by CT, 76
indeterminate by CT, 76 → proven benign, 12
indeterminate by CT, 76 → proven malignant, 64

All of the 24 nodules diagnosed as benign were found to be benign by tissue diagnosis or by prolonged follow-up showing no change. Tissue diagnosis was obtained on all 76 nodules wich did not meet the criteria for benignancy, and 12 of the 76 were also found to be benign. We have very similar statistics for our second group of 100 patients. Our experience, therefore, based upon 200 cases, is that if a nodule is benign, the CT examination will provide the diagnosis of a benign lesion in two out of three cases.

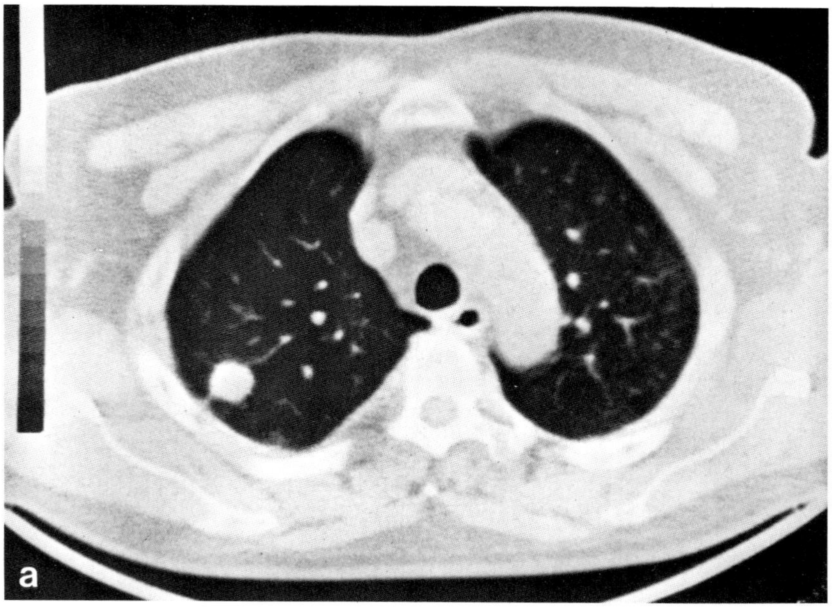

b

-809	-798	-792	-780	-766	-744	-741	-734	-749	-785	-817	-840	-822	-796	-813	-805	-788	-747	-706	-658	-638
-765	-770	-781	-781	-805	-793	-781	-755	-756	-784	-798	-803	-799	-778	-787	-788	-818	-813	-783	-764	-788
-763	-760	-764	-783	-790	-771	-743	-744	-760	-779	-802	-800	-788	-779	-783	-773	-788	-803	-798	-813	-839
-721	-741	-747	-771	-783	-753	-722	-737	-767	-794	-817	-817	-795	-779	-792	-796	-795	-790	-801	-797	-794
-723	-738	-763	-771	-766	-744	-727	-736	-767	-790	-788	-787	-815	-829	-808	-795	-797	-814	-809	-793	-779
-755	-736	-754	-764	-760	-722	-687	-703	-712	-730	-751	-771	-792	-787	-800	-803	-814	-824	-808	-799	-803
-762	-729	-714	-729	-742	-707	-647	-640	-651	-690	-721	-726	-743	-757	-776	-801	-799	-761	-742	-759	-765
-754	-702	-678	-681	-716	-722	-694	-674	-658	-651	-682	-700	-699	-735	-780	-787	-766	-736	-745	-721	-721
-779	-715	-667	-669	-695	-703	-657	-639	-642	-649	-625	-621	-631	-649	-664	-691	-726	-740	-736	-696	-682
-769	-746	-698	-639	-598	-580	-568	-534	-505	-494	-489	-503	-538	-585	-619	-653	-672	-671	-657	-633	-609
-735	-739	-680	-589	-490	-437	-407	-395	-362	-360	-332	-366	-436	-508	-577	-630	-636	-591	-568	-549	-523
-683	-673	-588	-485	-359	-273	-259	-262	-231	-173	-183	-210	-269	-340	-411	-458	-443	-436	-458	-463	-492
-513	-447	-363	-275	-194	-146	-97	-73	-53	-49	-62	-96	-128	-184	-259	-314	-348	-358	-381	-443	-505
-387	-244	-143	-67	-19	2	16	24	45	45	30	16	-30	-55	-103	-128	-144	-184	-291	-368	-484
-332	-153	-28	46	83	81	66	50	67	57	48	37	33	26	34	23	-6	-39	-94	-223	-404
-307	-132	5	84	85	45	48	89	97	73	63	66	42	40	47	83	66	69	16	-101	-275
-243	-81	7	36	73	91	91	66	49	48	58	81	83	72	84	88	78	61	30	-50	-202
-126	-8	59	63	88	111	107	77	54	54	71	85	112	106	97	81	60	29	28	-12	-130
-22	73	132	136	127	109	79	71	63	65	81	82	105	94	94	101	87	72	101	24	-21
22	112	121	122	110	77	71	61	61	46	55	68	58	36	26	21	47	83	87	80	40
13	63	63	66	51	71	73	80	65	56	46	15	21	29	26	29	36	53	50	73	43
98	95	79	64	56	20	11	51	80	80	77	45	37	38	34	49	31	16	19	43	33
107	116	96	84	81	48	38	30	33	42	40	14	-8	6	27	47	21	20	20	14	24
40	32	40	43	53	57	70	43	45	20	-4	-16	-2	26	47	45	43	67	61	53	29
-9	1	27	14	8	18	39	49	38	3	-10	9	30	44	73	78	75	78	76	63	12
13	18	15	-5	-12	2	30	38	29	16	9	7	13	19	15	17	34	29	38	1	-60
30	33	11	7	10	-18	6	27	29	35	39	24	25	13	8	19	0	-6	-5	-25	-92
13	10	24	31	44	24	37	39	39	0	5	5	28	47	47	23	3	6	14	0	-88
-7	8	12	35	41	36	23	10	19	25	26	24	37	37	28	11	10	19	20	-13	-138
-54	-19	0	36	31	0	-23	8	31	39	21	13	1	-19	-15	6	-5	-19	-100	-183	-275
-175	-129	-112	-56	-21	-3	11	11	25	42	37	41	27	-18	-8	17	3	-94	-252	-410	-505
-284	-236	-205	-162	-95	-46	-26	-2	21	38	37	31	12	-13	-4	-17	-63	-207	-391	-530	-605
-372	-349	-316	-277	-220	-141	-74	-46	-19	-6	28	35	15	-29	-65	-102	-173	-323	-504	-645	-698
-472	-481	-466	-461	-402	-320	-264	-216	-171	-117	-50	-41	-74	-141	-198	-249	-327	-415	-578	-720	-796
-584	-589	-574	-583	-533	-510	-480	-437	-357	-271	-206	-215	-247	-298	-345	-399	-439	-498	-606	-713	-757
-651	-669	-688	-662	-642	-642	-640	-606	-554	-482	-399	-347	-367	-410	-474	-508	-492	-497	-567	-665	-739
-638	-683	-700	-702	-683	-673	-651	-636	-652	-622	-566	-511	-486	-482	-526	-531	-521	-527	-563	-654	-734
-660	-697	-699	-677	-654	-654	-642	-662	-685	-687	-656	-614	-598	-609	-609	-581	-558	-532	-554	-620	-714
-624	-687	-722	-705	-675	-668	-664	-679	-703	-701	-690	-684	-678	-677	-694	-698	-646	-626	-640	-681	-720
-576	-682	-740	-724	-681	-656	-651	-658	-669	-686	-683	-694	-716	-742	-770	-765	-746	-736	-720	-724	-747
-501	-596	-649	-657	-629	-629	-640	-644	-650	-657	-687	-716	-726	-728	-748	-738	-750	-744	-732	-717	-744
-392	-522	-613	-639	-658	-645	-644	-652	-663	-689	-725	-731	-722	-697	-676	-683	-715	-733	-723	-710	-716
-329	-467	-571	-611	-630	-639	-655	-664	-670	-717	-730	-718	-723	-714	-702	-730	-748	-772	-755	-730	-719
-264	-387	-487	-563	-606	-621	-638	-673	-713	-754	-773	-765	-776	-760	-757	-785	-818	-844	-849	-834	-792
-146	-210	-317	-455	-529	-593	-622	-665	-699	-728	-777	-802	-812	-824	-831	-820	-814	-808	-809	-819	-800

Fig. 3a, b. A 60-year-old man with a 1.5 cm adenocarcinoma in the right lung. **a** CT scan showing the lesion as a sharply defined intraparenchymal mass with a tiny strand extending to the pleural surface. **b** Computer printout. Representative CT number of the 32 highest voxels is 90 HU. Note that there are voxels with CT numbers of 136, 132, and 127. This computer printout is very typical for a malignant lesion

Technique

Technical details are extremely important in any reliable method of assessing CT numbers of small pulmonary nodules. A number of items must be properly managed.

1. *The X-ray Beam.* Since CT numbers are determined by absorption of X-rays, it is important to periodically monitor kVp calibration, mA calibration, and actual scan time.
2. *Slice Thickness.* Slice thickness is determined by collimation of the X-ray beam. It is important to measure the actual slice thickness which corresponds to the control panel settings. We have achieved this simply by using a phantom composed of plastic sheets of 1 mm thickness with one hole in each sheet at a different level. When the phantom is scanned, the effective slice thickness can be measured from the number of holes visualized.
3. *Spatial Uniformity.* This parameter may be tested by scanning a water bath and recording

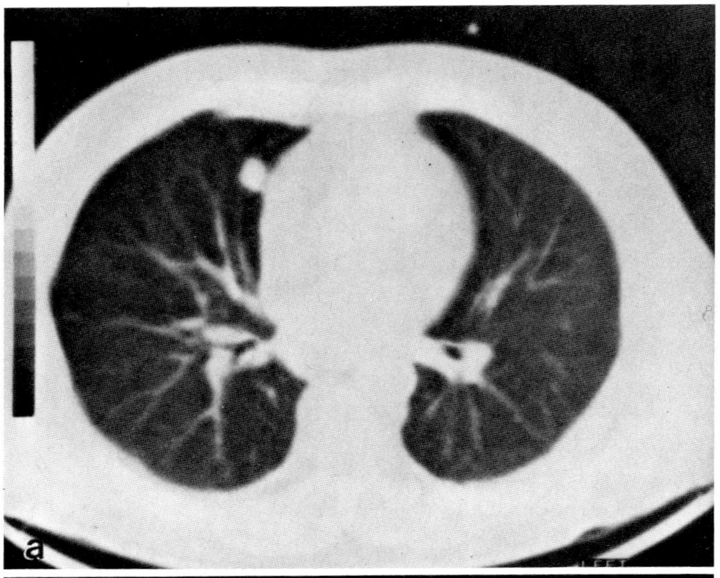

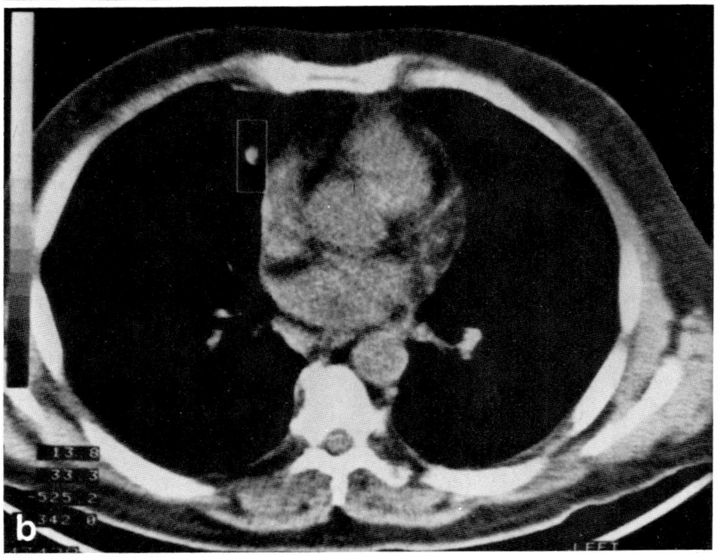

c

5	-849	-871	-881	-872	-867	-884	-901	-898	-911	-922	-900	-867	-870	-905	-908	-885	-859	-832	-782
0	-835	-847	-867	-874	-857	-872	-894	-886	-907	-925	-910	-864	-857	-889	-906	-878	-836	-813	-792
5	-838	-842	-864	-875	-860	-860	-871	-868	-883	-917	-922	-890	-861	-866	-901	-887	-854	-829	-825
9	-862	-863	-860	-874	-877	-880	-870	-838	-832	-863	-882	-875	-871	-863	-881	-878	-867	-857	-856
5	-844	-851	-846	-861	-894	-905	-879	-845	-831	-852	-847	-839	-868	-889	-893	-875	-876	-879	-876
9	-857	-858	-849	-859	-880	-894	-894	-864	-829	-856	-868	-847	-850	-897	-899	-878	-887	-915	-904
0	-868	-874	-862	-864	-863	-872	-883	-878	-839	-844	-853	-865	-865	-882	-876	-876	-878	-910	-913
3	-872	-861	-843	-850	-861	-863	-850	-857	-842	-825	-831	-843	-843	-863	-868	-874	-873	-892	-904
7	-880	-846	-804	-805	-825	-829	-809	-812	-787	-764	-788	-807	-821	-842	-866	-896	-899	-901	-898
3	-862	-855	-804	-768	-758	-741	-729	-740	-719	-689	-694	-731	-757	-794	-832	-883	-918	-931	-930
1	-822	-802	-758	-705	-677	-655	-613	-598	-601	-578	-581	-620	-659	-720	-784	-845	-877	-919	-945
4	-810	-764	-701	-637	-574	-519	-484	-452	-442	-430	-455	-498	-562	-635	-708	-812	-861	-876	-883
0	-782	-727	-652	-556	-477	-380	-318	-319	-328	-315	-334	-384	-443	-530	-616	-714	-804	-823	-803
2	-756	-686	-602	-472	-376	-301	-232	-214	-224	-217	-242	-315	-348	-407	-510	-599	-687	-772	-758
8	-756	-647	-550	-414	-300	-234	-192	-159	-145	-128	-150	-228	-275	-315	-402	-510	-585	-640	-685
9	-723	-610	-500	-392	-266	-195	-148	-96	-86	-89	-88	-137	-196	-241	-308	-425	-530	-582	-615
6	-669	-584	-451	-339	-222	-128	-101	-67	-44	-68	-85	-99	-128	-176	-247	-342	-452	-527	-580
9	-621	-522	-386	-258	-180	-103	-61	-41	-23	-41	-51	-65	-85	-115	-187	-282	-367	-459	-524
0	-578	-446	-316	-181	-94	-50	-18	-13	1	-6	-13	-23	-59	-83	-127	-224	-315	-397	-473
3	-518	-383	-239	-120	-37	9	32	50	45	29	9	2	-29	-52	-86	-177	-294	-373	-435
8	-449	-323	-182	-52	12	49	59	91	89	66	34	28	-12	-46	-99	-175	-272	-353	-386
6	-390	-260	-136	-20	35	51	73	82	90	97	76	60	16	-38	-108	-171	-254	-300	-337
8	-356	-230	-111	-5	66	82	88	86	79	81	88	63	9	-43	-78	-123	-176	-218	-271
8	-344	-234	-125	-22	74	104	93	85	92	83	75	55	12	-47	-68	-107	-145	-179	-200
3	-327	-221	-121	-36	40	102	118	103	105	88	59	42	20	-33	-77	-129	-175	-202	-186
8	-329	-237	-136	-42	20	95	134	116	75	76	63	18	-10	-53	-104	-151	-179	-190	-185
6	-369	-265	-173	-64	-3	66	130	127	77	54	27	-12	-44	-100	-152	-175	-186	-180	-171
0	-438	-312	-219	-120	-57	12	90	124	100	66	16	-39	-75	-127	-196	-218	-222	-202	-160
2	-501	-385	-285	-197	-114	-39	30	79	79	57	11	-36	-86	-145	-212	-230	-226	-193	-159
3	-548	-463	-374	-294	-210	-117	-36	10	35	33	5	-41	-103	-171	-239	-227	-207	-179	-123
2	-630	-576	-506	-418	-335	-244	-139	-65	-16	-19	-9	-39	-128	-175	-203	-199	-171	-148	-108
4	-701	-671	-617	-541	-460	-363	-251	-170	-118	-114	-112	-107	-145	-170	-169	-159	-136	-123	-113
1	-737	-733	-720	-659	-582	-483	-398	-315	-269	-252	-249	-249	-224	-202	-189	-155	-124	-92	-81
0	-785	-772	-785	-740	-668	-588	-553	-505	-464	-439	-405	-421	-392	-322	-257	-194	-121	-82	-69
7	-819	-793	-804	-781	-733	-691	-659	-638	-617	-623	-596	-588	-555	-491	-387	-279	-144	-60	-62
8	-820	-800	-790	-780	-768	-753	-749	-754	-731	-742	-751	-716	-670	-603	-503	-371	-212	-94	-47
0	-800	-815	-808	-800	-786	-774	-790	-818	-800	-806	-837	-804	-733	-635	-534	-417	-268	-128	-55
2	-796	-829	-843	-845	-816	-808	-833	-851	-844	-852	-870	-841	-762	-654	-535	-414	-287	-143	-53
7	-787	-827	-853	-853	-826	-844	-871	-864	-862	-879	-873	-859	-786	-662	-546	-401	-251	-119	-47
8	-803	-829	-839	-842	-825	-843	-863	-861	-848	-852	-838	-835	-797	-693	-569	-407	-241	-110	-32
8	-831	-860	-871	-866	-840	-833	-864	-876	-856	-837	-809	-789	-770	-688	-578	-420	-253	-118	-32
7	-821	-854	-876	-881	-877	-867	-843	-856	-881	-872	-849	-812	-763	-660	-542	-421	-253	-97	-27
1	-818	-849	-866	-876	-893	-892	-845	-852	-884	-877	-873	-844	-767	-661	-527	-387	-230	-79	-5
8	-836	-867	-885	-894	-881	-873	-869	-856	-870	-882	-873	-843	-779	-665	-524	-369	-217	-74	-16
2	-824	-872	-898	-904	-881	-855	-851	-837	-842	-864	-879	-832	-776	-679	-530	-372	-215	-75	-34
0	-807	-845	-876	-902	-889	-854	-837	-840	-856	-865	-866	-832	-752	-652	-503	-330	-181	-66	-26
6	-801	-832	-848	-873	-868	-886	-880	-865	-858	-865	-866	-810	-703	-589	-450	-266	-114	-14	5
5	-789	-831	-850	-855	-861	-885	-895	-880	-853	-865	-864	-799	-669	-515	-384	-243	-99	5	12
3	-812	-842	-859	-854	-870	-885	-879	-868	-881	-893	-872	-806	-665	-501	-357	-223	-89	17	46

Fig. 4a – c. A 67-year-old man with a 1.2 cm poorly differentiated small cell carcinoma adjacent to the heart in the right middle lobe. **a** CT scan (WL, – 300 HU; WW, 1800 HU). **b** CT scan (WL, 30 HU; WW, 360 HU). The cursor surrounding the lesion indicates the area from which a computer printout was obtained. **c** Computer printout from which a representative CT number of 94 HU was calculated

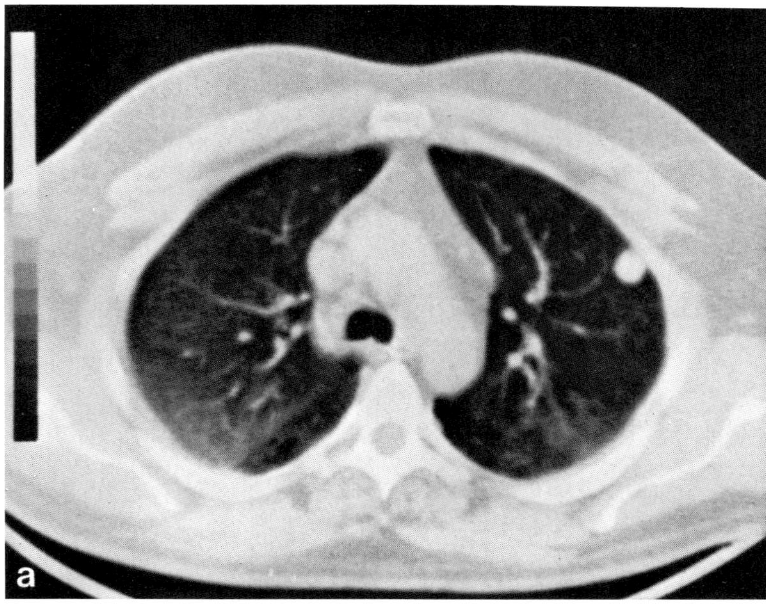

b

-548	-418	-289	-174	-111	-108	-122	-122	-78	-30	0	1	6	4	34
-472	-325	-166	-73	-56	-74	-80	-86	-76	-34	1	8	-7	-23	-10
-369	-199	-68	-1	13	8	10	-18	-22	-11	17	25	16	1	-14
-242	-90	-9	45	56	41	27	16	17	28	40	56	43	27	-1
-143	-15	76	131	120	112	86	76	68	69	69	72	62	21	3
-42	51	105	149	157	160	159	143	126	122	127	115	112	95	46
5	92	129	137	152	173	194	188	176	162	148	164	136	119	69
9	84	125	144	149	158	189	206	198	186	159	153	133	110	73
59	108	121	130	151	175	197	216	209	203	179	165	142	131	92
110	138	163	161	150	157	184	205	214	200	183	177	161	114	42
68	123	167	183	191	185	183	188	197	194	193	194	177	140	52
-3	97	155	178	192	196	203	210	203	186	177	168	140	86	-19
13	103	142	164	168	178	196	194	194	181	162	145	123	56	-75
-46	71	134	159	174	182	175	172	174	188	184	165	128	19	-158
-161	-22	63	121	145	170	191	202	193	185	177	147	61	-80	-257
-320	-162	-47	34	91	135	173	179	164	162	145	83	-8	-195	-395
-473	-315	-179	-73	-5	55	105	126	118	92	36	-68	-158	-297	-475
-549	-410	-298	-195	-119	-81	-54	-30	-28	-39	-95	-201	-314	-445	-589
-618	-528	-452	-377	-320	-282	-248	-220	-236	-236	-291	-391	-507	-613	-690
-688	-655	-622	-565	-506	-466	-446	-434	-436	-445	-513	-586	-641	-710	-759

Fig. 5a, b. A-48-year-old man. **a** CT scan showing a 1.1 cm subpleural parenchymal mass in the anterior aspect of the left upper lobe. **b** Computer printout showing a representative CT # of 196 HU. A needle biopsy showed evidence of benign inflammation. A follow-up chest roentgenogram showed no change after 1 year

CT numbers in various positions of the image. The mean CT number should be the same in all positions of the water bath to ensure that measurements of CT number are independent of spatial position of the nodule. Computer programs can be used for correction if there is a significant shift in CT number as a function of position.

4. *Daily Variations.* The mean CT number for water may vary by as much as ±15 HU. This shifting must be considered. A water-box phantom should be scanned each morning to determine the CT number for water with the same kV, mA, scanning time, and slice thickness that is used for examining nodules.
5. *Pixel Size.* Our study was carried out using a 6 in. radius of reconstruction and a 512 × 512 matrix. Each pixel element measured 0.6 × 0.6 mm. Because of partial volume effect there is a sharp fall in the number of utilizable pixels as pixel size increases. The technique is not feasible with a pixel size above 1 mm × 1 mm.

The most likely source of technical error is related to partial volume effect. The technique described should yield thin sections through the nodule which do not incorporate surrounding lung. Almost all solid nodules should show a representative CT number of at least 50 HU with several voxels which measure at least 90 HU. If a representative CT number of zero is recorded for a nodule, a technical error is likely. Slice thickness may be too large or the thin section was not taken sufficiently close to the center of the nodule.

Discussion

A significant portion of the population of benign pulmonary nodules can be recognized as benign because the nodules are distinctly denser than lung cancers. The perception that small granulomas are denser than small carcinomas has been previously

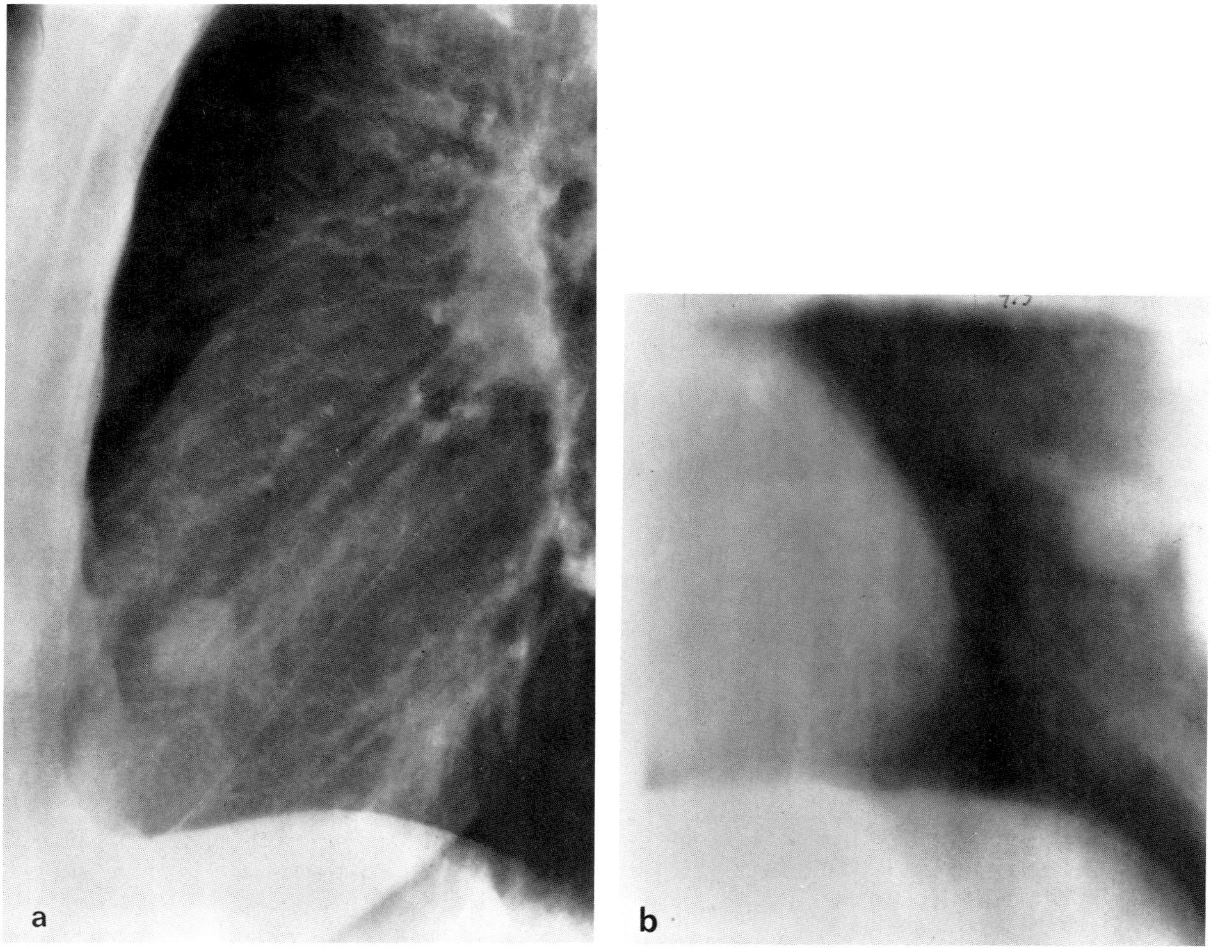

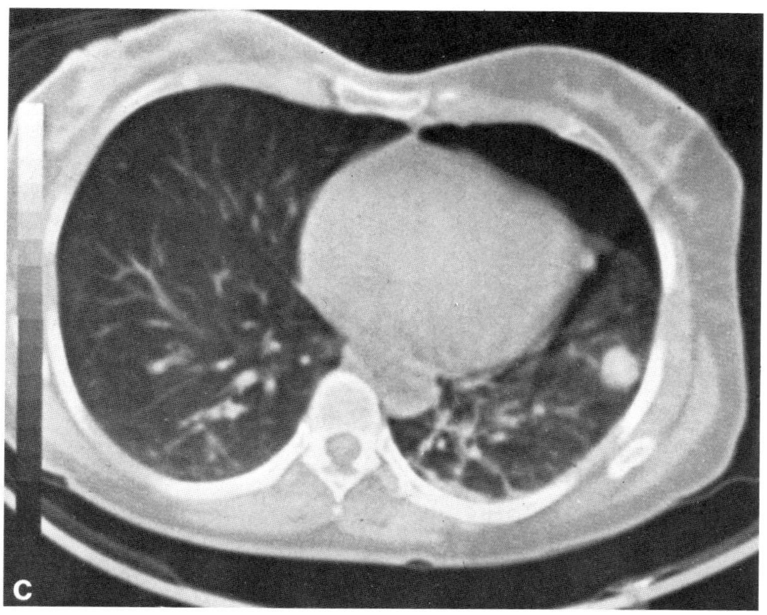

Fig. 6a – d. A 55-year-old women with a left lung nodule. The patient has been followed up for 2 years after the CT examination and the lesion is unchanged in size or appearance. **a** Lateral chest roentgenogram showing SPN in the lingula. **b** Standard tomogram interpreted as possible calcification, but no definite evidence of calcification. **c** CT scan (WL, – 700 HU; WW, 1800 HU). Prior to the CT scan, the patient had an unsuccessful attempt at needle biopsy of the lesion. Note the pneumothorax in the anterior portion of the left chest. **d** Computer printout which shows a representative CT number of 223 HU d

-576	-553	-558	-520	-456	-408	-369	-339	-294	-257	-184	-165	-198	-268	-361	-445	-518	-580	-620	-613	-614
-586	-540	-505	-446	-370	-295	-232	-191	-137	-107	-68	-58	-115	-198	-304	-415	-500	-545	-577	-553	-530
-543	-485	-403	-295	-197	-128	-83	-57	-30	-5	32	29	-22	-108	-207	-312	-425	-512	-548	-536	-518
-503	-421	-306	-161	-64	14	59	80	78	71	78	65	37	-7	-88	-195	-321	-450	-509	-506	-477
-452	-335	-202	-55	31	86	129	148	141	115	109	94	78	51	14	-68	-191	-321	-408	-415	-396
-366	-214	-77	20	71	83	121	149	163	149	131	133	130	107	69	-4	-90	-192	-274	-295	-302
-322	-138	14	74	106	122	139	142	161	161	160	138	122	119	100	56	-2	-59	-118	-171	-229
-238	-74	33	87	109	132	137	146	164	147	135	136	127	110	113	105	83	35	-19	-100	-185
-144	1	76	100	117	130	151	167	165	177	166	153	153	125	121	113	102	83	39	-122	-158
-101	46	108	111	104	107	139	173	197	217	237	224	189	155	138	116	112	112	79	0	-112
-78	56	116	123	127	119	125	157	214	245	262	253	218	163	141	133	118	107	89	29	-55
-35	60	104	134	143	133	138	175	224	250	251	234	216	178	142	129	112	87	69	38	-27
-10	95	122	133	146	145	161	206	249	275	272	227	187	160	142	117	107	107	85	42	-41
-9	104	148	159	146	136	151	188	233	260	258	239	204	161	141	116	89	85	83	60	-47
-12	91	164	187	152	149	169	173	204	235	223	213	199	167	138	136	130	114	105	81	2
-43	56	111	147	149	152	172	169	157	183	198	205	197	168	141	127	138	140	121	93	26
-51	20	40	67	95	102	114	143	144	152	175	197	206	184	148	130	127	123	117	88	28
-91	-6	23	31	40	58	82	114	137	152	168	178	194	184	155	151	134	116	116	91	8
-161	-59	-6	11	29	44	70	112	132	154	153	149	174	165	139	133	120	102	84	49	-42
-223	-114	-44	7	21	32	68	89	97	117	154	168	177	177	155	129	97	69	35	-22	-159
-272	-175	-101	-26	17	39	42	64	88	93	111	133	142	137	142	126	85	54	-1	-127	-309
-336	-221	-130	-74	-25	-8	-13	1	26	54	72	86	106	113	114	99	42	-15	-123	-289	-501
-403	-310	-215	-138	-90	-80	-76	-77	-43	-2	28	44	56	58	50	4	-48	-128	-272	-459	-634
-518	-419	-334	-264	-211	-164	-133	-131	-100	-74	-50	-24	-27	-34	-46	-96	-160	-267	-428	-609	-715
-573	-504	-415	-362	-312	-265	-225	-188	-168	-157	-150	-156	-133	-124	-138	-187	-284	-421	-585	-713	-715
-606	-559	-505	-465	-433	-406	-374	-313	-269	-253	-264	-282	-274	-238	-225	-285	-392	-527	-667	-751	-679
-634	-585	-552	-501	-490	-489	-492	-458	-394	-360	-358	-361	-361	-335	-329	-380	-488	-607	-685	-681	-512

Fig. 6d. Legend see p. 118

recognized [13], but no objective method was available for reliably documenting this phenomenon. It has been our observation prior to CT that granulomas acquire increasing density over a period of years. Granulomas which can be recognized as definitely calcified by standard chest radiography almost invariably have been present for at least 4 years. Granulomas present for a shorter period may be calcifying, but diffuse calcium deposits cannot be recognized. We found that nodules which are perceived as calcified by standard tomography always had a CT number of 450 HU or higher. Nodules with CT numbers of 164 – 450 HU are benign, but the calcium deposits generally will not be detectable.

Some time is required for a granuloma to acquire sufficient density for the lesion to be recognized as benign by CT. This time is variable, but it appears to be at least 1 year. We have had several patients with newly discovered SPNs in whom a chest roentgenogram obtained 3 – 9 months earlier was distinctly normal. In this circumstance the benign lesions have not been certifiable as benign by CT. Thus, the availability of prior chest roentgenograms is of some importance in establishing the probable contribution of CT analysis. CT is most useful when there are no prior chest roentgenograms (the lesion may have been present for several years) or if the only prior chest roentgenogram is 3 – 6 months old and shows no change.

Current Status

We have continued to accumulate personal data on patients with solitary pulmonary nodules evaluated by CT. At the present time (June 1980) we have had the following experiences:

1. One hundred and twenty proven malignant SPNs have been studied. No cases had a representative CT number greater than 150 HU.
2. In our initial 58 malignancies, no case had more than one voxel which measured more than 175 HU. Subsequently, we have encountered four cases with clusters of three to five voxels above 175 HU on one edge of the lesion. No case had a representative CT number greater than 150 HU. All such cases were adenocarcinomas with extensive scarring.
3. More than 50 patients have had SPNs which met our criteria for benignancy. We follow patients in the following manner:
   a) CT number greater than 200, follow-up chest X-ray in 1 year.
   b) CT number 164 – 200 HU, follow-up chest X-ray in 6 months.
   c) CT number 150 – 164 HU, but with clusters of voxels in the center of the lesion with CT numbers greater than 175 HU, follow-up chest X-rays at 3 and 6 months.

Tissue diagnosis is available in only 5 of our 50 patients with presumed benign disease. The remaining patients are being followed up at regular intervals and will be the subject of subsequent reports.

References

1. Siegelman SS, Stitik FP, Summer WR (1979) Management of the patient with a localized pulmonary lesion. In: Siegelman SS, Stitik FP, Summer WR (eds) Practical approaches to pulmonary diagnosis. Grune and Stratton, New York, pp 339 – 358
2. Davis EW, Peabody JW Jr, Katz S (1956) The solitary pulmonary nodule. A ten-year study based on 215 cases. J Thorac Surg 32:728 – 770

3. Good CA, Hood RT, McDonald JE (1953) Significance of a solitary mass in the lung. AJR 70: 543–554
4. Steele JD (1963) The solitary pulmonary nodule. J Thorac Cardiovasc Surg 46:21–39
5. Taylor RR, Rivkin LN, Salyer JM (1956) The solitary pulmonary nodule. A review of 236 consecutive cases, 1944 to 1956. Ann Surg 147: 197–202
6. Walske BR (1956) The solitary pulmonary nodule. Dis Chest 49:302–304
7. Good CA (1963) The solitary pulmonary nodule: a problem of management. Radiol Clin North Am 1:429–438
8. Holin SM, Dwork RE, Glaser S, Rikll AE, Stocklen JB (1959) Solitary pulmonary nodules found in a community-wide chest roentgenographic survey. A five-year follow-up study. Am Rev Tuberc 79: 427–439
9. McClure CD, Boucot KE, Shipman GA, Gilliam AG, Milmore BK, Lloyd JW (1961) The solitary pulmonary nodule and primary lung malignancy. Arch Environ Health 3:127–129
10. Good CA, Wilson TW (1958) The solitary circumscribed pulmonary nodule. JAMA 166: 210–215
11. Bloch RG (1948) Tuberculous calcification. A clinical and experimental study. AJR 59:853–864
12. Siegelman SS, Zerhouni EA, Leo FP, Khouri NG, Stitik FP (1980) CT of the solitary pulmonary nodule. AJR 135:1–13
13. Vivas JR, Crabtree SF (1955) The significance of size and radiographic density of solitary lesions in the lungs. Am Pract 4:857–861

Intensive Care

H. Pokieser

Universität Wien, Zentrales Institut für Radiodiagnostik, Allgemeines Krankenhaus, Alser Strasse 4, A-1090 Wien

Intensive care and therapy save critically endangered lives through the use of special therapeutic techniques managed by highly qualified personnel. Radiological methods have been integrated into the multidisciplinary regimes since the introduction of intensive care units (ICU) in the early 1950s. Started as improvised bedside radiography using discarded and reactivated single-phase machinery, radiodiagnosis has developed along with ICUs. At present, recently developed mobile machines yield chest and abdominal X-rays of a quality comparable to the standard of those produced in an X-ray department.

Many publications have dealt with the diagnosis of complex thoracic pathomorphology in critically ill patients. Literature published about specific radiological bedside techniques and the diagnostic capabilities of contemporary, mobile X-ray machines has, however, been limited [11, 12, 16, 17]. This contribution will, therefore, focus on the responsibilities of the radiologist to guide and supervise radiological imaging techniques and to seek clinical co-operation. In this connection, the radiological control of life support techniques will be stressed.

The Task of the Radiologist

In many ICUs roentgenology is performed without a radiologist. Unless this is caused by lack of personnel, the specific qualification of a radiologist and the technical capacity of a well-organized X-ray department should be utilized for the following tasks:

1. Special training of the radiological personnel and organization of the technical demands for prompt bedside roentgenology in order to yield images of constant high quality and ensure radiation protection;
2. Organization of an immediate reporting system and of film storage;
3. Radiological advice concerning indication and performance of special investigations such as angiography, computed tomography, scintigraphy and ultrasound.

The Need for Cooperation

Image interpretation based upon clinical information constitutes a general principle of radiodiagnostic work and is of special importance in the field of intensive care radiology. Daily film reading sessions with the referring clinical physicians guarantees fast information and is just as important as the radiologist's knowledge of the specified techniques of patient treatment and survey including their risks (vascular catheters, pacemaker, electrodes, intubation devices etc.).

The relevant clinical data for film interpretation are as follows:

Case History

Type and date of previous operations, traumata, endoscopies, bleeding episodes, aspirations, transfusions, stages of shock.

Special reference to the puncturing of or inserting of catheters into organs, body cavities or vessels *even if the attempts have failed.*

Unsuccessful puncturing of the right subclavian or internal jugular vein is of particular interest since it is often complicated by bleeding or lesions of the pleura. A left-sided superior caval catheter should raise suspicion of an unsuccessful right-sided puncture.

Radiology Today 1. Ed. by M. W. Donner and F. H. W. Heuck

Present Patient Status

State of consciousness, shock, cardiopulmonary, renal or cerebral insufficiency (including data of blood pressure, blood gas analysis, type of respiration, type of circulation assistance etc.).

Imaging Techniques

The main criteria of good quality bedside X-rays and their diagnostic implications are shown in Table 1 and demonstrated in Fig. 1.
In order to obtain sharp resolution of interstitial structures or cardiovascular contours under such difficult circumstances as lack of patient co-operation, tachypnoea, tachycardia etc., the shortest possible exposure time (20 ms or less) is required. The additional demand for good penetration of mediastinal structures implies the use of *high kV technique* (100 kVp or more).
Tungsten grids focussed on 100 or 110 cm, integrated into cassettes or cassette containers, are absolutely required to reduce scattered radiation. Table 2 lists the available mobile X-ray machines, including technical and exposure data. When comparing these data, it is obvious that only capacity discharge or battery-operated constant potential generators with a power of 20 kW are sufficient for the aforementioned demands. Single phase generators still used in many ICUs may be considered reserve machines if they are operated in combination with rare earth screens.
The mode of film exposure has to be taught in such a way that the proper positioning of the patient requires only a minimum of time. This procedure

Table 1. Quality demands of portable chest X-rays

Criteria of Imaging	Pathomorphology
Sharp imaging of peripheral interstitial structures	Early detection of interstitial oedema and emphysema
Detection of minor absorption differences	Pneumothorax; pneumatocele; miliary pattern; Westermark sign; mediastinal pathology
Good penetration and resolution (of heart and mediastinum, thorax in lat. projection)	Retrocardiac pathology; trachea, central airways; tracheal tubes and cuffs; intra-arterial and intravenous catheters

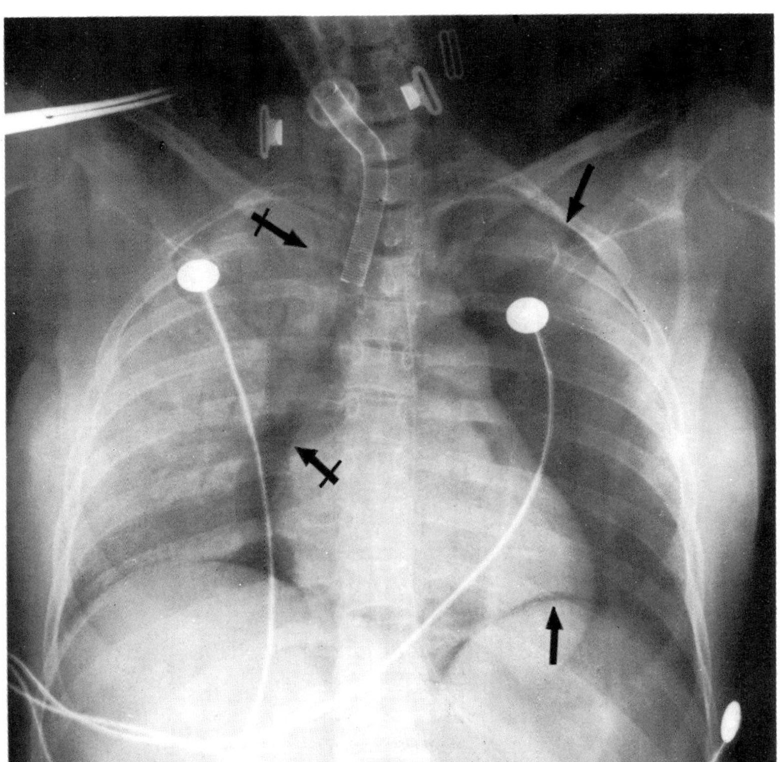

Fig. 1. Bedside radiograph: 120 kV, 400 mA, 0.02 s. High information content: small pneumothorax (↑), pneumomediastinum (⇞), air-bronchograms are visible retrocardially and in the periphery (Adult respiratory distress syndrome in a 23-year-old female patient after a suicide attempt)

Table 2. X-ray generators, power – exposure values

Generator type	Power supply	kW	kV	mA	Exposure time (s)[a]	
					Thorax AP	Lat.-lat.
One-pulse	Normal mains	1.25	60 – 90	18 – 20	0.3 – 1.2	Impossible
Two-pulse	Special mains	4.75	125	50 – 100	0.02 – 0.05	1.2
Capacitor Direct current	Normal mains Cable connection	20	100 or 125	250	0.01 – 0.05	0.05 – 0.1
Battery power Direct current	Line independent for approx. 700 exposures	20	133	400	0.01 – 0.02	0.02 – 0.03

[a] Approximation values: Average patient – tube distance, 120 – 150 cm; scattered radiation grid usage

commences with the setting up of the machinery, selecting the exposure time and observing the rules of radiation protection. This is followed by correct patient positioning, installing of the cassette, final adjustments and immediate exposure thereafter. The standard AP chest radiograph should be taken, if possible, with the patient sitting at a 60° angle (Fig. 2).

This position can be achieved with most types of ICU beds even if the patient is unconscious. (The base of the lungs is difficult to interpret when the patient is in a supine position. Furthermore, small pneumothoraces and pleural effusions remain undetected.)

Lateral projections of the patient in a supine position with horizontal beam as well as lateral projections of the patient in decubitus position with vertical beam are not performed routinely, but may be of great assistence in the further evaluation of uncertain findings in the standard AP chest X-ray. Special indications are: detections of small pneumothoraces and precise location of pulmonary or mediastinal opacities and of pacemaker electrodes.

Special Diagnostic Problems

A discussion of the various radiological manifestations of inflammatory lung diseases, cardiopulmonary insufficiency and the adult respiratory distress syndrome would extend beyond the scope of this contribution. These subjects have been well covered in the monographs by Goodman and Put-

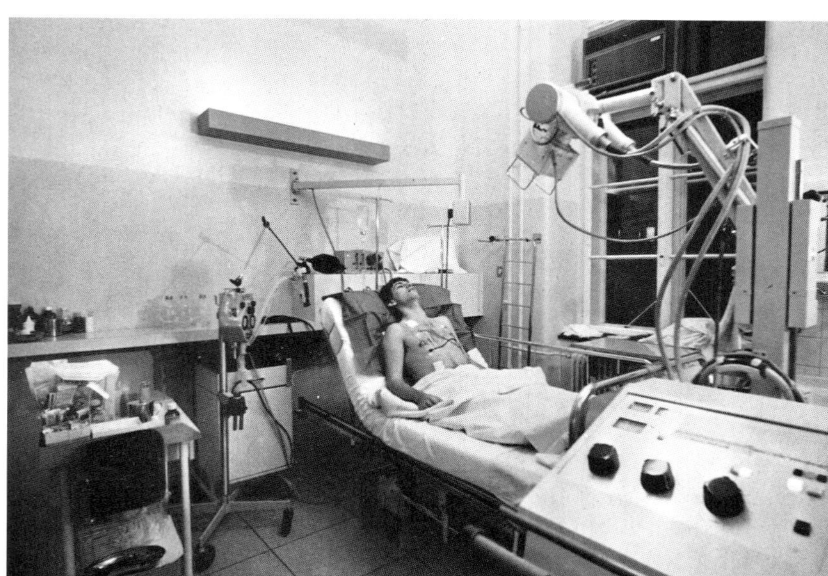

Fig. 2. Positioning of patient and tube for standard AP chest X-ray

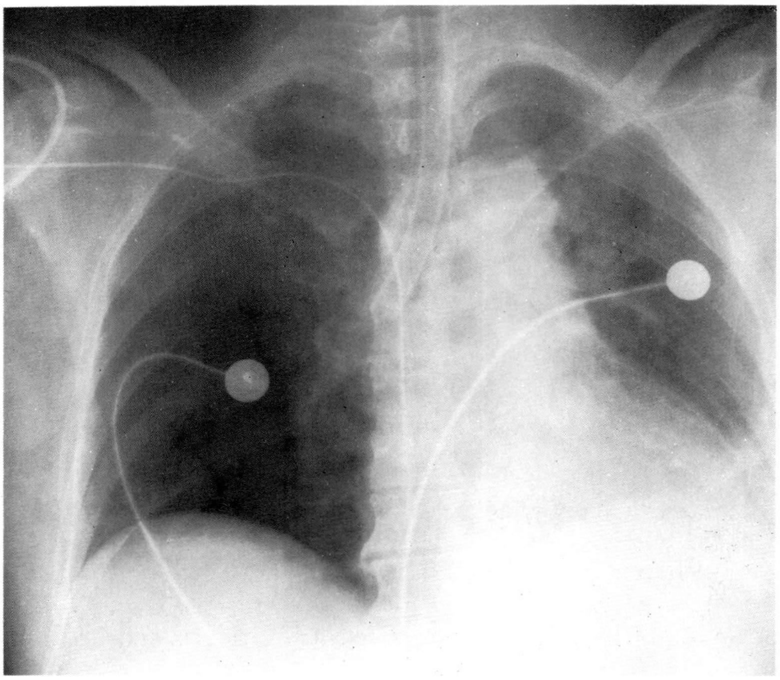

Fig. 3. Film obtained 2 h after right main stem bronchus intubation shows beginning atelectasis of the left lung with a shift of the mediastinum to the left, elevation of ipsilateral hemidiaphragm and a hyperinflated right lung

man [8], Ayella [1], Fraser and Pare's textbook and in many other publications [7, 10, 12, 15]. The topics selected here deal with the control of respiratory tube and vascular catheter position, detection of their aberrant positions and complications through the use of chest radiology. The chest X-ray is often the only source of precise information concerning the above. Furthermore, the superiority of high kVp technique for these purposes is evident.

Endotracheal Tubes

Aberrant positioning of endotracheal tubes in the right stem bronchus occurs in 10% – 15% of cases [7, 8, 18]. Recognition of incorrect positioning in the superior trachea or the larynx as well as of hyperinflation of the cuff is of equal importance in order to reduce the incidence of acute risks and late sequelae.

Proper Tube Positioning. With the head in midposition, the tip of the tube should be located 5 – 7 cm above the carina tracheae; the round or oval lucency of the cuff should lie within the tracheal band.

Flexion or extension of the cervical spine shifts the tip of a naso- or orotracheal tube 2 cm cranial or caudal respectively. Deep positioning of the tube results in lesion of the carina tracheae or in right main stem bronchus intubation when the head is moved forwards. If the tube is in a high position, extension of the cervical spine may cause damage to the vocal cords by the cuff [3].

Aberrant positioning in the right main bronchus causes hyperinflation of the right lung, mediastinal shift and partial collapse of the left lung (Fig. 3). Other aberrant positions are the right upper lobe bronchus, the larynx, the pharynx and the oesophagus.

If the cuff is hyperinflated, the lucency of the balloon extends beyond the tracheal band (Fig. 4). A resulting complication is pressure necrosis (bleeding, fistula formation, tracheomalacia, scarring, stenosis) [9].

Superior Caval Catheters

In 1977 Burri and Ahnefeld [2] presented an extensive study on the techniques of inserting central venous catheters, giving special attention to the type and incidence of incorrect positioning and complications. Our own experience supports the suspicion of these authors that the percentage of serious complications is generally underestimated. Immediate radiographic confirmation of the catheter position after insertion is obligatory. Prompt detection of aberrant positioning or complications of puncturing may be of vital importance. If the tip of the opaque catheter is not visible, a repeat

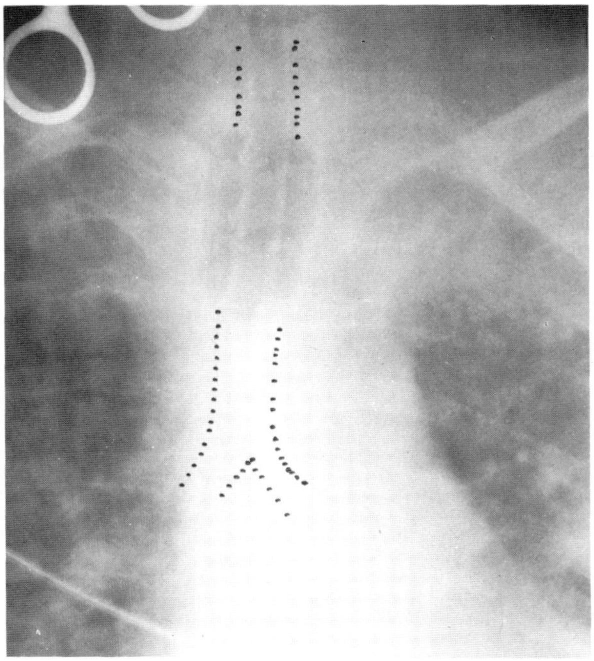

Fig. 4. Overinflation of the cuff

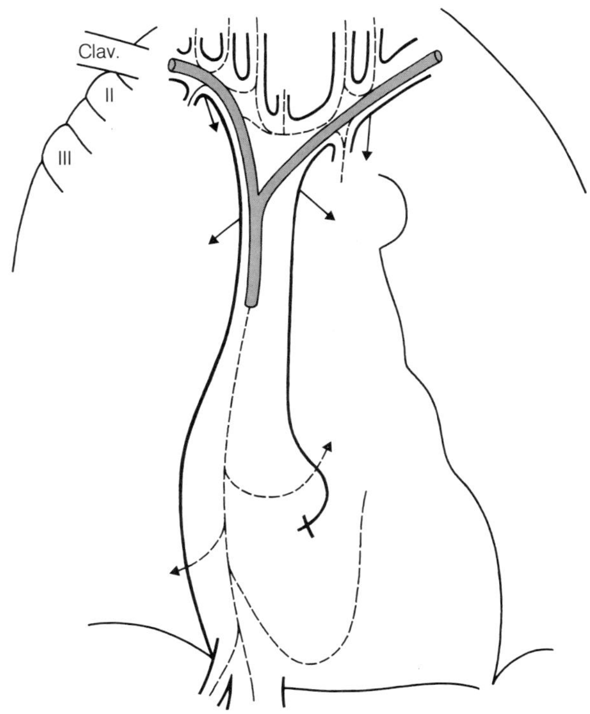

Fig. 5. Aberrant routes and location of potential perforations (↑) of superior caval catheters

exposure after injection of a small amount of contrast medium (5 ml) is necessary.

Proper Positioning of the Catheter Tip. – The tip should be positioned 2 cm above the right atrium and close to the right border of the mediastinal shadow. The location of the superior vena cava is defined by the distance between the sternal junction of the first and third ribs. Aberrant positioning occurs in 6% of cases of subclavian puncture and in 0.85% after catheter insertion into the internal jugular vein [2] and takes various forms:

1. Intravascular cranial positioning (Fig. 5): the catheter tip occupies a cranial position in the subclavian or jugular vein (with or without loop formation). Potential complications are: (a) movement of head or shoulder may result in dislocation of the catheter and (b) incorrect pressure monitoring.
2. Caudal positioning in the heart, hepatic veins or inferior vena cava, which may lead to lesions of valves or of the endocardium or to thrombosis.
3. Positioning in contralateral (subclavian, brachiocephalic, internal jugular) or ipsilateral (internal thoracic, inferior cervical, inferior thyroid) veins (Fig. 6), resulting in an increased risk of thrombosis.
4. Extravascular positioning (Fig. 7). Perforation of the vessel wall more commonly occurs by a puncturing needle (with ensuing paravascular catheter positioning) rather than by the catheter tip being pushed forwards (5). However, the catheter itself may occasionally penetrate the wall of a vein or even of the heart (right atrium).
5. Inadvertent intravascular positioning, which is easily detected by chest X-ray.
6. Paravascular or intramural positioning in the subclavian or brachiocephalic vein – more difficult to diagnose. The slightest suspicion of incorrect placement or impaired infusion in an apparently correct position necessitates the additional use of contrast medium (10 ml) followed by another radiograph.

Sequelae of extravascular catheter positioning are bleeding or infusion into the mediastinum, pericardial or pleural cavities, resulting in typical roentgenologic findings.

A pitfall is catheter positioning in a persistent left superior vena cava, mimicking mediastinal aberrant positioning along the left sternal margin.

The complications of venipuncture (Fig. 8) are less serious and occur less frequently if the internal jugular vein is punctured. According to the 20451 cases studied by Burri and Ahnefeld, lesions in the pleura or the subclavian artery occur in 1.08% – 1.39% if the subclavian route is chosen.

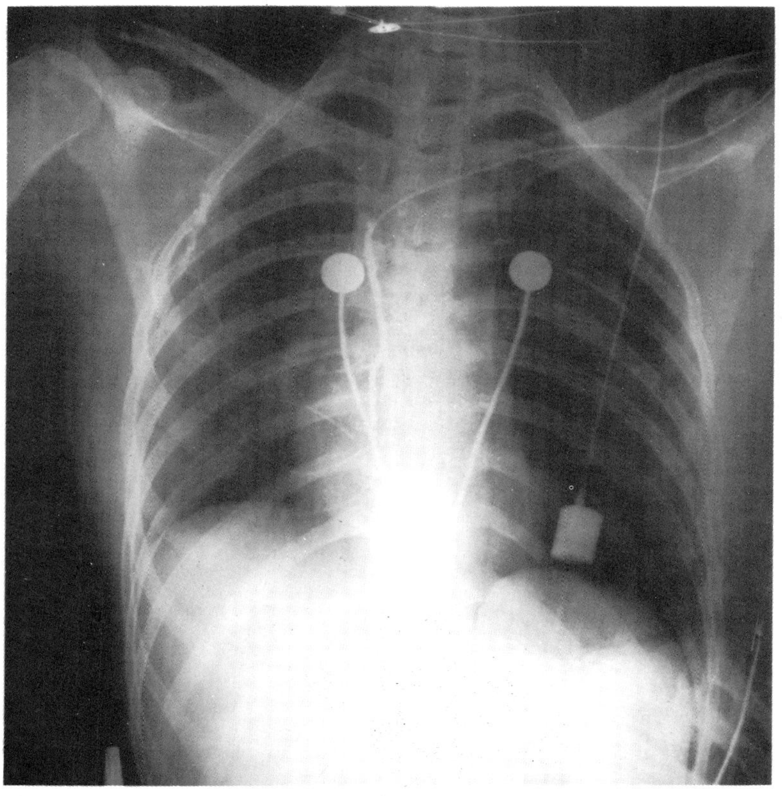

Fig. 6. Aberrant position of catheter tip in the right internal thoracic vein Film obtained after injection of 5 ml contrast medium. Pneumothorax on the left side

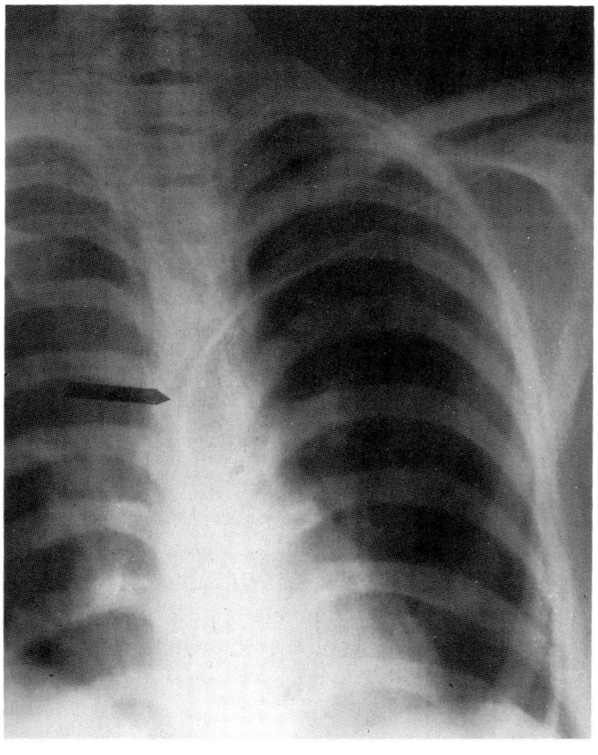

Fig. 7. Perivascular position of a left subclavian catheter with the tip in the mediastinum (this situation was followed by ectopic infusion)

According to our own results, occurrence is 2% – 3%. Subclavian artery bleeding causes asymmetrical widening of the superior mediastinum and is similar to substernal thyroid enlargement but without displacement of the trachea. Restitution is usually completed within 2 – 4 days. Peri-apical opacification is less commonly seen. Our experience indicates that a narrow, unilateral pneumothorax is the most common complication, whereas tension pneumothoraces or haemothoraces rarely occur.

Catheter Tear or Rupture (Fig. 9)

A tear in the catheter wall may be caused by bending or by the tip of the puncturing needle. This may result in haematomas or paravascular infusions. Embolisation of whole catheters, catheter fragments or guide wires are serious complications. Burri and Ahnefeld reported 315 cases [2].

Radiological location of embolised opaque material is not a problem. More skill is required for interventional transvenous extraction, which should always be attempted before operation is considered [4, 6, 13].

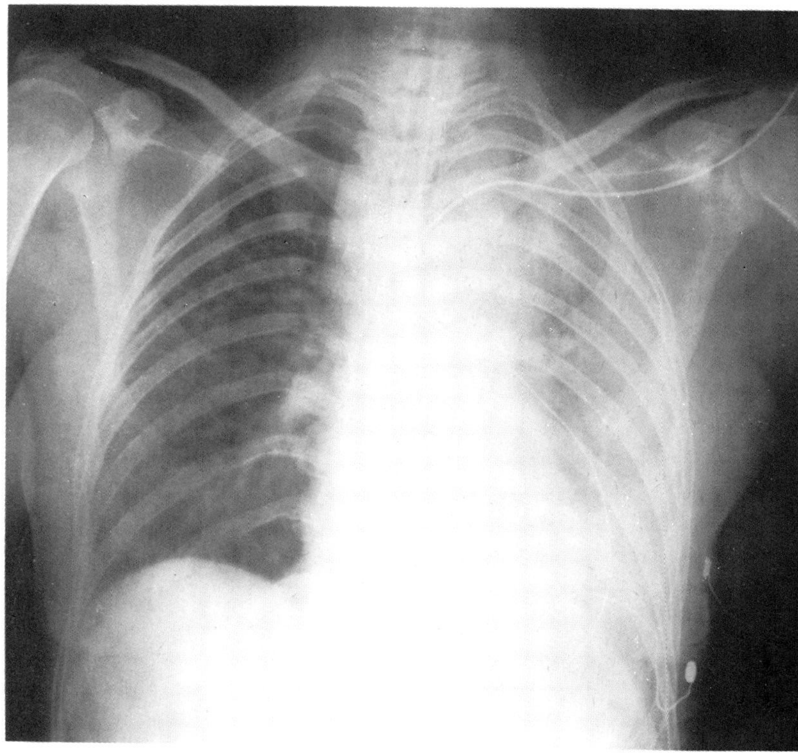

Fig. 8. Mediastinal haematoma and leftside Haemothorax after undesigned puncture of subclavian artery. Correct position of catheter

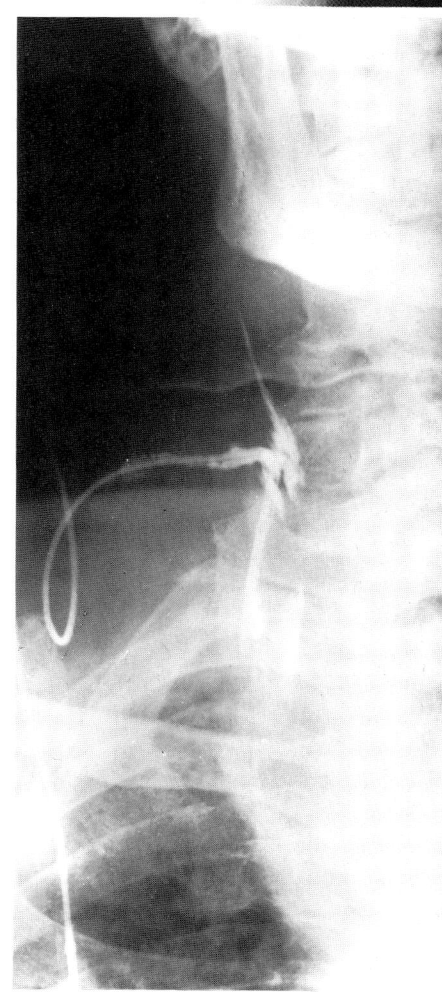

Fig. 9. Subcutaneous tear of a internal jugular catheter. Film obtained after instillation of 5 ml contrast medium, which spread along catheter and outside the internal jugular vein

References

1. Ayella RJ (1978) Radiologic management of the massively traumaticed patient. Wilkins & Wilkins, Baltimore
2. Burri C, Ahnefeld FW (1977) Cava-Katheter. Springer, Berlin Heidelberg New York
3. Conrardy PA, Goodman LR, Laing F et al. (1976) Alteration of endotracheal tube position. Crit Care Med 4:8
4. Dotter CHT, Rösch J, Bilbao MK (1971) Transluminal extraction of catheter and guide fragments from the heart and great vessels: 29 collected cases. AJR 111:467
5. Erbe W, Bücheler E (1979) Fehlerdaufdeckung durch die Röntgenuntersuchung in der Intensivmedizin. Prakt Anaesth 14:148
6. Fisher RG, Ferreyro R (1978) Evaluation of current techniques for nonsurgical removal of intravascular iatrogenic foreign bodies. AJR 130:541
7. Fraser RG, Pare JAP (1978) Diagnosis of diseases of the chest. 2nd edn, Vol I–IV. Saunders, Philadelphia London Toronto
8. Goodman LR, Putman CHE (1978) Intensive Care Radiology. Imaging of the critically ill. Mosby, St Louis
9. Kucher R, Lechner G, Pokieser H, Steinbereithner K (1967) Spätschäden der Trachea nach Tracheotomie. Anaesthesist 16:157
10. Pokieser H (1972) Röntgenologische Überwachung und Ergebnisse von Verlaufskontrollen. In: Kucher R, Steinbereithner K (eds) Intensivstation – Pflege – Therapie. Möglichkeiten, Erfahrungen, Grenzen. Thieme, Stuttgart, pp 380–408
11. Pokieser H (1974) Radiologische Diagnostik im Rahmen der Intensivmedizin Langenbecks Arch Chir 337:259
12. Pokieser H (to be published) Röntgendiagnostik an der Intensivbehandlungsstation (Bed-side-Radiology). In: Benzer H, Frey R, Hügin W, Mayrhofer O (eds) Lehrbuch der Anaesthesiologie, Reanimation und Intensivtherapie, Springer, Berlin Heidelberg New York
13. Porstmann W (1975) Fremdkörper im Herz-Kreislaufsystem und ihre transvasale Extraktion mittels Kathetertechnik. Dtsch Gesundh Wes 30:1201
14. Ravin CE, Putman CE, McLoud TC (1976) Hazards of the Intensive Care Unit. AJR 126:423
15. Rommelsheim K, Stoeckel H, Thelen M (1979) Indikation und Stellenwert der Röntgenthoraxaufnahme bei Patienten mit respiratorischer Insuffizienz. Prakt Anesth 14:102
16. Stender HS, Mellmann J, Trentz OA (1979) Fehlermöglichkeiten bei der Interpretation der Röntgenthoraxaufnahme in der Intensivmedizin. Prakt Anaesth 14:154
17. Thelen M, Franken T, Rommelsheim K (1979) Apparative Voraussetzung einer standardisierten Röntgendiagnostik in der Intensivmedizin. Prakt Anaesth 14:97
18. Zwillich CW, Pierson DJ, Creagh CE et al. (1974) Complications of assisted ventilation; a prospective study of 354 consecutive episodes. Am J Med 57:161

Gastrointestinal Radiology

Advances in Gastrointestinal Radiology

I. Laufer

Hospital of the University of Pennsylvania, 3400 Spruce Street, Philadelphia, PA 19104 (USA)

Introduction

The past few years have seen dramatic changes in the practice of gastrointestinal radiology, primarily because of the development of new techniques and their application to the solid organs, hollow viscera and functional evaluation of the gastrointestinal tract. Some of these technical developments have been spawned by a new breed of aggressive and involved radiologists practising what is now called "interventional radiology." [1] The application of the needle and catheter to the solid organs of the abdomen has led to more complete and more streamlined investigation and treatment in many abdominal conditions.

This review will highlight some of the more dramatic changes in gastrointestinal radiology considered under the headings of pancreas and biliary tract, needle and catheter, and hollow viscera.

Pancreas and Biliary Tract

Advances in this field will be discussed in detail in a separate presentation in this symposium. Clearly, the new imaging modalities have had a dramatic effect on our approach to these organs. As a result, many of the examinations which were standard procedure several years ago are no longer performed. Intravenous cholangiography is almost never performed for evaluation of the common bile duct, having been replaced by ultrasound for evaluation of duct size and by transhepatic cholangiography for precise morphological evaluation. Barium studies are now rarely used for evaluation of suspected pancreatic masses, having been replaced by the combination of diagnostic ultrasound and computerized tomography. One of the commonest of clinical problems, the investigation of patients with suspected cholelithiasis, has been particularly affected by these modalities. Although oral cholecystography is still performed in many cases as the initial investigation, most institutions have abandoned intravenous cholangiography in patients with nonvisualization of the gallbladder following two doses of contrast material. In many cases, even a second dose of contrast is bypassed in favor of diagnostic ultrasound. Since this study has been shown to be more than 90% accurate in the diagnosis of cholelithiasis, there are now those who advocate ultrasound as the initial diagnostic investigation for these patients [2].

Needle and Catheter

The needle and catheter techniques developed for angiographic studies have been applied very successfully to the diagnosis and treatment of abdominal disorders. In general terms, the needle and catheter can be used for imaging, biopsy, and treatment. The utilization of these techniques is best illustrated in the investigation of a patient suspected of having obstructive jaundice. Following an ultrasound examination to evaluate the state of the intrahepatic bile ducts, a percutaneous transhepatic cholangiogram is performed with the skinny neddle. If an obstructed lesion is demonstrated, a second skinny needle is introduced into the lesion to obtain material for cytologic study. Finally, the skinny transhepatic needle is removed and is replaced by a larger bore, sheathed needle. Through the sheath, a catheter is introduced into the biliary tree for drainage. At the same sitting, several other procedures may also be done. If the patient is suspected of having a benign stricture, the transhepatic catheter can be utilized to dilate

Radiology Today 1. Ed. by M. W. Donner and F. H. W. Heuck

the stricture. A catheter with multiple side holes can be left in place through the area of stricture so that internal drainage is accomplished from the biliary tree into the duodenum [3]. If the patient is suspected of having a pancreatic carcinoma, a transhepatic portogram can also be done to assess resectability of the tumor.

The needle and catheter have been used in a variety of other situations in the gastrointestinal tract. This includes drainage of pancreatic pseudocysts, abscesses, biopsy of lymph nodes and other masses, balloon dilatation of mesenteric vessels, and intestinal anastomoses.

Hollow Viscera

The development of fiberoptic endoscopy in the last decade has rekindled interest in the radiologic examination of the hollow viscera of the gastrointestinal tract. Many studies correlating radiologic diagnoses with endoscopic findings suggested that conventional single contrast studies were woefully inaccurate [4]. The search for improved techniques has largely been responsible for the resurgence of interest in double contrast examinations. The potential value of double contrast studies throughout the gastrointestinal tract has been recognized for many years. However, such studies could not be performed quickly, efficiently, and reproducibly because of the absence of adequate barium suspensions and techniques for gaseous distention. In recent years, these materials have become available and have made it possible to routinely perform good double contrast examinations of the gastrointestinal tract from the esophagus to the rectum [5, 6]. The availability of endoscopic correlation has accelerated our understanding of the interpretation of these studies by permitting constant radiologic – pathologic correlation.

Colon

The concepts of double contrast were first developed for examination of the colon. The technique for the double contrast enema was refined and popularized by Welin of Malmo [7]. This technique was described primarily in relation to the detection of polyps and cancer of the large bowel. The development of endoscopic polypectomy has added greater urgency and relevance to the detection of small polypoid lesions since these lesions can now be removed with a very low morbidity and virtually nonexistent mortality [8].

The radiologic signs suggestive of malignancy in a polyp are well known [9]. These include absence of a pedicle, lobulation of the surface, and puckering of the base (Fig. 1a). In addition, the incidence of malignancy rises dramatically with increase in size. Unfortunately, in many of the very small carcinomas these features of malignancy are very difficult to detect (Fig. 1b) [10]. Furthermore, these features are frequently present in benign polyps as well (Fig. 1c). Therefore, we feel that the safest approach is to have all polyps greater than 1 cm in diameter removed through the endoscope. Polyps of 5 – 10 mm in diameter will very rarely be malignant. In younger patients, it may be prudent to remove these polyps as well.

Although the double contrast enema was developed for the detection of polypoid lesions in the colon, this technique has proved particularly valuable in the evaluation of patients with inflammatory bowel disease [11, 12]. The method is useful for the detection of disease, in evaluating the extent of the disease, and for differential diagnosis [13]. The basic characteristics of ulcerative colitis include rectal involvement and mucosal granularity reflecting diffuse symmetric and confluent mucosal inflammation (Fig. 2a) [14]. Even in more advanced cases with deeper ulcers, the granular appearance of the mucosa remains and facilitates the distinction from granulomatous colitis (Fig. 2b). It has also been suggested that it may be possible to recognize severe epithelial dysplasia or "precancer" on double contrast study [15]. These areas appear as small, faceted filling defects during the quiescent phase of ulcerative colitis. The clinical utility of this observation remains to be confirmed.

In Crohn's disease, the characteristic early lesion is the "aphthous" ulcer [16]. Pathologically, this is a shallow, punched-out ulcer with an elevated margin on a background of normal mucosa. On double contrast study this is seen as a central collection of barium surrounded by a radiolucent halo with normal mucosa intervening between the ulcers (Fig. 3a). These lesions may be the only manifestation of involvement by Crohn's disease or they may be seen adjacent to segments of more severe involvement. These lesions are most commonly seen in the colon, but they may also be seen in the small bowel, stomach, and duodenum. In the stomach they are manifest basically as gastric and duodenal erosions (Fig. 3b) [17]. Indeed, the combination of erosive gastritis and duodenitis under the age of 35

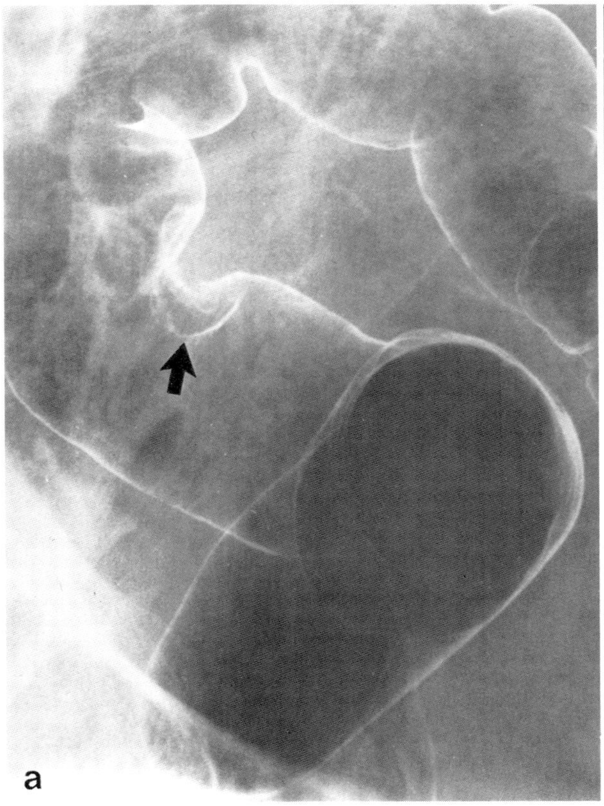

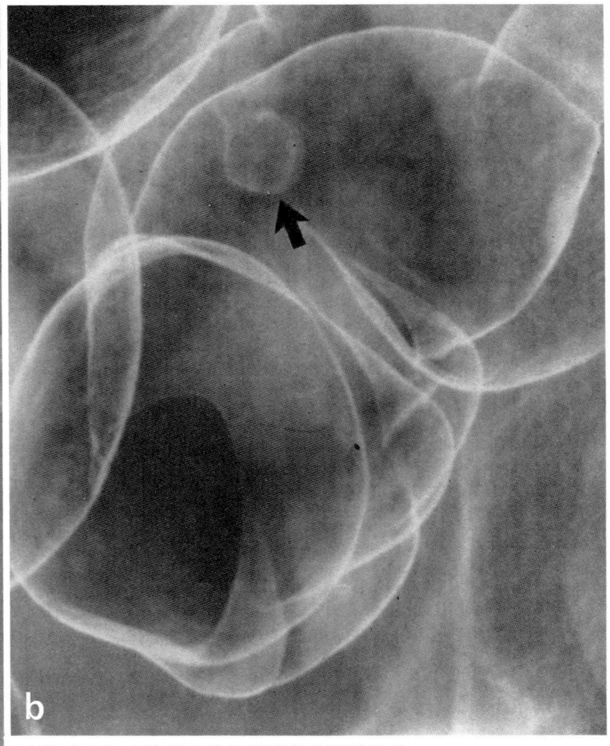

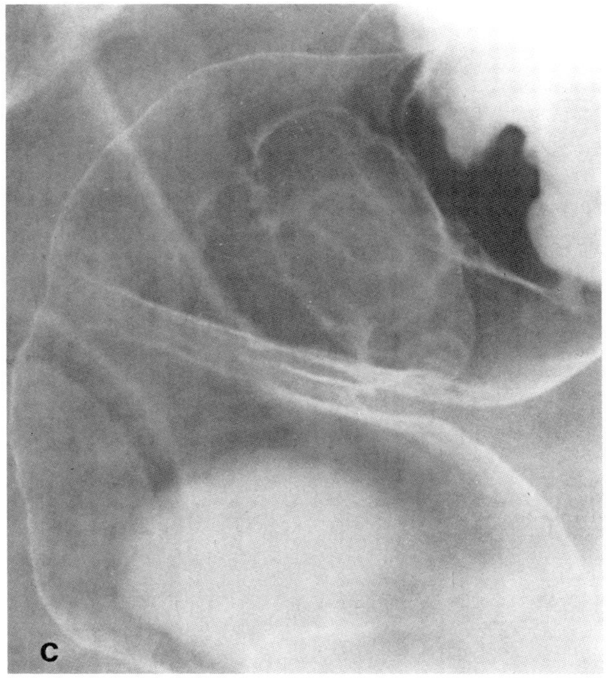

Fig. 1. a Typical early polypoid carcinoma. There is a 1.5 cm polypoid lesion in the sigmoid colon. The polyp has a slightly irregular surface with retraction of the base [5]. **b** This is a small polypoid carcinoma in the sigmoid colon. There is a relatively short, broad stock, but there is no other radiologic evidence to suggest that this is a carcinoma [5]. **c** Large, benign polyp. There is a large polypoid lesion at the rectosigmoid. The lesion is not pedunculated and the surface is very irregular. Nevertheless, this was a benign tubulovillous adenoma

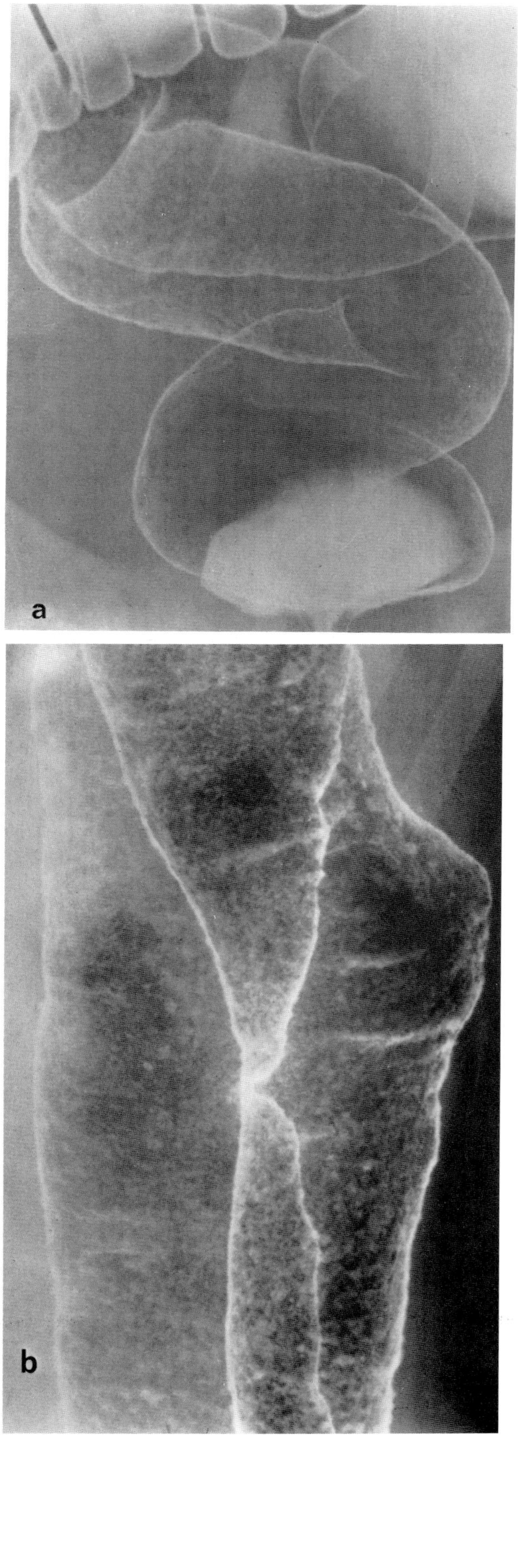

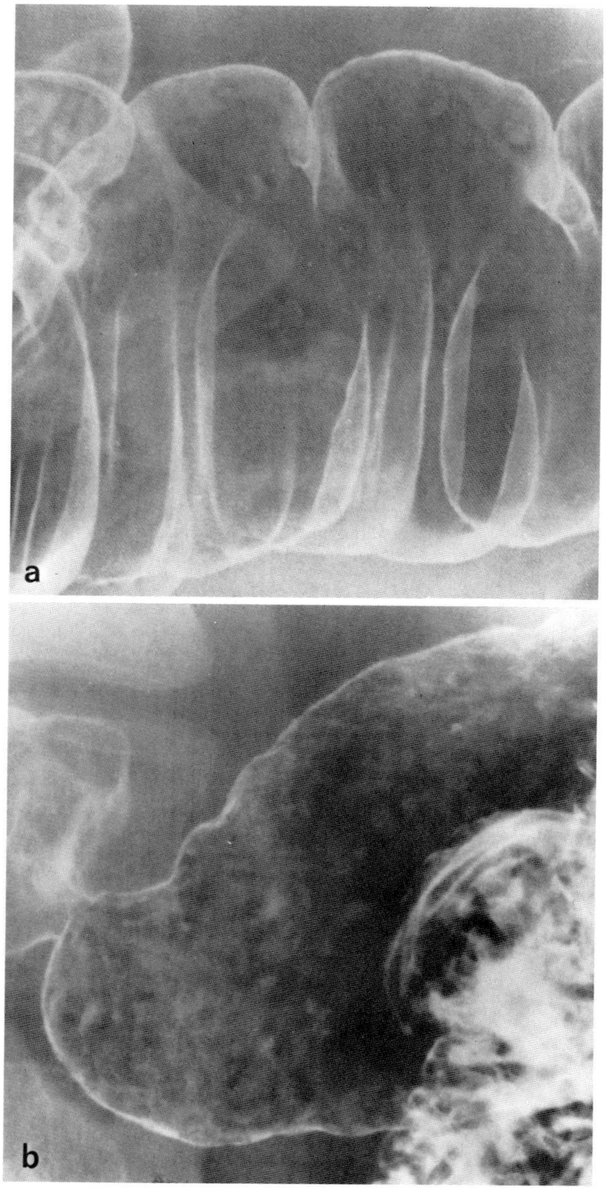

Fig. 3a, b. Crohn's disease. **a** Early lesions of Crohn's disease in the transverse colon manifest as aphthous ulcers. **b** Aphthous ulcers due to Crohn's disease in the stomach. The appearance is indistinguishable from nonspecific erosive gastritis [5]

◀ **Fig. 2. a** Early changes of ulcerative colitis with fine granularity of the mucosal surface in the rectosigmoid. **b** More advanced changes. In addition to the background granularity there are larger barium collections representing areas of ulceration on a background of diffuse mucosal inflammation [5]

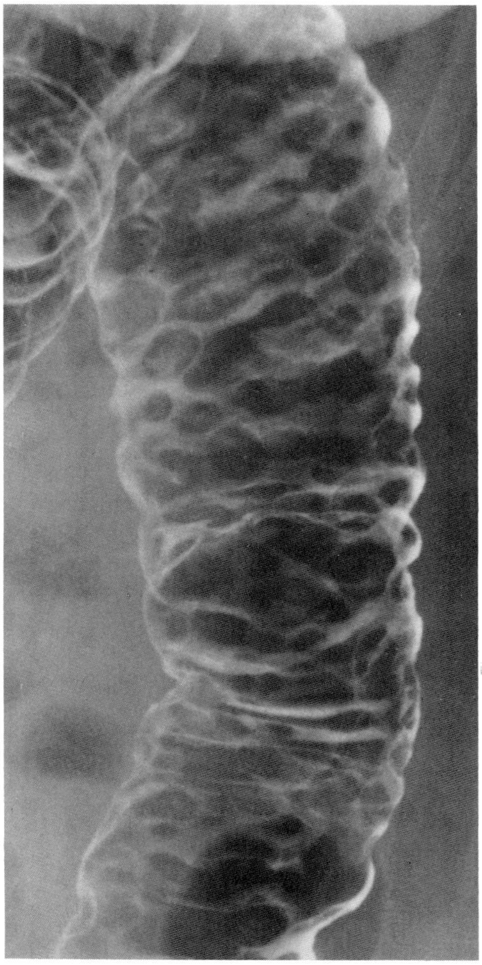

Fig. 4. Pseudomembranous colitis. Large polypoid filling defects in the descending colon represent plaques of necrotic mucosa secondary to pseudomembranous colitis [5]

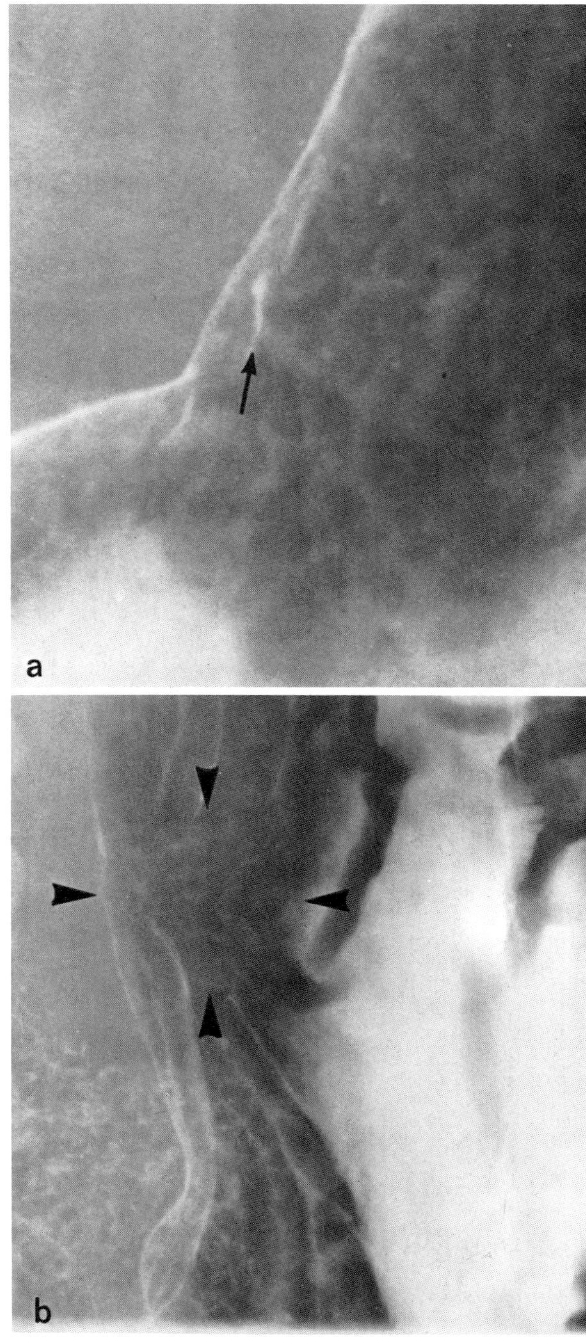

Fig. 5. a Linear ulcer; **b** ulcer scar. There are radiating folds to a point near the lesser curvature. This is a benign ulcer scar [5]

is very suggestive of Crohn's disease. We have found gastroduodenal involvement in 20% – 40% of patients with Crohn's disease.

Aphthous ulcers are not specific for Crohn's disease since they may also be seen in conditions such as amebic colitis, tuberculosis, ischemia, and Yersinia colitis [18]. Pseudomembranous colitis [19] has a fairly specific appearance with plaque-like filling defects representing islands of necrotic mucosa (Fig. 4). Contrast studies should be avoided or postponed in patients with pseudomembranous colitis and in any patient with fulminating colitis. Specifically, the double contrast examination should not be performed in patients with diverticulitis and ischemic colitis [20]. In the latter condition, in addition to the risk of perforation, gaseous distention may efface the characteristic thumbprinting, rendering diagnosis more difficult.

Upper GI Tract

Double contrast examination of the stomach was developed in Japan for the detection of early gastric cancer [21, 22]. Even in areas where gastric cancer is less common, the double contrast method

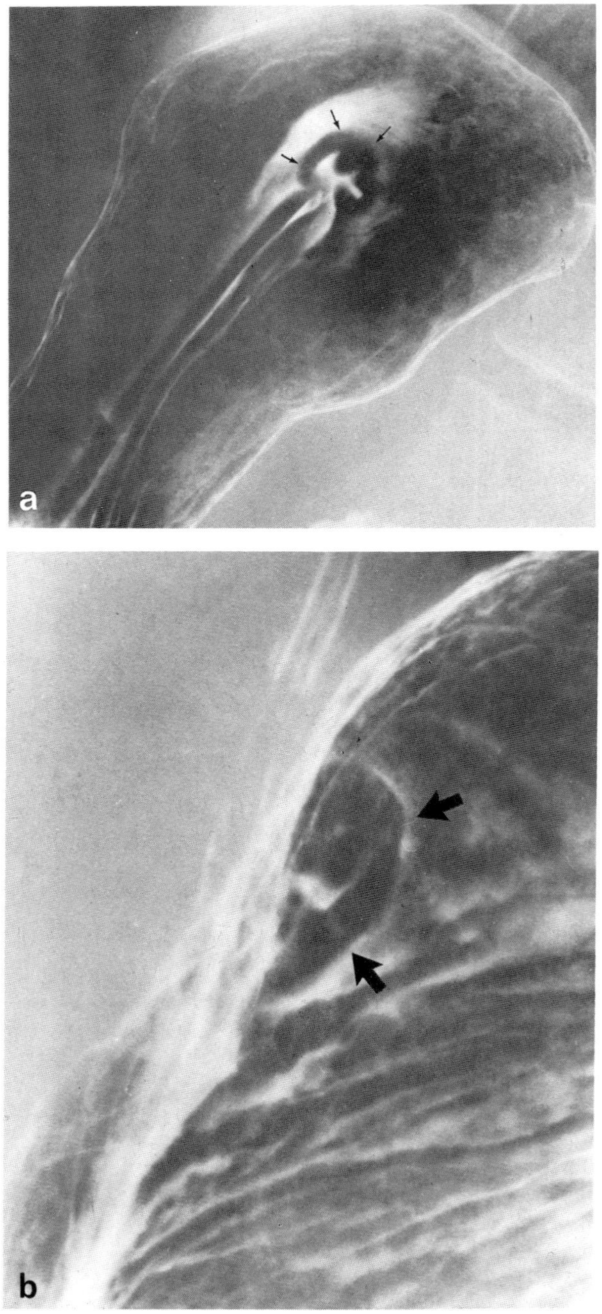

Fig. 6. a Normal cardia seen en face [5]. **b** Tumor adjacent to the cardia. There is a polypoid filling defect *(arrows)* which is not symmetric around the esophageal orifice. There is an additional small barium collection which represents an ulcer. This lesion represents a lymphoma deposit at the cardia

has been useful in the diagnosis of nonneoplastic lesion such as gastric erosions (Fig. 3b) [23], linear ulcers (Fig. 5a) [24], and ulcer scars (Fig. 5b). Gastric polyps are found in almost 2% of all double contrast gastric examinations [25]. The vast majority of these polyps are nonneoplastic in nature and are of no clinical consequence.

The double contrast method is particularly valuable for the examination of the gastric cardia and fundus. In normal patients, the cardia may have a variety of appearances including a filling defect, radiating folds, and a central barium collection (Fig. 6a) [26]. These normal appearances should not be mistaken for pathologic lesions. Deviations from these normal appearances should raise the possibility of a lesion in the region of the cardia (Fig. 6b).

The double contrast examination can also be extended to the duodenum to show the normal anatomy very clearly (Fig. 7a). There is a very delicate, velvety surface pattern in the duodenal bulb. In the descending duodenum, there is some complex anatomic detail with the major papilla on the medial surface and longitudinal and oblique folds on the posterior surface. With the patient in the prone position the minor papilla representing the opening of the accessory duct of Santorini may be seen on the anterior surface slightly lateral and cephalad from the major papilla (Fig. 7b) [27]. The minor papilla is generally smaller, but in some patients it is larger than the major papilla, presumably because of anomalies of the ductal system with the major ducts draining through the accessory papilla [28].

More recently the double contrast method has been applied to the esophagus [29]. In the upright position, the patient gulps a high density barium suspension as quickly as possible. The high density barium coats the mucosal surface. With rapid, repetitive swallowing air is ingested and the peristaltic sequence in the esophagus is interrupted (Fig. 8a). Rapid, serial spot films are obtained with the esophagus in varying degrees of distention. Occasionally, an oroesophageal tube can be used to obtain detailed double contrast studies of the esophagus (Fig. 8b) [30]. In our experience, this technique is of most value in the diagnosis of inflammatory changes in the esophagus in patients with reflux or ineffective esophagus due to candida albicans or herpes simplex [31]. Yamada [32] has also described in detail the radiologic features of small and early esophageal carcinomas. The findings usually include mucosal elevation, central ulceration, and infiltration (Fig. 8d) [33]. Other authors have also described the difficulty in detecting small esophageal carcinomas and the value of double contrast views in these cases [34].

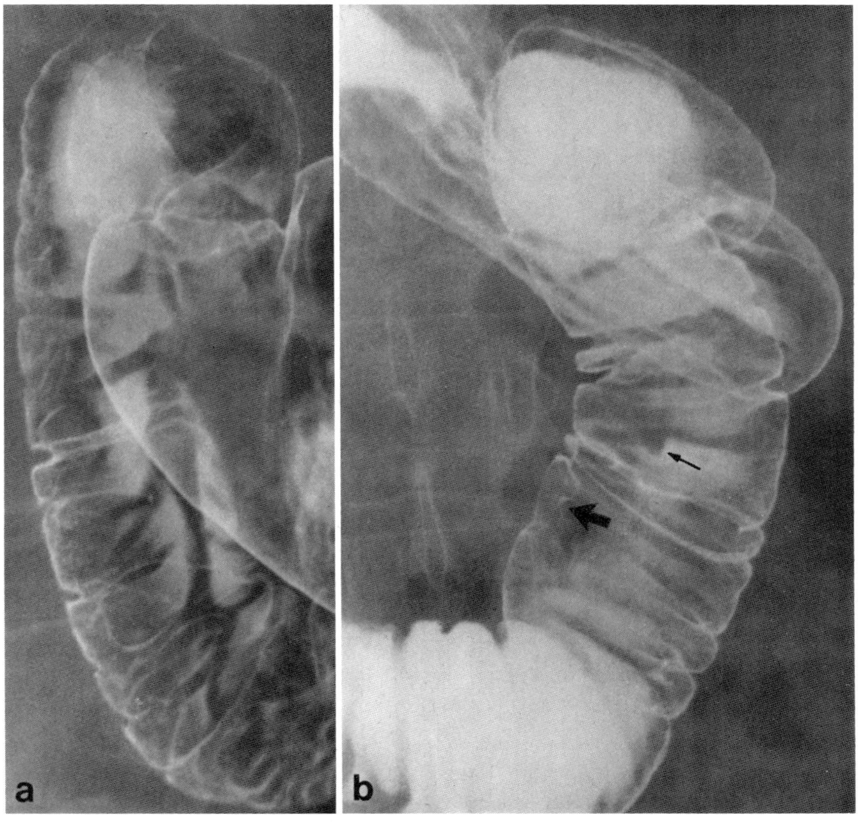

Fig. 7. a Double contrast view of the descending duodenum shows complex configuration of the papilla, longitudinal, oblique, and hooding folds. **b** A prone film of the duodenum shows the major papilla along the medial wall *(large arrow)*. Slightly lateral and cephalad is a smaller filling defect representing the minor papilla *(small arrow)*

Small Bowel

The technique of enteroclysis is described in detail by Sellink [35]. In the past, attempts to obtain a double contrast effect have utilized air or water following the barium infusion [36]. However, air enhances motor activity in the small bowel, resulting in suboptimal visualization. Water tends to wash the barium off the mucosal surface, resulting in poor mucosal coating. We have used methylcellulose as the double contrast agent as described by Herlinger [37, 38]. Following the infusion of 85% w/v micropaque, approximately 1 liter of methylcellulose is infused. The methylcellulose pushes the barium through the small bowel leaving the bowel coated with barium suspension and distended with the translucent methylcellulose (Fig. 9a). The methylcellulose and barium are immiscible. Therefore, the mucosal coating remains intact for 30 min or more. This technique is useful in the investigation of patients with unexplained abdominal pain (Fig. 9b), gastrointestinal bleeding, and symptoms of partial or intermittent bowel obstruction (Fig. 9c). It is also used for the evaluation and staging of patients with pelvic malignancy and for the preoperative evaluation of patients with Crohn's disease.

Lower Gastrointestinal Bleeding

Angiography has resulted in improvement in the diagnosis and treatment of lower gastrointestinal (GI) bleeding [39]. However, this is an invasive procedure and can only demonstrate active arterial bleeding at the rate of 0.5 ml per minute or greater. Alavi et al. [40] have developed an isotopic method for the detection of GI bleeding. Technetium sulfur colloid is injected into the actively bleeding patient. The sulfur colloid is cleared from the blood stream by the reticuloendothelial system except for isotope which extravasates at the site of hemorrhage. Thus, after a few minutes, accumulations of radioactivity outside the RE system and the blood vessels indicate the site of hemorrhage (Fig. 10). In animal models, this method has been found to be very sensitive, detecting rates of hemorrhage as low as 0.05 ml per minute. This technique has the advantage of being noninvasive, requiring only an intravenous injection of isotope. Scans can even be performed with a portable gamma camera on the wards or in the intensive care unit. Furthermore, serial studies can be obtained to document the continuation or cessation of bleeding. Once the site of hemorrhage is localized, it may be difficult to be

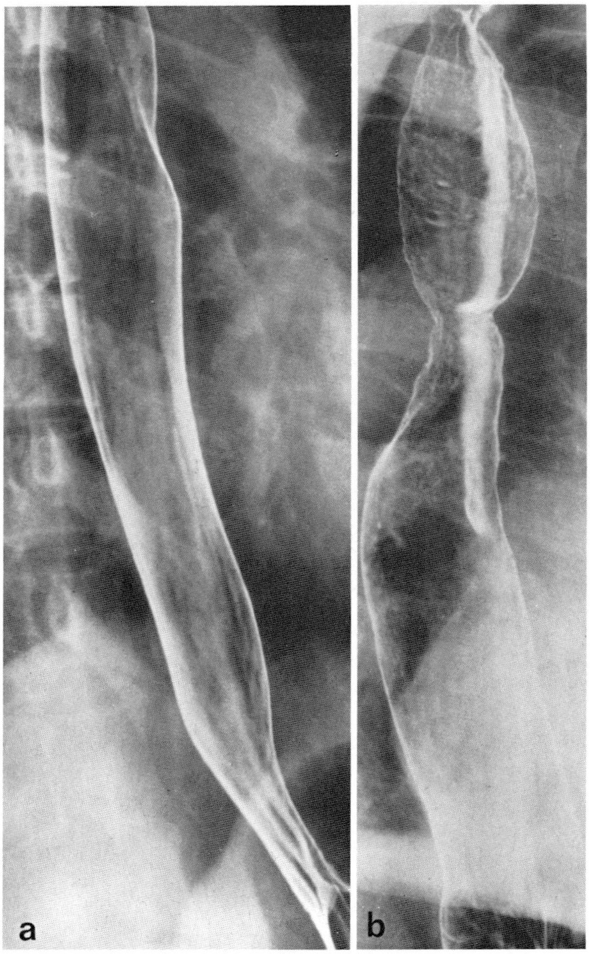

Fig. 8. a A normal double contrast esophogram. This study is performed with the patient in the upright position gulping a high density barium suspension. **b** Tube study of the esophagus. Excellent double contrast views of the esophagus can be obtained by means of intubation with a very small caliber oroesophageal tube. There is a mild stricture in the midesophagus due to Barrett's mucosa. **c** Reflux esophagitis. There is minimal narrowing in the symmetry at the gastroesophageal junction. There are small punctate collections of barium representing erosions. **d** A small carcinoma of the esophagus seen as an ulcerated plaquelike lesion

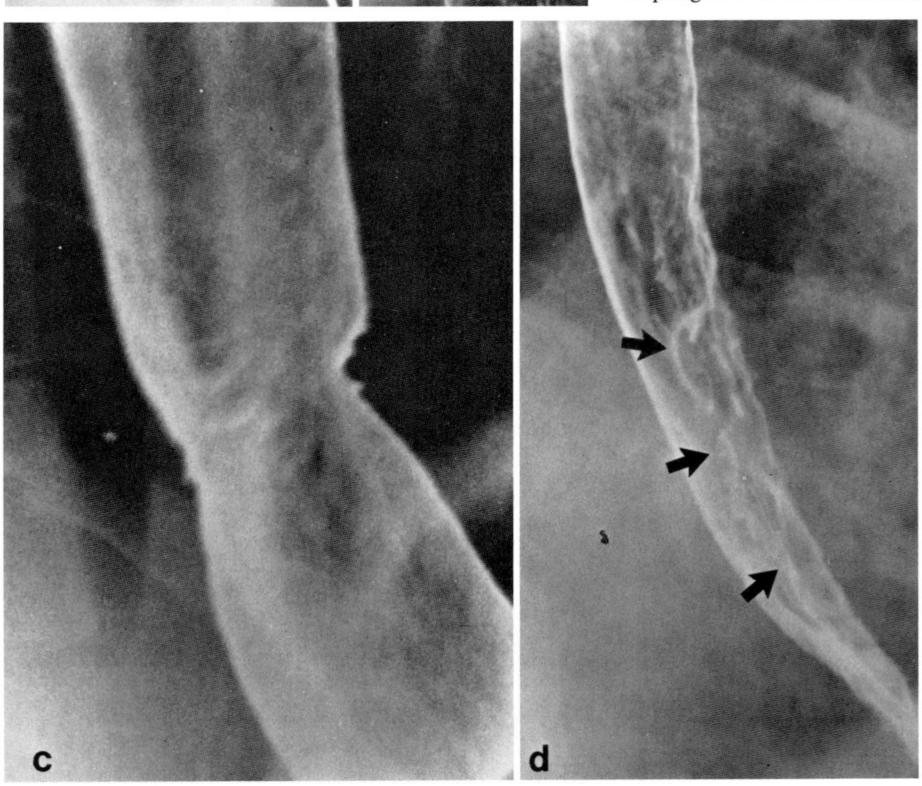

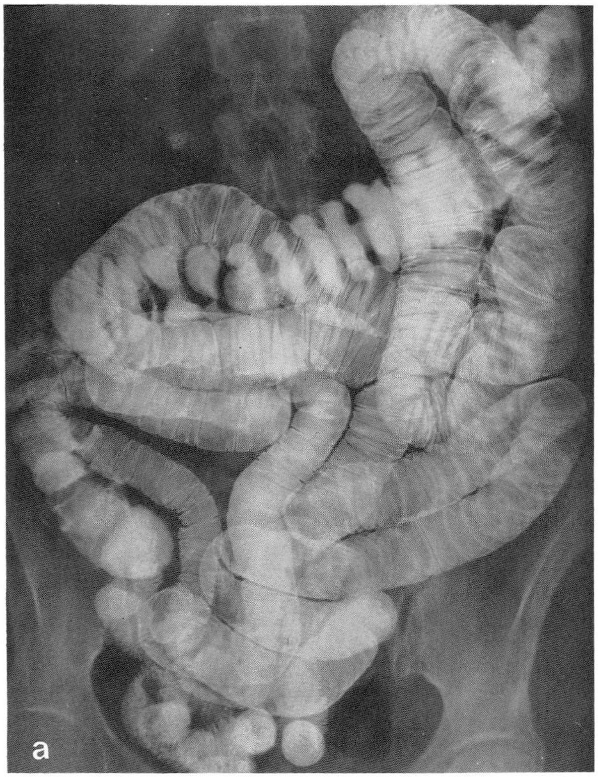

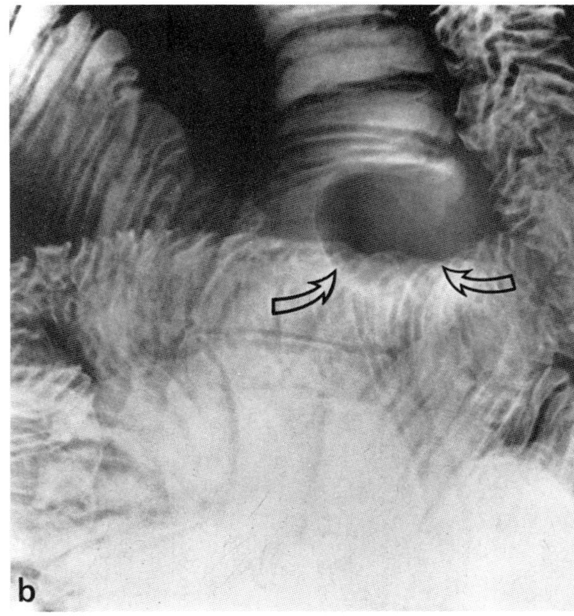

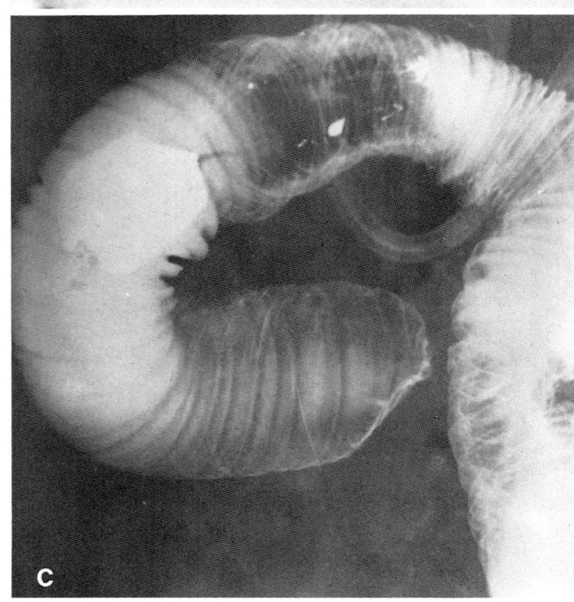

Fig. 9a – c. Double contrast examination of the small bowel. **a** Normal study. **b** Lipoma of the small bowel. A 69-year-old female presenting with intermittent abdominal pain. The double contrast small bowel enema shows an intramural tumor in the mid-small bowel. This was resected and proved to be a lipoma which presumably caused episodes of intussusception. **c** High-grade obstruction due to a band

certain whether it is arising from the small or large bowel. The later scans may demonstrate the movement of isotope which may be characteristic of either the small or large bowel.

This method is applicable mainly for bleeding from the small and large bowel. However, it may be difficult to detect bleeding sites in the hepatic or splenic flexures because of the accumulations of isotope in the liver and spleen. For the same reason, this method has not been useful for active upper GI bleeding.

The isotope scan shows only the site of bleeding, giving no information regarding its cause. Thus an angiogram may be performed following a positive isotope scan to confirm the site of bleeding, to determine the nature of the bleeding lesion, and, in many cases, to attempt angiographic control of bleeding.

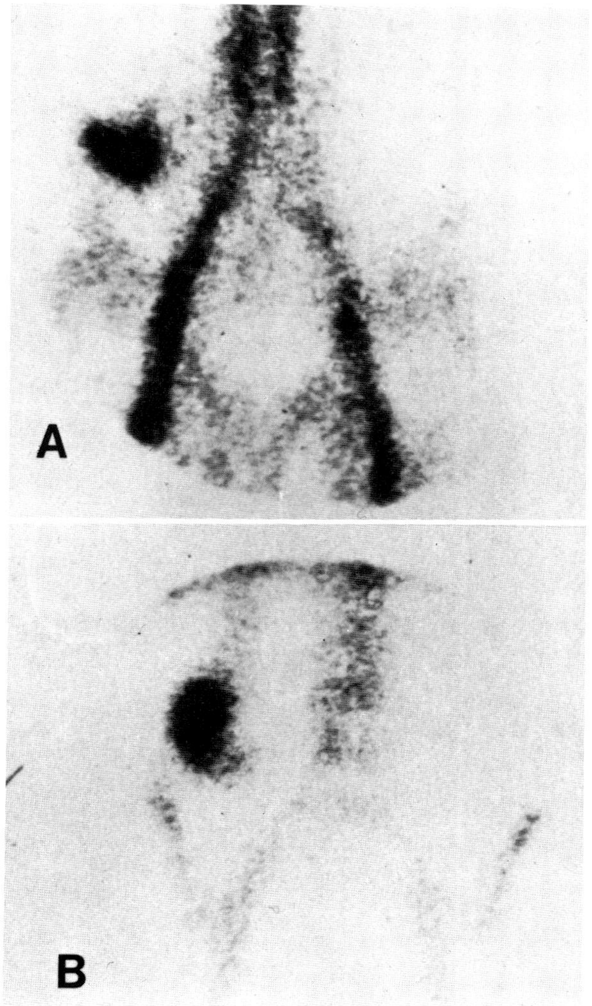

Fig. 10A, B. Rectal bleeding due to ischemic colitis demonstrated by technetium sulfur colloid scan (**A**). There is accumulation of isotope in the right lower quadrant. With later scans (**B**) the isotope is carried into the more proximal colon. (Courtesy of A. Alavi, University of Pennsylvania, Philadelphia)

References

1. MacIntosh PK, Thomson KR (1979) Symposium on interventional radiology. Radiol Clin North Am 17:369–647
2. Cooperberg PL, Burhenne HJ (1980) Real time ultrasonography. Diagnostic technique of choice in calculous gallbladder disease. N Engl J Med 302:1277
3. Ring EJ, Oleaga JA, Freiman DB, Husted JW, Lunderquist A (1978) Therapeutic applications of catheter cholangiography. Radiology 128:333
4. Laufer I, Mullens JE, Hamilton J (1975) The diagnostic accuracy of barium studies of the stomach and duodenum-correlation with endoscopy. Radiology 115:569
5. Laufer I (1979) Double Contrast Gastrointestinal Radiology with Endoscopic Correlation. Saunders, Philadelphia
6. Gelfand DW (1978) High density, low viscosity barium for fine mucosal detail on double-contrast upper gastrointestinal examinations. AJR 130:831
7. Welin S (1967) Results of the Malmö technique of colon examination. JAMA 199:369
8. Williams CB, Hunt RD, Loose H (1974) Colonoscopy in the management of colon polyps. Br J Surg 61:673
9. Youker JE, Welin S, Main G (1968) Computer analysis in the differentiation of benign and malignant polypoid lesions of the colon. Radiology 90:794
10. Ekelund G, Lindstrom C, Rosengren JE (1974) Appearance and growth of early carcinomas of the colon-rectum. Acta Radiol (Stockh) 15:670
11. Welin S, Brahme F (1961) The double contrast method in ulcerative colitis. Acta Radiol (Stockh) 55:257
12. Laufer I (1977) Air contrast studies of the colon in inflammatory bowel disease. CRC Crit Rev Diagn Imaging 9:421
13. Laufer I, Hamilton JD (1976) The radiological differentiation between ulcerative and granulomatous colitis by double contrast radiology. Am J Gastroenterol 66:259
14. Laufer I, Mullens JE, Hamilton J (1976) Correlation of endoscopy and double contrast radiography in the early stages of ulcerative and granulomatous colitis. Radiology 118:1
15. Frank PH, Riddell RH, Feczko PJ, Levin B (1978) Radiological detection of colonic dysplasia (precarcinoma) in chronic ulcerative colitis. Gastrointest Radiol 3:209
16. Laufer I, Costopoulos L (1978) Early lesions of Crohn's disease. AJR 130:307
17. Laufer I, Trueman T, deSa D (1976) Multiple superficial gastric erosions due to Crohn's disease of the stomach. Radiologic and endoscopic diagnosis. Br J Radiol 49:726
18. Lachman R, Soong J, Wishon G, Maenza R, Hanelin L, St. Geme J (1977) Yersinia colitis. Gastrointest Radiol 2:133
19. Stanley RJ, Melson GL, Tedesco FJ (1974) The spectrum of radiographic findings in antibiotic-related pseudomembranous colitis. Radiology 111:519
20. Bartram CI (1979) Loss of thumbprinting with double contrast barium enemas in acute ischemic colitis. Gastrointest Radiol 4:85
21. Shirakabe H, Ichikawa H (1973) Early gastric cancer. In: Stein N, Finkelstein AK (eds) Atlas of tumor radiology. Year Book Medical Publishers, Chicago, pp 277–357

22. Maruyama M (1979) Early gastric cancer. In: Laufer I (ed) Double contrast gastrointestinal radiology with endoscopic correlation. Saunders, Philadelphia, pp 241–371
23. Laufer I, Hamilton J, Mullens JE (1975) Demonstration of superficial gastric erosions by double contrast radiography. Gastroenterology 68: 387
24. Poplack W, Paul RE Jr, Goldsmith M et al. (1977) Linear and rod-shaped peptic ulcers. Radiology 122:317
25. Gordon R, Laufer I, Kressel HY (1980) Gastric polyps found on routine double-contrast examination of the stomach. Radiology 134:27–30
26. Herlinger H, Grossman R, Laufer I, Kressel HY, Ochs RH (1980) The gastric cardia in double-contrast study: Its dynamic image. AJR 135:21
27. Op den Orth JO (1978) Radiologic visualization of the normal duodenal minor papilla. ROEFO 128: 572–576
28. Stevenson GW, Laufer I (1979) Duodenum. In: Laufer I (ed) Double contrast gastrointestinal radiology with endoscopic correlation. Saunders, Philadelphia, pp 331–371
29. Goldstein HM, Dodd GD (1976) Double-contrast examination of the esophagus. Gastrointest Radiol 1:3
30. Suzuki H, Kobayashi S, Endo M, Nakayama K (1972) Diagnosis of early esophageal cancer. Surgery 71:99
31. Skucas J, Schrank WW, Meyers PC, Lee CS (1977) Herpes esophagitis: A case studied by air-contrast esophagography. Am J Roentgenol 128:497
32. Yamada A, Kobayashi S, Kawai B, Fujimoto A, Nakayama K (1972) Study on X-ray findings of early oesophageal cancer. Australas Radiol 16:238
33. Laufer I, Yamada A (1979) Tumors of the esophagus. In: Laufer I (ed) Double contrast gastrointestinal radiology with endoscopic correlation. Saunders, Philadelphia, pp 129–153
34. Koehler RE, Moss AA, Margulis AR (1976) Early radiographic manifestations of carcinoma of the esophagus. Radiology 119:1
35. Sellink JL (1976) Radiological atlas of common diseases of the small bowel. Stenfert Kroese, Leiden
36. Ekberg O (1977) Double contrast examination of the small bowel. Gastrointest Radiol 1:349
37. Herlinger H (1978) A modified technique for the double-contrast small bowel enema. Gastrointest Radiol 3:201–207
38. Herlinger H (1979) Small bowel. In: Laufer I (ed) Double contrast gastrointestinal radiology with endoscopic correlation. Saunders, Philadelphia, pp 423–494
39. Baum S, Athanasoulas CA, Waltman AC, Ring EJ (1973) Gastrointestinal hemorrhage: angiographic diagnosis and control. Adv Surg 7:149
40. Alavi A, Dann RW, Baum S, Biery DN (1977) Scintigraphic detection of acute gastrointestinal bleeding. Radiology 124:753

Enteroclysis or Small Bowel Enema of the Small Bowel – Some Technical Remarks

J. L. Sellink

Rijnsburgerweg 17, NL-2334 BC Leiden

Preparation

Over the past 10 years the enteroclysis examination, i.e., the administration of contrast medium via a tube directly into the distal duodenum, has become increasingly popular in Europe and beyond. Right at the beginning it was established on the basis of literature studies and practical experience that if one wishes to reach the cecum using the least amount of contrast medium, then the cecum must be empty. This ist also true for a follow through carried out in the conventional peroral fashion.

Contrast Fluid

Another well-known fact is that a cool contrast fluid enhances peristalsis, thus leading to a reduction of the total dosage required. On the other hand, a cool contrast medium also enhances nausea and vomiting, a tendency which increases as the rate of flow increases [1]. Obviously the most favorable combination will be the lowest temperature which the patient can endure without problems at the optimum rate of flow. The exact value of this temperature is yet to be determined; it is expected to lie between 15° and 20 °C. It has already been established that between the infusion bag and the distal end of the tube, the temperature of the contrast medium will increase by at least 5 °C [2].

Flow Rate

In the course of time it has been found that a rate of flow of 75 ml/min is the most favorable (Table 1). At this rate of flow, an average of almost 700 ml contrast medium is required to reach the cecum and to achieve the best evaluation of the motility. When the rate of flow exceeds 100 ml/min, a large segment of the intestine is stretched too quickly and paralysis develops so that the motility can no longer be evaluated. The amount of contrast fluid then required is much greater, and the examination will last considerably longer, partly because of the time-consuming special compression techniques which must be applied.
When the rate of flow is 50 ml/min or less, the intestine is insufficiently filled and the mucosal pattern is as disorderly as in a conventional transit examination. As listed below, in addition mild and/or local disturbances of the motility, a very important symptom of numerous diseases (see Fig. 1) and other conditions, are not visualized at all:

Table 1. Dose infusion rate for enteroclysis examinations [2]

	50 ml/min	75 ml/min	100 ml/min	125 ml/min
Average dose needed to reach the cecum	655 ml	695 ml	745 ml	835 ml
Cecum reached with 650 ml in:	65%	52%	45%	10%
1000 ml needed to reach the cecum	15%	15%	22%	33%
Examination time	± 15 min	≦ 15 min	≦ 30 min	≧ 30 min

Radiology Today 1. Ed. by M. W. Donner and F. H. W. Heuck

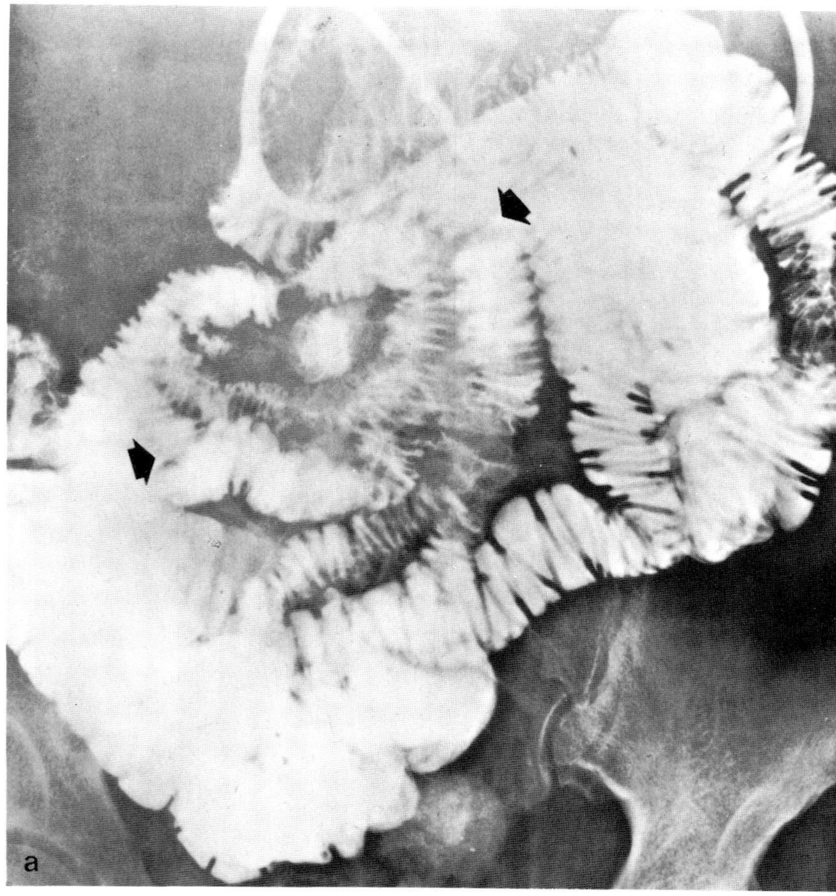

Fig. 1. a Centrally located local hypermotility caused by **b** carcinoid lesions in the mesentery in this area

Hypermotility can be symptomatic of:

1. Ischemia
   a) Adhesions or bands
   b) Vasculitis
   c) Arteriosclerosis
   d) Abdominal angina
   e) Radiation
2. Fear and emotion
3. Carcinoid syndrome
4. Thyrotoxicosis
5. Allergic reactions

Local hypermotility can be symptomatic of:

1. Slight anoxia
   a) Irradiation
   b) Fusion or bands
   c) Internal herniation
2. Carcinoid syndrome
3. Collagen diseases

Like the higher rates of flow, although to a lesser extent, a rate of flow of less than 75 ml/min will lead to a prolongation of the examination (Table 1).

The only cases in which a rate of flow of 75 ml/min is not sufficient to obtain adequate evaluation of the mucosa are pronounced hypermotility and demonstration of a subtle atrophy of the mucosa in the proximal jejunum of a patient with celiac disease (Fig. 2). Once the cecum has been reached, the rate of flow must be increased to 150 ml/min until the relevant loops are adequately filled.

A factor which also requires close attention is the density of the contrast medium. If the density is too high, small lesions will not cause a change in the intense white of the barium column; if it is too low, the changes will be so slight that they often will not be observed. Tests with a phantom have shown that at a voltage of 120 kV, the most favorable density is 40% w/v, which is comparable to a sp. gr. of 1.3.

A widespread misconception is the belief that the compression technique should only be applied to

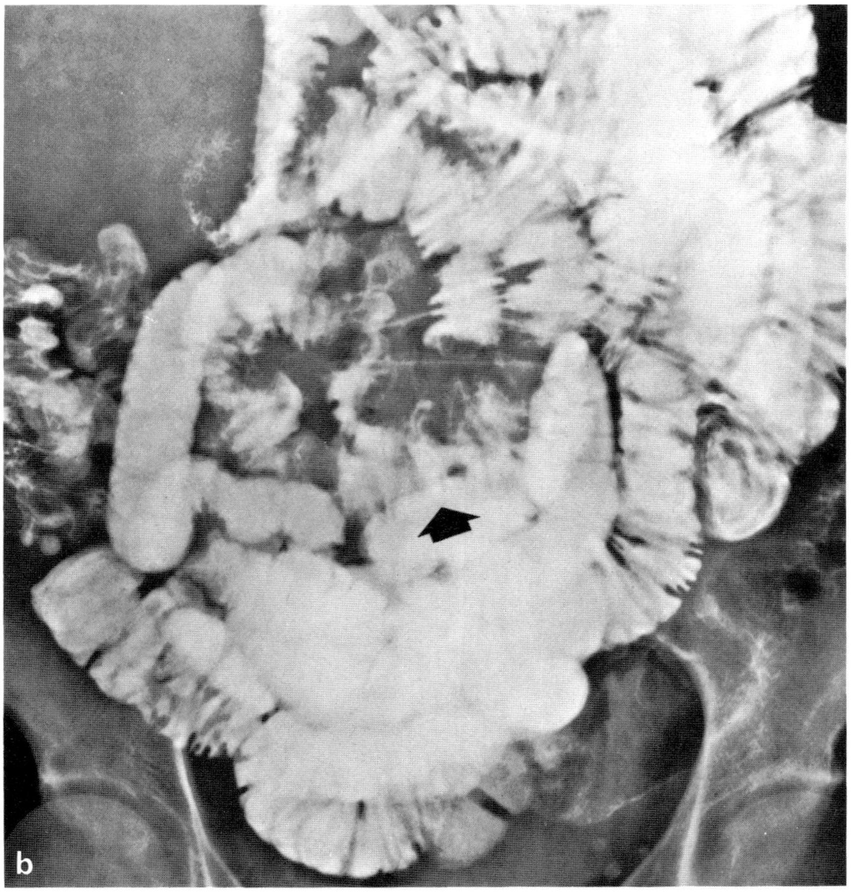

Fig. 1b. Legend see p. 143

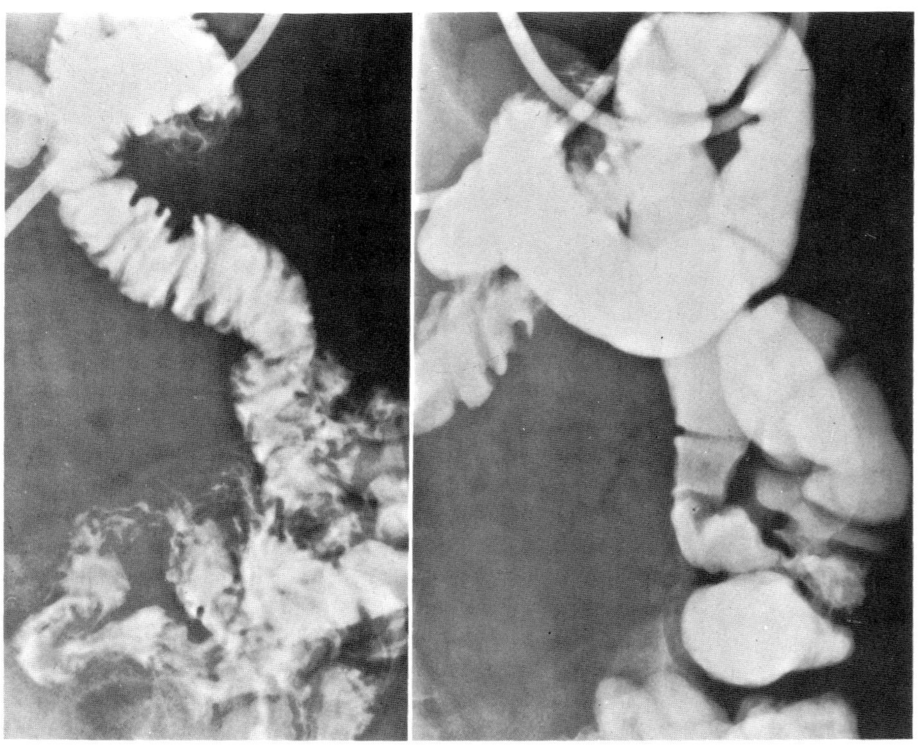

Fig. 2. Disappearance of mucosal folds, only visible when the wall of the bowel is sufficiently stretched by raising the flow rate of the contrast medium *(right)*

the distal ileum. A study of our material, however, has revealed that the number of abnormalities in the rest of the intestine is 4–5 times greater than that in the distal ileum. In the proximal third of the small bowel there are about twice as many abnormalities as in the middle third.

Where the intestine has few mucosal folds and every loop can be freely projected, for example in the ileum, the clear visualization of small abnormalities can be enhanced by a double contrast examination with air. As in the double contrast examinations of the stomach and colon, one should remember that the lowermost wall of the intestine is always visualized and thus that films should be taken of the patient in the prone and the supine positions. When the standard examination is extended to include air insufflation via the tube, an additional 10–15 min is required, depending on the motility of the intestine. Moreover it should be noted that a separate double contrast examination,

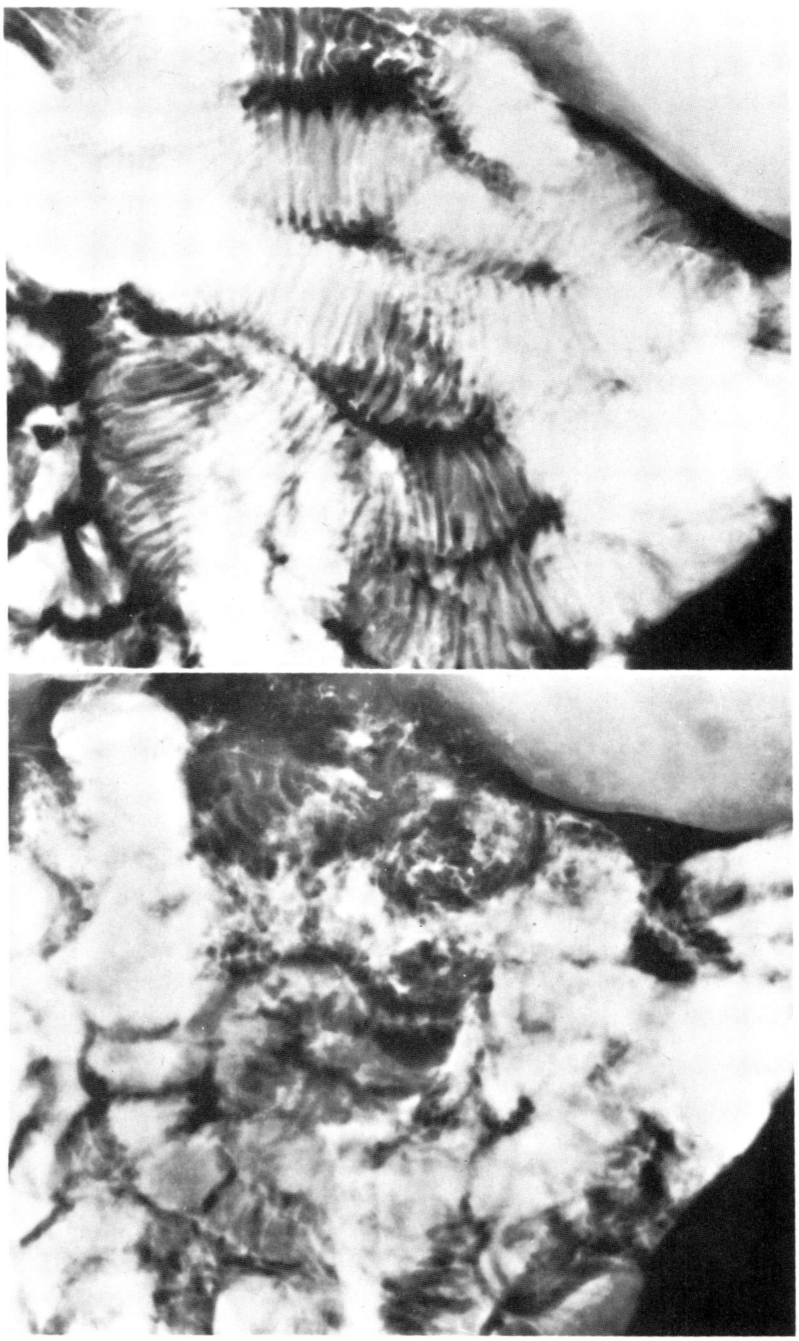

Fig. 3. Mucosal fold pattern in a 5-month-old baby (*top*). The pattern disappears as soon as infusion of the contrast medium stops (*bottom*)

in which at the most 200 – 300 ml contrast fluid of a higher sp. gr. (1.6 – 2.0) are administered, provides considerably better results [3].

Another method has become popular here and there during the past few years: the double contrast examination with methylcellulose [4]. However, this procedure not only fails to yield any gain as far as diagnosis is concerned, it also leads to drastic prolongation of the examination; in fact this method signifies an actual impoverishment of radiologic diagnostics. A slightly viscous water column is used to propel a fairly small amount of barium suspension with a higher specific gravity forward so that a film of barium remains on the walls of the intestine. It is clear that literally as well as figuratively this method implies "marginal line" diagnosis. Numerous abnormalities, including Meckel's diverticula, are far less clearly visualized than when the intestine is well-filled. Abnormalities of the wall of the intestine – both upper and lower – are often not visualized at all with this technique, in contrast to the double contrast method with air.

Disturbed motility, an important symptom for the diagnosis of numerous abnormalities which together account for about 10% of the pathology of the intestine, is not demonstrated at all with the methylcellulose method.

The enteroclysis examination of babies and patient with (sub)ileus requires special care and a slightly different procedure. These two techniques will be described briefly.

Enteroclysis Examination of Babies

For adults the administration of drugs that retard passage, such as sedatives, tranquilizers, and antispasmodic agents, is to be avoided; in contrast it is as a rule not possible to carry out the examination of babies without this type of medication. The hypomotility caused by these drugs can be compensated for by the administration of 2 – 3 ml metoclopramide.

The tendency toward flocculation of the contrast medium is so marked in babies that a relatively high rate of flow as well as a relatively large dose is required.

For babies the rate of administration should be 30 – 40 ml/min, which without a doubt will result in an abundant reflux into the stomach. In order to prevent regurgitation into the lungs, constant suction of the gastric contents by means of a second tube introduced via the other nostril is absolutely essential.

The specific gravity of the contrast medium should be about 1.15, which is also relatively high with respect to the 1.3 for adults. The reason is that the tendency toward flocculation of the barium suspension increases markedly as the dilution increases. Because of the expected reflux into the stomach it is necessary that an excess of contrast medium be prepared beforehand since interruption of the examination of a baby directly leads to failure. The following doses of contrast fluid are recommended:

a) 3 – 5 months – 200 ml,
b) 5 – 8 months – 300 ml,
c) 8 – 12 months – 400 ml.

In the case of an adult, there is almost always time to evaluate the results obtained at the end of the examination, in order, if necessary, to plan and take supplementary films; this is impossible with babies. Because of the marked tendency toward flocculation of the barium suspension, it is necessary to take all the X-rays during the infusion of the contrast medium, or at the very latest immediately thereafter (Fig. 3). There is no time to evaluate the exposures acquired since 2 – 3 min after termination of the infusion, flocculation will already be so pronounced that the mucosal relief is no longer visible.

Compression must be applied with extreme care and is only possible in a limited number of cases; unfortunately this means that the diagnostic yield is so limited that, for example, a Meckel's diverticulum is rarely or never visualized in a baby.

Enteroclysis Examination of a Patient with (Sub)Ileus

Before considering the technical details of the examination itself, several points should be mentioned:

It is at all times essential to know whether the ileus is due to mechanical obstruction or to paralysis since in the event of the former surgical intervention is usually necessary whereas in the latter case the patient's condition will deteriorate as a result of the anesthesia. It is interesting to note that within the first few minutes of the examination the probable cause of the ileus, i.e., either an obstruction or a paralysis, can often be surmised.

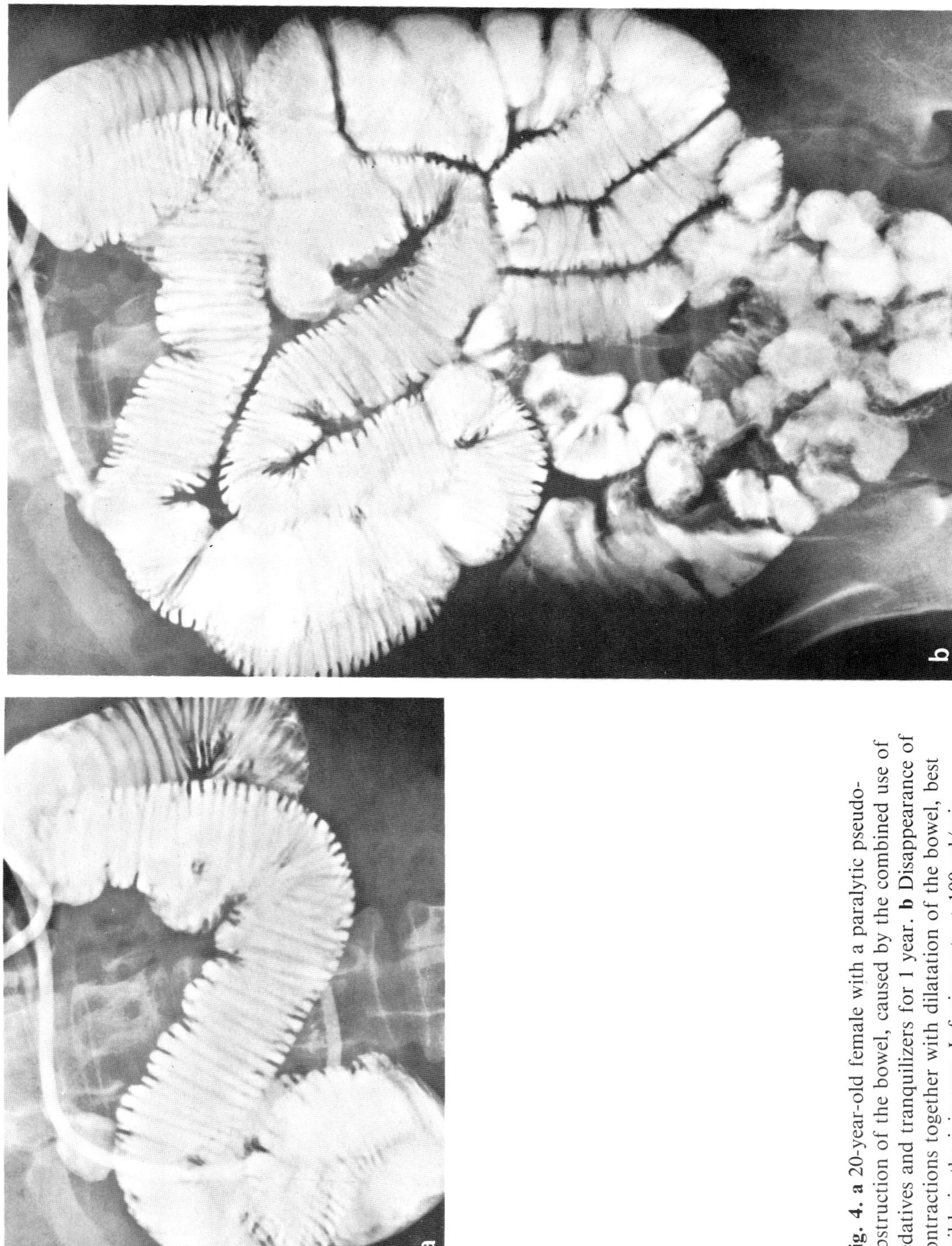

Fig. 4. a 20-year-old female with a paralytic pseudo-obstruction of the bowel, caused by the combined use of sedatives and tranquilizers for 1 year. **b** Disappearance of contractions together with dilatation of the bowel, best visible in the jejunum. Infusion rate ± 100 ml/min

If it is an obstruction, and if it is fairly recent, motility in the proximal jejunum will still be more or less intact. Distalward motility will decrease and dilatation of the intestine will increase. In the case of paralysis, the most pronounced disturbance of the motility will be seen in the jejunum, where dilatation will also be the greatest. Distalward dilatation will decrease and motility will increase (Fig. 4).

In contrast to statements in the literature, there is never any danger of thickening of the barium suspension in the small bowel; this occurs in the colon. As a rule the barium suspension will pass through the small intestine within 8 – 24 h – even if there are stenoses several millimeters wide; in our most severe case it took 1 week (Fig. 5). The surgeon must be aware of the fact that in the event of an operation after a radiologic examination, it may be necessary to suction off the residual contrast fluid during surgery.

As far as the technical procedure is concerned, this examination is characterized as follows:

Because of the large quantities of barium which ultimately end up in the colon and can cause serious clumping, laxation is recommended fairly soon after the examination. Moreover the contrast medium should be administered in three portions of 800 ml, each containing a lower barium concentration. We administer the contrast fluid as shown below:

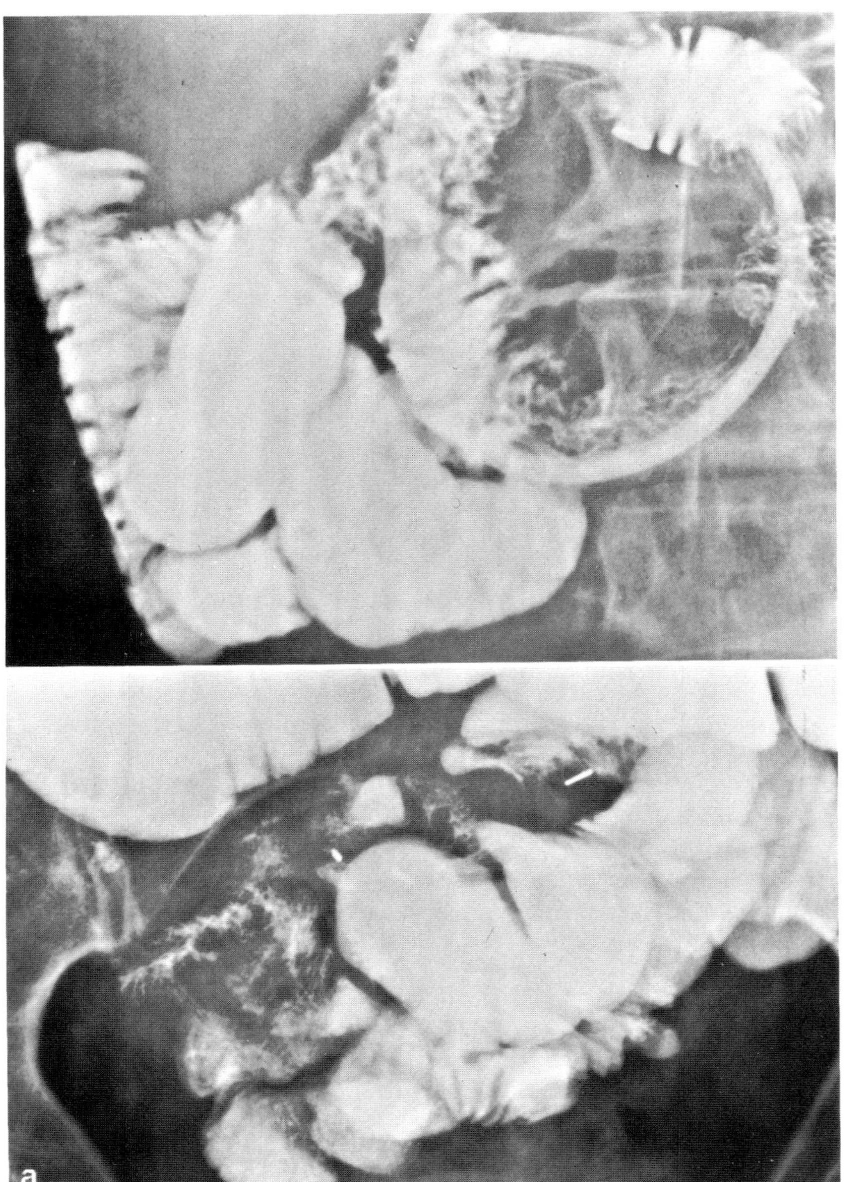

Fig. 5. a Severe mechanical obstruction of the distal ileum, caused by metastasis of an ovarian carcinoma. Note that there are still contractions in the first minutes of the examination, in contrast to the patient in Fig. 4. **b** The site of the obstruction was reached after 5 h, and the contrast medium completely passed the stenosis after 1 week

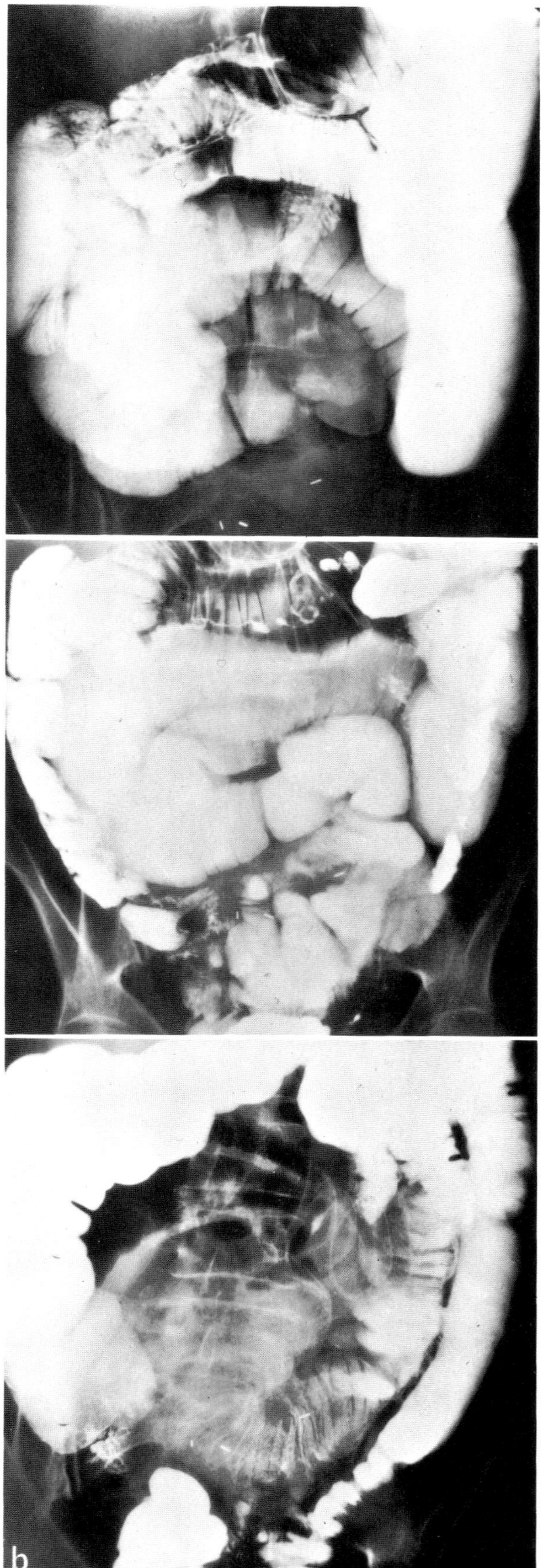

Phase a:
800 ml, sp. gr. 1.3 (= 40% w/v) – 75 ml/min,
Phase b:
800 ml, sp. gr. 1.15 (= 20% w/v) – 50 ml/min,
Phase c:
800 ml, tepid water (±35 °C) – 25 ml/min.

Because of the highly disturbed motility and the increased risk of a rapid reflux into the stomach, it is recommended that the rate of flow of the contrast medium be decreased gradually during the course of the examination, for example, as indicated above. Except in the case of extreme proximal stenoses, it is almost always necessary to reactivate the motility once or twice during the examination by administering metoclopramide via the tube. Our procedure is to administer 30 ml between phase a and phase b or phase b and phase c or 20 ml metoclopramide between a and b as well as b and c. In general the site of the obstruction will be reached within 1–2 h, or several hours in rare cases such as the previously mentioned patient of Fig. 5.
As in babies, but due in this case to the highly impeded passage, reflux of the contrast medium into the stomach almost always occurs; this contrast fluid should be removed regularly by means of a second tube.

Conclusion

Examination of the small intestine – when carried out according to the methods described in this review and avoiding the numerous errors that can be made [5] – has a high diagnostic yield with little change of overlooking important abnormalities.
Some physicians believe that, from the standpoint of practicality, enteroclysis is only worthwhile when there is strong clinical evidence of abnormalities or when better visualization of known abnormalities is desired; this is, of course, ridiculous.
On the other hand, one can understand the viewpoint that an enteroclysis examination should only be carried out after an unsuccessful conventional passage examination.

Fig. 5b. Legend see p. 148

References

1. Hippéli R, Grehn S (1978) Untersuchungen zur Intensivdiagnostik des Dünndarmes mit der Sondenmethode. ROEFO 129/6:713 – 723
2. Oudkerk M (to be published) Infusionsrate in enteroclysis examination. Thesis, Leiden University
3. Ekberg O (1977) Double contrast examination of the small bowel. Gastrointest Radiol 1/4:349 – 353
4. Herlinger H (1978) A modified technique for the double-contrast small bowel enema. Gastrointest Radiol 3/2:201 – 207
5. Miller RE, Sellink JL (1979) Enteroclysis: The small bowel enema. How to succeed and how to fail. Gastrointest Radiol 4/3:269 – 283

The Colon: Air Contrast Versus Endoscopy

R. E. Miller

Indiana University Medical Center, Department of Radiology,
1100 West Michigan Street, Indianapolis, IN 46223 (USA)

Proctosigmoidoscopy (PSS) and the barium enema (BE) have historically been extremely valuable diagnostic tools in the study of colon disease. Since the BE provided an examination far beyond the capability of PSS, and PSS could be used to examine directly the more difficult areas for radiologic evaluation (rectum and rectosigmoid), the two techniques were obviously complementary. The recent advent of colonoscopy (CS) (examination of the entire colon by fiberoptic techniques) is basically an extension of PSS.

Current evidence supports the contention that CS and the BE are also complementary. Each technique has its distinct advantages and disadvantages. The clinician must be fully aware of the relative merits of each method so as to utilize these tools most effectively [19, 20].

Just as it is true for the BE and all other diagnostic modalities, including the examining finger and PSS [1, 2], CS also has limitations [3, 4]. The colonoscope is limited in its ability to make extremely acute bends or curves, and because of this mechanical restriction, lesions can be missed. There are blind areas in all patients. These occur where there are sharp angles, acute bends, flexures, or folds in the colon. The blind areas encountered most frequently are in the rectosigmoid colon, in the splenic and hepatic flexures, and near the ileocecal valve in patients with a redundant cecum (Fig. 1). Fixation and constriction of the colon from adhesions, inflammation, neoplasms, and other problems cause CS to be further limited. Although success rates vary with the skill of the examiner, the splenic flexure is reached in about 95% of the patients, the hepatic flexure in approxi-

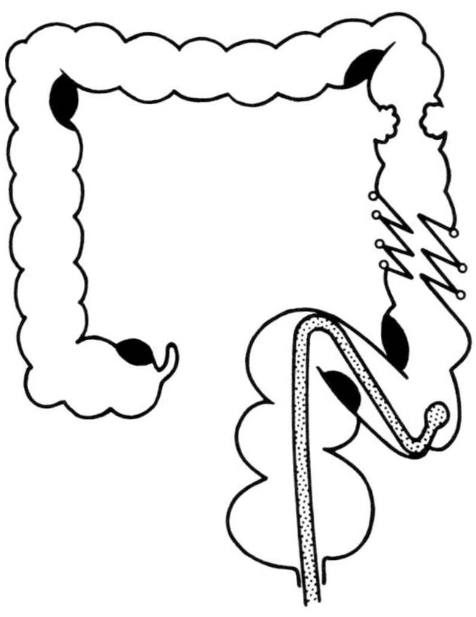

Fig. 1. Colonoscopy is blind or limited in areas of sharp angulation, constriction, and fixation. Dark areas show most frequent areas of difficulty. Colonoscope tip, acutely angled at sigmoid descending colon junction, is a frequent blind spot for viewing and snaring during CS

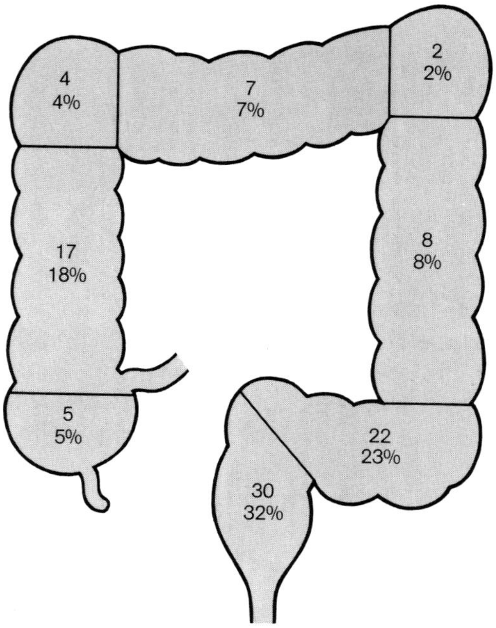

Fig. 2. Location of synchronous carcinomas in 95 patients, occurring in all parts of colon. Of these carcinomas, 60% occur in single or adjacent segments; 40% are separated by one or more segment

Radiology Today 1. Ed. by M. W. Donner and F. H. W. Heuck

mately 90%, and the cecum in only about 85% [5, 6]. Therefore, in approximately 15% of CSs, the ascending colon will not be examined. The examination of the entire colon is mandatory to detect synchronous carcinomas or other coexistent lesions. Synchronous carcinomas occur in approximately 4% – 7% of patients who have carcinoma of the colon [7, 8] (Fig. 2).

Colonoscopy requires considerably more time per examination than does the BE. It is not uncommon for CS to require 1 h to examine an entire colon from cecum to rectum. In most areas, the cost of examining the cecum by CS is at least three times that required for a BE. Patient discomfort is greater, more medication is required, and the recovery period is longer for CS than for a quality air contrast BE. Though the risks of either diagnostic or therapeutic CS are small, they clearly outweight the minor risks of the BE [9].

The BE is far superior to CS in an emergency for suspected bowel obstruction or massive bleeding, because no preparation is required on these patients. Large quantities of fecal material or blood will predictably obscure the lens of the colonoscope. Although the quality of the BE is often limited, barium sulfate suspensions may flow around fecal material and blood clots to permit localization of the site of the pathologic condition. Occasionally, the enema shows that there is only fecal impaction and no organic obstruction at all.

The BE is often superior for localizing a lesion prior to surgery. The distance measurements on the colonoscope cannot simply be transferred to the patient at laparotomy. "Bowing" and "telescoping" the colon on the colonoscope account for this discrepancy.

The diagnostic strong points of CS are that it can detect mucosal change, small polyps, and vascular lesions too subtle for BE detection. The BE in early ulcerative colitis is often normal, whereas CS or proctoscopy shows obvious changes. Williams et al. [4] reported that only 18% of colonscopically diagnosed polyps of less than 1 cm were seen by conventional BEs, although 78% of such polyps were seen by air contrast BE. Similarly, Miller [10] reported that 40% more colon polyps were seen by air contrast BE than conventional BEs. Williams et al. [4] also reported that the air contrast BE identified a very respectable 98% of colonoscopically diagnosed polyps greater than 1 cm. Additionally, up to 25% of all colonic cancers are missed by initial full column BEs [10, 11, 12]. Wolff et al. [12], using largely, although not exclusively, air contrast BEs, roentgenographically visualized 48% of colonoscopically visualized polyps greater than 1 cm. Therefore, CS has a distinct advantage in the diagnosis of small polyps and a small, though important, advantage in the detection of larger polyps. Occasionally, however, the air contrast enema will detect large polyps and even a 4-cm malignant neoplasm of the cecum missed at endoscopy [2, 12].

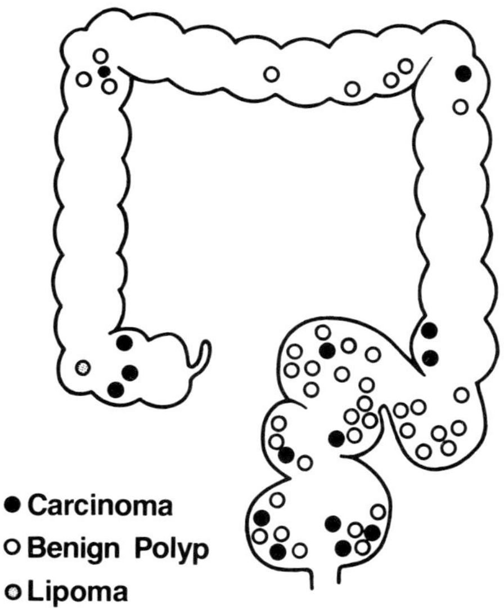

Fig. 3. The distribution of 55 cases of polypoid colonic lesions missed by endoscopy. In each case, the endoscopist reached or passed beyond the area of the lesion. In several cases, a repeat BE study or repeat endoscopy revealed the lesion. The lesions grouped as carcinoma include in situ to invasive categories and total 15

Figure 3 demonstrates the distribution of these 55 cases of polypoid colonic lesions. Colonoscopy failed to identify 32 of the 55 lesions, whereas 24 lesions were initially missed by PSS. One polypoid tumor or the rectosigmoid junction was missed by both. Most undetected lesions ranged from 0.5 to 1.5 cm. Histologic proof of each lesion was subsequently obtained by repeat endoscopy with biopsy, polypectomy, or surgery. The unusually high incidence of carcinomas in this series may reflect the failure to report benign, seemingly less serious lesions under these circumstances.

An incomplete examination may obviously account for failure to identify colonic lesions by colonic endoscopy. However, if the endoscopist reaches or passes the areas in question and identifies no lesion, an endoscopy report of "normal" ensues. Such a report must be interpreted within the limitations of the procedure. Failure to appreciate these limitations may result in inappropriate patient management.

Colonoscopic errors can be reduced by using a quality air contrast barium enema study to guide the subsequent endoscopic examination. It is generally agreed that CS should remain the secondary examination to clarify biopsy or remove lesions identified by the BE study.

Failure to apply good air contrast BE technique will result in missing 33% – 43% of colon polypoid lesions [2, 4, 10, 13, 14]. Preferably, radiographs should be reviewed by both the endoscopist and radiologist.

We believe the greatest assets of CS are those of combined biopsy or polypectomy. With minimal additional time, cost, and patient risk, lesions can be biopsied or polypoid lesions removed by electrocautery. Laparotomy and colonic polypectomy carry 0.5% mortality [15] and 20% morbidity [16]. Colonoscopic polypectomy has a morbidity of approximately 0.5% (perforation, hemorrhage) and only extremely rare mortalities are reported [9]. Polypectomy subsequently spares the patient time, cost, and radiation exposure of annual repeat BE for following polyp size change.

With rare exceptions, such as polyps of less than 0.5 cm, aged patients, or technically difficult examinations (diverticular disease, redundancy) expectant BE observation of polyps appears unwarranted [3, 4].

After complete polypectomy, a repeat air contrast BE or CS is suggested at yearly intervals initially, but these may be discontinued or restricted to every 3 – 5 years if no new polyps are found. Such a program, combined with annual clinical follow-up and PSS, avoids both unnecessary CSs and BEs [4].

Postoperative evaluation of the anastomotic site for recurrent colon cancer is difficult for the BE, as surgical changes may appear nodular, narrowed, or otherwise deformed. Similarly, patients with ureterosigmoidostomies need careful evaluation of their anastomotic site, as they are prone to develop colon cancer [17]. Colonscopy offers direct visualization with biopsy; however, extramural tumor is not excluded by a normal appearing mucosal surface [3].

Despite the assets of CS, most colonoscopists [3] agree that the BE, especially air contrast BE, and PSS should remain the primary examinations for patients with suspected colonic disease. Wolff and Shinya [18] believe "colonoscopy serves as a back-up procedure to the contrast enema." Errors of interpretation of BE roentgenograms are more common than failure of the air contrast technique itself. With cooperative feedback, the colonoscopist's findings make a careful review of the X-ray films an enlightening and beneficial learning experience for both the radiologist and the colonoscopist. Improved patient care should result from such interchange.

In the study of colonic disease, endoscopy and roentgenography are clearly complementary. Each diagnostic technique has its assets and limitations. Colonoscopy has recently made great diagnostic and therapeutic advances. However, the BE, especially the air contrast type, remains an extremely valuable tool. If results of the two methods conflict, one or both should be repeated. If both initial diagnostic studies are "normal" or unrevealing and the clinical signs or symptoms persist, repeat examinations should be performed.

References

1. Carlile T (1967) Cancer of the gastrointestinal tract. Year Book Medical Publishers, Chicago, pp 187 – 211
2. Miller RE (1975) Examination of the colon. Curr Probl Diagn Radiol 5:3 – 40
3. Marks G (1974) Flexible fiberoptic colonoscopy: A guide for its use in the management of diseases of the colon. JAMA 228:1411 – 1413
4. Williams CB, Hunt RH, Loose H et al. (1974) Colonoscopy in the management of colon polyps. Br J Surg 61:673 – 682
5. Gaisford W (1974) Fiberendoscopy of the cecum and terminal ileum. Gastrointest Endosc 21:13 – 18
6. Sakai Y (1974) Further progress in colonoscopy. Gastrointest Endosc 20:143 – 147
7. Ekelund GR, Pihl B (1974) Multiple carcinomas of the colon and rectum. Cancer 33:1630 – 1634
8. Peabody CN, Smithwick RH (1961) Practical implications of multiple tumors of the colon and rectum. N Engl J Med 264:853 – 855
9. Berci G, Panish JF, Schapiro M et al. (1974) Complications of colonoscopy and polypectomy. Gastroenterology 67:584 – 585
10. Miller RE (1974) Detection of colon carcinoma and the barium enema. JAMA 230:1195 – 1198
11. Saunders CG, MacEwen DW (1971) Delay in diagnosis of colonic cancer: A continuing challenge. Radiology 101:207 – 208
12. Wolff WI, Shinya H, Geffen A et al. (1975) Comparison of colonoscopy and the contrast enema in 500 patients with colorectal disease. Am J Surg 129:181 – 186
13. Laufer I, Smith NCW, Mullens JE (1976) The radiological demonstration of colorectal polyps undetected by endoscopy. Gastroenterology 70:167 – 170

14. Theoni RF, Menuck L (1977) Comparison of barium enema and colonoscopy in the detection of small colonic polyps. Radiology 124:631 – 635
15. Turell R (1969) Disease of colon and rectum. 2nd edn. Saunders, Philadelphia, Vol 1, p 359
16. Kleinfield G, Gump FE (1960) Complications of colostomy and polypectomy. Surg Gynecol Obstet 111:726 – 728
17. Preissig RS, Barry WF Jr, Lester RG (1974) The increased incidence of carcinoma of the colon following ureterosigmoidostomy. Am J Roentgenol Radium Ther Nucl Med 121:806 – 810
18. Wolf W, Shinya H (1974) Modern endoscopy of the alimentary tract. Curr Probl Surg 1:30 – 52
19. Miller RE, Lehman G (1978) Polypoid colonic lesions undetected by endoscopy. Radiology 129:295 – 297
20. Miller RE, Lehman G (1976) The barium enema: Is it obsolete? JAMA 235:2842 – 2844

Radiology of the Liver: Overview

A. Gebauer, M. Kessler, and J. Lissner

Ludwig-Maximilians-Universität München, Klinikum Großhadern, Radiologische Klinik und Poliklinik, Marchioninistraße 15, D-8000 München 70

Introduction

The various liver diseases listed in Table 1 require different diagnostic techniques. Standard examinations have included X-ray, radionuclide imaging using technetium sulfur colloid or technetium phytate, and, as an invasive method, angiography.

The diagnostic value of X-ray has been and remains low, because one can detect only calcified lesions. For many years angiography has been the only method capable of directly detecting intrahepatic lesions after suspicious findings have been diagnosed by the "screening method" of liver scintigraphy [14, 15, 17].

Ultrasound (US) and computed tomography (CT) have considerably enlarged the diagnostic spectrum of examination of the liver. This fact necessitates a review of the various methods. First I should like to point out the diagnostic value of the different methods with regard to the various liver diseases before proposing the best diagnostic procedure for each case.

Table 1

Diffuse liver diseases	*Methods*
– Inflammatory disease	– X-ray
– Cirrhosis	
– Fatty infiltration	*Radionuclide imaging*
– Haemochromatosis	
	Angiography
Circumscribed liver diseases	– Arteriography
	– Venography
Neoplastic disease	– Hepatic veins
– Hepatoma	– Portal vein
– Metastases	
Benign tumors	*Ultrasound*
– Cysts	*CT*
– Echinococcosis	
– Angioma	*Interventional methods*
– Adenoma	
– Focal nodular hyperplasia	
Abscesses	
Trauma	

Diffuse Liver Diseases

Inflammatory liver diseases are diagnosed by the specific liver function tests. Diagnostic radiology has been required only in severe cases to exclude a complication. Neither CT nor sonography nor angiography is helpful. Liver scintigraphy is able to document the known hepatic dysfunction in the form of reduced or delayed activity enhancement of the liver with increased background activity.

Liver Fibrosis/Cirrhosis

Sonography. Hepatic cirrhosis involves progressive disruption of liver architecture with replacement by fibrous tissue. This fibrous tissue causes a considerable increase in the number and the intensity of the intrahepatic boundary surfaces [13, 25]. As a result the intrahepatic structural echoes are multiplied and the liver gives a picture that is lighter and more dense (Fig. 1). This liver pattern is termed the "bright liver" [11]. The intrahepatic vessels cannot be detected easily in the peripheral parts of the liver. Often the "tramline" pattern of the portal vein is lost, and it is difficult to distinguish between the portal and the hepatic veins. The probability of diagnosis of cirrhosis increases with the identification of an enlarged spleen and ascites.

Nodular changes in cirrhosis show a lucency and may erroneously be taken for a malignant neoplasm.

Radiology Today 1. Ed. by M. W. Donner and F. H. W. Heuck

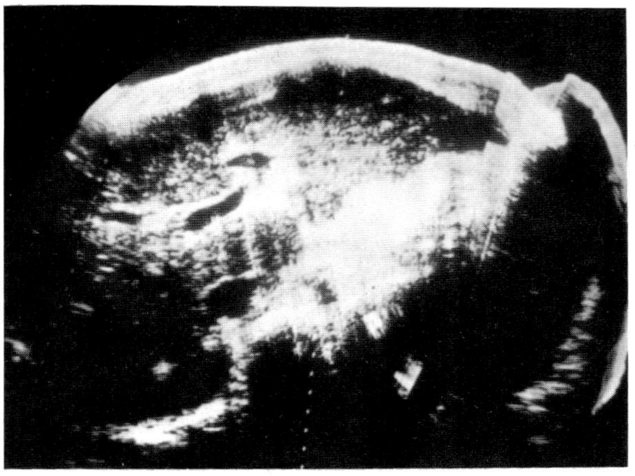

Fig. 1. Liver cirrhosis. The echoes are more dense and brighter. The "tramline" sign of the portal vein is lost

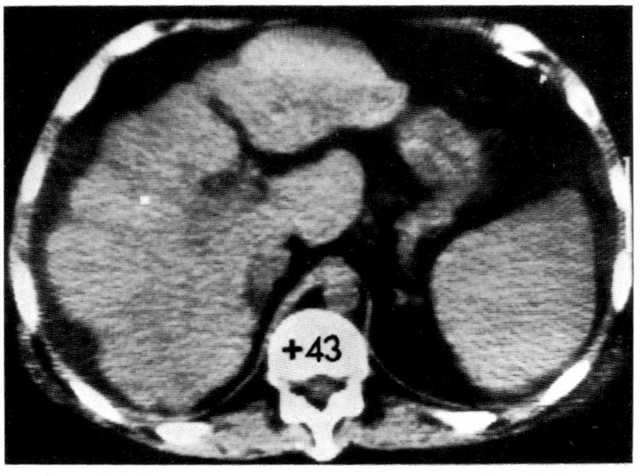

Fig. 2. CT in cirrhosis. The left and caudate lobes are particularly enlarged

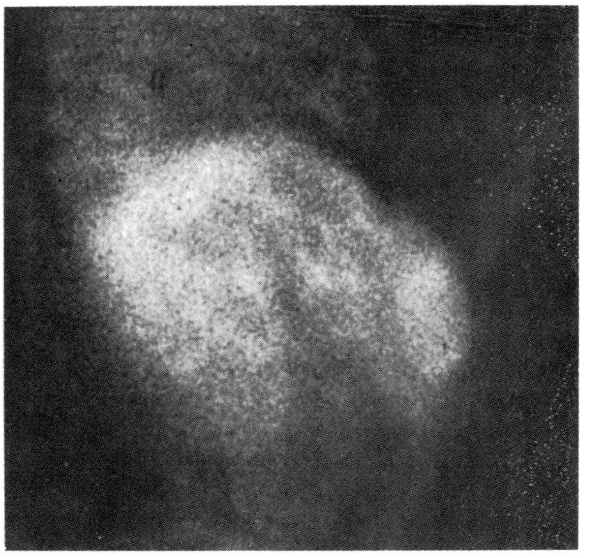

Fig. 3. Scintigraphy in cirrhosis (*lateral view*). The isotopic enhancement in the liver is decreased with increased enhancement in the liver is decreased with increased enhancement in the spleen and the bone marrow (*ribs*)

To sum up, sonography gives a typical picture but not a pathognomonic one [7, 8, 11, 13, 25].

Computed Tomography. Computed tomography of a hepatic cirrhosis shows a clear lobular picture, in which particularly the left hepatic lobe, the caudate lobe, and the quadrate lobe are enlarged (Fig. 2). The density values do not differ significantly from the normal hepatic tissue. Again, in CT an enlarged spleen and the identification of ascites make the diagnosis of cirrhosis more probable [9, 11, 22].

Radionuclide Imaging. Scintigraphy of the liver using technetium sulfur colloid or technetium phytate results in a rather typical picture: corresponding to the defect of the hepatic cells the capacity for phagocytosis of the Kupffer cells is reduced and the isotopic enhancement of the spleen and bone marrow is higher (Fig. 3). In early stages of cirrhosis the accuracy of radionuclide imaging is about 40% – 60% [3, 9, 29].

Angiography. During the early stage of cirrhosis the vascular pattern is normal because neither an increase in portal hypertension nor a decrease in liver size can be observed. During increasing portal hypertension and collateral hepatofugal circulation the coiling of the intrahepatic arteries is striking. Quite often it is accompanied by vasodilatation of the arteries. During the end-stage of cirrhosis the vascular tree is folded up as if too large for the shrunken liver. The intrahepatic arteries are twisted like a corkscrew.
The arteriographic findings in diffuse liver diseases are as nonspecific as the photographic findings. As a result, angiography is in no way pathognomonic for cirrhosis or chronic hepatitis [14].

Diagnostic Procedure. The diagnosis of cirrhosis of the liver is a histologic one. US, CT, and scintigraphy are not effective in the early diagnosis of the cirrhotic liver. But these methods may suggest this diagnosis when the replacement by fibrotic tissue is quite advanced. The accuracy of these methods is about 50% [3, 5, 8, 9, 22]. Angiography does not identify the replacment of the liver by fibrous tissue, but does diagnose the resulting hemodynamic conditions like portal hypertension

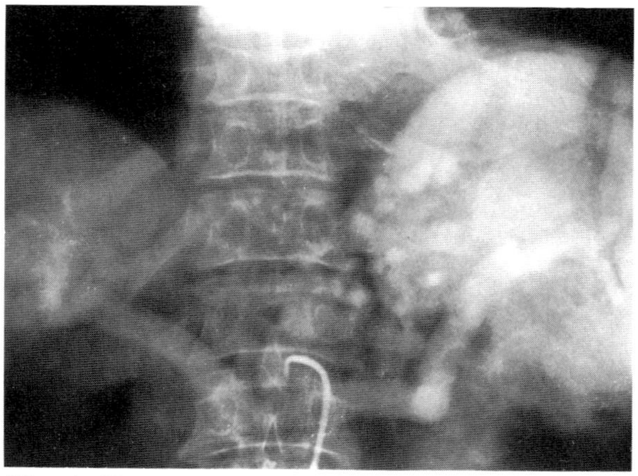

Fig. 4. Hepatofugal circulation in cirrhosis. Enlarged coronary vein and esophageal varices are outlined

and hepatofugal circulation (Fig. 4). Angiography is necessary before planning shunt surgery. Additionally, in the case of nonspecific CT and US findings, arteriography can be an essential method when looking for a postcirrhotic carcinoma.

Fatty Infiltration

Sonography. Diagnostic US shows compact echogenic structures which have a more uniform and less coarse pattern than those in cases of cirrhosis (Fig. 5). Sonography does not reliably distinguish between fatty infiltration and cirrhosis [8, 9, 11].

Computed Tomography. With CT fatty degeneration (70% – 80% of hepatocytes containing fat droplets) will demonstrate a pathognomonic picture: there is a so-called reversed density between the portal vein and its branches, which show a higher density, and the liver parenchyma, which shows a reduced density (Fig. 6). The density of the fatty liver is below 40 – 45 HU [3, 21, 22].

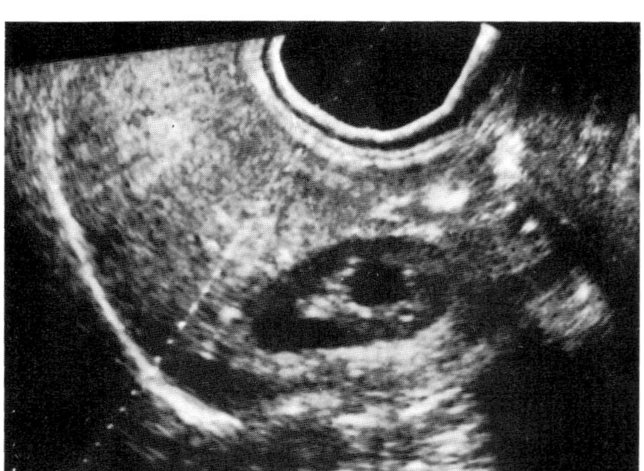

Fig. 5. Fatty infiltration. The echoes are more dense but less coarse compared with cirrhosis

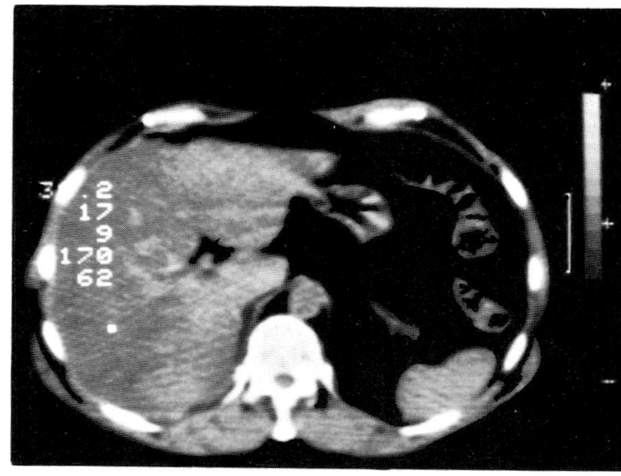

Fig. 6. CT in fatty infiltration. Reduced density of parenchyma (below 40 – 45 HU)

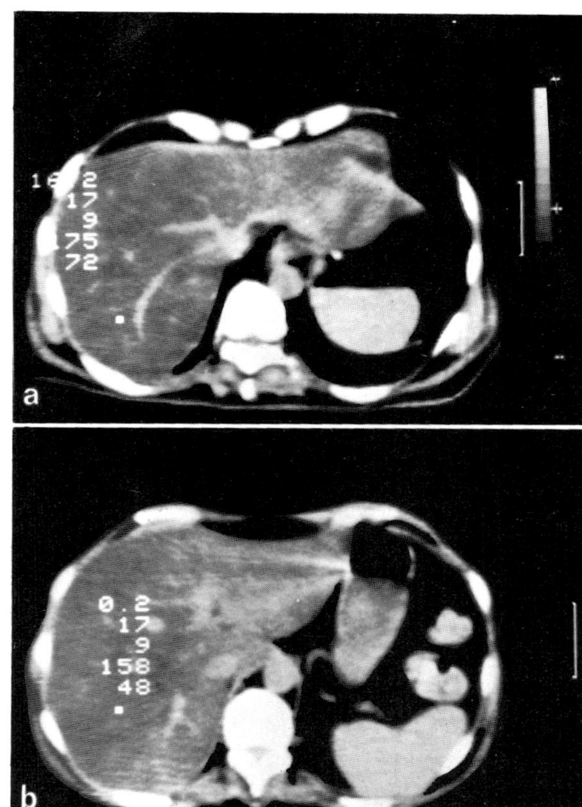

Fig. 7a, b. Fatty infiltration, when using hepatotoxins. **a** At the beginning of the therapy (16 HU). **b** 5 months later: density is reduced (1 HU), fatty infiltration increased

Radionuclide Imaging. If, in the case of fatty infiltration, damage to the liver cells exists, the capacity for phagocytosis will be limited. Correspondingly an increased activity of the spleen and bone marrow is recognizable.

Angiography. Angiography will demonstrate only a nonspecific picture, with the exception of attenuated vessels, which are stretched out. Angiography is not indicated in fatty infiltration [14].

Diagnostic Procedure. Although fatty infiltration is a histologic diagnosis, CT is the radiologic method of choice because by measuring hepatic density one can directly quantify the degree of fatty infiltration. This is important, particularly when following the course of liver disease or when using liver toxic medication (Fig. 7). US and scintigraphy are not specific.

Circumscribed Liver Diseases

Table 1 shows the most important focal diseases of the liver.

X-ray. Echinococcus, hemangiomas, hepatoblastomas and a few other have calcifications in about 3 – 33% [19] and can be detected by X-ray (Fig. 8). With regard to all circumscribed liver diseases, calcified focal lesions are very uncommon. Therefore X-ray is not a screening method to diagnose focal liver defects.

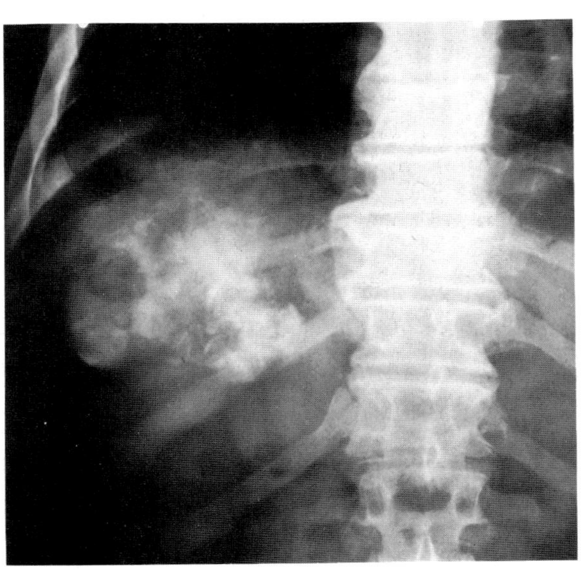

Fig. 8. X-ray shows calcified echinococcal cysts

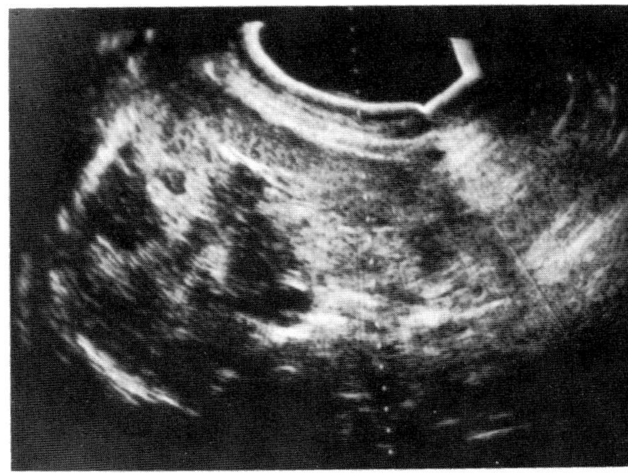

Fig. 9. Hepatic metastases usually yield reduced echoes

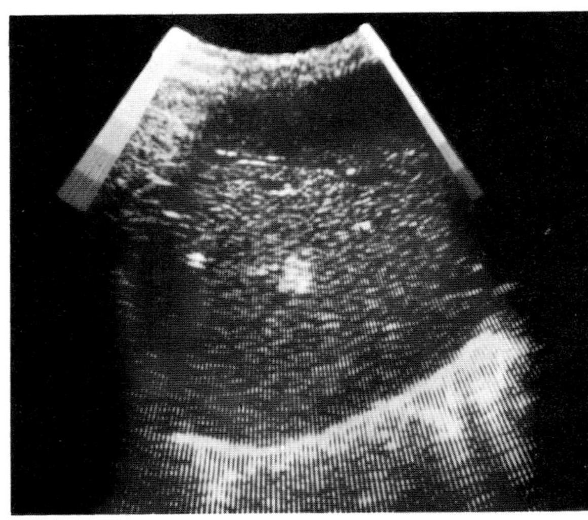

Fig. 10. Echogenic metastases from gastrointestinal tract

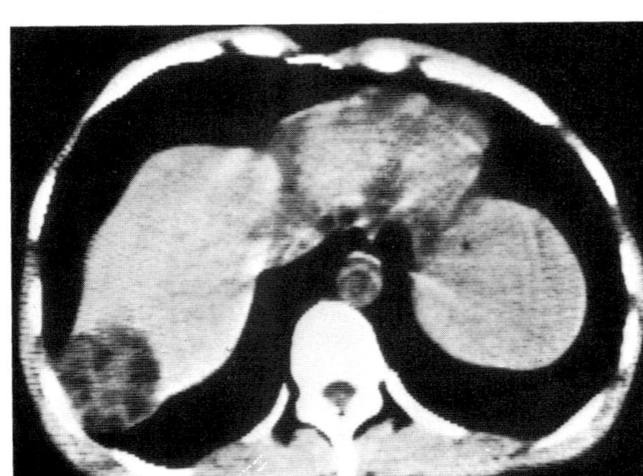

Fig. 11. Multiple secondary cysts in hydatid disease

Sonography. Focal liver alterations normally yield reduced echoes (Fig. 9). This is true for an overwhelming majority of metastatic tumors, which in addition often show a well-defined marginal border [13, 20, 25]. Echogenic focal lesions of the liver (Fig. 10) occur primarily in metastases from the gastrointestinal tract [20]. Also, hemangiomas and focal nodular hyperplasia are echogenic due to the numerous vascular walls and fibrous tissue septa [6, 10, 26]. Areas without echo correspond to hepatic cysts. The existence of multiple secondary cysts is characteristic of hydatid disease (Fig. 11) [23].

Abscesses often cannot be differentiated with certainty from a necrotic decaying tumor [30]. According to the literature, diagnostic accuracy for ultrasonic detection of focal liver alterations lies between 72% and 90% [2, 7, 8, 9, 12, 13, 17, 24]. Correct differential diagnosis is much more difficult and will be accurate only when differentiating between cystic and solid masses.

Radionuclide Imaging. Focal defects larger than 2 cm in diameter will be demonstrated by liver scintigraphy. True positive findings are normally supported with high accuracy, according to various authors in the vicinity of 96% [2, 3, 5, 7, 17, 24]. False positive findings are rather frequently mainly due to a deep gallbladder fossa, costal grooves, or aberrant formations.

Computed Tomography. The most exact diagnosis of focal hepatic alterations is possible with CT; sensitivity varies between 81% and 96%, and specificity, between 80% and 90% [2, 3, 6, 9, 21, 22]. A correct differential diagnosis is possible in about 69% of focal liver diseases [22]. This high accuracy is possible by measuring the density before and after administration of the contrast medium and by computed tomographic arteriography of the liver [18]. This technique is recommended in the evaluation of selected patients, especially when there is a discrepancy between findings by other methods. Depending on the density of the process one can recognize focal alterations from the size of 0.5 to 1 cm (Fig. 12). Intrahepatic calcifications are easily detected.

Even with density measurements correct differential diagnosis between necrotic metastases, abscesses, and cysts can be difficult. In the case of similar density values, analysis of the border is often decisive (Fig. 13).

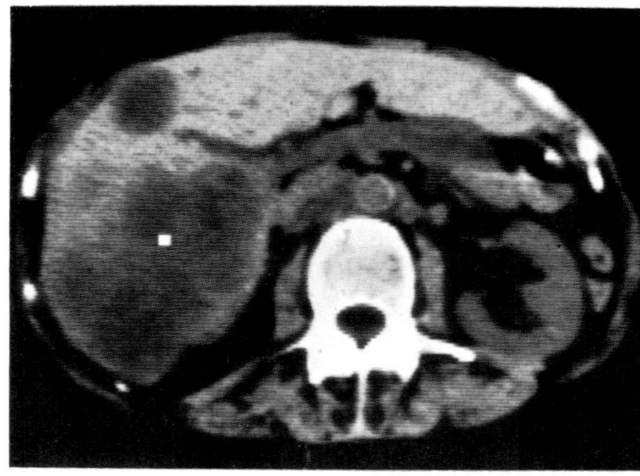

Fig. 12. CT findings in hepatic metastases: multiple areas of decreased density

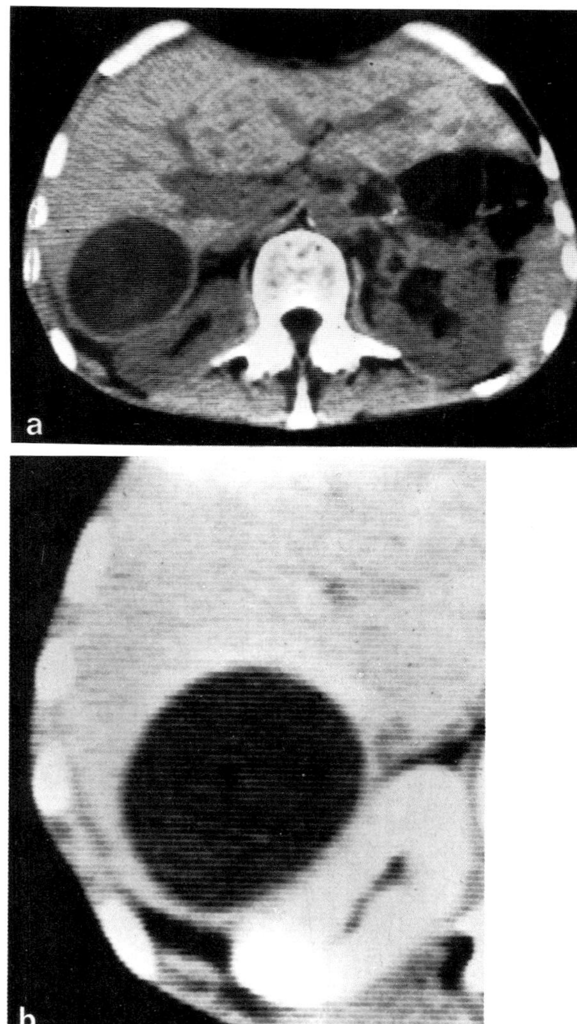

Fig. 13a, b. Pyogenic liver abscess: A decreased density (18 HU). Enhancement shows a border of increased density due to inflammatory hypervasculisation

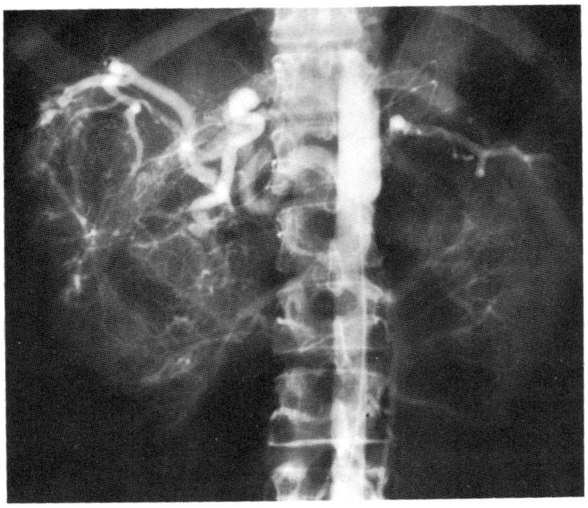

Fig. 14. Hypervascularization in FNH demonstrated by angiography

Angiography. Prior to the introduction of CT and US the task of angiography was to clarify defects shown on the liver scintigram [15, 17]. According to the literature (listed in [14]) the accuracy of diagnosing hepatic metastases is between 80% and 85%, the average value for sensitivity being 90% and for specificity, 80%.

Tumors of the liver are always supplied by the hepatic artery. Positive finding of tumorous vessels is possible only by direct catheterization of the hepatic artery (Fig. 14).

Portography permits the indirect diagnosis of focal alterations only by observing vascular displacement, which means that only focal processes larger than 2 – 3 cm are detectable [4].

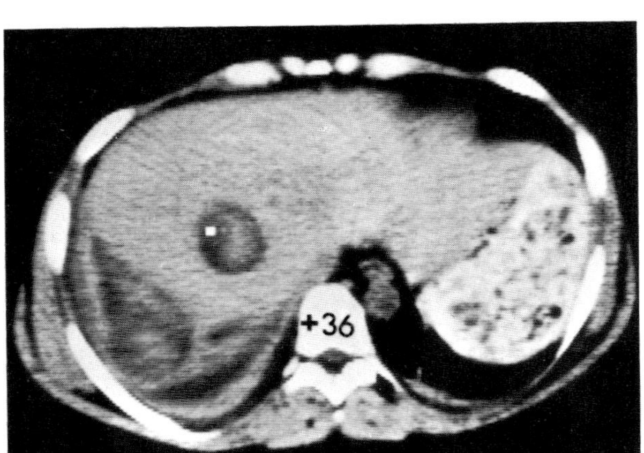

Fig. 15. Intrahepatic bleeding causes an increased density and can be evaluated by CT, as can the perihepatic hematoma

Diagnostic Procedure. There are different plans for the diagnosis of focal liver disease. The value of liver scintigraphy as a noninvasive screening method is well known, because of its high sensitivity (literature is listed in [2, 9]).

Some authors prefer a combination of scintigraphy and sonography [2, 9], others a combination of scintigraphy and CT [7, 24]. We prefer diagnostic US as a screening method because of the low costs. If there is discrepancy between the findings, CT should be used.

Because of its invasiveness, arteriography is ruled out as a screening method for focal liver diseases. Before an operation arteriography is most important to depict the vascular anatomy of the liver circulation.

Hepatic Trauma

Sonography. Sonography is a suitable method for the visualization of bleeding ruptures. A few days after the trauma, the size and the extent of the hematoma and of the perihepatic fluid collection can be measured.

Often ultrasonography cannot be used in recently traumatized patients because of excessive intestinal gas and dressings or incisions of the abdominal wall.

CT is the best method for these patients, because it depicts not only the hepatic rupture but the bleeding itself and also the size of the perihepatic hematoma [1] (Fig. 15). If CT is not available, scintigraphy can visualize the defect of parenchyma corresponding to rupture.

Arteriography displays ruptures of the parenchyma with an accuracy similar to that of CT. The advantage of liver arteriography consists in the identification of the vascular anatomy, for example, before resection of part of the liver, and also in the identification of traumatic arteriovenous, arterioportal, or arteriobiliary fistulae not detectable by CT.

Interventional Radiology

In recent years CT and US, as noninterventional methods, have been increasingly used. Nevertheless invasive methods are becoming more and more important, for example, the percutaneous

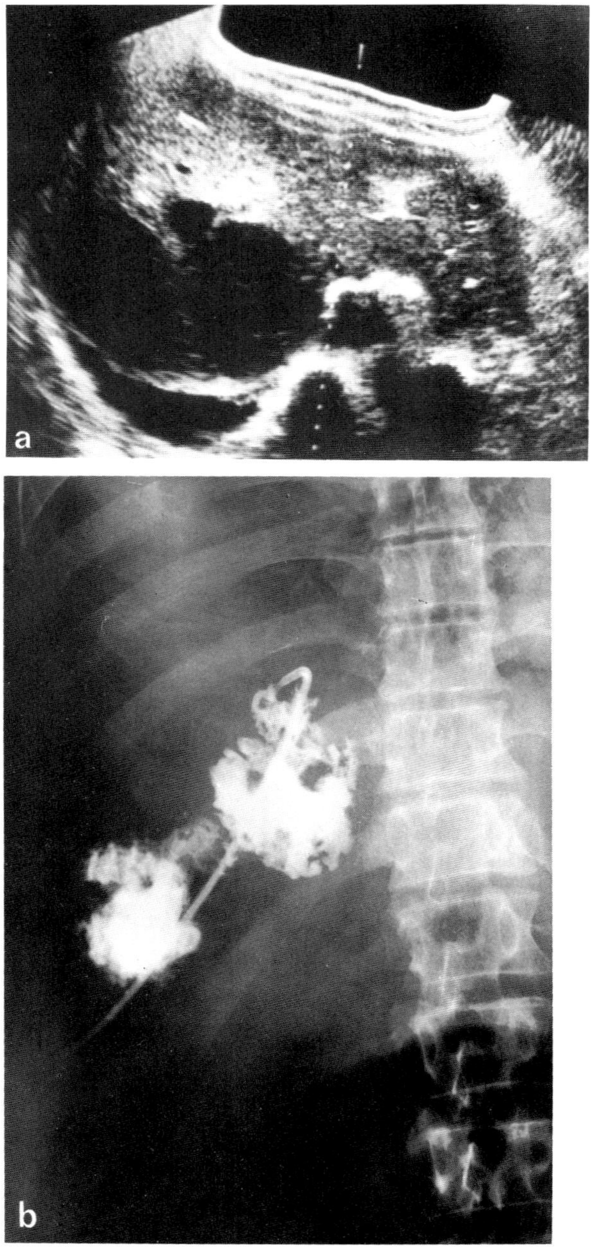

Fig. 16. a Pyogenic liver abscess; **b** percutaneous transhepatic drainage guided by US

transhepatic obliteration of esophageal varices and the embolization of angiomatous liver processes or percutaneous abscess drainage. Let us demonstrate a case (Fig. 16): Through transcutaneous drainage and instillation of antibiotics into the abscess cavity, laparotomy was rendered unnecessary. These methods have become possible by the use of needle puncture guided by US or CT.

Conclusions

CT and US have brought about a change in radiologic diagnosis of the liver. Until a few years ago, arteriography had been the decisive method to verify parenchymal defects diagnosed by scintigraphy. Increasingly the two methods, CT and US, have made possible accurate differential diagnosis. US with less costs and personnel should be used in the first instance. Our own experience shows that in cases where CT is not possible a combination of scintigraphy and US will yield the same good results as CT.
The value of angiography lies in the preoperative visualization of the vascular supply and in the visualization of the hepatocentral or hepatofugal circulation in cases of portal hypertension. The importance of interventional-therapeutic radiology will increase, e.g., transcutaneous abscess drainage guided by US or CT, transhepatic obliteration of esophageal varices, and US- or CT-guided biopsy of focal liver defects.

References

1. Brecht G, Lackner K, Janson R, Thurn P (1980) Die Computertomographie in der Notfalldiagnostik. ROEFO 132:282
2. Bryan PJ, Dinn WM, Grossman ZD, Wistow BW, McAfee JG, Kieffer StA (1977) Correlation of computed tomography, gray scale ultrasonography and radionuclide imaging of the liver in detecting space-occupying processes. Radiology 124:387
3. Büll U, Scherer U (1979) Statische und dynamische Szintigraphie der Leber versus Computertomographie. In: Bessler W, Schaub W (eds) Jahrbuch der Gesellschaft für Radiologie und Nuklearmedizin. Wintherthur
4. Burcharth F (1979) Percutaneous transhepatic portography. I. Technique and application. AJR 132:177
5. Chafetz N, Taylor A, Alazraki NP, Gosink B (1979) The heterogeneous liver scan: Ultrasound correlation. Radiology 130:201
6. Freeny PC, Vimont TR, Barnett DC (1979) Cavernous hemangioma of the liver. Ultrasonography, arteriography and computed tomography. Radiology 132:143
7. Frick MP, Knight LC, Feinberg SB, Loken MK, Gedgaudas E (1979) Computer tomography, radionuclide imaging and ultrasonography in hepatic mass lesions. Comput Tomography 3:49

8. Gebauer A, Scherer U (1978) Differentialindikation für die Computertomographie und die Ultraschalluntersuchung. Internist (Berlin) 19:568
9. Grossmann ZD, Wistow BW, Bryan PJ, Dinn WM, McAfee JG, Kieffer StA (1977) Radionuclide imaging, computed tomography and gray-scale ultrasonography of the liver: A comparative study. J Nucl Med 18:327
10. Jaschke W, Kaick G (1979) Echographische Diagnostik eines kavernösen Hämangioms der Leber. ROEFO 130:721
11. Joseph AEA, Dewbury KC, McGuire PG (1979) Ultrasound in the detection of chronic liver disease (the "bright liver"). Br J Radiol 52:184
12. Kamin PD, Michael MD, Bernardino E, Green B (1979) Ultrasound manifestations of hepatocellular carcinoma. Radiology 131:459
13. Lutz H, Katterle D, Petzoldt R (1975) Ultraschalldiagnostik von Lebermetastasen. Leber Magen Darm 5:223
14. Münster W (1976) Arteriographische und portographische Diagnostik der Lebererkrankungen. Springer, Berlin Heidelberg New York, Handbuch der Medizinischen Radiologie, vol 12/1, p 59
15. Nebesar RA, Pollard JJ, Stone DL (1966) Angiographic diagnosis of malignant disease of the liver. Radiology 86:284
16. Novy SB, Wallace SW, Goldman AM, Ben-Menachem Y (1974) Pyogenic liver abscess. Radiology 1/121:388
17. Pokieser H, Czembirek H, Mayrhofer M, Urbanek A, Kahn P, Weiss W, Base W (1977) Einsatz und Leistungsbreite von Szintigraphie, Sonographie und Angiographie bei umschriebenen Leberprozessen. Roentgenblaetter 30:53
18. Prando A, Wallace S, Bernardino ME, Lindell MM (1979) Computed tomographic arteriography of the liver. Radiology 130:697
19. Rupp N (1976) Die Nativdiagnostik der Lebererkrankungen im Röntgenbild. Springer, Berlin Heidelberg New York, Handbuch der Medizinischen Radiologie vol 12/1, p 3
20. Scheibe W, Gosink BB, Leopold GR (1977) Gray scale echographic patterns of hepatic metastatic disease. AJR 129:983
21. Scherer U (1978) Computertomographische Untersuchungen der Oberbauchorgane. Internist (Berlin) 19:579
22. Scherer U, Lissner J, Brall B, Eisenburg J, Zrenner M, Schildberg FW (1979) Computertomographie der Leber. ROEFO 130:531
23. Schulze K, Hübener K-H, Klott K, Jens H, Bähr R (1980) Computertomographische und sonographische Diagnostik der Echinokokkose. ROEFO 132:514
24. Snow JH, Goldstein HM, Wallace S (1979) Comparison of scintigraphy, sonography and computed tomography in the evaluation of hepatic neoplasms. AJR 132:915
25. Taylor KJW, Carpenter DA, Hill CR, McCready VR (1976) Gray scale ultrasound imaging. Radiology 119:415
26. Treugut H, Klott H, Hübener KH (1980) Fokale noduläre Hyperplasie der Leber. ROEFO 132:216
27. Triller J (1979) Ultraschallgezielte abdominelle Punktion. Radiologe 19:173
28. Vock P (1979) Computertomographisch gezielte Nadelpunktion. Radiologe 19:182
29. Wolf F, Krönert E (1978) Leber und Gallenwege. Springer, Berlin Heidelberg New York, Handbuch der Medizinischen Radiologie, vol 15/2, p 765
30. Wooten WB, Green B, Goldstein HM (1978) Ultrasonography of necrotic hepatic metastases. Radiology 128:447
31. Zornoza J, Wallace S, Ordonez N, Lukeman J (1980) Fine-needle aspiration biopsy of the liver. AJR 134:331

The Biliary System: Overview

W. Frommhold

Universität Tübingen, Medizinisches Strahleninstitut, Röntgenweg 11, D-7400 Tübingen

Graham and Cole [1] introduced their epoch-making study on oral cholecystography with the following words: "The revolutionary effect on the diagnosis of gastrointestinal conditions which was made possible by the use of the opaque meal has given rise repeatedly to the idea that if, by some means, an opaque substance could be safely introduced into the gall-bladder so that its contour could be seen with the roentgen ray, the diagnosis of many obscure and doubtful cases of cholecystitis might be easy and accurate."

Today, more than 55 years later, it seems that another methodologic revolution has brought about fundamental changes in the diagnosis of the biliary tract system.

Examination procedures like intravenous cholangiography, which back in 1953 [2] seemed to herald completely new diagnostic possibilities for the assessment of the biliary tract system, are loosing ground and are now more being replaced by the noninvasive, complication-free methods of computed tomography (CT) and sonography. Besides that, the technique of endoscopic retrograde cholangiopancreatography (ERCP) has well established itself in the diagnosis of jaundice, and percutaneous transhepatic cholangiography (PTC) already reaches beyond the border between diagnosis and therapeutic measures. There are, furthermore, procedures in nuclear medicine which, since recently, offer possibilities which contribute to an assessment of pathophysiologic functional conditions at the sphincter of Oddi.

The aim of the following survey is to give a critical review of the various examination techniques of the biliary tract, to define the position and value they have today and to give recommendations as to their reasonable tactical use. It is only logical that it should also consider the relationship between cost and benefit in each case.

Today, as in the past, *oral cholecystography* continues to be *the* basic radiologic examination technique [3, 4, 5].

We still find today that a survey film of the right upper abdomen without contrast medium should be taken before the contrast agent is applied, but this does not at all mean that we are unaware of the opinions of other authors [6], who, following retrospective evaluation of a large number of gallbladder examinations, were led to conclude that sensibility in oral examinations performed without first obtaining the survey decreases by only 0.43%. For the individual patient, however, we consider the identification of tiny concrements which are not visualized after application of the contrast agent and the demonstration of a limy bile, porcelain gallbladder or a circumscribed calcification in the wall too important to not have the survey taken.

Such findings obviously do not constitute an indication for CT, a much too costly and sophisticated measure. Let me, however, even at this stage point out that today, whenever there is a suspicion of a disease of the biliary duct system, *ultrasound examination* maintains its position as the first differential diagnostic method after case history, clinical examination and required laboratory examinations have been completed [3]. In the hands of an experienced examiner it constitutes a diagnostic procedure that can also be applied in critical situations, can be repeated as often as necessary, does not put any strain on the patient, and can be considered a totally safe examination. The rapid localization of the gallbladder, which can be readily differentiated by means of the amplified echo of the back wall due to diminished sound wave absorption of the liquid content, the delineation of its shape and size as well as the safe identification of concrements measuring more than 3 – 5 mm are all unquestioned advantages of sonography.

Typical criteria for the identification of stones within the gallbladder are intravesical lucent areas in a dorsal or central position with the characteristic dorsal bandlike acoustic shadows, which are

Radiology Today 1. Ed. by M. W. Donner and F. H. W. Heuck

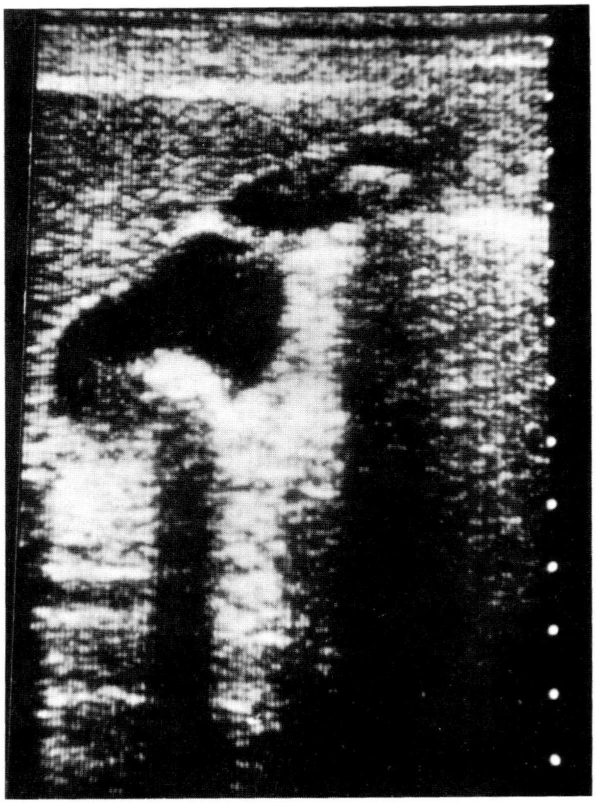

Fig. 1. Ultrasound examination of the gallbladder: Intravesical lucent area with characteristic dorsal bandlike acoustic shadow: cholelithiasis

produced by the reflection of sound waves from the concrements and result in blanks in the contours of the wall at the back side of the gallbladder (Fig. 1). With the rate of success varying between 90% and 99% [7, 8, 9] according to the experience of the examiner, the sonographic examination is at least equal to all the other radiologic examination techniques as far as the diagnosis of stones in the gallbladder are concerned.

Since the identification of calculi is definite by means of sonography, further radiologic differentiation also of the bile ducts becomes unnecessary, knowing that intraoperative cholangiography is performed as a routine measure. On the other hand, additional X-ray imaging is required if a medicamentous litholysis is taken into consideration. This is, however, only possible in the case of noncalcified concrements and if the organ has maintained its ability to contract [10].

It is still a disadvantage of oral cholecystography that it allows a primary assessment of the large bile ducts in no more than 10% of cases. Due to the emptying of the contrast bile after a stimulating fatty meal the percentage of visualization of the common bile duct can be raised to about 20% of the positive fillings of the gallbladder. We cannot approve Hoeffels's point of view according to which a stimulating fatty meal becomes unnecessary in cases of normal visualization of the gallbladder because pathologic findings concerning the bile ducts can only be expected in 0.47% of cases [11].

On the other hand, we share the opinion that disorders in the upper intestinal tract concerning motility and resorption can have an impact on the release of cholecystokinin from the duodenal mucosa and the upper jejunum. That is why the failure of the gallbladder to contract after a stimulating fatty meal is of no pathognomonic significance, all the more so since, vice versa, gallbladders with operatively and histologically secured inflamed lesions of the wall may still respond with good contraction.

In comparison with a fatty meal the use of cholecystokinin-related synthetic substances produces a more reliable and rapid effect. Since the intramuscularly administered substance (dosage, 0.4 μg per kilogram body weight) attacks the muscular apparatus of the wall of the gallbladder directly, the contraction of the gallbladder is performed in less than half the time. A contraction to 60% of the initial size can be observed within 15 – 20 min, whereas the same process after a fatty meal requires 40 – 50 min. The rate of successful visualization of the common bile duct could thus be raised from 10% [12] to 86% [13]. This is of special significance because pathologic changes in the wall of the gallbladder become evident only after intensive contraction. The more frequent diagnosis of adenomyomatoses (in 6% of cases as compared with 0.8% with the conventional application of a fatty meal) is of special significance here [14] (Fig. 2).

Keeping in mind that (a) segments of the wall of the gall bladder with high contractility alone may be the cause of pain symptoms typical of the biliary tract system and (b) that the role they play in the formation of concrements is no longer discussed, parenteral stimulation of the gallbladder seems to be indicated in certain cases even after intravenous or infusion cholecystography which did not respond to the fatty meal or which showed clinical symptoms suggesting a disease of the biliary tract. Basically speaking, the morphological diagnosis of the entire biliary tract cannot be considered complete unless the main bile duct has also been satisfactorily assessed.

The main indications for the application of injection or infusion cholecystangiography can be summarized as follows:

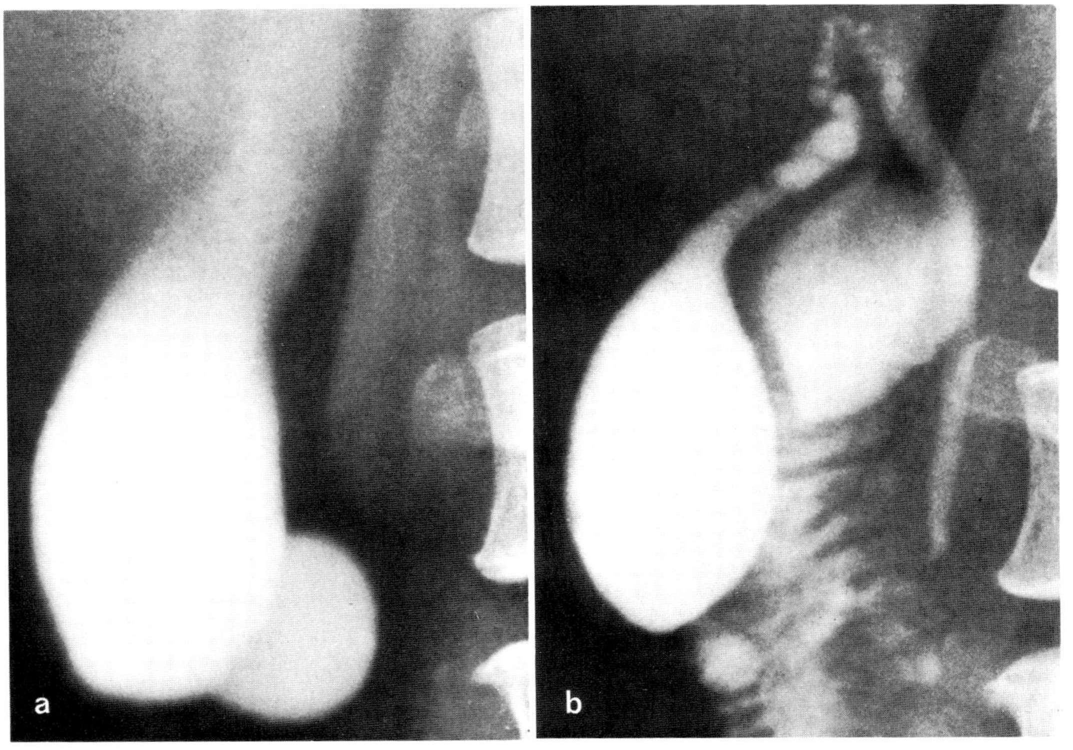

Fig. 2a, b. Oral cholecystography. **a** Before contraction; **b** intensive contraction after intramuscular application of synthetic cholecystokinin (Takus): adenomyomatosis at the fundus of the gallbladder

1. In the case of a normal gallbladder and lack of visualization of the main bile duct on oral cholegraphy, if the presence of clinical symptoms require further investigation. In this context it has to be noted, however, that in contrast to our own experience, some authors hesitate to perform an intravenous examination immediately after completing an unsatisfactory oral cholegraphy, even when the patient is in a sufficiently hydrated condition [15].
2. Preoperatively, after diagnosis of cholecystolithiasis, to exclude or manifest concrements in the bile ducts if intraoperative cholangiography is not determined.
3. For an assessment of the main bile duct after diagnosis of a porcelain gallbladder or of limy bile in the survery film.
4. In cases of lacking or only faint visualization of the gallbladder on oral cholegraphy. In 75% to 80% of these cases visualization of the bile duct system can be achieved by intravenous application of the contrast medium.
5. For an assessment of the bile ducts after cholecystectomy or in cases of cystic duct obstruction [5].

The complication rate of intravenous application of the current commercial preparations is doubtlessly overrated; in this context it is worth noting that the risk of inducing a probably transitory hyperthryroidism in endemic goiter areas is far greater (27.9%) with orally applied contrast media than with intravenous contrast media (15.8%) [16, 17]. Discussions about the pretesting of a contrast agent before the examination have been closed; such pretesting is of no clinical value, and the decision against it has no legal consequences.

General experience shows that tolerance increases considerably if the infusion technique is applied. This method is furthermore characterized by the advantage that even in patients with moderately increased serum bilirubin it produces sufficient diagnostic information in the majority of cases and gives the examiner enough time for additional zonographic or tomographic examinations. The upper limit for a successful visualization of the biliary tract in patients with an increased bilirubin level is estimated today at 4–6 mg % [5]. More recent animal studies carried out by Burgener and Fischer [18] in 1975 and confirmed in a clinical study by Fuchs [19] have shown that only in cases

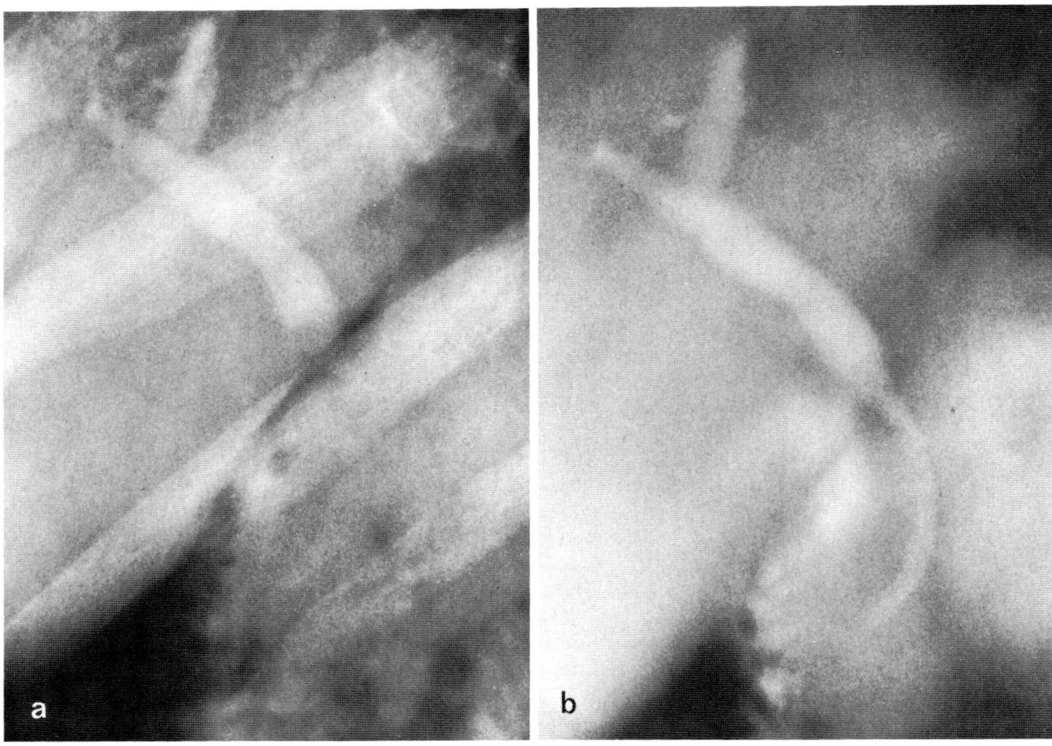

Fig. 3a, b. Intravenous cholecystangiogram. **a** "High blockage" of the common bile duct; **b** tomogram: stenosis of the intrapancreatic part of the common bile duct caused by enlargement of the head of the pancreas in chronic pancreatitis

of incomplete choledochal stenosis will the infusion of higher doses of contrast agents result in higher iodine levels in the hepatic bile and improve visualization of the large bile ducts. Parting from the basic assumption of an "optimum supply of the contrast medium" [20], to the functional activity of the hepatic cell and to the prehepatic transport capacity of the albumin vehicle [21], the rate of excretion of the contrast agent decreases as obstruction of the common bile duct increases. In cases of complete obstruction, the iodine concentration required for radiographic visualization of the bile ducts is never attained. Prolonged infusion time does not improve results. Burgener's observations on animal experiments seem to be quite interesting in this context; he found the alkaline phosphatase level to be a better parameter to determine the probability of successful visualization of the gallbladder than the traditionally used serum bilirubin level and liver enzyme values [22]. Recently these findings have been proven clinically [23].

With the help of zonography and tomography [24, 25], on the other hand, the evaluation of the common bile duct is raised to 80%–85% of all cases examined. Apart from the identification of inflammatory, scarred and tumorous processes in the common bile duct, there may also be indications of space-occupying lesions in the area of the head of the pancreas (Fig. 3). Intravenous cholangiography serves in particular to demonstrate concrements in the bile duct. Large-scale surgical statistics have shown that cholecystolithiasis is associated with choledocholithiasis in 25% of all cases. Therefore residual stones are the most common cause (36%) of "second-look" operations of the biliary tract [26]. The preoperative detection of stones in the common bile duct is complicated by the fact that the clinically particularly relevant tiny concrements float freely in the biliary ducts and may possibly evade detection by temporary intrahepatic location.

The diameter of the common bile duct after cholecystectomy may only partially be seen as an indication of mechanical obstruction. From a diameter of 10 mm upward, however, a bilidynamically effective obstruction becomes more and more probable [27] and can be postulated above 15 mm [28]. It has to be noted, however, that not all mechanical obstructions at the papilla provoke dilatation of the common bile duct. In the tomogram, the nonopaque concrement can be recognized easily by the sharp semicircular contours of the contrast agent.

A papillary stenosis as secondary cholangitis of the terminal choledochal segment is represented by a prolonged rigid and extended papillary canal with mostly irregular contours and without displacement of other choledochal segments. In the majority of cases, it is caused by irritation and bacterial flora due to disorder of the bile flow and can be attributed to cholangiolithiasis in roughly 90% of cases.

Although this type of disorder usually results in an only moderate dilatation of the common bile duct, cases with extreme dilatation have also been observed, which might falsely be interpreted as a tumorous process. On a survey radiograph, stones in the pancreatic duct are in nearly all cases interpreted as concrements in the choledochal segment close to the papilla, especially in the presence of cholelithiasis, although there are no clinical signs indicating an obstruction of the bile flow. Only cholangiography will give full information on the topographic situation [25].

Especially in cases of patients with complaints after cholecystectomy without demonstration of calculi, i.e., in cases of so-called postcholecystectomy syndrome, technical progress in radiology and nuclear medicine in addition to new morphological findings has given us great insight into the dynamic functions of the bile ducts.

The introduction of the *hepatobiliary sequential scintigraphy* with the use of 99mTc-marked HIDA derivatives like diethyl-IDA facilitated the procurement of new information on the bile flow [29]. The substance administered in a dosage of 0.06 mCi per kilogram body weight is excreted via liver and bile into the intestine within 1 h as a rate of 95%. The extension and approximate localization of posthepatic obstruction can be diagnosed with the help of photoscintigrams taken at 30–60 min after injection and with late scans. Investigations into the quantitative aspects of disorders of the bile flow have become possible with the calculation of the hilar passage curve [30]. The analysis of time and activity periods in representative areas of the liver parenchyma and at the hilum of the liver (regions of interest) and subtraction of the parenchyma graph from the hilar graph provided information on the posthepatic, i.e., exclusively biliary, passage of the substance through the liver or the bile-conducting system (Fig. 4). This curve of the hilar passage is characterized by the time needed to reach the maximum level (T_{max}), by the time taken up by the regression from the maximum down to 50% of the maximum ($T_{1/2}$) and the continuity of the bile flow in the phase of exretion.

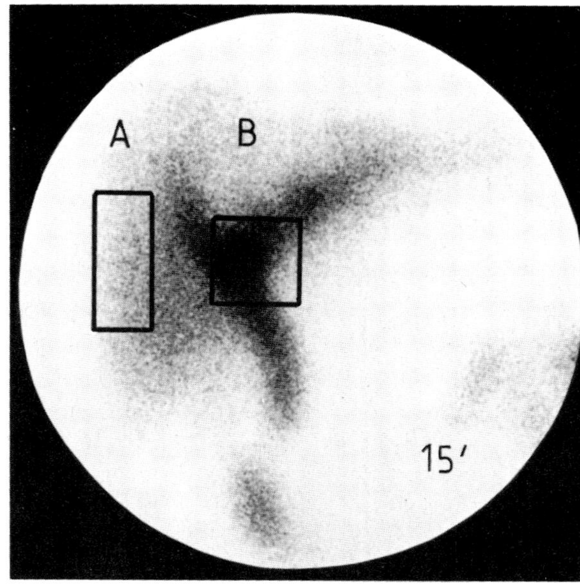

Fig. 4. Hepatobiliary sequential scintigraphy (99mTc-IDA) Regions of interest for evaluating the hilar passage curve. *A,* liver parenchyma; *B,* hilum of the liver

A cholestasis can be diagnosed from a retarded bile passage into the duodenum and a suspected dyskinesia in the papillary area from a discontinuity of the bile flow. Such findings are characteristic above all for patients suffering from the typical complaints of disorders of the bile ducts after cholecystectomy which did not reflect any pathologic changes in laboratory tests or in the morphological appearance as visualized by means of traditional radiologic techniques. We believe they can be associated with a preclinical stage of a bile flow obstruction; further clarification of such findings and the need for therapeutic measures in particular should be orientated on the severity of the symptoms (Figs. 5, 6).

In the case of a lower choledochal obstruction with prestenotic dilatation of the proximal segments, differential diagnosis must include the possibility of a papillary carcinoma and also an inflammatory swelling of the papilla in the presence of concrements. *Hypotonic duodenography* can be of great diagnostic value in many cases. If a high blockage of the common bile duct is observed a carcinoma of the head of the pancreas must also be taken into consideration. If one considers that due to the fact that opacification of the biliary ducts in these cases is poor anyhow, one can readily recognize the limits of the common radiologic examination techniques [25].

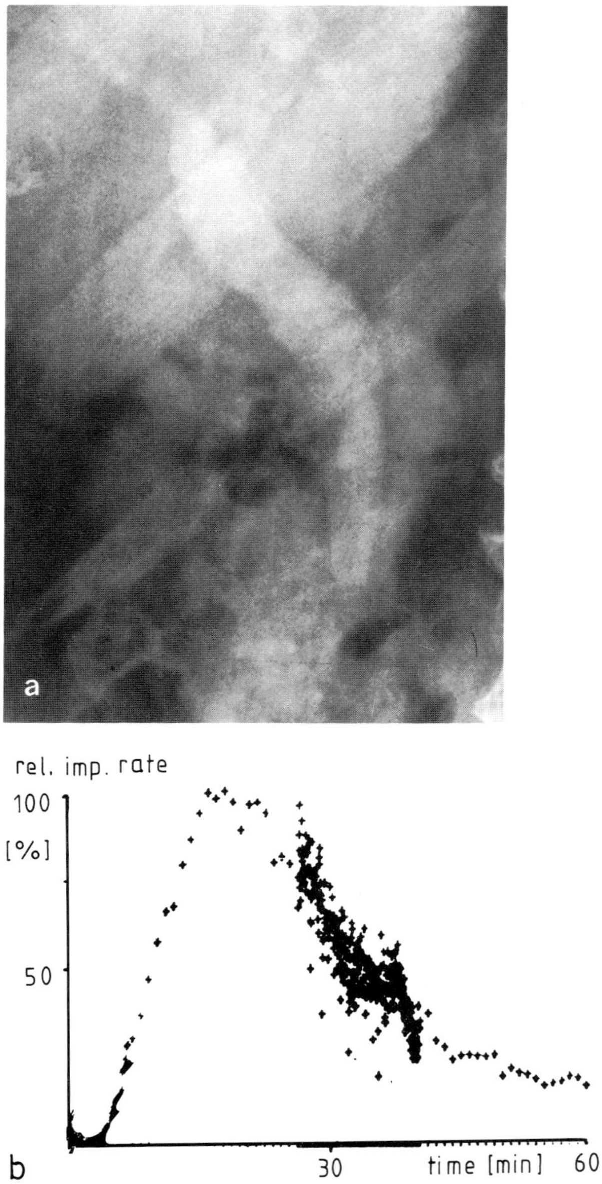

Fig. 5a, b. Quantitative hepatobiliary cholescintigraphy. **a** Intravenous cholangiogram after cholecystectomy: moderate dilatation of the common bile duct. **b** Hilar passage curve: rapid and continuous decrease of the activity: normal flow (4 mCi 99mTc-IDA)

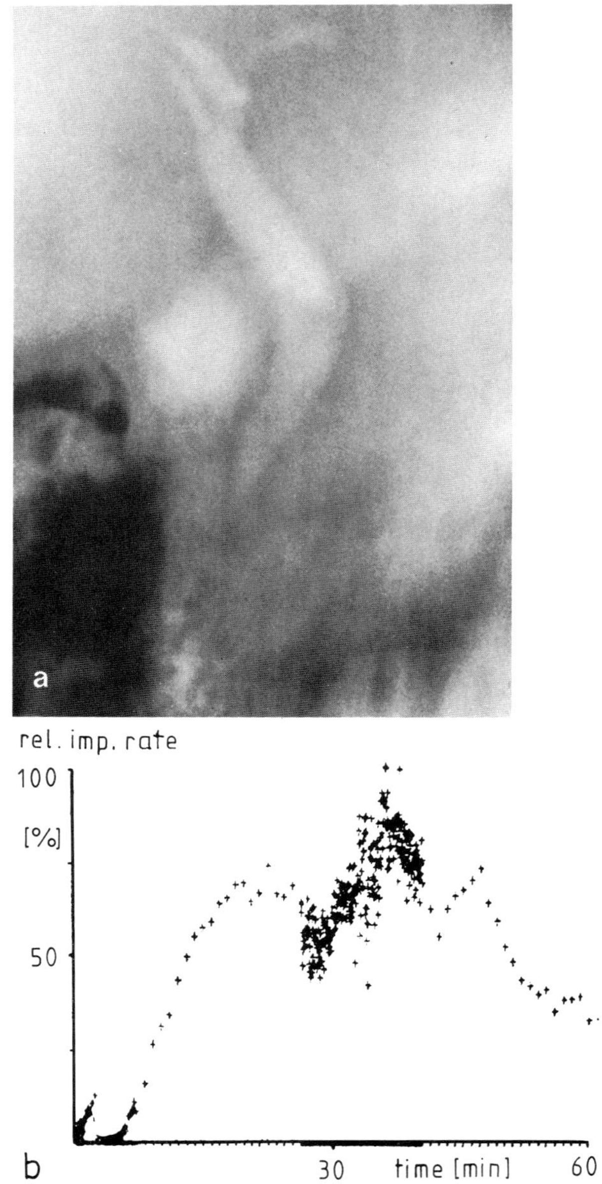

Fig. 6a, b. Quantitative hepatobiliary cholescintigraphy. **a** Intravenous cholangiogram after cholecystectomy; tomogram: mild dilatation of the common bile duct, elongated terminal choledochal segment. **b** Hilar passage curve: delayed and discontinuous decrease of the activity: dyskinesia and partial obstruction of the common bile duct caused by a papillary stenosis

Cases like these are typical indications for ERCP or PTC. The two methods do not compete with but supplement each other, with the main indication for PTC being jaundice. Consistently, the indications for ERCP can be derived from the routine examination methods discussed so far; main criteria are, apart from an intolerance of contrast agents, a suspected disease of the bile ducts on negative or inadequate cholangiogram or suspected pathologic changes in the distal choledochus or the papilla of Vater.

Jaundice patients should undergo ERCP only if there are consequences to be drawn from the endoscopic diagnosis. In the case of an extrahepatic obstruction, the type of stenosis is very likely to be clarified by ERCP (Fig. 7). One has, however, to

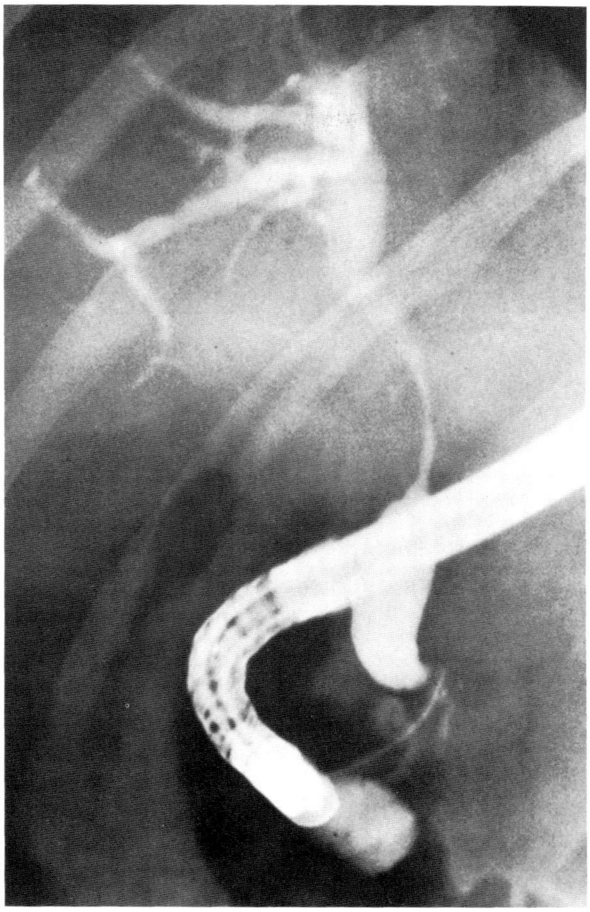

Fig. 7. ERCP: stenosis of the midportion of the common bile duct in a 55-year-old icteric patient. Operation revealed carcinoma of the common bile duct

reckon with the real danger that in cases of incomplete obstruction the obstructed passage of the contrast agent after retrograde administration may pave the way for the development of cholangitis [31]. On the other hand, the method allows endoscopic sphincterotomy, drainage of the bile ducts by means of inserting a catheter for lower choledochal obstruction, and extraction of stones from the choledochal duct.

In cases where ERCP is unsuccessful or if, in jaundiced patients, there is reason to suspect a more or less total blockage of the biliary tract caused by a tumor in the bile ducts or at the head of the pancreas or by an occlusive prepapillary concrement, PTC is the method of choice (Fig. 8). With growing dilatation of the intrahepatic bile ducts to be established by sonography [32, 33] or CT, the rate of success in evaluating the topographic – anatomic localization and in demonstrating the morphology of a bile duct obstruction increases to between 82% and 99% [34, 35]. Moreover there is the possibility of an external bile drainage and of internal recanalization by means of a catheter in inoperable cases.

The complication rate in PTC has been defined merely by a 0.5% mortality rate and by bile extravasation or bile peritonitis in 2% – 5% of cases. By using the Chiba needle extravasation of bile can be lowered to 2%.

The improvement of methodologic aids and the reduction in risk this involved raises the point whether the new, noninvasive methods like *sonography* or *CT* if they produced equally valuable diagnostic information, would not allow the abandonment of invasive examination procedures. In the differential diagnosis of disorders of the biliary tract, just as in connection with other organic diseases, there are voices to be heard who, after critical evaluation of the different examination procedures, conclude that for identification of the cause of obstruction in mechanical jaundice PTC is superior to sonography and to CT [36].

On the other hand, centers with profound experience in CT draw attention to the danger of underrating the possibility of complications in PTC. It has been shown in angiography [37] and in the refined CT diagnosis that using PCT considerable intrahepatic bleeding, partly with bile extravasation, occurs in about 15% of cases. Therefore, they conclude, the application of PTC is only justified if the therapeutic consequences of external bile drainage determine the method [38].

Thus beyond any doubt *sonography* is to be considered the primary diagnostic procedure in cases of obstructive jaundice; at least its results determine further action toward a more precise diagnosis [39, 40]. The rate of success of a sonographic examination as regards the identification of the type of jaundice reaches 97%, whereas the exact etiology can only be determined in roughly 60% of cases [7, 39]. More than in any other examination technique, however, the success rate in sonography is strongly dependent on the experience of the examiner.

The diagnostic advantages of *CT* become clearly evident if an increased bilirubin level makes intravenous or infusion cholangiography impossible or if further differentiation by sonography cannot be achieved due to overshadowing of air in the intestinal loops. This is especially true for the evaluation of the common bile duct, which passes behind the duodenum and is unidentifiable in 20% of cases because of overshadowing by air. Since the density resolution of CT is very sensitive it is possible to differentiate the wall of the gallbladder in inflammatory processes from the mostly thick-

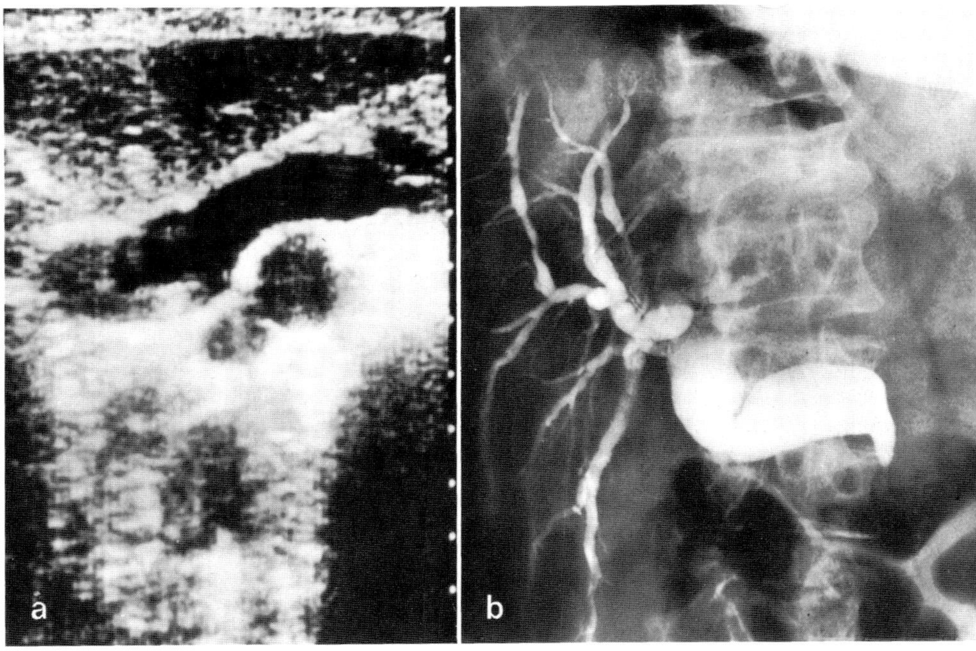

Fig. 8a, b. 70-year-old icteric female patient. **a** Sonography: considerably dilated common bile duct. **b** PTC: complete stenosis of the common bile duct. Operation revealed carcinoma of the head of the pancreas

ened vesical bile and to determine the localization of neoplasms together with their extension and relations to neighboring organs. This applies in particular to malignant tumors in the large bile ducts. Moreover, it is possible to differentiate an obstruction caused by a lower concrement from an obstruction caused by tumorous growth, and even differentiation from a carcinoma of the pancreas is possible in the majority of cases (Fig. 9). A hydrops of the gallbladder, which can be differentiated from the empyema by a considerable thickening of the wall of the gallbladder and high density values of the bile, can mostly be identified by CT with the demonstration of the course of the large bile ducts by means of thin contiguous cross sections (Fig. 10). Valuable information can also be obtained in cases of so-called excluded gallbladder and cholestasis [41]. Inoperability of tumors can be detected if the invasive growth of the tumor into other organs can be recognized. Thus, it is possible to save severely ill jaundiced patients from unnecessary invasive diagnostic procedures and from operations (Fig. 11).

Computed tomography is always justified for patients whose prior case history, diagnostic and laboratory findings and sonographic examination did not definitively determine the cause of jaundice. After inadequate sonographic results it has certainly to be preferred to invasive examination techniques.

The critical, rather restrictive attitude toward CT, in which we differ from the approach taken by other authors [42], is among other things also based on cost-benefit estimations, which simply have to be taken into consideration today (Table 1). It is especially in this context that we must see the indications for the costly diagnostic procedure

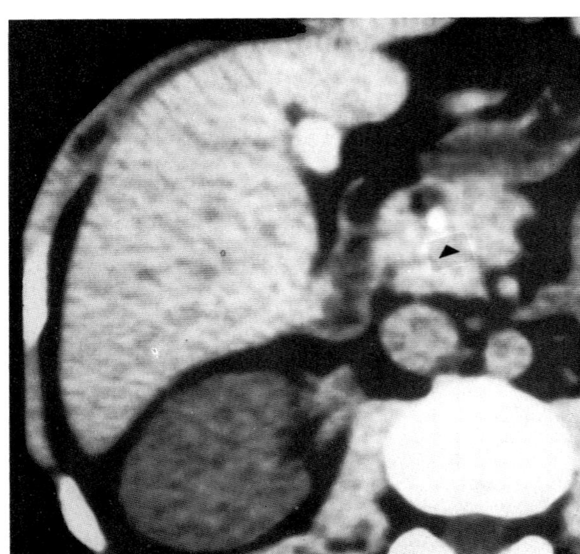

Fig. 9. CT in 36-year-old patient with pain in the right upper abdomen. Small concrement in a moderate dilated common bile duct. Cholelithiasis

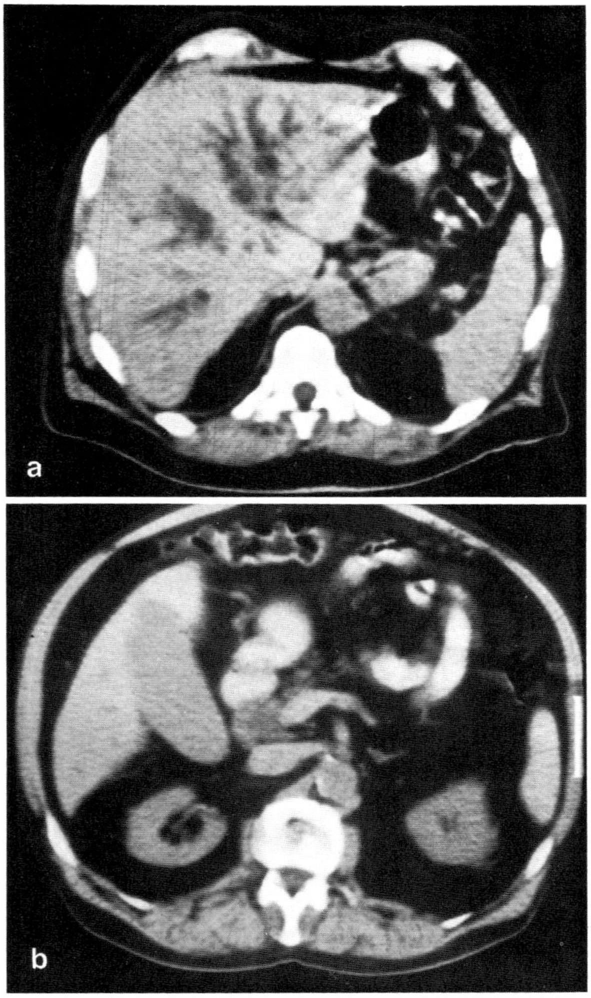

Fig. 10a, b. CT. Extrahepatic cholestasis in a 62-year-old patient. **a** Dilated intrahepatic bile ducts. **b** Hydrops of the gallbladder. Operation revealed papillary carcinoma

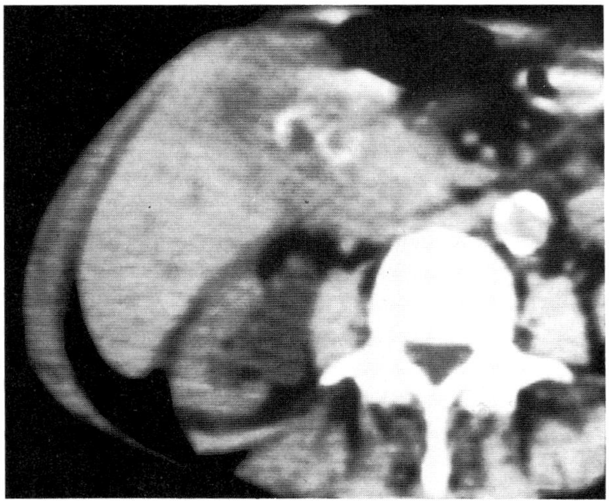

Fig. 11. CT in 72-year-old female patient. Carcinoma of the gallbladder with infiltrative growth in the liver parenchyma. Cholelithiasis. Hydronephrosis caused by lymph node metastasis

Table 1. The cost of various diagnostic procedures (based on figures provided by the German insurance company, AOK, in April 1980)

Procedure	Cost DM
Sonography (two organs)	50. –
Oral cholecystography (four films)	61. –
Intravenous cholangiography (four films)	61. –
Scintigraphy	89. –
PTC (four films)	86. –
ERCP	150. –
Computed tomography	300. –

of CT not only in the light of professional criteria but also in terms of the social responsibility which we have to accept in our profession as long as no disadvantages arise for our patients.

References

1. Graham EA, Cole WH (1924) Roentgenologic examination of the gallbladder: preliminary report of a new method utilizing the intravenous injection of tetra-brom-phenolphthalein. JAMA 82:613
2. Frommhold W (1953) Ein neuartiges Kontrastmittel für die intravenöse Cholezystographie. ROEFO 79: 283
3. Berk RN, Leopold GR (1978) The present status of imaging of the gallbladder. Invest Radiol 12/6:477
4. Suramo I, Lanning P, Lahti R (1979) Comparison of ultrasound and roentgen examination of biliary tract. Diagn Imaging 48:138
5. Whalen JP (1979) Caldwell lecture. Radiology of the abdomen: Impact of new imaging methods. AJR 133:585
6. Andersen JF, Madsen PER (1979) The value of plain radiography to oral cholecystography. Radiology 133:309
7. Triller J, Fuchs WA (1980) Abdominale Sonographie. Thieme, Stuttgart
8. Braun B, Schwenk W (1978) Ultraschalldiagnostik der Cholelithiasis. Ein Vergleich mit röntgenologischen Untersuchungsverfahren. Dtsch Med Wochenschr 103:1101
9. Crade M, Taylor KJW, Rosenfield AT, de Graaff CS, Minihan P (1978) Surgical and pathologic correlation of cholecystosonography and cholecystography. AJR 131:227
10. Wolpers C (1976) Auswahl der Gallensteinträger zur Litholyse. Leber Magen Darm 6/1:43
11. Hoeffel J-C, Burger G, Senot P, Claudon M (1980) Oral cholecystography: Is the fatty meal always necessary? Radiologe 20:24

12. Hippéli R, Eibach E (1979) Rationelle kombinierte Röntgenuntersuchung von Gallenblase und Magen. Leber Magen Darm 9:111
13. Schindler G, Pirschel J, Grehn S (1979) Optimierung der peroralen Cholezyst-Cholangiographie mit Ceruletid. ROEFO 130:423
14. Strik WO, Züchner F, Fleischer K, Longin F (1976) Ergebnisse von 11699 Cholezysto- und Cholangiographien. Therapiewoche 26:7462
15. Ansell G (1976) Complications in diagnostic radiology. Chapter II: Oral and intravenous cholegraphy. Blackwell, Oxford London Edinburgh Melbourne
16. Steidle B, Grehn S, Seif FJ (1979) Jodinduzierte Hyperthyreose durch Kontrastmittel. Dtsch Med Wochenschr 104:1435
17. Seif FJ, Stöckle G, Grehn S, Steidle B (1980) Changes of thyroid hormones, thyrotropin, and prolactin after application of iodinated radiographic media in patients of an endemic goiter area. J Mol Med 4:211
18. Burgener FA, Fischer HW, Adams JT (1975) Intravenous cholangiography in different degrees of common bile duct obstruction. An experimental study in the dog. Invest Radiol 10:342
19. Fuchs WA, Preissig R (1975) Prolonged drip-infusion cholangiography. Br J Radiol 48:539
20. Mayer-Burg J, Wilhelmi U (1969) Die Infusions-Cholecysto-Cholangiographie. Eine Verbesserung der röntgenologischen Ergebnisse durch Applikation optimaler Kontrastmitteldosen. ROEFO 111:641
21. Kölling K, Schoen D (1970) Über den Einfluß der Serumbindungskapazität auf den Kontrast im Cholangiocystogramm. ROEFO 113:372
22. Burgener FA (1981) Biliary iodipamide and iodoxamate excretion as function of basal bile flow in normal, common bile duct obstructed and liver-damaged dogs. ROEFO 134:40
23. Zeman R, Taylor KJW, Burell MI, Gold J (1980) Ultrasound demonstration of anicterie dilatation of the biliary tree. Radiology 134:689
24. Frommhold W (1977) The biliary tract system-A challenge to diagnostic radiology. J Belg Radiol 60:411
25. Frommhold W, Frommhold H (1974) Leistungsfähigkeit und Grenzen der intravenösen Cholangiografie in der Pankreasdiagnostik. Leber Magen Darm 4:212
26. Hess W (1977) Nachoperationen an den Gallenwegen. Enke, Stuttgart
27. Sparkman RS, Lovett VF (1961) Preoperative cholangiography. Ann Surg 154:75
28. Schindler G, Küper K (1979) Lecture at IV. European Congress of Radiology, Hamburg 1979
29. Rosenthall L, Schaffer EA, Losbona R, Pare P (1978) Diagnosis of hepatobiliary disease by 99m-TC-HIDA cholescintigraphy. Radiology 126:467
30. Schindler G (1980) Habilitationsschrift, University of Tübingen
31. Wienbeck M, Ley HG, Miller B, Lenz W, Hausamen TU (1975) Cholangitis als tödliche Komplikation der endoskopischen retrograden Cholangio-Pankreatikographie (ERCP). Fortschr Gastroenterol Endoskopie 6:143
32. Conrad MR, Landay MJ, Janes JO (1978) Sonographic "parallel channel" sign of biliary tree enlargement in mild to moderate obstructive jaundice. AJR 130:279
33. Weill F, Eisencher A, Zeltner F (1978) Ultrasonic study of the normal and dilated biliary tree: "shotgun" sign. Radiology 127:221
34. Ferucci JT, Wittenberg J (1977) Refinements in chiba-needle transhepatic cholangiography. AJR 129:11
35. Jorge A, Lorenzo J, Baro JL, Diaz M, Sanchez D (1979) Perkutane Cholangiografie mit der Chiba-Nadel. Leber Magen Darm 9:131
36. Gold RP, Casarella WJ, Stern G, Seaman B (1979) Transhepatic cholangiography: The radiological method of choice in suspected obstructive jaundice. Radiology 133:390
37. Hoevels J, Nilsson W (1980) Intrahepatic vascular lesions following nonsurgical percutaneous transhepatic bile duct intubation. Gastrointest Radiol 5:127
38. Boijsen E (1980) V. CARVAT-Symposium. Rome, May 1980
39. Dewbury KC, Joseph AEA, Hayes S, Murray C (1979) Ultrasound in the evaluation and diagnostic of jaundice. Br J Radiol 52:276
40. Koenigsberg M, Wiener SN, Walzer A (1979) The accuracy of sonography in the differential diagnosis of obstructive jaundice: A comparison with cholangiography. Radiology 133:157
41. Levitt RG, Sagel SS, Stanley RJ, Jost RG (1977) Accuracy of computed tomography of the liver and biliary tract. Radiology 124:123
42. Heuck F, Buck J (1980) Der Informationswert der Röntgen-Computer-Tomographie für die Beurteilung von Gallenwegen und Gallenblase. Radiologe 20:6

Liver Circulation

H. D. Piroth

Marienhospital, Onkologische und Radiologische Abteilung, Rochusstrasse 2, D-4000 Düsseldorf 30

Introduction

Knowledge of the liver blood flow is an important parameter as far as the clinical evaluation of liver function is concerned. Especially the degree of seriousness and the life-threatening danger of the alterations of liver haemodynamics have to be seen in a direct connection with liver blood flow.
According to Brünner [1] a strong relationship exists between the chance of survival after portovenous shunt operation (Fig. 1) and the kind of anastomosis. Thirty-three percent of patients with a splenorenal shunt and only 14% with a portocaval shunt live 10 more years. This shows that the practically complete diversion of the portal blood flow into the vena cava is compatible with life in only a few cases. Survival for 10 years in patients undergoing splenorenal shunt therefore has to be attributed, at least in some cases, to the existing portal blood flow. However, also in the case of portocaval shunt a small percentage of patients do live longer than 10 years. Therefore we have to assume that – and we find this in the relevant literature – the reduction of the total liver blood flow because of partial or a complete elimination of the portal flow will be compensated by an increase of the flow in the hepatic artery.
Therefore preoperatively the total liver blood flow with the relationship of the arterial and portal flow besides the morphology of the vessels as shown in the angiogram has to be known.

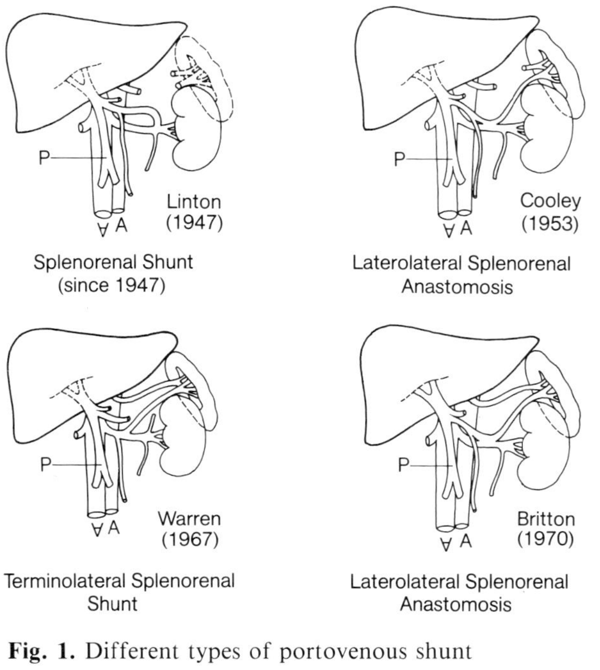

Fig. 1. Different types of portovenous shunt

Methods for Determining Liver Haemodynamics

Electromagnetic Procedures

Electromagnetic registration of flow velocity is one of the methods which have been known for many years and it is occasionally still used today. In its original form it can only be performed at the open vessel. Only recently have Kolin [2] and Mills [3] described a technical improvement of this principle (Fig. 2). Here a tiny wire loop is introduced into the vessel through catheters. After the positioning of an extracorporeal magnetical field, measurement of the intra-arterial flow velocity can be made.

Nuclear-Medical Procedures

Biersack et al. [4] and Thelen et al. [5] have reported a nuclear-medical study of perfusion by which the relationship of the portal to the arterial liver blood flow can be determined. The advantage of this method (Fig. 3) is its simple feasibility without any risk, which makes it possible to repeat

Radiology Today 1. Ed. by M. W. Donner and F. H. W. Heuck

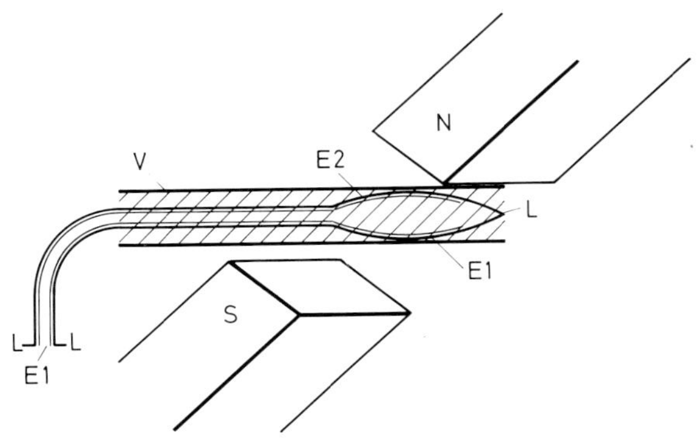

Fig. 2. Principle of electromagnetic flowmeter E1/E2, electrodes; *L,* wire loop; *N* and *S,* magnetic fields; *V,* vessel

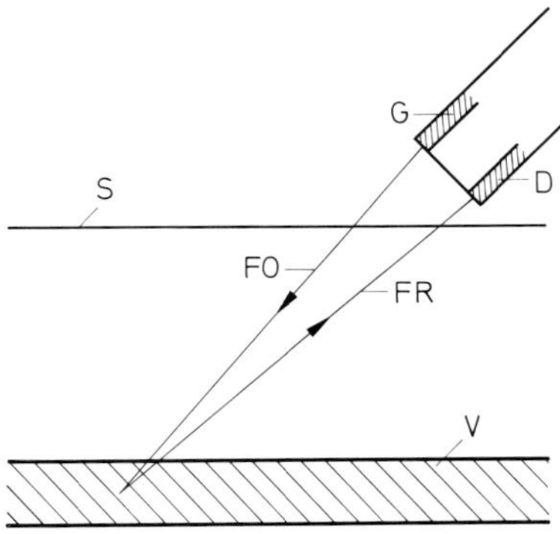

Fig. 4. Principle of Doppler sonography. *S,* body surface; *FO/FR,* emitted and reflected frequencies; *G,* generator; *D,* detector; *V,* vessel

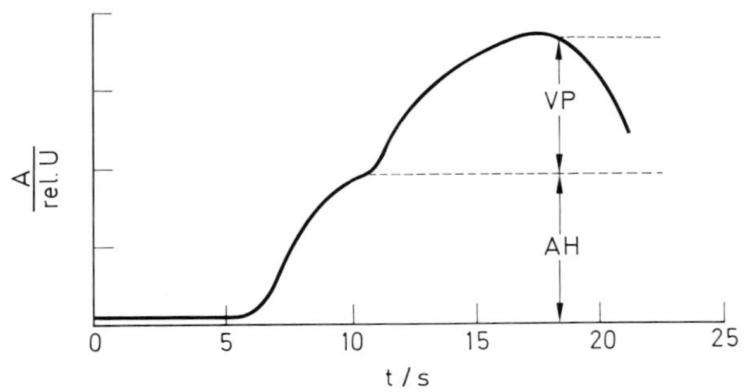

Fig. 3. Nuclear medical perfusion study performed with a gamma-camera. *A,* activity; *VP,* vena portae; *AH,* arteria hepatica; *t,* time

control measurements over a long period. However, an essential disadvantage is the lack of absolute values as far as the blood flow is concerned.

Doppler Sonography

This clinical diagnostic procedure is an already well-known method (Fig. 4) which makes possible measurement of the flow velocity without surgical intervention.

The sound is reflected (by moving blood particles) and the alteration of the frequencies caused by this movement is proportional to the flow velocity. The disadvantages of this method are: penetrance to only a limited depth in the body, dependence of the measurement upon the angle of the vessel to the body surface and the limitation of measurements to vessels wider than 6 mm.

Besides these disadvantages, we are faced with the fact that without any knowledge of the diameter of the vessels it appears impossible to determine the blood flow apart from the clinically less important flow velocity. According to Ulrich et al. [6] the measurements of the vessels with an ultrasound reflector cannot be considered sufficient.

Angiodensitometry

Angiodensitometry is a completion of angiography. This method is exercised as cine- or video-densitometry, depending on whether X-ray cinematography or X-ray videorecording is used for the densitometric measuring of contrast medium in the blood.

Figure 5 demonstrates the principle of measurement: the variation of the light intensity of the X-ray cinematography or video-picture, which is caused by the bolus of contrast medium at the points of measurement, can either be measured by opto-electronic systems or by an electronic video-window in the video-monitor. In this way at both points of measurement typical curves of contrast motion can be registered.

As a first result of angiodensitometric measurement the time "Δt" is determined; this is the time which the blood takes inside the concerned field of vessels for the passage from one point of measurement to the other. In the angiogram the distance between the points of measurement "s" and the diameter of the vessel "d" can be established. Thus it is possible to calculate the flow "F" according the formula:

$$F = \left(\frac{d}{2}\right)^2 \cdot s \cdot 60/\Delta t\,.$$

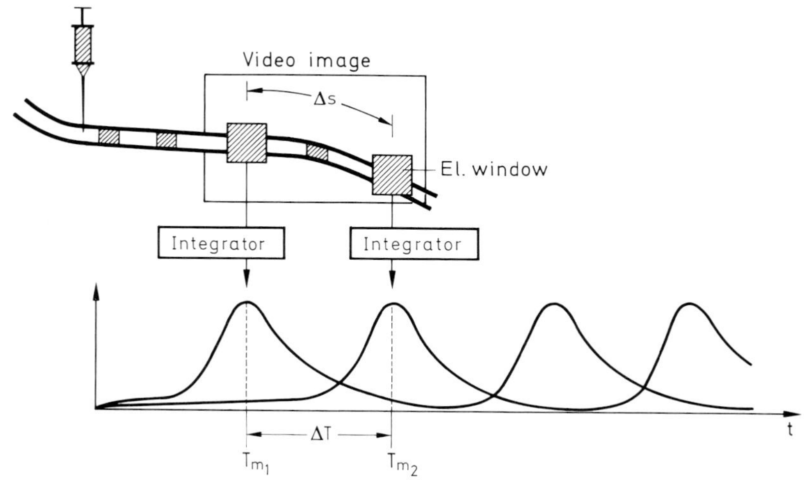

Fig. 5. Principle of angiodensitometric flow measurement

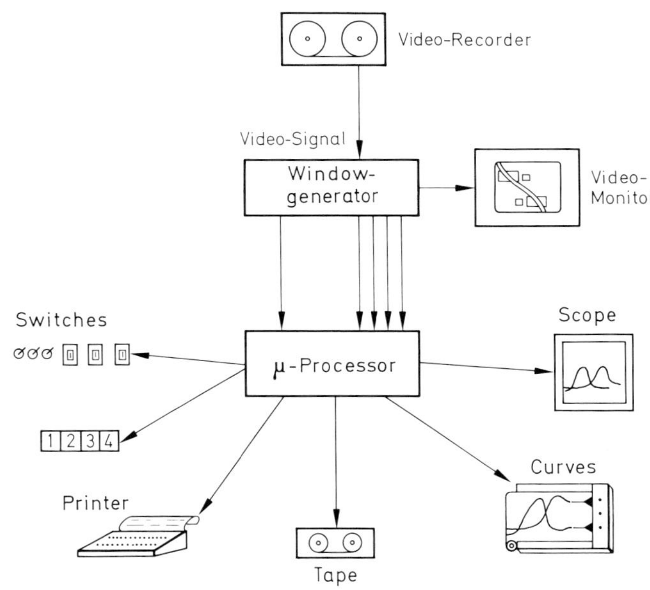

Fig. 6. Videodensitometric system with an integrated microprocessor

The flow is obtained in millilitres/minute when the diameter and the distance are measured in centimetres and time in seconds.
Experimental research with circulation models according to Busch [7] and theoretical studies by Vanselow et al. [8] have demonstrated that especially in the situation of pulsating flow velocity one has to work with small boli of contrast medium. In this way the momentaneous flow velocities of different phases of a heart action and thereby the medium flow value can be determined.
Different parameters have been used as criteria for the running time of the contrast medium between the points of measurement. Vanselow and Heuck [9] work with a contrast medium appearance time, while Rutishauser [10], Lantz [11] and Heintzen et al. [12] calculate the difference of the mean transit time at both points of measurement.
The advantage of determining the appearance time is the simplicity of the method and the invariance of the measuring area. A disadvantage is the systematic overestimation of the flow velocity, which, on the basis of the experimental studies of Vyska [13], can be considered relatively constant. Besides this, the exactitude of the appearance time directly depends on the picture frequency and therefore on the cinematographic equipment.
In contrast to determination of appearance time, determination of the mean transit time is an integral measurement, which considers the various flow profiles of the laminar flow in a blood vessel. On the basis of research with a circulation model,

Busch and Piroth [14] developed a videodensitometric system with an integrated microprocessor (Fig. 6). Besides the background-corrected videodensitometric registration of the passage curves this system permits:

1. A direct video-presentation of the normalized and corrected curves;
2. The automatically and optically directed calculation of the difference of the mean transit time;
3. The calculation and processing of the application of contrast medium depending on the phases of heart action.

Especially Busch [6] demonstrates that a reliable measurement is possible with a few, however, at least four, boli of contrast medium in the case of heart phase-triggered application.

Thus it can be ensured that an acceptable mean value of the various momentaneous velocities of an arterial flow is determined.

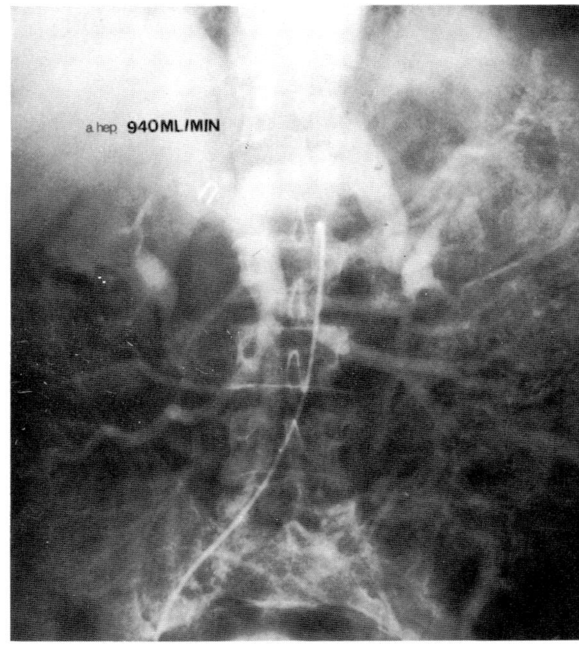

Fig. 7. Splenorenal shunt increasing arterial flow

Results of Angiodensitometric Determination of Liver Haemodynamics

So far only a few reports exist on results of the determination of liver haemodynamics. Felix et al. [15] found good agreement with results given in the literature after cinedensitometric measurements in the vena portae. However, the measurements only concern the vena portae. Widrich et al. [16] made semiquantitative estimations of the portal and arterial liver blood flow by visual evaluation of cinematographic records. Even though these examinations only give information in an orientating way, the authors did observe an increase of the arterial flow within 22 – 36 months after shunt operation. In a similar way Zimmon and Kessler [17] report an increase of the arterial blood flow in the postoperative phase.

As yet there are hardly any reports on the results of simultaneous determinations of arterial and portal flow of an awake patient.

In our own investigations densitometric measurements of arterial and portal flow were carried out in routine splenoportography. In 17 normal patients we found flow values (ml/min) of 540 (s = ± 110) for the a. hepatica communis and 1160 (s = ± 190) for the vena portae. In 51 patients with Liver cirrhosis these values were 660 (s = ± 180) and 590 (s = ± 310) respectively. The results are normalized to a body surface area of 1.73 m^2. We applied about 35 ml (8 ml/s) in the truncus coeliacus or 25 ml in the a. lienalis for the portal flow and five boli of contrast medium with 6 ml (22 ml/s) each in the aorta abdominalis 10 cm above the truncus coeliacus.

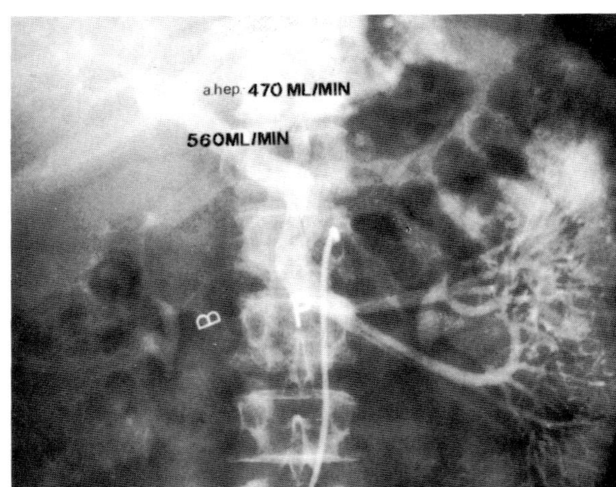

Fig. 8. Mesenterical portography and measurement of arterial and portal flow

The results show the expected reduction of the portal flow, depending on the degree of the cirrhosis, and the increase of the arterial flow (see Fig. 7) as compensation for the portal flow.

By experimental and comparative studies it has been demonstrated that determination of flow by videoangiodensitometry is correct within 15% (see Fig. 8).

Because of the known streamlining phenomena in the vena portae, successive applications of contrast media in the a. mesenterica superior and in the truncus coeliacus were carried out to control the measurements in this special situation. The results with eight patients showed that the measurements are reliable within 15%.

With seven patients it was possible to make a control measurement postoperatively within 6 weeks. In all cases an increase of arterial flow was observed in instances of reduced portal flow (on average, more than 85% over the basic value).

The clinical importance of angiodensitometry can be summarized as follows:

1. The degree of reduction of liver haemodynamics and the relationship of arterial to portal flow can be determined.
2. In the case of reduced portal flow no shunt operation should be performed if the arterial flow is reduced too, for a lack of ability to compensate must be expected.

References

1. Brünner H, Schmidt HD (1977) Möglichkeiten der splenorenalen Anastomose bei portaler Hypertonie. Dtsch Med Wochenschr 102:219 – 222
2. Kolin A, Macalpin R, Steckel R (1978) Electromagnetic rheangiometry-an extension of select angiography. AJR 130:13 – 23
3. Mills CJ (1977) The electromagnetic flowmeter. Med Instrum 11
4. Biersack HJ, Janson R, Malothi D, Thelen M, Winkler C (1977) Sequentielle Hepatospleno-Szintigraphie mit 99mTc-Pertechnetat beim experimentellen posthepatischen Block. ROEFO 127:572 – 574
5. Thelen M, Schutz D, Schild H, Biersack HJ, Frommhold H (1978) Änderungen der Leberhämodynamik nach mesenterikokavaler Dacron-Prothesen-Anastomose (sog. "H-Shunt") bei portaler Hypertension. ROEFO 128/4:423 – 431
6. Ulrich B, Leriot J (1977) Experimentelle Befunde der Leberdurchblutungsmessungen mittels eines Ultraschall-Doppler-Flußgerätes. Z Exp Chir 910
7. Busch HP (1980) Aufnahme und Auswertung videodensitometrischer Durchflußmessungen mittels einer Prozeßrechner gesteuerten Anlage. Thesis, University of Mainz
8. Vanselow K, Heuck F, Deininger KH (1975) Neue Grundlagen und Theorien zur Verbesserung der Angio-Cine-Densitometrie IV. ROEFO 123/5: 468 – 478
9. Vanselow K, Heuck F (1975) Neue Grundlagen und Theorien zur Verbesserung der Angio-Cine-Densitometrie III. ROEFO 123/4:358 – 363
10. Rutishauser W (1969) Kreislaufanalyse mittels Roentgendensitometrie. In: Aktuelle Probleme der Angiodensitometrie, vol 6. Huber, Bern Stuttgart Vienna
11. Lantz B (1973) A methodological investigation of roentgen videodensitometry, a comparison between theoretically computed and experimentally measured contrast. Acta Radiol [Diagn] (Stockh) 14
12. Heintzen R, Malercyk V, Pilarcyk J (1971) Neue Verfahren zur Videodensitometrie und Videometrie. In: Heuck F (ed) Densitometrie in der Radiologie. Thieme, Stuttgart
13. Vyska K, Profant M, Schicha H, Becker V, Freundlieb C, Feinendegen LE (1974) Theoretische Grundlagen der Anwendung der minimalen Transitzeiten für die Bestimmung der Ejektionsfraktion in Herzkammern. 10. Intern. Jahrestagung der Gesellschaft für Nuklearmedizin, 11. – 14. Sept. 1974, Munich
14. Busch HP, Piroth HD (1978) Video-Angio-Densitometrie mittels mikroprozessorgesteuerter Meßwerterfassung und Meßwertverarbeitung. Biomed Tech [Suppl] (Berlin) 24:160
15. Felix R, Bücheler E, Vanselow K, Schulz D, Bayerl W, Schneider H (1972) Cinedensitometrie des Portalkreislaufes. ROEFO 117/5:570 – 586
16. Widrich WC, Robbins AH, Johnson WC, Nabseth DC (1980) Long-Term Follow-up of Distal Splenorenal Shunts. Radiology 134:341 – 345
17. Zimmon DS, Kessler RE (1971) Regulation of portal pressure in man. Gastroenterology 60:169

Radiology of the Pancreas: Overview

A. L. Baert, E. Ponette, and G. Marchal

Katholieke Universiteit Leuven, Universitaire Ziekenhuizen, Diagnostische Radiologie, Capucijnenvoer 35, B-3000 Leuven

Non-invasive Conventional Radiological Methods

Of the many non-invasive conventional radiological methods used for indirect evaluation of the pancreas, the main modalities still used today include: plain film of abdomen and thorax, intravenous cholangiography and gastro-intestinal barium studies including hypotonic duodenography.

In acute pancreatic conditions the main importance of the signs visible on the plain film of the abdomen lies in the differential diagnosis with other frequent causes of "acute abdomen" such as intestinal occlusion and gastroduodenal perforation. Specific signs indicating acute pancreatitis, such as sentinel loop or the "colon cut off" sign, are present in only about 50% of the cases or even less.

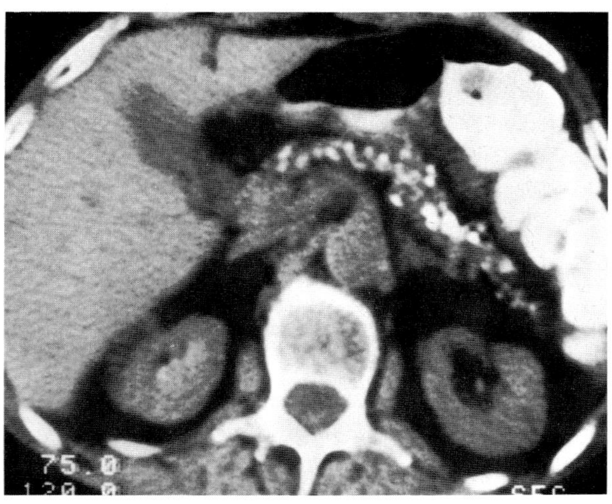

Fig. 1. Chronic calcifying pancreatitis. CT scan of the upper abdomen. Numerous nodular type calcifications disseminated throughout body and tail of the pancreas. Note extreme parenchymal atrophy

The configuration and characteristic distribution of pancreatic calcifications as visible on the plain film may, in some instances, identify them easily as being of pancreatic origin, either parenchymatous or located in a dilated main pancreatic duct, but recent studies clearly indicate the superiority of computed tomography (CT) for detecting pancreatic calcifications, which were seen in all cases using CT, but in only 72% on plain film [8]. Moreover, CT permits easy and correct intra- or extrapancreatic localization of upper abdominal calcifications, such as calcified nodes in the hepatic hilum, which on the plain AP film may erroneously be seen as situated within the pancreatic head (Fig. 1).

One should, however, be aware that pancreatic calcifications, although strongly suggestive of chronic pancreatitis, may be observed in pancreatic adenocarcinoma and in other more exceptional primary pancreatic neoplasms, such as cystadenocarcinoma, mucoid adenocarcinoma and in calcified islet cell tumours.

Intravenous cholangiography may detect abnormalities of the main bile duct in about 60% of the cases of chronic pancreatitis [16]. However, in many cases endoscopic retrograde cholangiopancreatography (ERCP) will provide better anatomical detail of the choledochus and visualization of the main pancreatic duct in the same procedure. Moreover, results of IV cholangiography tend to become poor in the presence of obstructive jaundice. For these reasons IV cholangiography should no longer be recommended as a routine screening procedure in the study of patients suspected of having pancreatic disease.

Gastroduodenal barium studies for evaluating pancreatic disease have become less important during recent years. The fundamental purpose of upper gastro-intestinal studies, namely to seek evidence for pancreatic enlargement, is better achieved by ultrasound and CT. Obvious extrinsic deformities of the stomach or duodenum will be

Radiology Today 1. Ed. by M. W. Donner and F. H. W. Heuck

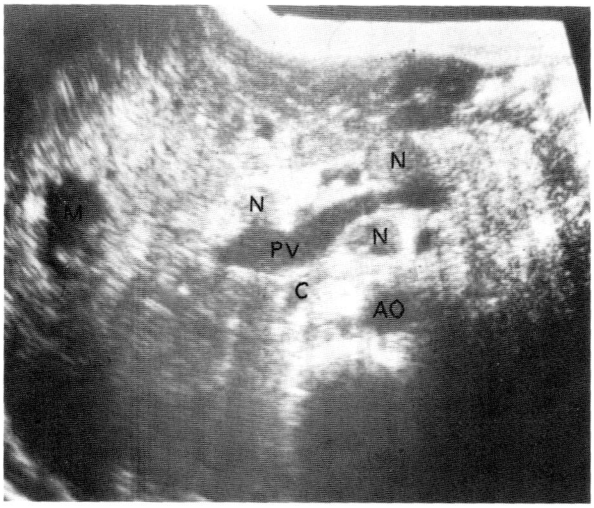

Fig. 2. Metastatic adenopathies surrounding the pancreas. Ultrasound study of the upper abdomen. Transversal cut. Three moderately enlarged lymph nodes (*N*) can be seen ventral and dorsal to the splenic vein and portal vein (*PV*). There is also a metastatic lesion (*M*) within the right hepatic lobe. *C*, inferior vena cava; *AO*, aorta

easily visualized by both methods, which also permit a more specific diagnosis between several pancreatic and extrapancreatic conditions which may cause enlargement of the duodenal loop on the gastro-intestinal barium study (Fig. 2).
Because of the intimate relationship between the internal border of the duodenum and the pancreatic head, hypotonic duodenography is able to visualize the mucosal relief in superb detail and may demonstrate subtle alterations of the pattern and lining of the mucosa of the descending duodenum, indicating pancreatic disease; however, objective evaluation of these alterations remains difficult. Moreover, the presence of barium may delay for several days other pancreatic imaging modalities, thereby increasing the cost of hospitalization. Upper gastro-intestinal barium studies therefore tend to be less and less used as primary diagnostic procedures for studying patients suspected of having pancreatic disease. However, the knowledge and correct interpretation of the signs on upper gastro-intestinal studies which may indicate indirect evidence of pancreatic disease remains important because many of these patients present with atypical vague abdominal complaints and a barium meal may be ordered by the clinician as a first procedure.

Non-invasive New Radiological Methods

Ultrasonography

A technically satisfactory ultrasound examination may beautifully display pancreatic anatomy as seen for the head and body in Fig. 2, but presence of air may adversely affect the quality of the image. Frequently the tail of the pancreas is not visible; for this reason real time apparatus by virtue of the pressure exercised through the transducer may allow to displace intestinal air and thereby produce a better anatomical demonstration.
In our experience ultrasound examination of patients with acute pancreatitis is not very useful. Frequently a lot of air is present in the distended abdomen and only a large hyporeflective area is seen in the pancreatic region, obscuring any anatomical detail. CT is here the procedure of choice (Fig. 3). Pancreatic tumours will be visualized either as hyporeflective or hyperreflective areas with or without contour deformity [9, 15, 20]. In optimal conditions ultrasound allowed us to diagnose tumours in the pancreatic head as small as 2.5 cm in diameter.

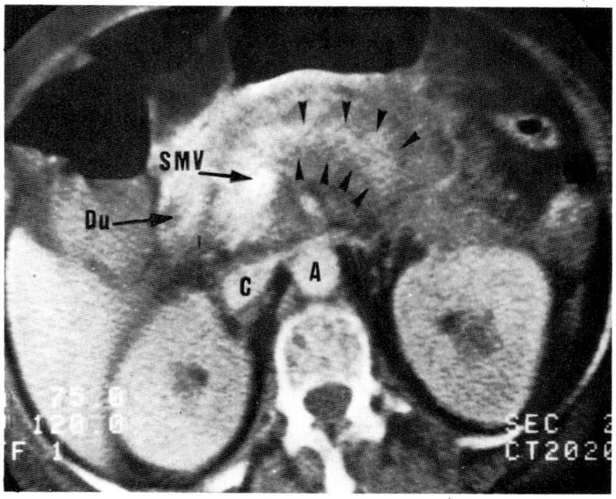

Fig. 3. Severe acute pancreatitis. CT scan of the upper abdomen, 45 s after IV bolus injection of contrast medium. Large hypodense area representing peripancreatic exudate surrounds the pancreas. Important reduction of the volume of the portion of the pancreas which is still vascularized (▶). *SMV*, superior mesenteric vein; *Du*, descending duodenum; *C*, inferior vena cava; *A*, aorta

Equally good results are obtained by ultrasound in pseudocyst of the pancreas presenting as a typical fluid-containing, sharply delineated mass without internal echoes but with amplification of the dorsal border.
In chronic calcifying pancreatitis ultrasound will visualize the pancreatic calcification in only a minority of patients [8].

Computed Tomography

Direct imaging of the pancreas by CT is now possible even in thin patients and children. Pancreatography by intravenous administration of uro-angiographic contrast media is now an easy practical modality. This method allows the study of the normal pancreatic anatomy, its variants, such as pancreatic lipomatosis, and various pathological conditions [11]. Separation of the vascular components within the pancreatic head (the superior mesenteric vein) and the pancreatic body (splenic vein) is also possible with contrast-enhanced CT [12].
In acute pancreatitis contrast-enhanced CT allows the perfect identification of the pancreatic tissue which is still well vascularized and therefore makes possible differentiation from the peripancreatic exudate surrounding the organ (Fig. 3). The appearance of air within the peripancreatic exudate indicates abscess formation and is an ominous prognostic sign in acute pancreatitis, indicating usually lethal complications. In more benign cases the exudate will become organized, a wall becomes visible and the absorption coefficient of the mass decreases.
In the study of chronic pancreatitis the possibilities of CT are more restricted and ERCP is the main radiological procedure on which diagnosis should be based. CT findings in chronic pancreatitis may include, beside calcifications, a moderately dilated pancreatic duct with varying degree of loss of pancreatic parenchyma (Fig. 4).
In our experience CT is the main procedure for the follow-up and control of pancreatic pseudocyst because of the superior anatomical detail provided by this method (Fig. 5).
Spontaneous evacuation of a pseudocyst of the tail into the small bowel is suggested by reduction in volume and the presence of a small amount of air on the control examination. Fine anatomical detail also allows identification of extension of the pseudocyst into the retroperitoneal region (pararenal space), posterior mediastinum, diaphragmatic pillar, mesocolon and abdominal wall.

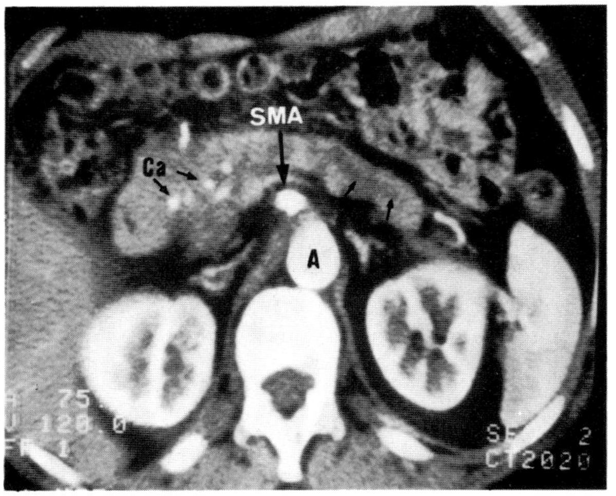

Fig. 4. Chronic calcifying pancreatitis. CT scan of the upper abdomen, 20 s after IV bolus injection of contrast medium. Several calcifications are situated within the pancreatic head. A moderately dilated pancreatic duct (→→) can be seen within the tail of the pancreas. *A,* aorta; *SMA,* superior mesenteric artery; *Ca,* calcifications

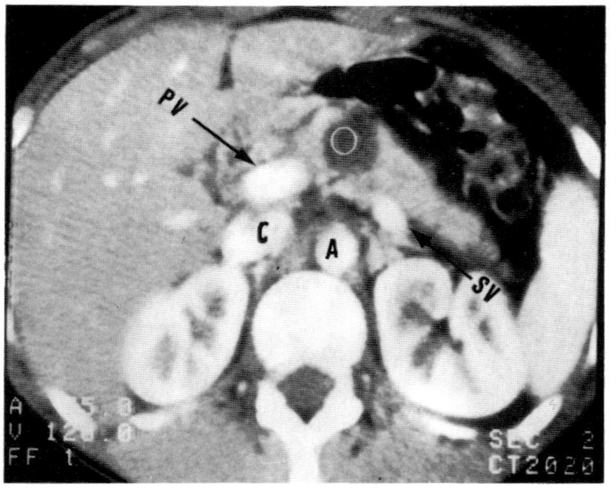

Fig. 5. Pancreatic pseudocyst. CT scan of the upper abdomen, 20 s after IV bolus injection of contrast medium. At the junction of the body and tail of the pancreas a spherical pseudocyst with diameter of ca. 4 cm can be seen. *PV,* portal vein; *SV,* splenic vein; *C,* inferior vena cava; *A,* aorta

Vascular complications of acute and chronic pancreatitis seen by CT are thrombosis of the confluence of the superior mesenteric vein and splenic vein, proven by a hypodense area during the early vascular phase after contrast administration as well as the demonstration of venous collaterals in the upper abdomen.

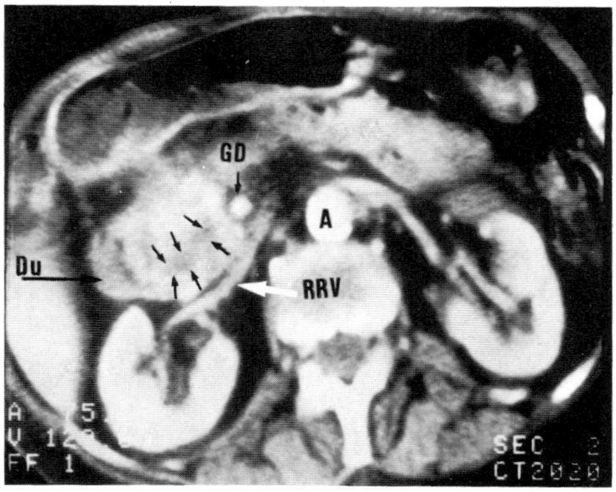

Fig. 6. Adenocarcinoma of the pancreatic head. CT scan of the upper abdomen, 45 s after IV bolus injection of contrast medium. Irregularly shaped hypovascular area (→→) becomes visible within the normal vascularized pancreatic head and corresponds to adenocarcinoma of the pancreas. Only slight bulging of the posterior aspect of the pancreatic head with slight posterior displacement of right renal vein (*RRV*) is seen. *Du,* descending duodenum; *GD,* gastroduodenal artery; *A,* aorta

A pseudo-aneurysm of the splenic artery due to erosion by pancreatic tail pseudocyst may be detected by CT. The false aneurysm is identified by the intense contrast accumulation within the fluid of the pseudocyst.

In our experience most adenocarcinomas of the pancreas present as hypodense areas after contrast enhancement, and even small tumours of 2 – 3 cm without contour deformity may be diagnosed in this way (Fig. 6).

The simultaneous finding during the CT examination of lymph node or hepatic metastasis allows evaluation of operability, but angiography should still be performed in order to assess the direct extension of the pancreatic tumour to surrounding structures, mainly vessels.

Present available studies on the diagnostic value of CT in pancreatic diseases [9, 14, 15, 18] were mainly performed with scanning times of 5 – 20 s or even more. Rapid improvement of CT apparatus and especially reduction of scanning time has lead to impressive improvement of image quality. It is therefore too early to fully evaluate the impact of CT on pancreatic diagnosis, but this method clearly emerges as the method of choice for the study of acute pancreatitis and pancreatic neoplasms.

Invasive Radiological Methods

Pancreatic Angiography

Until recently angiography was considered one of the most accurate examinations for evaluation of the pancreas. Optimum results require, however, considerable skill involving superselective catheterization of the different afferent vessels of the pancreas, and even in experienced hands and on films of high technical quality diagnostic errors did occur. In some instances arteriography of even large tumours was completely normal; in others subtle changes in the calibre of the vessels did not allow differential diagnosis between chronic pancreatitis and pancreatic carcinoma. One therefore has to re-assess the role of pancreatic angiography, as done recently by Freeny [6].

Concerning diagnosis of pancreatic lesions, arteriography remains the primary procedure for the detection of endocrine active tumours of the pancreas, because of:

1. The high degree of vascularity of a majority of these lesions, at least the insulin-producing variety (Fig. 7);
2. The smallness of some of these tumours, which causes them to escape detection by either ultrasound or CT.

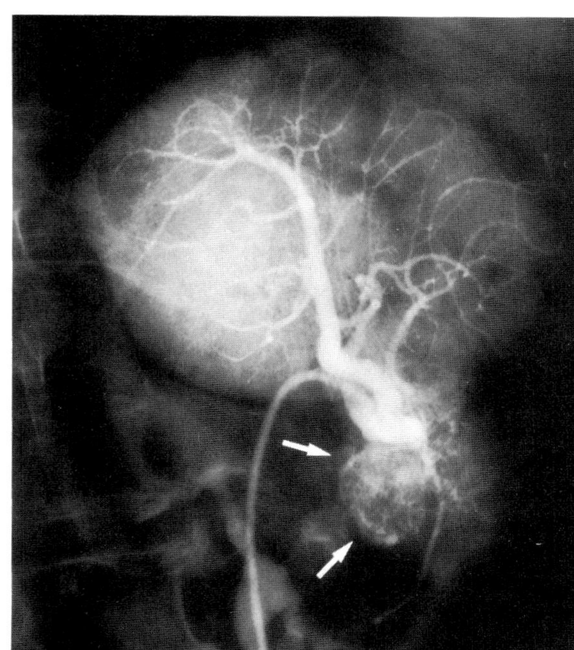

Fig. 7. Insulinoma. Selective arteriography of the splenic artery. Left posterior oblique view. A well-vascularized nodular opacity (→) measuring 3 by 3 cm is situated within the pancreatic tail very close to the splenic hilum

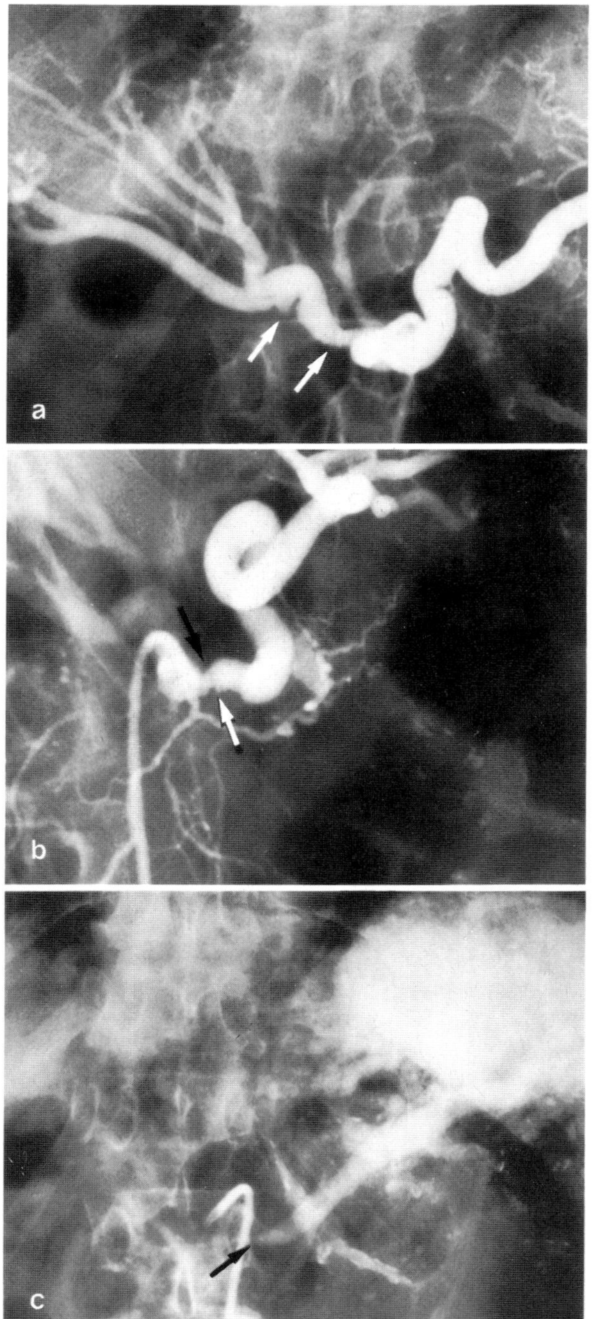

Fig. 8a–c. Inoperable adenocarcinoma of pancreatic head and body. **a** Coeliac arteriography, arterial phase, AP view. Occlusion of gastroduodenal artery (→) and irregular outline of inferior aspect of common hepatic artery (→) caused by tumoral invasion. **b** Selective splenic arteriography, arterial phase, left posterior oblique view. Irregular outline (→) of inferior aspect of the splenic artery becomes visible on this additional oblique view and allows a more correct evaluation of the real extent of the tumour. **c** Coeliac arteriography, venous phase, AP view. Progressive narrowing and complete occlusion (→) of the splenic vein near to the body midline

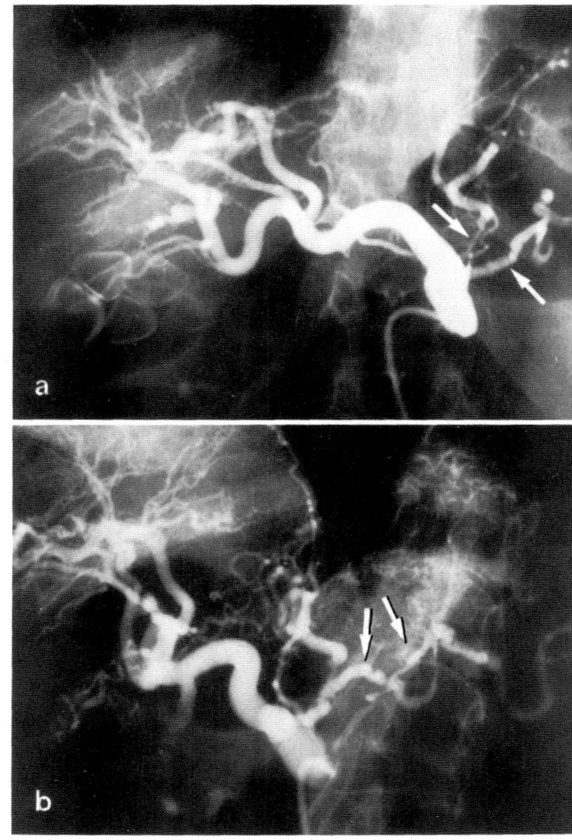

Fig. 9a, b. Inoperable adenocarcinoma of the pancreatic body and tail. Coeliac arteriography. **a** Arterial phase, AP view. Irregular narrowing and indentations of the proximal portion of left gastric (→) and splenic arteries (→). **b** Arterial phase, right posterior oblique view. The distal extent (→) of the invasion of the splenic artery by the pancreatic tumour is better visible on this additional view

In addition, pancreatic arteriography for the diagnosis of pancreatic carcinoma may be considered if previous studies, including ERCP, are negative. Angiography was still considered essential by Freeny [6] for the diagnosis of adenocarcinoma in 11 out of 35 patients. Furthermore, arteriography still has a main role in diagnosing nonresectable tumours, obviating exploratory laparatomy by revealing invasion of major vascular structures (Fig. 8a, b, c). Careful technique and additional views may be very useful here (Figs. 9a, b, 10).

In addition, in cases of resectable tumours arteriography will be most useful to the surgeon as a "vascular road map." Arteriography in patients with severe chronic pancreatitis or pseudocyst is also considered by many surgeons as essential for a proper pre-operative evaluation.

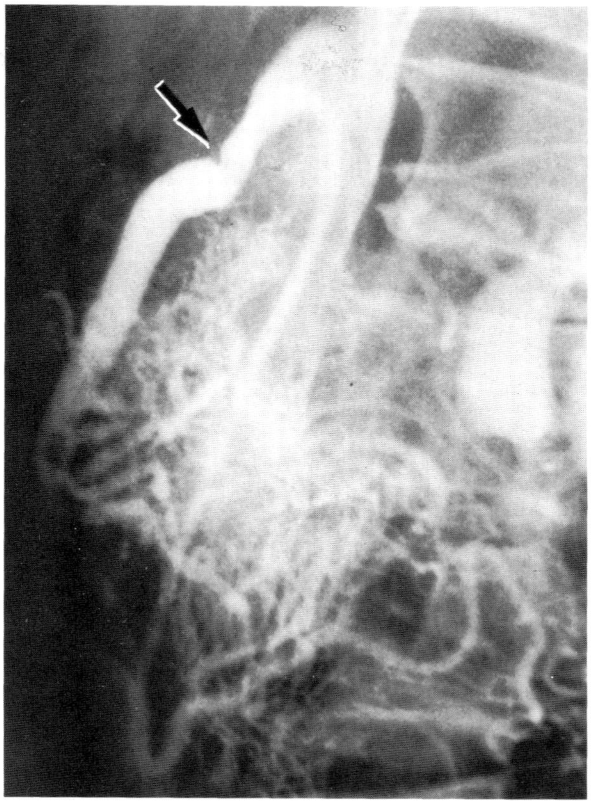

Fig. 10. Inoperable adenocarcinoma of the pancreatic head. Superior mesenteric arteriography. Arterial phase, right posterior oblique view. Tumoral invasion (→) of the proximal portion of the superior mesenteric artery is evident on this additional projection

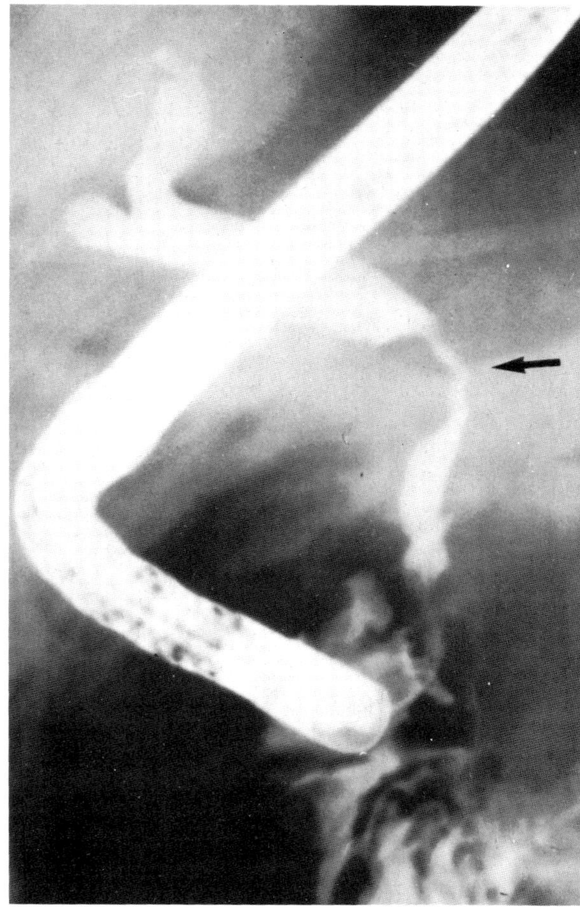

Fig. 11. Adenocarcinoma of the pancreatic body. ERCP, right posterior oblique view. Stenotic segment (→) of about 3 cm length is visible on the mid-portion of the pancreatic duct; proximal to the stenosis, the pancreatic duct is extremely dilated

Endoscopic Retrograde Cholangiopancreatography

Success rates for retrograde opacification of the pancreatic duct is now situated at 95% or more and of the main bile duct, at 85% [1, 17]. The complication rate is estimated at 2%–3% [2]. This method will visualize directly the pancreatic ductal system and will therefore be most useful when the pancreatic ducts are primarily involved, as in pancreatic carcinoma, or if diseases of the parenchyma secondarily involve the ductal system, as in chronic pancreatitis. After ultrasound and CT, ERCP is therefore the method of choice for investigation of those two conditions.

The most characteristic ERCP findings in chronic pancreatitis are dilatation and tortuosity of the main pancreatic duct, with dilatation and blinding of the lateral branches.

Irregularly lined stenotic segments are typical for carcinoma (Fig. 11). In some cases percutaneous transhepatic cholangiography (PTC) and ERCP may be mutually complementary in indicating site and appearance of a stenotic lesion (Fig. 12). ERCP findings in 252 pancreatic carcinomas, reported in ten different series from three continents, were published by Stewart [19]. Obstruction or stenosis of the main pancreatic duct was present in 91% of the cases, but the common bile duct was abnormal in 68 of 75 cases when it was cannulated and visualized. No patient proved to have a carcinoma had a normal ERCP. The diagnostic accuracy was 98.4%, but the series contained only cases with successful duct cannulation.

ERCP is especially useful for the study of periampullary tumours (Fig. 13). Those tumours are frequently not directly visualized by CT owing to their small size. CT will mostly indicate the site but not the cause of an obstruction on the terminal

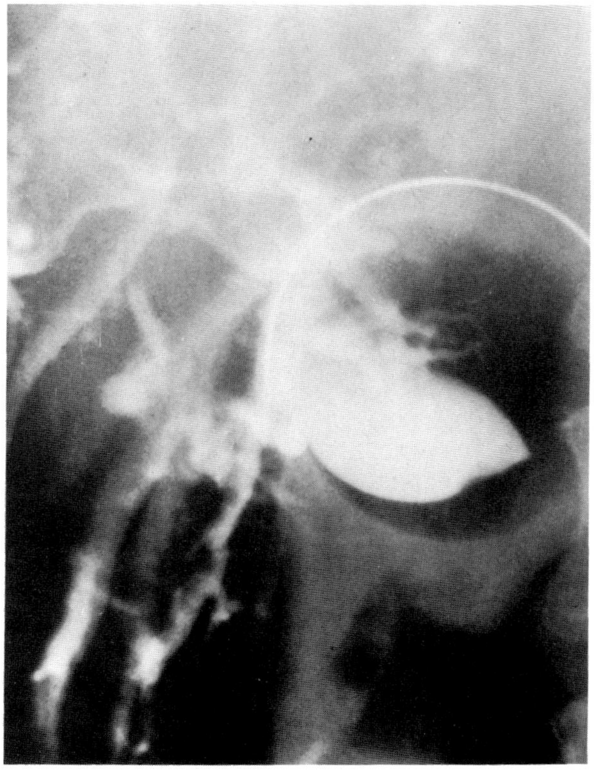

Fig. 12. Adenocarcinoma of the pancreatic head. Percutaneous transhepatic cholangiography (PTC). Dilatation of the intrahepatic bile ducts and of the common bile duct. Progressive narrowing and complete occlusion of the distal portion of the common bile duct due to extrinsic compression by pancreatic tumour

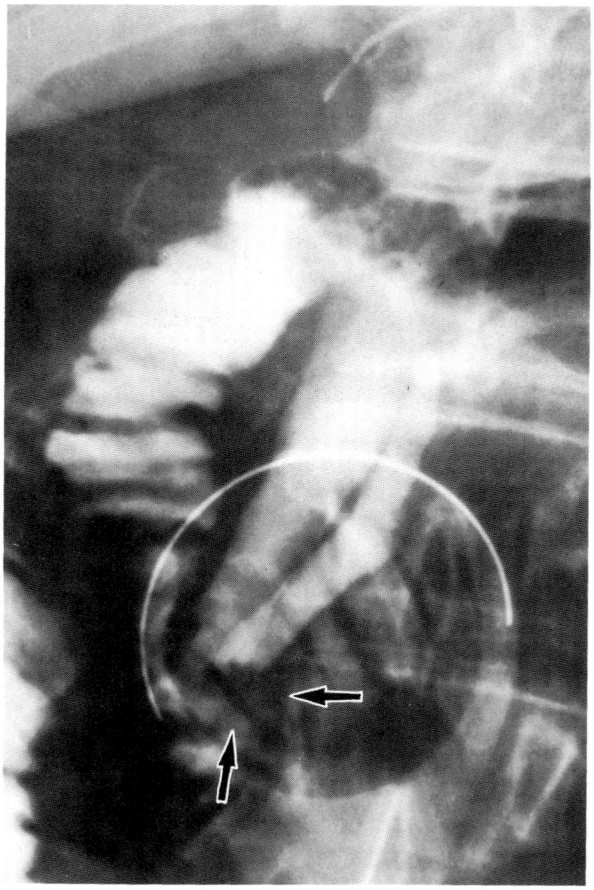

Fig. 13. Ampulloma. ERCP, right posterior oblique view. Moderately dilated common bile duct and pancreatic duct caused by a small tumour of the ampulla hepatopancreatica visible as a lacunar filling defect (→) in the distal segment of the pancreatic duct

portions of the main bile and pancreatic duct (Fig. 14).

In some cases, however, ERCP findings will not allow differentiation between carcinoma and pancreatitis; useful complementary information may be obtained by cytological examination of the aspiration fluid obtained from the pancreatic duct [1, 17].

Percutaneous Cytodiagnosis of Pancreatic Carcinoma

During recent years it became clear that the expectation of diagnosing early small carcinomas of the pancreas by ERCP was not being realized. In order to reduce or eliminate endless expensive work-ups and procedures in patients suspected to have pancreatic carcinoma, where prognosis is poor at best, needle aspiration biopsy has increasingly become an established technique in many departments for study of pancreatic lesions discovered by ultrasound or CT. Evander [4] obtained correct cytological diagnosis in 60% of patients with pancreatic carcinoma, and Triller [21] recently reported success in 20 of 31 patients. Dekker and Lloyd [3] performed 15 biopsies in 13 patients with positive findings of carcinoma in 11 patients. With only 2% – 5% of patients with pancreatic carcinoma alive after 5 years, this approach has gained much in appeal. The complication rate of diagnostic abdominal puncture is extremely low, and only one report of malignant seeding of the tract after needle aspiration of pancreatic carcinoma has been published [5].

Pancreatic Vein Catheterization for Hormone Assay

Although pancreatic angiography is probably the best imaging method for detecting pancreatic

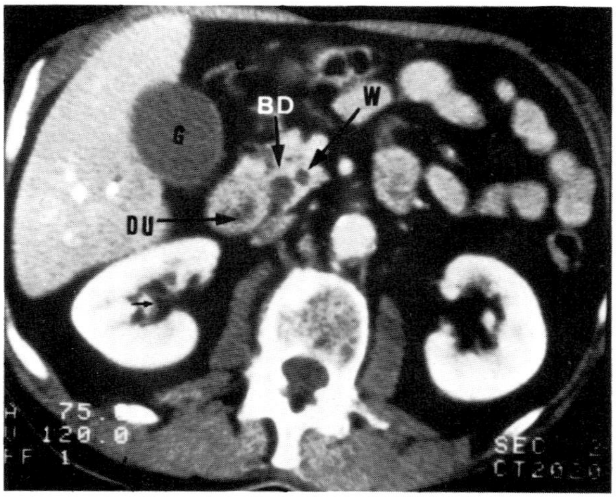

Fig. 14. Ampulloma. CT scan of the upper abdomen, 45 s after IV bolus injection of contrast medium. Two small spherical hypodense areas juxtaposed within the pancreatic head correspond to the dilated distal portion of the common bile duct (*BD*) and dilated pancreatic duct (*W*). The lesion itself, responsible for the obstrucion of both canals, was not visualized on the CT images. *Du,* descending duodenum; *G,* gall bladder

insulin-producing tumours, it only detects 40% – 60% [7]. In Zollinger Ellison syndrome a recent paper by Mills [13] stated that only three patients out of 20 had unequivocally positive angiographic studies.

Scandinavian authors [7, 10] reported a high rate of success by radio-immunoassay of subselective vein branch samples in patients with islet cell tumours and hyperplasia. The accuracy of this test was higher than any other localization technique, sensitive enough to identify even microscopic islet cell hyperplasias.

References

1. Anacker H, Weiss HD, Kramann B, Rupp N, Grünberg G, Lanz W (1975) Die Pankreaticographie und ihre Korrelation mit der Angiographie und der Ultrasonographie in der Pankreasdiagnostik. Radiologe 15:183 – 190
2. Bilbao MK, Dotter CT, Lee TG, Katon RM (1976) Complications of endoscopic retrograde cholangiopankreaticography (E.R.C.P.). Gastroenterology 70:314 – 320
3. Dekker A, Lloyd JC (1979) Fine needle aspiration in ampullary and pancreatic carcinoma. Arch Surg 114:592 – 596
4. Evander A, Ihse I, Lunderquist A, Tylen U. Akerman M (1978) Percutaneous cytodiagnosis of carcinoma of the pancreas and bile duct. Am Surg 188:90 – 92
5. Ferrucci J, Wittenberg J, Margolis MN, Carey RW (1979) Malignant seedling of the tract after thin needle aspiration biopsy. Radiology 130:345 – 346
6. Freeny PC, Ball TJ, Ryan J (1979) Impact of new diagnostic imaging methods on pancreatic angiography. AJR 133:619 – 624
7. Ingemansson S, Kühl C, Larsson LI, Lunderquist A, Lundquist I (1978) Localisation of insulinomas and islet cell hyperplasias by pancreatic vein catheterisation and insulin assay. Surg Gynecol Obstet 146:725 – 734
8. Lackner K, Frommhold H, Grauthof H, Mödder U, Heuser L, Braun G, Buurman R, Scherer K (1980) Wertigkeit der Computertomographie und der Sonographie innerhalb der Pankreasdiagnostik. ROEFO 132:509 – 513
9. Lee JTK, Stanley RJ, Melson GL, Sagel S (1979) Pancreatic imaging by ultrasound and computed tomography. Radiol Clin North Am 16:1
10. Lunderquist A, Eriksson H, Ingemansson S, Larsson LI, Reichard W (1978) Selective pancreatic vein catheterisation for the hormone assay in endocrine tumor of the pancreas. Cardiovasc Radiol 1:117 – 124
11. Marchal G, Baert AL, Wilms G (1979) Intravenous pancreaticography in computed tomography. J Comput Assist Tomogr 3:727 – 732
12. Marchal G, Wilms G, Baert A, Ponette E (1980) Applications of specific vascular opacification in CT of the upper abdomen. ROEFO 132:45 – 48
13. Mills SR, Doppman JL, Dunnick NR, McCarthy DM (1979) Evaluation of angiography in Zollinger-Ellison syndrome. Radiology 131:317 – 320
14. Mödder U, Friedman G, Bücheler E, Baert A, Lackner K, Brecht G, Buurman R, Rupp N, Heller HJ (1979) Wert und Ergebnisse der Computertomographie bei Pankreaserkrankungen. ROEFO 130:57 – 61
15. Partain CC, Staab EV, McCartney WH (1979) Multiple imaging modalities for the study of pancreatic disease. Semin Nucl Med 9:36 – 41
16. Pringot J, Ponette E, Goncette L, Baert A, Dautrebande J (1976) Contribution des examens radiologiques classiques et angiographiques au diagnostic de la pancreatite chronique. Acta Gastroenterol Belg 39:426 – 457
17. Salmon PR (1978) Re-evaluation of endoscopic retrograde cholangiopancreatography as a diagnostic method. Clin Gastroenterol 7:651 – 663
18. Sheedy PF, Stephens DH, Hattery RR, MacCarty RL (1977) Computed tomography in the evaluation of patients with suspected carcinoma of the pancreas. Radiology 124:731
19. Stewart ET, Vennes JA, Geenen JE (1977) Atlas of endoscopic retrograde cholangiopancreatography. C. V. Mosby, St Louis
20. Triller J (1978) Sonographische Diagnostik des Pankreas. Radiologe 18:255
21. Triller J (1979) Ultraschall gezielte abdominale Punktionen. Radiologe 19:173 – 182

Abdominal Abscesses

M. A. Meyers

State University of New York at Stony Brook, Health Sciences Center, Department of Radiology, Stony Brook, NY 11794 (USA)

Intraperitoneal abscesses are now seen most commonly as a postoperative complication and are particularly frequent following cholecystectomy and gastric operations. *Escherichia coli* and other gram-negative bacteria are the dominant organisms cultured, but streptococci and staphylococci still play an important role. Many cases of postoperative abscesses are secondary to anastomotic leaks [1, 2]. Intra-abdominal abscesses are often clinically insidious, presenting with mild abdominal pain, malaise, and a slight fever. Early radiologic identification and localization is of extreme importance, since morbidity and mortality increase with delay in treatment.

Intra-abdominal abscesses may be indicated by conventional radiologic techniques by the demonstration of (a) a soft-tissue mass, (b) a collection or pattern of extraluminal gas, (c) viscus displacement, (d) loss of normally visualized structures, (e) fixation of a normally mobile organ, or (f) opacification of a communicating sinus or fistulous tract [3]. Secondary signs include scoliosis, elevation or splinting of a diaphragm, localized or generalized ileus, and pulmonary basilar changes. Except for the demonstration of a sinus tract, the primary signs are often very subtle and difficult to ascertain early in the course of the process. The secondary signs are nonspecific and merely supportive.

Recent progress in radiologic capabilities has been centered on two fronts:

1. A more refined concept of the pathogenesis of the disease, involving an understanding of the spread and localization of intraperitoneal infections. In this way, the specific intraperitoneal recesses for the development of abscesses remote from the primary site of origin of the infection may be anticipated, leading to more prompt diagnosis and management.
2. The application of the sophisticated modalities of ultrasonography, computed tomography (CT), and isotopic imaging. These not only have permitted earlier and precise diagnosis, but have also led to treatment by guided drainage.

Dynamic Anatomic Considerations and Localizing Features

Recent anatomic-radiologic correlations by Meyers have established the preferential pathways by which a remote abscess develops from a primary site of infection [1]. The posterior peritoneal attachments and associated recesses serve as watersheds directing the spread and compartmentalization of contaminated material (Fig. 1). Table 1 outlines the localizations of intraperitoneal abscesses most commonly encountered as postoperative complications.

The most common site for a localized intraperitoneal abscess is the pelvis, particularly its central cul-de-sac (pouch of Douglas) (Fig. 2). From the pelvis, contaminated fluid ascends the paracolic gutter (on the right preferentially) to the subhepatic spaces (Figs. 3 – 5), seeking especially the posterior subhepatic space (hepatorenal fossa). This site, lying in the paravertebral groove, is also

Table 1. Radiologic-anatomic classification of intraperitoneal abscesses (adapted from Meyers and Whalen [3])

Supramesocolic	Inframesocolic
Right subphrenic	Pelvic
Anterior	Paracolic
Posterior	Right
Right subhepatic	Left
Anterior	Infracolic
Posterior	Right
(Morison's pouch)	Left
Left subphrenic	
Lesser sac	

Radiology Today 1. Ed. by M. W. Donner and F. H. W. Heuck

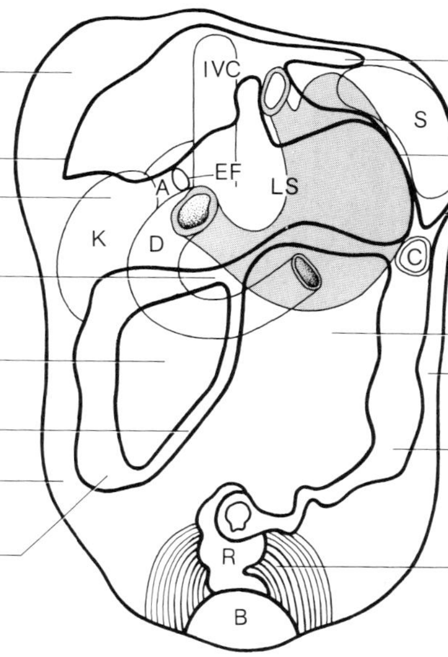

Fig. 1. Posterior peritoneal reflections and recesses. *S,* spleen; *LS,* lesser sac; *IVC,* inferior vena cava; *EF,* epiploic foramen of Winslow; *K,* right kidney; *D,* duodenum; *A,* adrenal gland; *C,* splenic flexure of colon; *R,* rectum; *B,* urinary bladder [1]

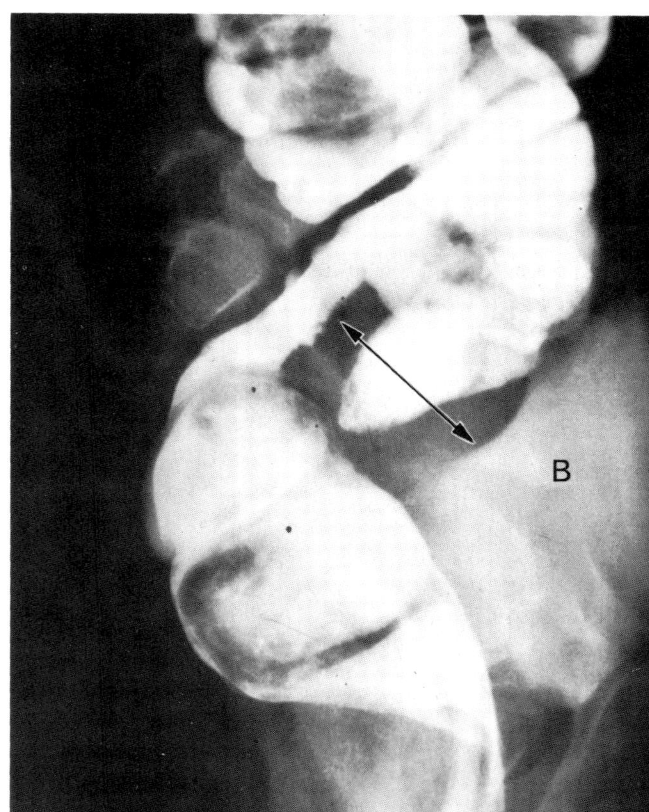

Fig. 2. Pelvic abscess in a child after appendectomy. Large soft tissue mass compresses and separates the rectosigmoid junction and the urinary bladder (*B*). A redundant sigmoid loop seen in this lateral view projects in this area but is truly off the midline

known as Morison's pouch and is the second most common intraperitoneal area for localized abscess formation. The contamination, however, may not coalesce here and the infection then may be contained in the right subphrenic space. In cases of generalized peritonitis, the lesser sac as a rule remains sterile, presumably because the epiploic foramen of Winslow is promptly sealed off by inflammatory adhesions.

Left subphrenic abscesses, in contrast, usually result from immediately contiguous sites and are seen following operations on the stomach, spleen,

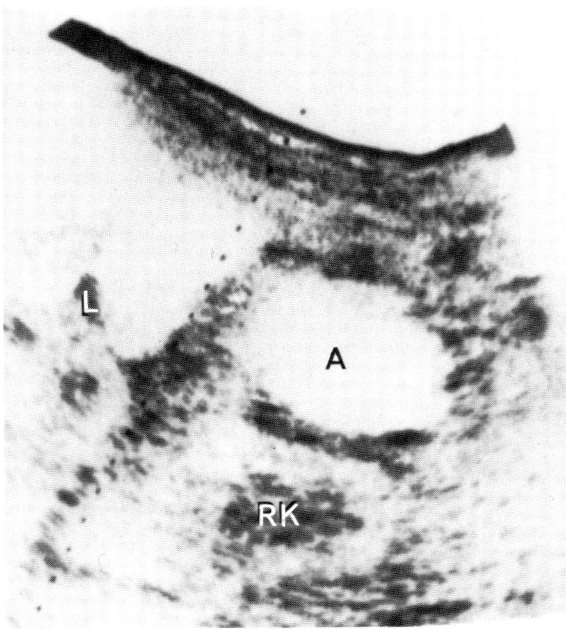

Fig. 3. Morison's pouch abscess shown by ultrasonography, in a patient following Whipple's procedure for pancreatic carcinoma. A large abscess (*A*) has coalesced immediately anterior to the right kidney (*RK*), beneath the liver (*L*)

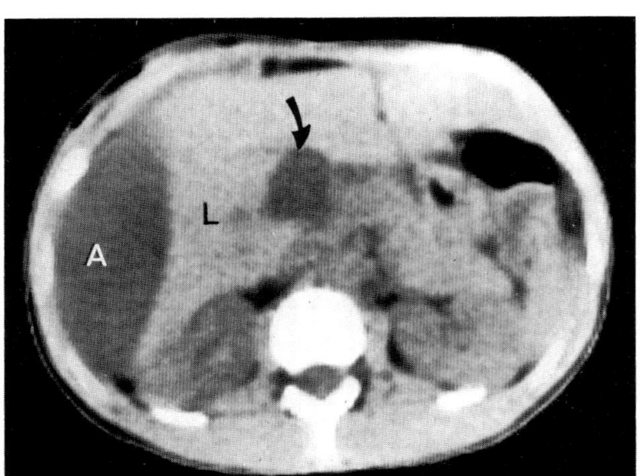

Fig. 4. Right subhepatic and right subphrenic abscess, after cholecystectomy, demonstrated by CT. An abscess occupies the anterior subhepatic space (*arrow*) and a larger one (*A*) has developed in the right subphrenic space, displacing and compressing the liver (*L*). (Courtesy of Leon Love, M. D., Loyola University School of Medicine, Maywood, Illinois)

or splenic flexure of the colon (Fig. 6). The left paracolic gutter, being narrow and shallow, is generally not a significant avenue for the transmission of infections; furthermore, the phrenicocolic ligament serves to disrupt continuity between this recess and the left subphrenic space. These pathways and localizing features are evident not only by conventional radiologic techniques, but have also been recently confirmed by ultrasonography, isotopic studies [4], and CT [5].

The Newer Imaging Modalities

Ultrasonography has a sensitivity of almost 95% and a specificity approaching 100% in the diagnosis and localization of intra-abdominal abscesses [6]. These present generally as irregular fluid collections with indistinct margins (Fig. 3). It is too time consuming, however, to serve as a survey evaluation of the entire abdomen in suspected abscesses; it is best used when localizing features have been indicated.

Computed tomography may reveal an abscess as a mass with low attenuation value displacing surrounding structures, occasionally with a peripheral rim of higher density which may show contrast enhancement; there may be thickening or obliteration of neighboring fascial planes, and the presence of gas bubbles or air-fluid levels usually allows definitive diagnosis (Fig. 4). CT may diagnose and accurately define the extent of involvement in at least 90% of cases, depending upon the size of the abscess [7]. The characteristic signs on ultrasonography and CT usually permit clear distinction from other postoperative fluid collections such as seromas and lymphocysts.

The overall accuracy for gallium-67 examination (Fig. 5) is highly dependent on the type of patient studied; the presence of a surgical incision may be confused with an abscess cavity as well as with nonspecific uptake in inflammatory but nonsuppurative lesions, bowel, and tumors [6]. It is particularly useful as an initial survey in suspected abscesses when there are no localizing clinical signs and plain film findings are negative or equivocal. Table 2 outlines our diagnostic algorithm in cases of abdominal abscesses.

Management

Not only the identification of the presence of an intra-abdominal abscess but also its precise localization by radiologic techniques dictate the

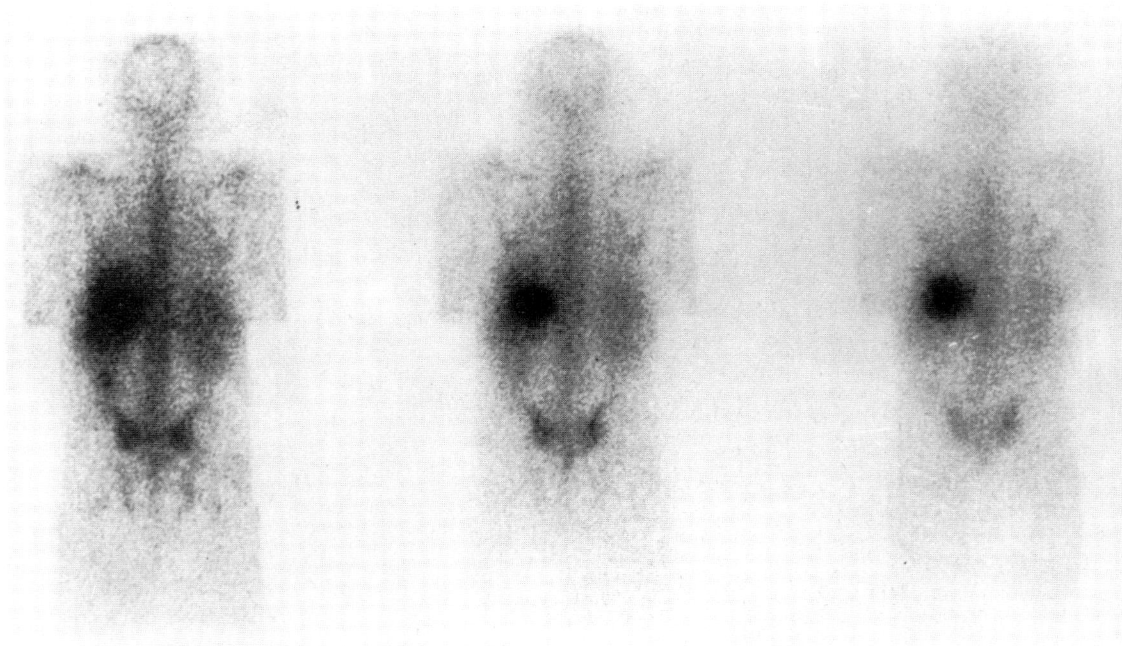

Fig. 5. Right subhepatic abscess. Gallium-67 scan demonstrates localized uptake in the right upper quadrant [6]

Table 2. Diagnostic algorithm for suspected abdominal abscess

Localizing clinical signs	No localizing clinical signs
Plain film ↓ → Positive and diagnostic: STOP; Negative or equivocal ↓	Plain film ↓ → Positive and diagnostic: STOP; Negative or equivocal ↓
Ultrasound ↓ → Positive and diagnostic: STOP; Negative or equivocal ↓	Gallium scan ↓ → Positive ↓ Computed tomography of suspicious area; Equivocal ↓ Ultrasound; Negative ↓ Computed tomography (xiphoid → pubis)
Gallium scan ↓ → Negative; Equivocal[a] ↓ Computed tomography of suspicious area; Positive → Computed tomography of suspicious area	Ultrasound → Positive and diagnostic STOP; Equivocal ↓ Computed tomography of suspicious area

[a] If equivocal or positive in area not already examined by ultrasound, ultrasound should be repeated prior to CT

most appropriate route of surgical drainage [1] (Fig. 7). Although antibiotics play an important role, operative drainage remains the cornerstone of therapy. A transperitoneal approach is generally employed for drainage of anterior subphrenic and subhepatic, left subphrenic, lesser sac, and multiple abscesses. An abscess compartmentalized to the right posterior subhepatic space is best drained

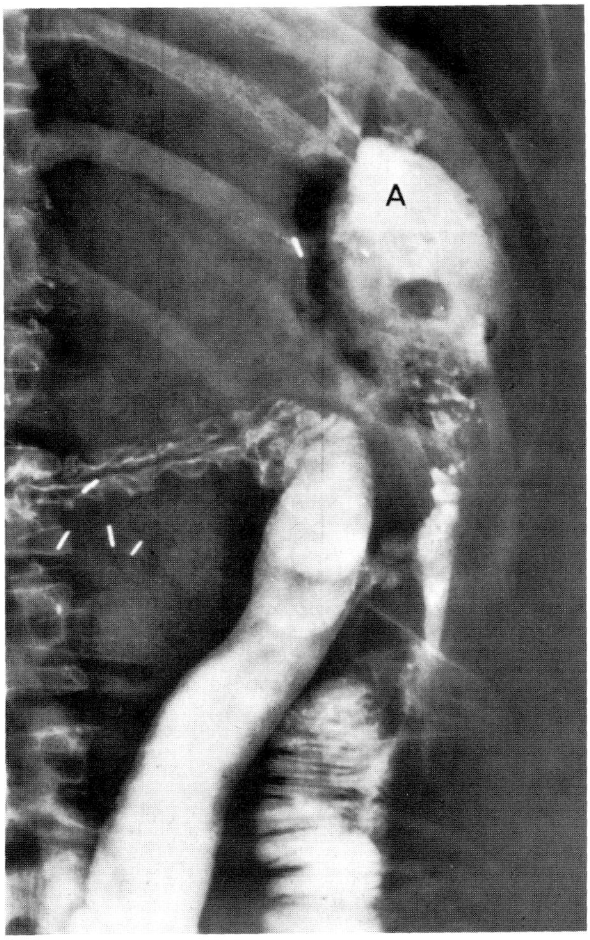

Fig. 6. Left subphrenic abscess. Following surgical resection of the splenic flexure of the colon, an anastomotic leak results in a left upper quadrant abscess (*A*) and fistulization to a small bowel loop

by Ochsner's extrapleural approach through the bed of the resected 12th rib. The right posterior subphrenic space is drained via Trendelenburg's transpleural route. Drainage of postsplenectomy abscesses is usually done posteriorly through the bed of the 12th rib to prevent contamination of the peritoneal cavity and provide the most dependent drainage [8]. Ultrasound- and CT-guided aspiration and drainage of intra-abdominal abscesses represent recent major advances in management [9, 10].

References

1. Meyers MA (1976) Dynamic radiology of the abdomen: Normal and pathologic anatomy. Springer, New York Heidelberg Berlin

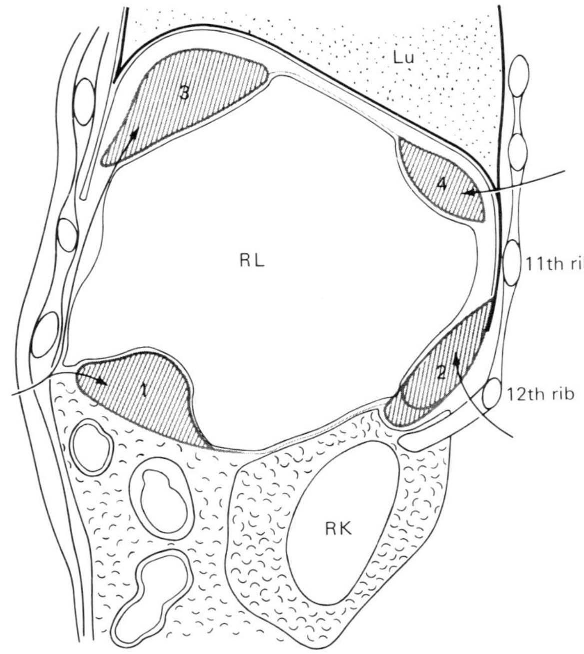

Fig. 7. The four sites of localized abscesses around the right lobe of the liver (*RL*) and surgical approaches [1]

2. Samuel E, Duncan JG, Philip T, et al. (1963) Radiology of the postoperative abdomen. Clin Radiol 14:133 – 148
3. Meyers MA, Whalen JP (1971) Radiologic aspects of intraabdominal abscesses, In: Ariel I, Kazarian K (eds) The diagnosis and treatment of intraabdominal abscesses. Williams & Wilkins, Baltimore, pp 87 – 127
4. Myerson PJ, Myerson D, Spencer RP (1977) Anatomic patterns of GA-67 distribution in localized and diffuse peritoneal inflammation: Case report. J Nucl Med 18:977 – 980
5. Churchill R, Love L, Reyes C, Moncade R (to be published) CT of intraperitoneal infections. Gastrointest Radiol
6. Taylor KJW, Sullivan DC, Wasson JF, Rosenfield AT (1978) Ultrasound and gallium for the diagnosis of abdominal and pelvic abscesses. Gastrointest Radiol 3:281 – 286
7. Aronberg DJ, Stanley FJ, Levitt RG, Sagel S (1978) Evaluation of abdominal abscess with computed tomography. J Comput Assist Tomogr 2:384 – 387
8. Jordan GL Jr (1975) Complications of Pancreatic and Splenic Surgery. In: Artz CP, Hardy JD (eds) Management of Surgical Complications, 3rd edn. Saunders, Philadelphia, pp 534 – 572
9. Haaga J, Alfidi RJ, Havrilla TR, Cooperman AM, Seidelmann FE, Reich NE, Weinstein AJ, Meaney TF (1977) CT detection and aspiration of abdominal abscesses. AJR 128:465 – 474
10. Gerzof SG, Robbins AH, Birkett DH (1978) Computed tomography in the diagnosis and management of abdominal abscesses. Gastrointest Radiol 3:287 – 294

The Value of Computed Axial Tomography in Acute Abdominal Emergencies

B. Mayr, G. Feifel, B. Sommer, U. Scherer, J. Doppman, and J. Lissner

Ludwigs-Maximilians-Universität, Klinikum Großhadern, Klinik für Radiologie, Röntgen A, Marchioninistraße 15, D-8000 München 70

A number of possible diagnoses must be considered in a patient presenting with an "acute abdomen." The workup of such a patient requires the appropriate selection of the most efficacious, most expeditious, and least invasive diagnostic tests. Computed tomography (CT) has established itself as a valuable diagnostic aid in the differential diagnosis of the acute abdomen. We have reviewed the CT findings in 83 patients with proven diagnoses of intra-abdominal abscess, bleeding, and acute pancreatitis to evaluate the contribution of CT in the workup of abdominal emergencies.

Method

All examinations were performed on a Siemens Somatom with a 5-s scan time, 8 mm slice thickness, and 125 kV. When the clinical condition of the patient permitted, up to 800 ml 2% oral Gastrografin were given to opacify the stomach and bowel. In selected cases (15%) intravenous contrast medium (Angiografin 65%) was administered to opacify pancreatic parenchyma or abscess wall.

Abscesses

Mortality caused by an untreated or inadequately treated abdominal abscess is high (untreated abscess: 80% – 100%; inadequate drainage: 48% – 63%; adequate drainage: 5% – 15%) [1, 4, 10]. Successful treatment, that is, adequate surgical drainage of all localized collections, depends upon early diagnosis of the lesion and exact localization of its extent [4].

The CT diagnosis depends upon the demonstration of a gas-containing hypodense mass, clearly separable from bowel (Fig. 1a). Postoperative air or gas from a bowel perforation must be distinguished from gas within an abscess [2, 8, 20]. In most instances (35 of 41) abdominal abscesses presented as hypodense masses without air and diagnosis depended upon correlating clinical and CT findings (Fig. 1b). Differential diagnoses included hematoma, necrosis, and infarction [2, 3, 8, 11, 20].

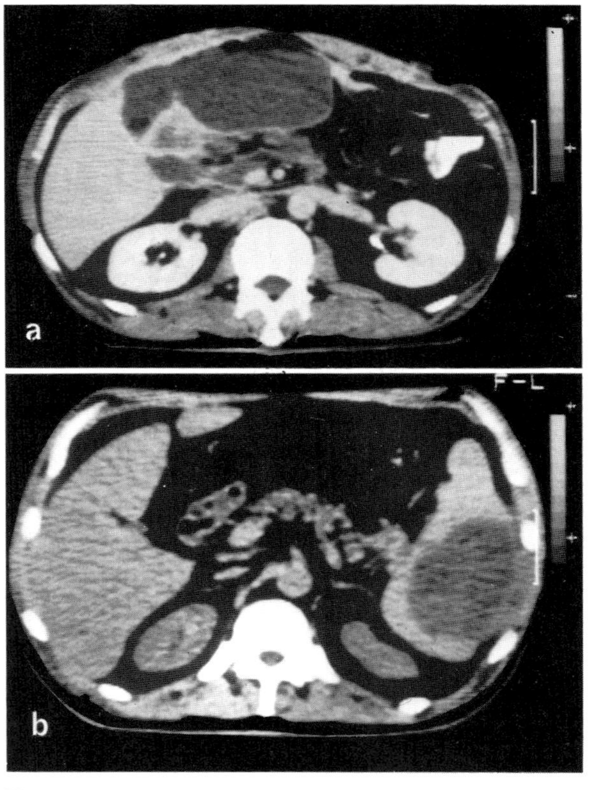

Fig. 1. a Parahepatic abscess following cholecystectomy CT shows an air-containing hypodense mass with an enhanced rim after intravenous contrast. **b** Splenic abscess: CT shows a hypodense mass within the enlarged organ

Radiology Today 1. Ed. by M. W. Donner and F. H. W. Heuck

Table 1. Influence of CT scanning on therapeutic decisions in 39 patients with proven abdominal abscess

Value of CT	Surgery	Conservative treatment
Essential	11	0
Helpful	21	1
Low contribution	3	0
No contribution	2	1
	37	2

Results

In 41 patients with abdominal abscesses proven by surgical drainage in 39 and serial studies in 2, 39 were visualized by CT. The location and the extent of the process were correctly predicted in all these patients. Two false negative diagnoses of abscesses were made by CT. A perirectal abscess in a patient with Crohn's disease was not identified, and a renal abscess was misdiagnosed as a necrotic tumor. In both patients the surgeon made his therapeutic decision on the basis of other diagnostic studies.

The referring physicians considered the contribution of CT to patient management essential in 11, helpful in 22, of low contribution in 3, and noncontributory in 2 (Table 1).

Pancreatitis

Acute pancreatitis is characterized by enzymatic necrosis of the pancreas. The extent of the necrosis and its rate of progression determine the severity of the attack [5, 17]. While the edematous stage without or with minimal necrosis responds to conservative therapy in 90% of patients, the progression to segmental or total necrosis requires operative intervention [5, 17]. The diagnosis of such progression by clinical and laboratory findings or by plain film is often uncertain and delayed [9, 19]. Therefore the clinician depends upon imaging modalities to demonstrate changes of necrosis and its extent, as well as secondary changes, such as abscess and pseudocyst formation. The CT findings in acute pancreatitis can be divided into three stages: Stage I is characterized by peripancreatic edema with enlargement of the gland and blurring of its margins. Small collections of retroperitoneal fluid are also seen at this stage,

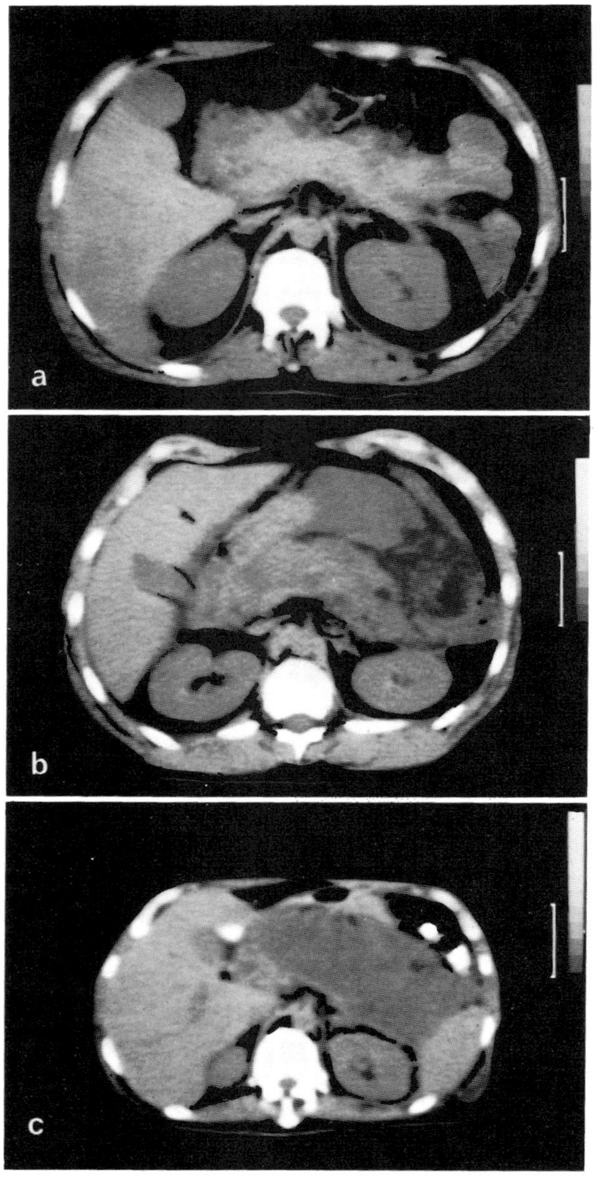

Fig. 2a–c. Acute pancreatitis. **a** Stage I; **b** stage II; **c** stage III

but CT signs of parenchymal necrosis are absent (Fig. 2a).

Progression to stage II is characterized by further pancreatic enlargement and larger collection of retroperitoneal fluid. Intraperitoneal fluid, usually confined to the lesser sac, can also be seen at this stage. In addition, focal hyperdense areas due to hemorrhage or hypodense areas due to necrosis appear in the pancreas (Fig. 2b). In stage III, necrosis extends to involve large segments or the entire gland (Fig. 2c) [7, 15].

Table 2. Influence of CT scanning on therapeutic decisions in 24 patients with acute pancreatitis

Value of CT	Surgery	Conservative treatment
Essential	3	1
Helpful	0	10
Low contribution	2	7
No contribution	1	0
	6	18

Results

Of 24 patients, the diagnosis of acute pancreatitis was established by typical clinical and laboratory findings in 18. The remaining six patients also had histologic confirmation of the diagnosis at the time of surgery. The influence of CT scanning on the decision to treat conservatively or surgically is shown in Table 2. In 14 of 24 patients, the CT findings were considered essential or helpful in making critical therapeutic decisions. A single patient with CT-demonstrated total glandular necrosis was initially treated conservatively because clinical symptoms did not correspond to extensive CT findings. When surgery was eventually performed, pancreatic necrosis was found.

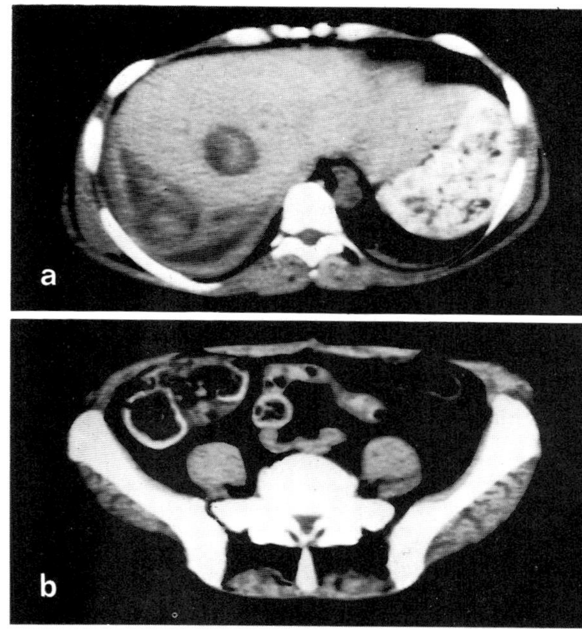

Fig. 3. a Subcapsular and intrahepatic hemorrhage following trauma. CT shows areas of high and low attenuation due to recurrent bleeding. **b** Diffuse intramural increase in density throughout the wall of the small and large bowel. Histology failed to confirm the presence of blood

Bleeding

The site of hemorrhage in a patient with presumed or known blood loss is the most important information for directing therapy [18]. The CT diagnosis of hemorrhage is particularly valuable where parenchymal organs such as the spleen, liver, kidney, or pancreas are involved, because it indicates the presence of a lesion as well as in many cases the source of blood loss.

On CT, clotted blood appears initially as an isodense or hyperdense mass, which gradually falls to fluid density (Fig. 3a). Rarely progressive increase in density is observed due to organization and fibrosis [6, 12, 13, 14, 16].

Results

Of 17 patients with abdominal hemorrhage, the diagnosis was established by surgery in eight patients and by follow-up in nine. In one patient diffuse intramural increase in density throughout the wall of the small and large bowel was interpreted by CT to be due to intramural bleeding, but histology failed to confirm the presence of blood (Fig. 3b). In 11 of 17 patients, the findings of CT strongly or moderately influenced the choice of therapy, particularly in two patients with ruptured spleen and one patient with hepatic rupture (Table 3).

Table 3. Influence of CT scanning on therapeutic decisions in 17 patients with confirmed abdominal bleeding

	Surgery	Conservative treatment
Essential	3	1
Helpful	2	5
Low contribution	3	3
No contribution	0	0
	8	9

Conclusion

Our investigation shows that in patients with an acute abdomen, CT can provide valuable diagnostic information which influences the course of therapy. Patients referred with clinical suspicion of abscess, acute pancreatitis, bleeding, and negative CT findings are not included in this study. The study was not randomized, but examined consecutive patients pro- or retrospectively in whom the influence of CT on therapeutic decision could be evaluated. The effect of CT on mortality or morbidity was not evaluated. In 83 patients with abscesses, pancreatitis, or bleeding, CT strongly or moderately influenced therapeutic decisions in 68%.

References

1. Ariel JM, Kazarian KK (1971) Diagnosis and treatment of abdominal abscesses. Williams & Wilkins, Baltimore
2. Aronberg DJ, Stanley RJ, Levitt RG, Sagel SS (1978) Evaluation of abdominal abscess with computed tomography. J Comput Assist Tomogr 2:384–387
3. Bydder GM, Kreel L (1980) Attenuation values of fluid collections within the abdomen. J Comput Assist Tomogr 4:145–150
4. Encke A (1979) Pathogenese, Klinik und Therapie der lokalisierten Peritonitis insbesondere des subphrenischen Abszesses. In: Höring R (ed) Peritonitis. TM, Bad Oeynhausen, p 219
5. Feifel G, Heberer G (1980) Der gastroenterologische Kommentar. Leber Magen Darm 10:6–7
6. Haertel M, Fuchs WA (1979) Computertomographie nach stumpfem Bauchtrauma. ROEFO 131: 487–492
7. Haertel M, Tillmann U, Fuchs WA (1979) Die akute Pankreatitis im Computertomogramm. ROEFO 130: 525–530
8. Halber MD, Daffner RH, Morgan CL, Trought WS, Thompson WM, Rice RP, Korobkin M (1979) Intraabdominal abscess: Current concepts in radiologic evaluation. AJR 133:9–13
9. Hartung H, Kirchner R (1980) Diagnostik und Therapie der akuten Pankreatitis. Leber Magen Darm 10:1–5
10. Hau T, Ahrenholz DH, Simmons RL (1979) Secondary bacterial peritonitis: The biologic basis of treatment. Curr Prob Surg 16/10:1–65
11. Hübener KH, Schmitt WGH (1979) Die computertomographische Diagnostik von Abszeßbildungen. ROEFO 130:53–57
12. Hübener KH, Schmitt WGH (1979) Computertomographische Densitometrie des menschlichen Blutes. Einfluß auf das Absorptionsverhalten von parenchymatösen Organen und Ergußbildungen. ROEFO 130:185–188
13. Korobkin M, Moss AA, Callen PW, DeMartini WJ, Kaiser JA (1978) Computed tomography of subcapsular splenic hematoma. Radiology 129: 441–445
14. Mall JC, Kaiser JA (1980) CT diagnosis of spenic laceration. AJR 134:265–269
15. Mödder U, Rosenberger J (1980) Befunde und Ergebnisse der Angio-CT bei Pankreatitiden. Deutscher Röntgenkongreß, Cologne 1980
16. Moss AA, Korobkin M, Price D, Brito AC (1979) Computed tomography of splenic subcapsular hematomas: an experimental study in dogs. Invest Radiol 14:60–65
17. Neher M (1977) Der derzeitige Stand der operativen Behandlung der akuten Pankreatitis. Z Gastroenterol 15:67–75
18. Oestern HF, Rehner M (1972) Bauchtrauma. In: Baumgartl F, Kremer K, Schreiber HW (eds) Spezielle Chirurgie für die Praxis, vol 2, part 2. Thieme, Stuttgart, p 561
19. Ranson JHG (1979) Acute Pancreatitis. Curr Prob Surg 16/11:1–84
20. Wolverson MK, Jagannadharo B, Sundaram M, Joyce PF, Riaz MA, Shields JB (1979) CT as a primary diagnostic method in evaluating intraabdominal abscess. AJR 133:1089–1095

Developments in Computerized Tomography Including Non-X-ray Techniques

M. Pfeiler

Firma Siemens AG, Unternehmensbereich Medizinische Technik, Henkestrasse 127, D-8520 Erlangen

Introduction

Computerized tomography (CT) employs a novel type of image buildup technique based on measured data obtained with a classic information carrier in the field of medicine, namely X-radiation. The rapid and impressive success attained by CT since its introduction in the first half of the 1970s has led to a number of attempts to combine its image reconstruction algorithm with other information carriers, most of which have also been tried and tested for medical applications, for example, the gamma radiation of nuclear-diagnostic indicators. To differentiate this from the "real" CT technique, namely roentgen (X-ray) CT, or RCT, we then speak of emission CT, or ECT. It is the aim of this article to provide an overview of such further cross-sectional imaging techniques with CT image reconstruction, the principle and the particular physical-technical problems receiving special attention. Furthermore, the attempt is also made – if only in outline – to assess the relevance and prospects of these techniques. Such an overview would also appear useful as background information for a discussion of the developmental tendencies in X-ray CT, since the knowledge and results gained with the other techniques might also be employed to advance the "real" or original (X-ray) CT technique.

X-ray Computerized Tomography – About the Principle and the State-of-the-Art

It is probably true to say that the principle of CT can best be outlined by these three characteristics: The transradiation of a section or slice (of the patient's body), distortion-eliminating image reconstruction, and digital-electronic acquisition and processing of data ("computer").

With respect to the essential idea of CT, the second feature is the decisive one. Without the distortion-eliminating image reconstruction stage, the images obtained (either with or without the computer) would retain the long-range blurring seen in the classic transversal planigraphic images. It is assumed that the CT algorithm employed is the so-called convolution method (Fig. 1), that is, the establishment of the radiation attenuation reliefs for individual projections, subsequent high-pass filtration ("subtraction of unsharpness"), and the superimposition of these thus modified radiation attenuation reliefs in the same projection direction ("back projection") [1, 2].

X-ray CT has now become well established both from the point of view of its clinical usefulness and the level of its physical technical development. Following the rapid development of the initial phase, CT technology has now become stabilized; this means that its further development follows a by and large constant path in common with the further development of other established techniques. Small, important, but not spectacular advances are seen in the further development of the technology with the aim of compensating for increasing costs and increasing both the reliability and operating convenience of the equipment. Also, in the case of the natural and understandable desire to extrapolate the specifications, that is, to provide even sharper images with even greater density resolution obtained with even shorter scan times, small steps forward are repeatedly taken. These steps normally remain unremarkable in the absence of a quite specific problem, for which such a small step can represent an appreciable advance. Figure 2 shows an example of how, by means of a further modification of the algorithm, the "fine depiction" of bony structures can be promoted. A rapid further development resulting in a considerable improvement of all features simultaneously, however, is limited by the question of cost and patient dose.

It is for this reason that, at the Mayo Clinic, a special CT unit is under development for dynamic

Radiology Today 1. Ed. by M. W. Donner and F. H. W. Heuck

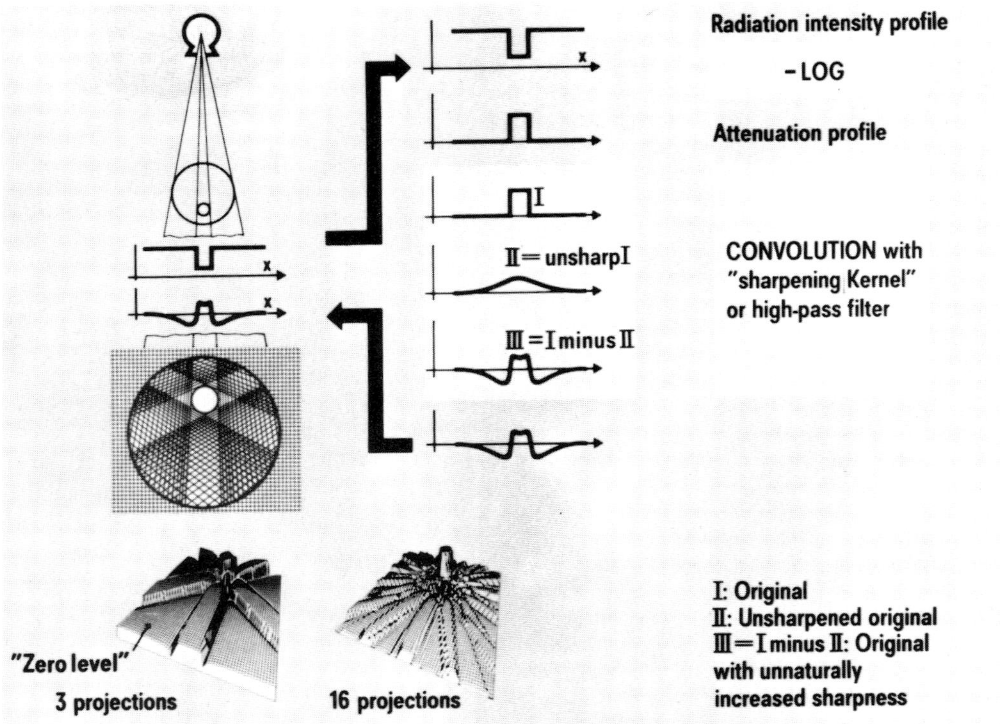

Fig. 1. X-ray CT: image reconstruction

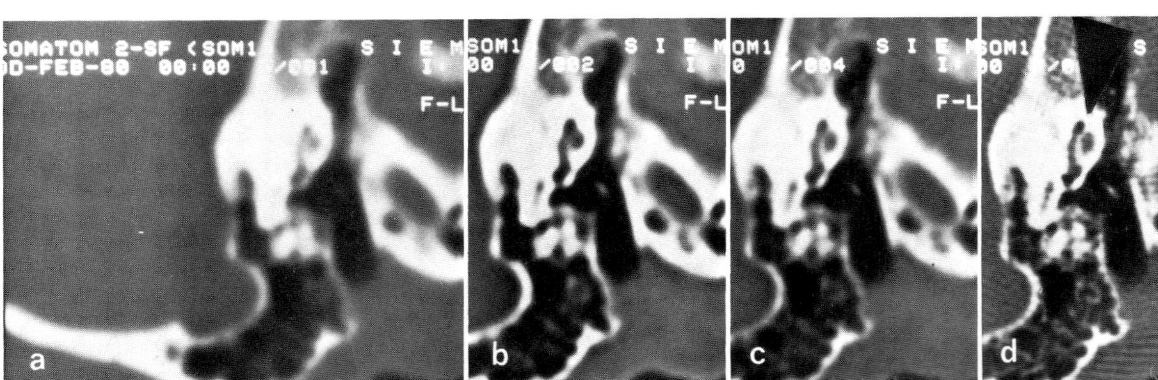

Fig. 2a – d. Increase in resolution and structure enhancement by "high definition algorithm" for the example of the inner ear (▶ cochlea); eightfold zooming; 2 mm slice thickness. **a** Normal mode. **b** Normal mode with "edge enhancement". **c** Special high definition. **d** Experimental high definition mode

heart CT: In order to obtain extremely short exposure times of, for example, 10 ms, for use in examinations of the heart, requirements with respect to spatial resolution and the differentiation of density differences have been quite drastically moderated [3]. In order to achieve such a short exposure time (at an image rate of a maximum of 60 exposures per second), the device employs 28 X-ray tubes arranged in a semicircle. Opposite these, there is a fluorescent screen, used as the detector, the light from which is received by 28 optical image intensifiers (aligned to the X-ray tubes opposite) each forming the first element of a television chain. The object is transirradiated not by a fan beam but by a conical beam: This means that attenuation values are measured not simply for a slice but for an extensive volume. Admittedly, however, the years of effort to find a "three-dimensional reconstruction algorithm," that is, to develop a "simultaneous multilayer technique,"

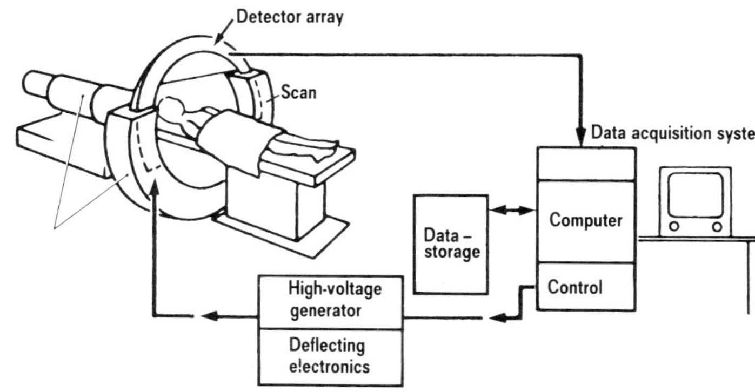

Fig. 3. Heart CT. The patient lies in the funnel system – open on top – of the radiation (X-ray) source. (Lines on the left point to X-ray source housing with funnel system. The electron beam of the X-ray tube is guided in the funnel walls from the cathode at the tip of the funnel to the ring anode.) Modified from Boyd [6]

have apparently not been crowned with any practically useful success. The project continues to appear plagued by a, rather theroretical, inconsistency: Even if one could be satisfied with 28 projections corresponding to the 28 X-ray tubes, these 28 projections are distributed only over 180° and not over 180° plus fan angle. This condition must, however, be met to satisfy the general CT condition, namely, that it must be possible, from the individual beams of all the fans, to put together parallel projections distributed over 180° and covering the whole object. In order to meet this requirement, however, the device, that is, its gantry, bearing 28 X-ray tubes and 28 image intensifiers, must move, although only for a single exposure, through the fan (or conical) angle of one of the emitters. An instructive photograph of a model of the device intended to carry 28 X-ray tubes can be seen in [4].

The concept of an absolutely movement-free CT device for use in dynamic heart studies is presented in [6]. Here, through the deflection of an electron beam the focal spot is made to run around the patient on a ring anode "open at the top," through 180° plus fan angle, which leads to an overlapping of the radiation source and detector areas (Fig. 3) which has to be taken into account both with respect to equipment construction and image reconstruction. Up to four focal spots on parallel paths, which function together with a double detector, produce the data needed for up to eight simultaneous CT images. The shortest exposure time is to be 50 ms at, in that case, a maximum of five exposures per second.

In addition to the advances in the area of technology and the just-described work on improving the specifications or "exposure parameters," a third point is of particular topicality: the development of techniques that permit special applications with the equipment of the present state of the technical art. An example of this is ECG-oriented image reconstruction [8]. Here, from a number of systematized scanning cycles, a complete series of such projection as belong to a given phase of the cardiac cycle are selected. In this way, for the heart, a computed tomogram having an effective scanning time for this cardiac phase of, for example, 200 ms can be reconstructed, although the actual scanning time of the equipment is a multiple of this. Clinical experience with this technique has, in the meantime, been gained [9].

A further example is the sequential scanning technique, e.g., for dynamic studies of blood flow [5] in which an additional control device and special programming involving the use of short repetition times permits a method of working such as is offered, for instance, by the programme selector of a cut-film angiographic system. As a rule, the associated software will also contain the evaluation possibilities tailored to this method, e.g., the establishment of time/density diagrams for selectable image areas ("regions of interest"), which, throughout the series of images, are always located at the same place of the organs under investigation (Fig. 4). The term "evaluation technique" concerns a further point which should also be mentioned quite generally when considering developmental tendencies. In this very area there is a constant development and, since, to a large extent only the evaluation program software is involved, this development is also taking place outside the laboratories of the CT manufacturers. The clinically active user of CT equipment does not need to take particular note of this development since, when it has been tried and tested, a new additional program is, as a rule, capable of being "retrofitted" to an existing CT machine over a considerable period of time.

As mentioned at the beginning, (X-ray) CT has led to a series of attempts to employ the CT reconstruction algorithm also to signals that can be obtained with information carriers other than X-rays. For this reason, in a consideration of the

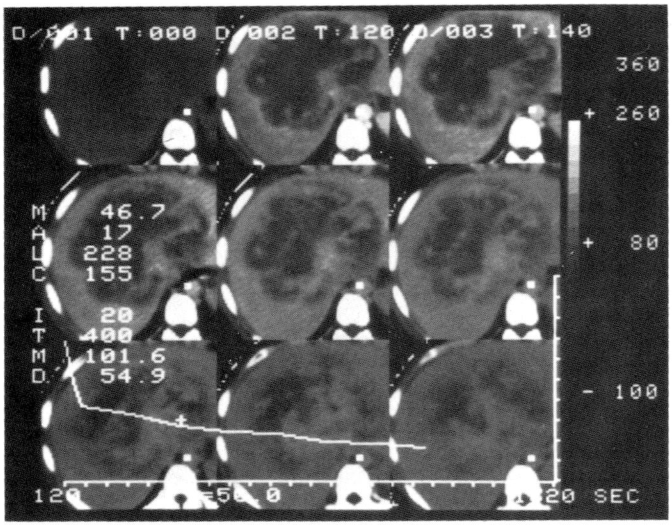

Fig. 4. Sequential or dynamic CT for studies, for example, of the temporal contrast medium flow ("dynamics"). Determination of time/CM density curves for a preselected area, here in the aorta

developmental tendencies in the field of CT, these techniques should be included, and not least since on the basis of considerations and results, repercussions may be expected for X-ray CT.

CT Procedures With Different Information Carriers

Emission CT (ECT)

CT imaging techniques of different information carriers are shown in the following lists. The first non-X-ray CT procedure in the list is emission CT (ECT).

X-ray CT or RCT (roentgen CT)
Dynamic heart X-ray CT
ECT (emission CT) with single photons
PECT (positron emission CT) with photon pairs
Nuclear magnetic resonance CT
Ultrasonic CT
Proton CT
Impedance (resistance) CT
Microwave CT

The technical origins of ECT, including initial clinical results, however, must be dated earlier than RCT, in particular on the basis of the publication [10] of Kuhl et al. in 1963. There is no doubt, however, that the work on the physics and technology of the emission cross-sectional image experienced a sort of renaissance induced by RCT.

What is the nature of the relationship between RCT and ECT with respect to the build-up of the image (Fig. 5)? In the case of RCT, during the acquisition of data, the line integral of the attenuation coefficient μ is measured along the individual rays of the projections which are used for image reconstruction. Such a line integral is nothing other than the sum of the attenuation exponents of the volume elements "hit" by the beam on its path from the source of radiation to the detector. This measured value is then employed in the reconstruction of the CT image.

The same procedure can also be employed in the cross-sectional image reconstruction of an activity distribution. The sum of activities is measured along a beam, the direction of which is determined by the detector collimator. If an ideal situation is assumed ("without μ," Fig. 5), the analogy to RCT is perfect; CT image reconstruction provides a cross-sectional image of the distribution of activity free from superimposition. In actual fact, however, the activity distribution is located within a medium that attenuates the radiation originating in the activity on its way to the detector.

The actual measured value as a line integral of the activity, "weighted" by the radiation attenuation, cannot be used for the application of an immediate CT reconstruction. The question now arises as to whether, by means of a correction, the desired line integral might be "split off" that expression, that is, computed in such a way as though the site of the activity on the measuring beam considered were without influence on the results of measurement. In the simple example selected (Fig. 6), it can be seen immediately that, for the *single photon ECT,*

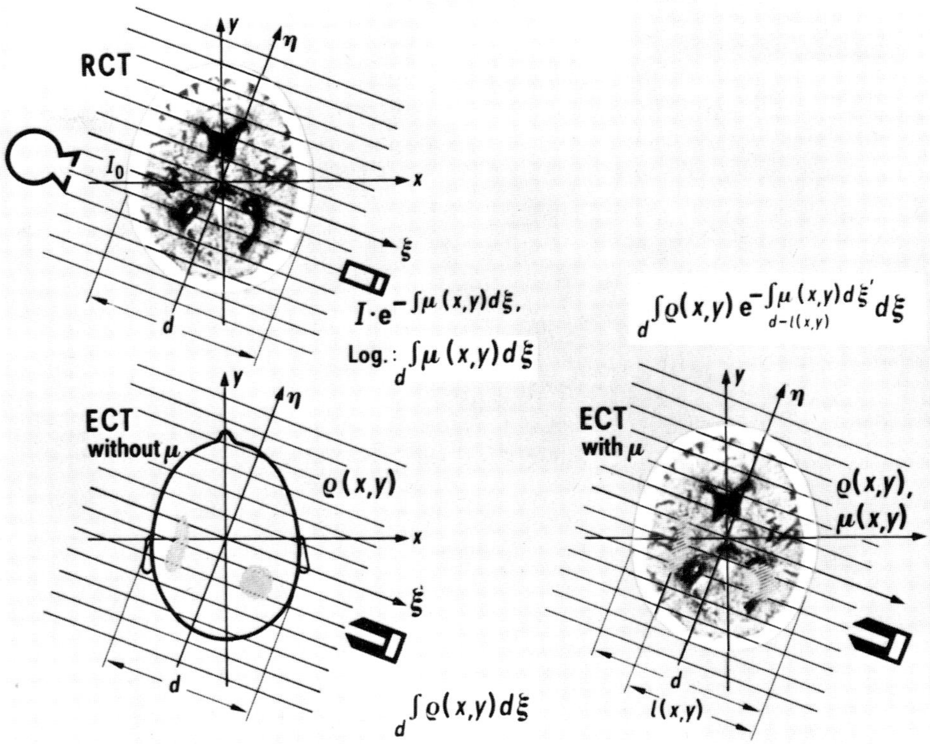

Fig. 5. X-ray CT (RCT) and ECT: Complete analogy obtains only in the ECT case of an activity distribution in the attenuation-free medium ("without μ")

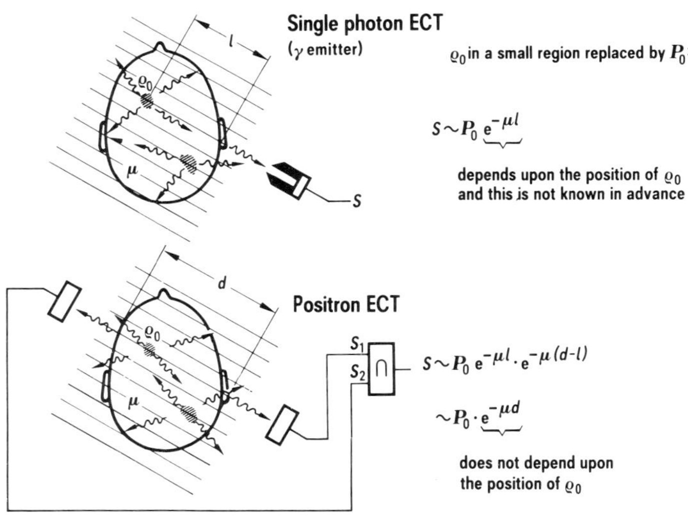

Fig. 6. ECT: Plausibility explanation on the influence of radiation absorption; a simple example

that is, the ECT with the isotopes emitting the usual gamma radiation, activity and attenuation do not combine in the measured result in isolation. Even if the distribution of the attenuation coefficient μ was completely known, e.g., by means of a separately obtained X-ray CT scan, and if, as in the present case, it were even homogeneous, the resulting signal still depends upon the position of the source of activity marked by the length l (which is not known in advance).

In the case of *positron ECT,* the situation is quite different, for it is not the radiation (here positrons) emitted by the marking isotope that is measured. Rather, after a short distance, e.g., 4 mm, an emitted positron, at an energy of 1 MeV, fuses with an electron and, in the course of mutual annihilation, these two particles are converted into two directly opposed 511 keV γ quanta. If this annihilation radiation is measured with two opposed detectors, the signals of which are only evaluated when they appear simultaneously, collimation of the radiation is, at first, obviated. An emission that is not along the line connecting the detectors can, after all, activate only a single detector, the signal of which alone will, however, not be evaluated by the coincidence circuitry of the input electronics.

Of decisive importance for a CT-conform cross-sectional imaging technique, however, is that the resulting signal of the activity along the detector-connecting line is independent of the position of the activity along this line. In the example shown, the radiation quantum emitted from the area of ϱ_0, arrives at the right detector with a probability reduced by the attenuation factor of its path, that is, $e^{-\mu l}$; for the radiation quantum moving to the left, the probability of arrival is reduced by the attenuation factor $e^{-\mu(d-l)}$. The probability of simultaneous arrival of the two quanta, or, in other words, the ratio of the recorded gamma quanta pairs to those emitted at the point in question, is the product of the individual attenuation factors. This product, however, no longer depends upon where along the detector-connecting line the annihilation radiation appears. It is always equal to the attenuation factor for a quantum which moves over the entire cross-sectional path d, which, with the aid of an external source of radiation – preferentially a source of positrons – can be measured in a simple manner.

While in the case of the single photon ECT the measured value delivered by the detector could not be corrected even with knowledge of the entire attenuation value distribution to the desired line integral of the activity, in the case of positron ECT the measurement of the radiation attenuation through the cross section of the object along the measuring line is adequate to permit the desired correction. This plausibility consideration in the simple example is confirmed by the discussion of a more complex example (Fig. 7). From this example it can also be seen that, in the case of the single photon emission, a second detector of similar construction, i.e., to that used in positron ECT, does not provide the prerequisites for an uncompromising application of the CT algorithm. Although in the case of relatively homogeneous object structures compromises certainly can be entered into for the correction, in general, iterative algebraic algorithms are given preference [11 – 14, M. M. Ter-Pogossian, personal communication]. One scanner of the (single photon) ECT type diverges entirely from the classic CT scanning principle (Fig. 8) and "scans" the cross section under observation in a meandering manner using collimators focused to a point [15, 16]. The collimators of six pairs of detectors distributed around the circumference of the device "share" the scanning work on the half of the cross section facing them so that, owing to the inherent absorption of the object, not too much useful radiation is lost. While one pair of detectors move toward each other in a meandering manner, the neighboring pair move away from each other. The scanning results from all directions are superimposed. The "raw image" obtained in this way can be subjected to further processing via a (high-pass) filtering process (somewhat similar to the "harmonization" employed in radiology). The

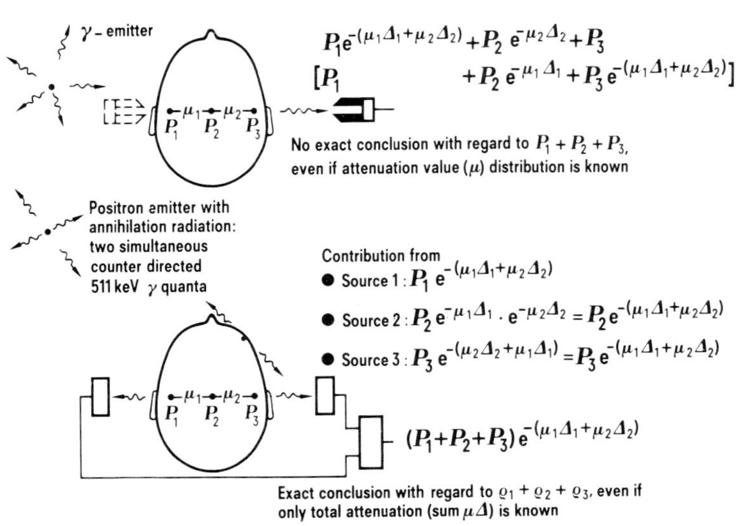

Fig. 7. ECT: Plausibility study on the influence of radiation absorption; a more complex example

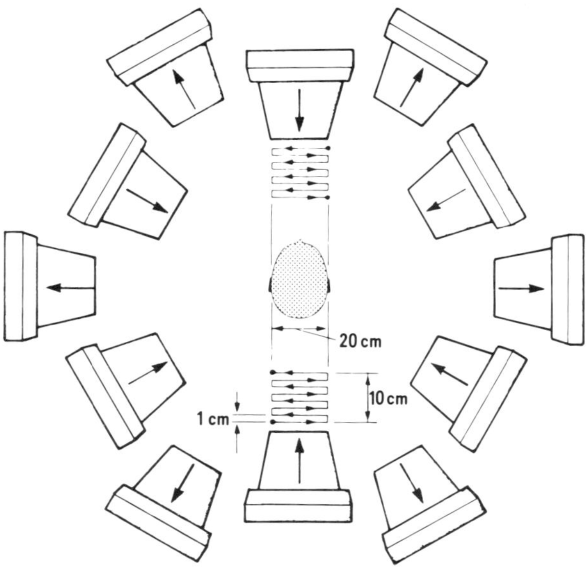

Fig. 8. ECT with focused collimators and "meandering" detectors. Figure modified from Strelzoff, A. [16]

scan time of, for example, some 5 min, of such a machine, and also the characteristics described by the image example (Fig. 9), can be considered representative, also for the other single photon techniques that are more strongly modeled on CT. The resolution is, today, at about 10 mm (in the sense of the half value width of the so-called line spread function) typical for the images in the field of nuclear diagnosis [17] but is comparatively favorable. The sensitivity, expressed in terms of short scanning time, is relatively high; for a machine such as that shown in Fig. 7 with two (opposing) single-channel detectors, some 30 min would be typical.

The techniques of single photon ECT are, at the moment, becoming highly topical since, for the acquisition of data, a conventional gamma camera – which is often already available – mounted on a rotating stand can be employed (Fig. 10); by employing the structure of the collimator channels as measuring lines for a number of simultaneously acquired complete projections, the additional translation movement which, in the case of, for example, single-channel collimators, is a necessity, can be obviated. In this way, during a single scan, the measured data for a number of parallel slices are obtained [19].

Despite years of research and development work, however, neither single photon ECT nor positron ECT has attained anywhere near the importance of CT in terms of clinical application. One reason for this – in the sense of an unconfirmed working hypothesis – may be found in the limited spatial resolution which does not permit utilization of the freedom from superimposition effects, which is in principle present, for a morphological evaluation. In other words: when fine structures are not visible, they are anyhow unable to exercise a mutually interfering effect with respect to recognition. If, however, the freedom from superimposition is to be employed for the quantitative determination in

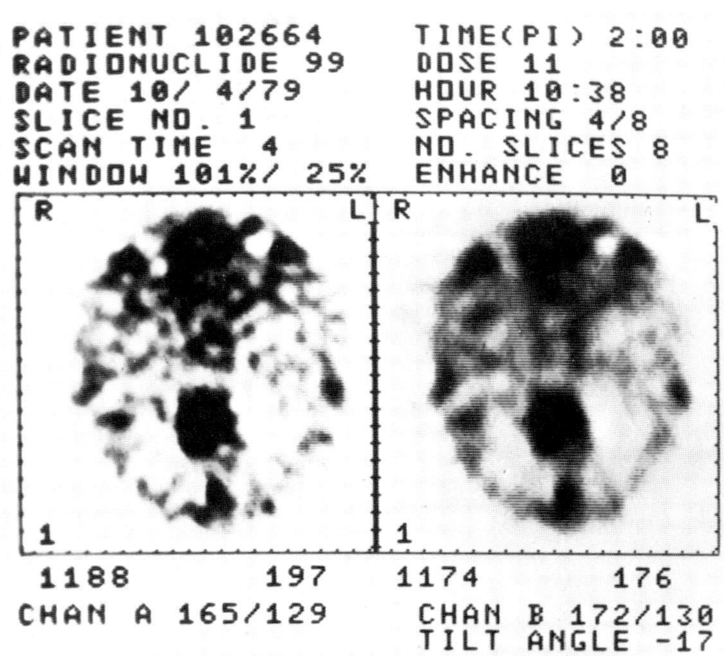

Fig. 9. ECT: Typical study taken with a unit having focused collimators: glioma of the brain stem and pons. (By courtesy of the Dept. of Stereotaxis and Nuclear Medicine of the University of Freiburg/FRG; medical head of dept.: Prof. F. Mundinger)

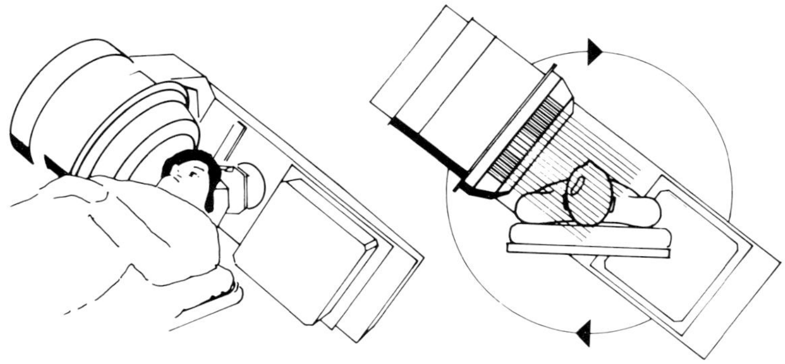

Fig. 10. ECT: Using a gamma camera for measuring complete projections (rotation only, no translation): left sketch modified from a photograph in Patton, J. A. [18]

a way similar to the measurement of CT numbers in roentgen CT, doubts are basically well founded with respect to single photon ECT. Here, after all, the influence of the attenuation of the radiation by the tissue itself can be corrected only to a certain degree. The positron ECT, on the other hand, *can* supply an superimposition-free image which is uninfluenced by the attenuation properties of the tissue. The half-life times of the positron-emitting radiopharmaceutical agents, however, are so short that positron ECT requires the presence of a cyclotron in the immediate neighborhood (preparation, transport). The indicator atoms essential for positron ECT have only short half-lives, e.g., carbon-11, 20 min; oxygen-15, 2 min – a fact, which, on the other hand, favors the application of high activities (which reduces the quantum noise in the picture).

An improvement of the ECT technique by enhancing the spatial resolution will scarcely be possible since the limitation to the quantum flow given by the restricted dose "loadability" of the patient applies every bit as much to the ECT procedure as it does to the established image-producing systems employed in nuclear medical diagnostic work.

The particular advantage of positron ECT is based on the possibility of displaying metabolic functions using "biologically similar" radionucleides or radiopharmaceuticals. The above mentioned positron emitting isotopes of carbon and oxygen as well as nitrogen are also isotopes of elements which play an essential part in the basic metabolic processes. From that stems the most effective motivation to continue the development of positron ECT. However, the goal of this research has to include the economic production of radionucleides and radiopharmaceuticals.

Proton CT

In the case of *proton CT,* protons or other heavy charged particles are employed to transradiate the object in place of X-rays. In contrast to X-ray radiation, in the case of which the number of gamma quanta penetrating the object constantly diminishes owing to photoabsorption or Compton scatter effects, the high-energy protons simply diminish in energy as a result of their interaction with the atoms of the object. That is to say that the information to be employed for the CT image takes the form of a loss of energy of the proton which, for example, can be measured by means of a highly pure germanium detector or a so-called plastic detector, that is, a scintillator made of transparent plastic, employed in conjunction with a photo-multiplier.

An obvious advantage of proton CT is the reduced dose: For 30 cm water, according to information contained in [20], a dose advantage of about a factor of 6 is obtained when using 230 MeV protons as compared with 100 keV X-rays. It must, however, be admitted that the diagnostic analogy to X-ray radiation is not complete; the contrast media commonly employed with X-rays, containing elements with a high atomic number, e.g., iodine, have a slight influence on the proton beam. Moreover, it is apparently not known whether and to what extent beams of protons "react" to pathologic tissue. A certain disadvantage in comparison with X-ray CT results from the fact that an originally well-collimated proton beam undergoes a spreading effect due to the small deflections experienced by the charged protons on moving past the atoms of the object and caused by the electrical nuclear fields of the latter: After all, after passing through 30 cm water, a 230 MeV proton beam spreads by about 14 mm. The attempt can be made, by taking into account this slightly curved path of the individual protons, to estimate the spread (considered macroscopically) of the proton beam and to compute a correction for the loss of resolution or, alternatively, to employ heavy particles that are less susceptible to deflection, e.g., helium nuclei ("α particles"), and in this way to achieve improved resolution. In such a case, however, the dose advantage over the X-ray technique might be lost.

The high costs for a proton CT installation which, after all, must contain a complicated and expensive particle accelerator and also a CT-appropriate beam tap-off facility (production of the beams forming a projection, for example, by means of magnetic deflection of the proton "pencil" beam), are certainly the major reason for proton CT not being a real option at present.

Nuclear Magnetic Resonance Imaging

The present objective of numerous working groups is the production of cross-sectional images with the aid of *nuclear magnetic resonance* (NMR). The principle of signal production is explained, taking the hydrogen atomic nucleus as an example, on the basis of the sketch shown in Fig. 11. The principle is represented in a strongly simplified form, using a macroscopic model to describe what is really a quantum-mechanical process [23].

The nucleus of the hydrogen atom rotates about its own axis, that is, it possesses a "spin," behaving like a mechanical gyroscope. Its positive charge also rotates. A moving charge, however, behaves like an electric current which, in this case, flows around the axis of the gyroscope. For this reason, this current produces a magnetic moment. In a piece of, for example, water-containing material, many such proton gyroscopes are present, depending upon the content of hydrogen or water, and their axes are randomly oriented. With the aid of a static, external magnetic field, a force can be exerted on these gyroscopes – on the basis of their magnetic moments – which results in the axes of all the gyroscopes being aligned in a single direction (second sketch from the left in Fig. 11). On switching on the field, the following processes occur until total alignment has been achieved: The proton gyroscopes have the tendency, shared in common with real gyroscopes, with their axes perpendicular to the force exercised upon them by the magnetic field, to take "avoiding action" as it were. They precess about the direction of the field lines of the external magnetic field, that is, their axes "dance" a cone-shaped pattern about a field line. The cone angle, which is initially equal to the angle between the original position of the gyroscope axis and the direction of the field lines, becomes smaller and smaller – in the case of solid or liquid material, owing to the influences of the surroundings ("friction") – until the axes of all the gyroscopes are all aligned in the direction of the external magnetic field lines.

If, for example, a laterally directed force now briefly acts upon these aligned gyroscopes – and such a force can, in the sketch, be produced with the aid of a lateral magnetic field – the gyroscopes tend to "take avoiding action," moving their axes perpendicularly to the direction of this force. That is, they begin, once again, to precess. The speed of this movement, the precession frequency, also referred to as the Larmor frequency, is determined by the strength of the static magnetic field first described and is higher the more powerful this magnetic field is (for protons, e.g.: 4.26 MHz at 1 kGauss). If, now, the laterally effective force "impinges" upon the gyroscopes in rhythm with the precession frequency, as shown in the sketch, then, with a magnetic alternating (lateral) field of identical frequency, even small field strengths of the alternating field suffice to "completely tilt over" the axes of the gyroscopes. For this procedure, energy is required, and this is obtained from the alternating field. If the high frequency generator, and thus the alternating magnetic field, are switched off, the proton gyroscopes return to their

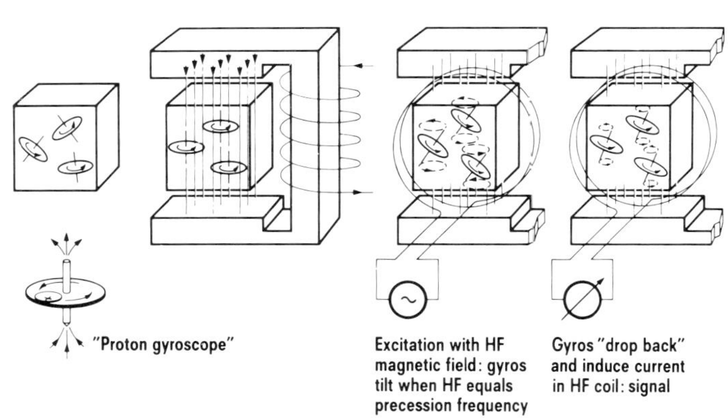

Fig. 11. NMR: Simplified representation with the aid of a macroscopic model instead of the actual quantum-mechanical procedure. (The plus sign on the "proton gyroscope" indicates its electrical charge, the lines entering and leaving its axis indicate its magnetic momentum.) (See p. 204, Fig. 12)

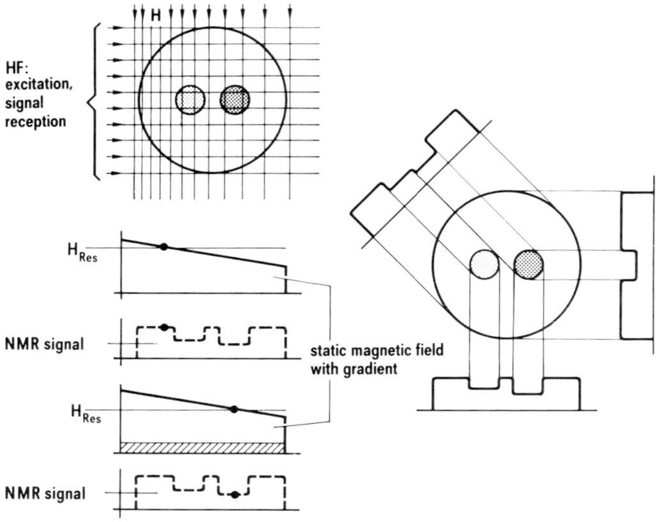

Fig. 12. NMR CT: Production of "projections" for the NMR signal by changing a magnetic gradient field

positions as determined by the static magnetic field. In so doing, with the aid of their own magnetic field, which is constantly changing due to precession, they induce a high frequency current in the coil, which can then be used as a signal current. This signal provides information as to the density of the collection of protons, and thus, for example, as to the water content of the material involved, for the more protons are present, the larger will be the signal.

The signal, however, also provides information as to the chemical nature of the material contained within the volume examined. Depending upon the degree of "fixation" of the proton in a molecule, the proton returns to its initial position more or less rapidly. This relaxation period ("relaxation time"), recognizable in the behavior of the signal is thus a characteristic of the nature of the material examined. But how can we now selectively examine and image a cross section of an examined object in the manner typical of CT? A model proposal by P. Lauterbur [24] shows the construction of a projection in the form required by CT: A magnetic gradient field (Fig. 12) ensures that the condition for NMR is met only for a single line through the represented cross section. If the uniform part of the magnetic field is made stronger, this line, for which the NMR signal can be called up, shifts further and further toward the right. Such signal projections are now established for various directions – the object in the example has two regions of varyingly diminished material density and shows, qualitatively, three different projections – and in analogy to CT, the cross-sectional image is reconstructed from them.

The described "gradient method" of generating locally selective signals using a time-variant gradient and a nonvariant signal frequency could be inverted: In case of a time-constant magnetic gradient field the NMR characteristics of selected locations could be picked by varying the frequency of excitation and therefore of the NMR signal.

P. Lauterbur has coined the term *"Zeugmatographie"* for nuclear magnetic resonance CT (Zeugma = "yoke," "bridge" – what belongs together; here, apparently, the strength of the static and the frequency of the alternating magnetic field).

But also in the case of, NMR a cross-sectional image build-up is possible which is not employed in CT image reconstruction. Using magnetic field focusing the attempt can, for example, be made to produce the resonance condition only for a single point and, using this point, to scan a cross section of the body [25]. This procedure is remotely similar to the already discussed technique of ECT employing focusing collimators. A further procedure excites the volume under investigation, as it were, line-wise or rod-wise [26] and then "scans" these lines or rods using the magnetic gradient field rotated through 90°, in a punctiform manner, to pick up the NMR signal. Pictures have been obtained both with the technique that employs the CT algorithm and also the other methods described. Sample pictures are, for example, shown in [26]; a more recent publication [27] demonstrates an image through the head.

The NMR picture shown in Fig. 13 is part of the results of the research group cited unter [35] and was added to this article during press.

On the basis of the example images published it is clear that, with respect to the morphology, despite numerous years of research work [28] a NMR image cannot fully compete, for example, with the image produced by roentgen CT, and that, in all

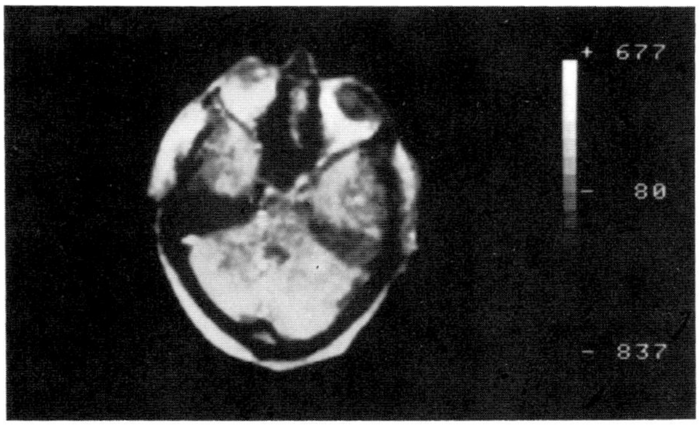

Fig. 13. NMR picture or NMR tomogram: In comparison to the (more water containing) soft tissue, bones are imaged black or darker. Data acquisition time, 1.5 min (sample from the research group cited under [35])

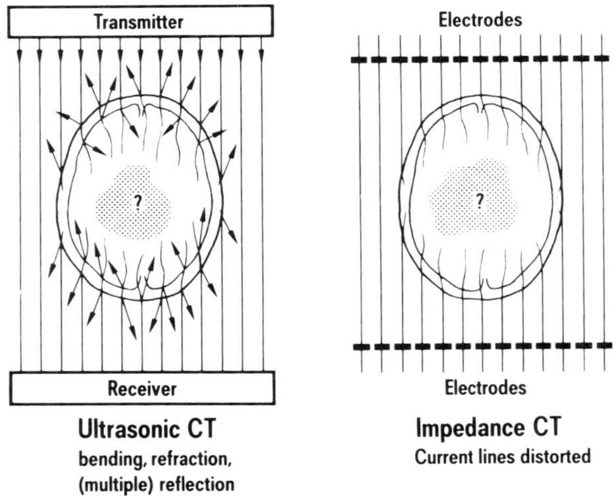

Fig. 14. Further physical attempts to use the CT algorithm. (Coupling medium in the measurement devices, e.g., water)

probability, it will not be able to do so in the future. The prospects for NMR images are to be seen in the representation of metabolic processes, for example, the special metabolism of a tumor, which they permit. Here, however, clinical research is obviously only at its beginning.

Possible biologic effects of NMR induced by the static magnetic field of high field strength, the high frequency applied, and the electric current induced by rapid temporal changes in the magnetic field (depending upon the technique involved, by switching of the static field) are discussed in [29] and a comprehensive list of references to other publications given. The high frequency and the static magnetic field do not seem to pose any threat to health; for the temporal changes in the magnetic field, however, restrictions are indicated.

Note:

The simplified model in this Figure demonstrates how the proton gyros aligned by the external static magnetic field and then disturbed return with decreasing precession amplitude to their original state or state of equilibrium. This procedure is characterized by the relaxion time mentioned (which has the meaning of a physical time constant) called spin-lattice relaxation time T_1 [30]. In addition to this relaxion time T_1 there is also a spin-spin relaxation time T_2. The reason for this is that the micro gyros synchronously and in the same way disturbed by the alternating magnetic field laterally, do not return synchronously precessing to their original position. They relatively quickly loose this synchronism, for which T_2 is the measure. T_2 is often much smaller, but in any case smaller than T_1, because after the return of the proton gyros to their original position precession no longer exist. For biological, say water containing tissue depending upon its type, the relaxation times lie between 50 and 1000 ms. Measurement techniques for T_1 and T_2 are described in [30].

It should also be mentioned that not every atomic nucleus has a spin and with it a magnetic momentum. Nuclei with an even number of the protons contributing to the nucleus as well as an even number of the neutrons do not have a spin. Therefore, the next element of interest for diagnostic purposes is phosphorus, which participates in the biological tissue and therefore metabolism. The nuclei of phosphorus, however, deliver a significantly smaller detectable signal than the protons as nuclei of hydrogenium.

Ultrasonic CT

In the list of cross-sectional imaging techniques (p. 196), a further three methods are to be found. There is well-founded research work on ultrasonic imaging from, for example, the Mayo Clinic [31]. The desire for an ultrasonic CT is based on its quantitative character: While the conventional ultrasound techniques represent, in the main, transitional areas between regions with differing acoustic properties – at interfaces at which the ultrasound waves are reflected – an ultrasonic tomographic technique employing transmission would show the sound power attenuation and possibly the velocity of sound in a CT image as "true" acoustic properties of the material under investigation. The difficulties associated with such transmission techniques, are, however, considerable, since the prerequisite, so necessary for a CT technique, of a straight-line course of the radiation of the information carrier, cannot be adequately met with ultrasound in complex acoustic structures such as we are dealing with in the human body (Fig. 14, left). In addition, "sound-empty" zones, for example, behind a bone, in an ultrasonic CT facility would lead to difficult-to-avoid artifacts or information-diminishing corrections in a manner similar to the interference in an X-ray CT image caused by metal inclusions.

There remain only *impedance and microwave CT*. In the case of the impedance image, too, the uncertainty as to the straightness of the course of field lines represents the main problem (Fig. 14, right). Examinations carried out to date [32] do not appear very encouraging. In the case of microwave CT, the problems that are generally applicable to a microwave imaging technique persist: If electromagnetic radiation of very high frequency, as is required for a high degree of spatial resolution, is selected, then the depth of penetration is small, as we can recognize in the example of the thermogram (electromagnetic radiation in the infrared range). If greater depth of penetration is permitted, that is, lower frequencies are selected, the degree of spatial resolution diminishes (*example:* 4 GHz microwave frequency, depth of penetration into body tissue approx. 20 mm, resolution in the body tissue approx. 5 mm). The question is yet to be answered as to whether compromise solutions may acquire clinical relevance [33, 34].

In this connection, it should be pointed out that in the case of NMR, which, after all, employs "high frequency," that is, the high-frequency magnetic alternating currents (e.g., 4 MHz), spatial resolution is not determined by the frequency of the alternating fields. Here, it is the spatial range of the resonance condition that determines resolution.

Conclusion

In conclusion, we shall attempt to assess the relevance and prospects of the techniques discussed (Fig. 15). The two ECT techniques are still partly at the experimental stage, but are already in clinical use in several areas. The particular usefulness in comparison with the conventional (emission) type of image is not so self-evident as in the case of roentgen (X-ray) CT; here, we must await further clinical experience, account also being taken of possibly required and complex additional equipment (e.g., cyclotron). The proton CT option appears simply too expensive for further research or developmental activities to be expected in the near future.

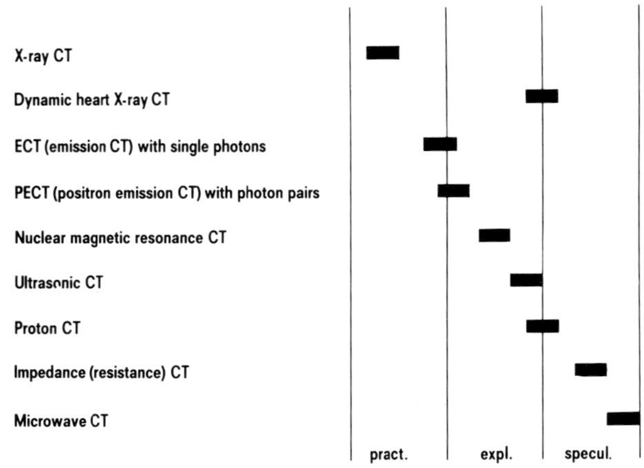

Fig. 15. Cross-sectional imaging techniques using the CT algorithm: an endeavor to assess the relevance and prospects

In the case of NMR in several areas functioning imaging devices exist at least as prototypes. Undergoing clinical tests still have to prove the diagnostic relevance, especially correlated to the question of biochemical characteristics of the examined tissue. The attempts to develop ultrasonic CT are – since the gain in information would, in principle, be very promising – obviously to be taken seriously only with respect to a possible compromise solution, while impedance and microwave CT may be relegated completely to the area of scientific speculation.

Summary

For the build-up of its images, X-ray (roentgen) CT employs not only a highly developed computer technology but also special CT algorithms (preprocessing of recorded "projections," followed by their "high-pass" filtration and back projection). The diagnostic success of X-ray CT provided, and still provides, the motivation, in addition to X-ray radiation, to try to make use also of other information carriers for the recording of cross-sectional images, employing the principle of CT image reconstruction. Examples are emission CT, proton CT, NMR CT, and "impedance" CT.

A synoptic presentation of the computerized tomographic principle, given at the beginning of the contribution, emphasizes three essential features – the transradiation of only a single layer (slice), distortion-eliminating image reconstruction, and digital electronic data processing. A discussion of the tendencies with respect to the further development of X-ray CT, from the point of view of improving the general properties of the system, then focuses particular attention on two projects of dynamic heart CT; in addition, the further expansion of present-day equipment for special applications is dealt with. The main part of the contribution is concerned with the overview of the above-mentioned non-X-ray techniques and includes a description of their fundamentals. Finally, an attempt is made to provide an assessment of the relevance and prospects of these techniques.

References

1. Pfeiler M (1980) Röntgen-Computertomographie; eine röntgentechnische Bestandsaufnahme. MTA 26:303–319
2. Pfeiler M, Linke G (1979) Computertomographie und konventionelle Radiologie, eine physikalisch-technische Gegenüberstellung. Radiol Diagn (Berl) 20:604–617
3. Ritman EL, Sturm RE, Wood EH (1977) Needs, performance requirements and proposed design of spatial reconstruction systems for diagnostic and investigative studies of cardio-pulmonary and circulatory dynamics. In: [7]
4. Ultra high-speed, multi-axial computerized X-ray Scanner developed by the Mayo Clinic. Radiology/Nucl Med Mag 9:49
5. Hacker H (1977) Time controlled computertomographic angiography. J Comput Assist Tomogr 4:405–409
6. Boyd DP, Gould RG, Quinn JR, Sparks R, Stanley JH, Herrmannsfeldt WB (1979) A proposed dynamic cardia 3-d densitometer for early detection and evaluation of heart disease. IEEE Trans Nucl Sci. Vol. NS-26, no. 2, part 2 of two parts
7. Ter-Pogossian MM, Phelps ME, Brownell JR, Cox JR Jr, Davis DO, Evens RG (eds) (1977) Reconstruction tomography in diagnostic radiology and nuclear medicine. University Park Press, Baltimore London Tokyo
8. Pfeiler M (1980) Röntgen-Computertomographie; Einführung und Überblick über den Stand der Technik. Biomed Tech (Berlin) 20:604–617
9. Lackner K, Thurn P (1980) EKG-gesteuerte Kardio-Computertomographie. ROEFO 132/2:164–169
10. Kuhl DE, Edwards RQ (1963) Image separation radioisotope scanning. Radiology 80:653
11. Budinger TF, Gullberg GT (1977) Transverse section reconstruction of gamma-ray emitting radionuclides in patients. In: [7] pp 315–342
12. Phelps ME, Hoffman EJ, Mullani NA, Higgins CS, Ter-Pogossian MM (1977) Some performance and design characteristics of PETT III. In: [7] pp 371–392
13. Ter-Pogossian MM, Phelps ME, Hoffman EJ, Coleman RE (1977) The performance of PETT III. In: [7] pp 359–369
14. Cho ZH, Eriksson L, Chan J (1977) A circular ring transverse axial positron camera. In: [7] pp 393–421
15. Stoddart HF, Stoddart HA (1980) A new development in single gamma transaxial tomography union carbide focused collimator scanner. In [21] pp 2710–2712
16. Strelzoff A (1978) The radionuclide brain imager. Union Carbide Imaging Systems, Norwood (Imaging systems, vol 1)
17. Budinger TF, Derenzo SE, Gullberg GT, Greenberg WL, Huesman RH: Emission computer assisted tomography with single-photon and positron annihilation photon emitters. J Comput Assist Tomogr 1:131
18. Patton JA (to be published) Emission tomography. In: [19]
19. Coulam C, Erickson JJ, Rollo FD, James AE (eds) (to be published) Basic principles of medical imaging. Appleton-Century-Crosts, New York
20. Hanson KM (1979) Proton computed tomography. In [22] pp 97–107
21. Workshop on physics and engineering in computerized tomography. Newport Beach, California, January 17–19, 1979. IEEE Trans Nucl Sci Vol. NS-26, No. 2, part 2 of two parts
22. Raviv J, Greenleaf F, Herman G (eds) (1979) Computer aided tomography and ultrasonics in medicine. Proceedings of the IFIP TC-4 Working Conference on Computer Aided Tomography and Ultrasonics in Medicine. North-Holland, Amsterdam New York Oxford
23. Male S (1979) How does NMR work? New Sci 81:875
24. Lauterbur PC (1973) Image formation by induced local interactions: Examples employing nuclear magnetic resonance. Nature 242:190
25. Damadian R, Minkoff L, Goldsmith M, Stanford M, Koutcher J (1976) Field focusing nuclear magnetic resonance (FONAR): Visualization of a tumor in a live animal. Science 194:1430
26. Morris PG, Mansfield P, Pykett JL, Ordidge RJ, Coupland RE (1980) Human whole body line-scan imaging by nuclear magnetic resonance. In: [21] pp 2817–2820
27. Holland GN, Moore WS, Hawkes RC (1980) NMR neuroradiography. Br J Radiol 53:255
28. Herman R (1979) A chemical clue to disease. New Sci 81:876–877
29. Budinger TF (1980) Thresholds for physiological effects due to RF and magnetic fields used in NMR imaging. In: [21] pp 2821–2825
30. Farrah THC, Becker ED (1971) Pulse and fourier-transform NMR. Introduction to theory and methods. Academic Press, New York San Francisco London

31. Greenleaf F, Johnson SA, Bahn RC, Rajagopalan B, Kenue S (1980) Introduction to computed ultrasound tomography. In: [22] pp 125 – 136
32. Price LR (1980) Electrical impedance computed tomography (ICT): A new CT imaging technique. In: [21] pp 2736 – 2739
33. Microwaves seek and help destroy cancers (1980) Microwaves 19:17
34. Jacobi JH, Larsen LE (1980) Microwave time delay spectroscopic imagery of isolated canine kidney. Med Phys 7:1 – 7
35. Ganssen A, Löffler W, Oppelt A, Schmidt F (to be published) Kernspin-Tomographie. CT, Sonographie

Urinary Tract Radiology

Urinary Tract Radiology: Overview

M. A. Bosniak

New York University, Medical Center, 550 First Avenue, New York, NY 10016 (USA)

Many new developments have occurred during the past few years in radiology of the urinary tract. Three of the more important areas are:

1. *Contrast media:* Increased awareness of the incidence of renal failure caused by the use of intravenous contrast agents.
2. *Imaging:* Further advances and more experience in the noninvasive imaging of the urinary tract by ultrasound and CT.
3. *Interventional techniques:* Increased use of interventional techniques in the management of disease associated with the urinary tract, including interventional angiography and percutaneous pyelonephrostomy techniques.

Contrast Media

It has become evident over the past few years that acute renal failure is a much more common event following the intravenous use of iodinated contrast media (wheter it be for urography, angiography, cholangiography, or contrast-enhanced CT) than had previously been appreciated. The identification of those patients who are at increased risk therefore is of great importance in decreasing the incidence of this complication.

Previous reports on the occurrence of acute renal failure following urography identified patients with multiple myeloma (and other dysproteinemic states) as being at increased risk as well as dehydrated patients and those with uric acid nephropathy. More recently it has become evident that diabetic patients, and particularly those with evidence of renal disease and juvenile onset diabetics, are especially at risk to develop renal failure following intravenous contrast studies [1, 2, 3]. There is considerable difference of opinion as to whether every patient with evidence of renal disease (as indicated by an elevated blood creatinine level) is at increased risk from intravenous contrast and whether the occurrence of acute renal failure is dose related [4, 5]. That higher doses of contrast are more likely to cause acute renal failure certainly appears to be true for patients with evidence of prior renal disease, but may not necessarily be true for those patients who develop acute renal failure without prior renal disease [6]. The mechanism for the development of renal failure in these patients is not clear and theories ranging from sludging of blood in small glomerular capillaries to direct toxic effect on the tubular cells have been advanced. However, the fortunate aspect of these cases is that the condition appears to be self limited and that if proper medical therapy is instituted following the onset of acute renal failure, the prognosis is good for return of renal function to the level that existed prior to the contrast-induced failure. On the other hand permanent deterioration of renal function has been noted, particularly in diabetics with preexisting renal failure, at levels of serum creatinine in excess of 5 mg/100 ml [1]. Also this deterioration in renal function in these patients may not be detected clinically.

A recent paper by Older et al. points out that the radiologist might be the first physician to realize that a patient is in renal failure following the use of intravenous contrast [7]. These authors have shown that a persistent nephrogram (or an increasing nephrogram) seen hours after an intravenous injection of contrast (in a patient who does not have urinary tract obstruction) is the earliest sign that acute renal failure is occurring (see Fig. 1). Follow-up studies over the next 12 – 24 h will confirm this finding along with appropriate urine and blood creatinine levels. Therefore a persistent nephrogram is a urographic finding seen not only in patients with preexisting acute renal failure but also in those with renal impairment caused by and developed during the urogram. With this information physicians can be alerted early on to this

Radiology Today 1. Ed. by M. W. Donner and F. H. W. Heuck

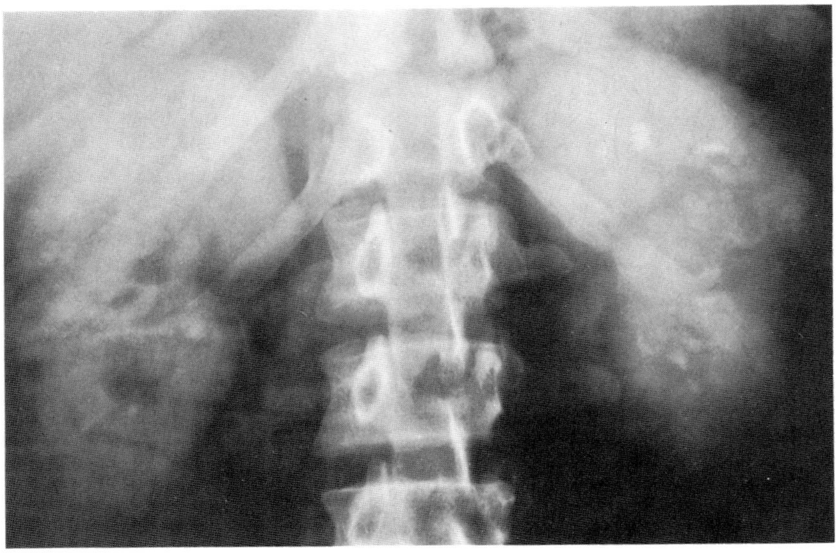

Fig. 1. Film of upper abdomen taken 24 h following arteriogram. Bilateral nephrograms are seen. Some contrast is seen in nonobstructed calyceal structures. The finding is that of acute renal failure secondary to contrast media. The patient was oliguric and the blood creatinine level rose to 6.3 mg/100 ml. Diuresis occurred 5 days later and blood creatinine level returned to normal

potential problem and further radiologic tests or scheduled surgery can be avoided until the acute renal failure has resolved.

In summary, it is important that physicians be aware that some patients are at increased risk to develop acute renal failure following the use of intravenous contrast agents. The high-risk group of patients include diabetics, including juvenile onset diabetics with laboratory identified renal disease (creatinine over 1.5 mg per 100 ml), uric acid nephropathy, multiple myeloma, and dehydrated patients. From the available literature it would certainly seem that in this high-risk group of patients certain extra precautions should be followed: (1) contrast media should be avoided and other tests be substituted when possible; (2) if the use of contrast is necessary for diagnosis, then the patient should be *well hydrated* and the smallest dose of contrast media possible should be used. Also, a prolonged and persistent nephrogram following the intravenous injection of contrast (in a patient with a nonobstructed collecting system) is the earliest clue to the development of acute renal failure.

Imaging

Sonography and CT have had a considerable impact on the diagnosis of urinary tract disease, including diagnosis of adrenal, renal, and perirenal disease as well as retroperitoneal and pelvic pathology. Aspects of sonography will be covered elsewhere in this symposium and will not be discussed here, but some applications of CT will be reviewed.

The contributions of CT in evaluation of urinary tract, adrenal, and retroperitoneal disease has greatly increased over the past few years as more equipment has become available to radiologists and because newer equipment has offered an improvement in detail over the earlier and slower scanners. Almost all areas of uroradiology have benefited from the use of CT in diagnosis. This presentation will not attempt to detail all of these areas, but will highlight a few of them.

Adrenal radiology (which is covered elsewhere in this symposium) has been greatly influenced by the availability of CT. In fact most radiologists who have the use of this equipment will use CT as the first (and often only) radiographic technique in the evaluation of many adrenal diseases. This is particularly true for the evaluation of functioning adrenal cortical and medullary tumors as well as for metastatic neoplasm to the adrenals. In patients with Cushing's syndrome, the demonstration of a unilateral tumor as the cause of the patient's symptoms rather than bilateral hyperplasia (Cushing's disease) can be performed easily and accurately [8]. Likewise the ability to detect an adrenal tumor in a patient with the clinical symptoms plus laboratory signs of pheochromocytoma makes detailed angiographic studies unnecessary in many cases [9, 10]. Likewise the assessment of adrenal pathology including other primary tumors as well as metastatic tumor to the adrenal has been greatly expanded and improved with the use of CT.

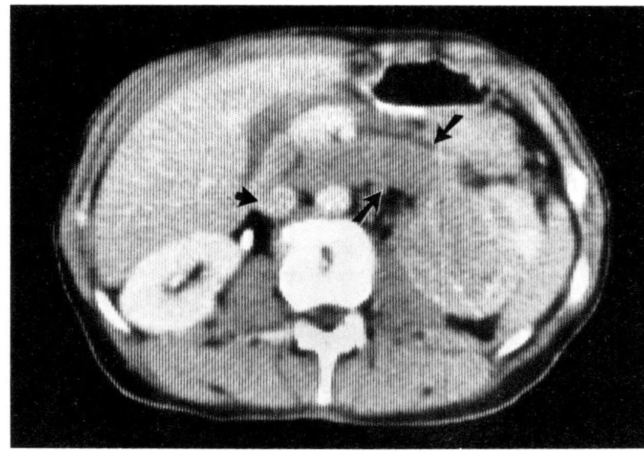

Fig. 2. Computed tomogram: Large carcinoma of the left kidney. Left renal vein (*arrow*) is enlarged and filled with tumor. Also, defect in inferior vena cava (*arrow head*) indicates caval involvement as well

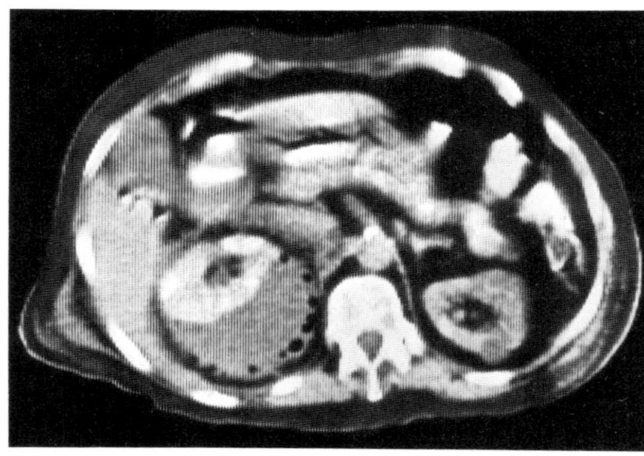

Fig. 3. Computed tomogram: Large perinephric abscess posterior and medial to right kidney. Air bubbles due to air-producing bacteria are present within the abscess. The right kidney is otherwise intact, while the left kidney contains two small cortical cysts. At surgery, drainage of perinephric abscess was accomplished

Computed tomography has had a great impact on the diagnosis of renal and perirenal diseases as well. The technique has been very successful in evaluating renal masses and avoiding the need for angiography and needle aspiration in many cases [11]. CT has been used successfully to stage renal malignancies [12], to show the extent of neoplastic involvement of the renal vein and the inferior vena cava [13] (Fig. 2), and to discourage surgery in nonresectable tumors. The technique has been able to detect the presence of fat in a renal tumor, thereby proving the diagnosis of angiomyolipoma and enabling kidney-saving surgery to be performed. The technique has been of great value in diagnosing perirenal bleeding and inflammatory condition with extreme accuracy, making possible proper identification and a correct surgical or drainage approach (Fig. 3). Stones that are radiolucent on routine radiography can be seen on CT, making possible easy differentiation from other filling defects within the collecting system, such as tumors [14].

The evaluation of the retroperitoneum has also been greatly enhanced by the use of CT [15]. The evaluation of lymph node enlargement both in the diagnosis and staging of lymphoma as well as its detection in metastatic disease has had a tremendous impact on the planning of treatment of these patients. The localization of disease for fine needle aspiration biopsy (or larger needle biopsy) has been greatly advanced by the addition of CT [16]. Abdominal surgery to obtain tissue for confirmation of metastatic malignancy has been increasingly avoided. The nature and extent of primary retroperitoneal malignancies can be clearly assessed with this technique, as can the differentiation of extrinsic from intrinsic ureteral obstruction. Diagnosis of abdominal aortic disease is usually well performed by sonography, but in obese patients or in confusing aortic problems CT is often able to outline the disease process with great reliability. The technique has also been of great value in assessing the results of chemotherapy and radiotherapy and has been used to detect tumor recurrence following surgery [17].

Sonography has the main role in evaluation of the female pelvis, but CT is most helpful in the older population to outline the spread of neoplastic disease, the involvement of pelvic lymph nodes, the staging of bladder neoplasms as well as the evaluation of the prostate and its staging [15, 18]. (Further discussion of CT in pelvic disease is offered in another section of this symposium.)

The improvement in the ability of CT to outline disease process in the urinary tract, adrenals, or retroperitoneum has not only improved diagnostic accuracy but has also caused a decrease in the need for diagnostic angiographic procedures.

Interventional Techniques

There has been a great increase in the number and performance of various percutaneous interventional techniques to treat disease of the urinary tract. These techniques can be divided into two categories: (1) angiographic techniques and (2) pyelonephrostomy techniques.

Angiographic techniques are discussed in more detail in other sections of this symposium and will not be covered here, but a partial listing of these angiographic techniques specifically applicable to the urinary tract is given below:

1. Renal artery angioplasty to:
   a) relieve renovascular hypertension;
   b) preserve renal function by increasing renal perfusion;
   c) dilate strictured anastomoses following renal transplantation.
2. Renal vascular occlusive techniques to:
   a) control renal bleeding (e.g., following injury) or pelvic bleeding following pelvic injury or fracture;
   b) occlude renal artery aneurysm or arteriovenous fistulas;
   c) occlude (embolization) blood supply to renal cell carcinoma; for aid in nephrectomy or as part of nonsurgical treatment of tumor;

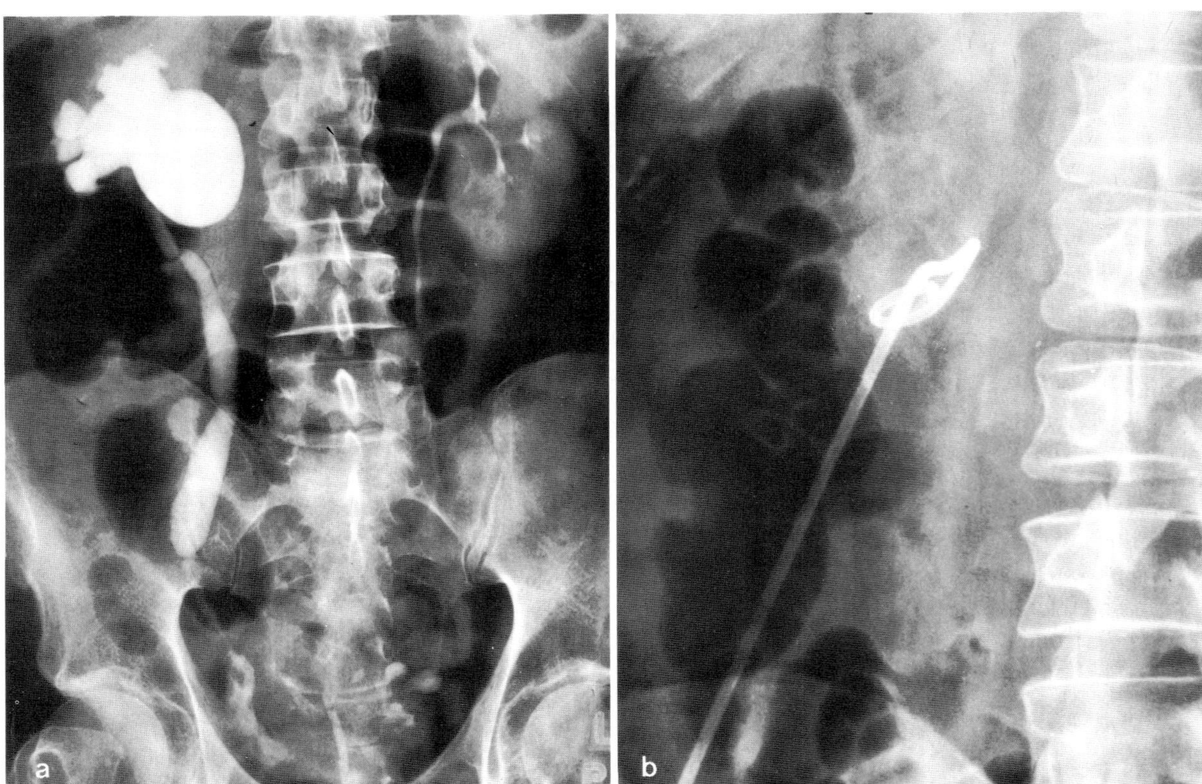

Fig. 4. a Intravenous urogram performed following pelvic surgery. Right hydronephrosis with leakage and obstruction at distal ureter. **b** Abdominal film following percutaneous pyelonephrostomy. A "pigtail" catheter is in place in the right renal pelvis, accomplishing temporary drainage of right kidney prior to surgical repair of the distal right ureter

d) occlude end-stage kidneys as a medical nephrectomy.

Percutaneous nephrostomy techniques have been increasingly used to treat a large number of conditions and diseases involving the urinary tract [19, 20]. A partial listing is given below:

1. To provide drainage of the obstructed renal collecting system, particularly when it cannot be accomplished in a retrograde fashion. This may be a temporary maneuver to tide the patient over until definitive surgery is performed (Fig. 4) or may be converted to a long-term drainage maneuver. By far the most common indications for percutaneous nephrostomy are in pyonephrosis and azotemia.
2. To enter the collecting system to:
   a) treat stone disease by displacment, basket extraction, dissolution with chemicals, or fragmentation [21];
   b) occlude the ureter to stop inoperable ureteral leaks or fistulas by balloon catheter or tissue adhesives [22];
   c) dilate ureteral strictures by balloon catheter;
   d) facilitate permanent internal drainage by bypassing obstruction with catheter stents [19];
   e) allow the installation of chemotherapy to treat urothelial tumors;
   f) make possible nephroscopy or biopsy techniques.
3. To enter and drain renal and perirenal abscess and fluid collections.

While some of the drainage techniques described above have been used for a considerable time, it is only recently that there has been a more widespread interest, acceptance, and appreciation of the value of these techniques in patient management. This is partly due to the availability of improved imaging techniques that have allowed better visualization and understanding of the disease process as well as to the improvement and diversification in catheter and needle technology [23, 24]. This has created the impetus for further extension of the nephropyelostomy procedure from simple external drainage techniques to treatment of obstructions (stones, strictures, etc.) as well as the introduction of more comfortable permanent internal drainage stents. It has been the experience of most workers in this field that these techniques have been increasingly accepted by the medical community because of their efficacy and relative safety.

References

1. Harkowman S, Kjellstrand CM (1977) Exacerbation of diabetic renal failure following intravenous pyelography. Am J Med 63:939
2. Van Zee BE, Hoy WE, Talley TE, Jonkie JR (1978) Renal injury associated with intravenous pyelography in non-diabetic and diabetic patients. Ann Intern Med 89:51
3. Shafi T, Chou S, Porush JE, Shapiro B (1978) Infusion intravenous pyelography and renal function – Effects on patients with chronic renal insufficiency. Arch Intern Med 138:1218
4. McClennan BL (1979) Current approaches to the azotemic patient. Radiol Clin North Am 17/2:197
5. Wagoner RD (1978) Acute renal failure associated with contrast agents. Arch Intern Med 138:353
6. Hayman LA, Evans RA, Fahr LM, Hinck VC (1980) Renal consequences of rapid high dose contrast CT. AJR 134:553
7. Older RA, Korobkin M, Cleeve DM, Schaaf R, Thompson W (1980) Contrast-induced acute renal failure: persistent nephrogram as clue to early detection. AJR 134:339
8. Korobkin M, White EA, Kressel HY, Moss AA, Montagne J (1979) Computed tomography in the diagnosis of adrenal disease. AJR 132:231 – 238
9. Stewart BH, Varvo EL, Haaga J et al. (1978) Localization of pheochromocytoma by computed tomography. N Engl J Med 229:460
10. Laursen K, Damgaard-Pedersen K (1980) CT for pheochromocytoma diagnosis. AJR 134:277
11. McClennan BL, Stanley RJ, Melson GL, Levitt RG, Sagel SS (1979) CT of the renal cyst: is cyst aspiration necessary? AJR 133:671
12. Love L, Churchill R, Reynes C, Schuster GA, Moncada R, Berkow A (1979) Computed tomography staging of renal carcinoma. Urol Radiol 1/7: 3 – 10
13. Marks WM, Korobkin M, Callen PW, Kaiser JA (1978) CT diagnosis of tumor thrombosis of the renal vein and inferior vena cava. AJR 131:843 – 846
14. Segal AJ, Spataro RF, Linke CA, Frank IN, Rabinowitz R (1978) Diagnosis of non-opaque calculi by computed tomography. Radiology 129:447
15. Korobkin M, Callen PW, Fisch AE (1979) Computed tomography of the pelvis and retroperitoneum. Radiol Clin North Am 17:301
16. Haaga JR (1979) New techniques for CT-guided biopsies. AJR 133:633
17. Bernardino ME, deSantos LA, Johnson DE, Bracken RB (1979) Computed tomography in the evaluation of post-nephrectomy patients. Radiology 130:183
18. Price JA, Davidson AJ (1979) Computed tomography in the evaluation of the suspected carcinomatous prostate. Urologic Radiology 1/1:39
19. Pfister RC, Newhouse JH (1979) Interventional percutaneous pyeloureteral techniques. Percuta-

neous nephrostomy and other procedures. Radiol Clin North Am 17:351
20. Stables DP, Ginsberg NJ, Johnson MD (1978) Percutaneous nephrostomy: a series and review of the literature. AJR 130:75
21. Smith AD, Reinke DB, Miller RP, Lange PH (1979) Percutaneous nephrostomy in the management of ureteral and renal calculi. Radiology 133:49
22. Gunther R, Marberger M, Klose K (1979) Transrenal ureteral embolization. Radiology 132:317
23. Gunther R, Alken P, Altwein J (1979) Percutaneous nephropyelostomy using a fine-needle puncture set. Radiology 132:228
24. Elyaderani MK, Dorn JS, Gabriele OF (1979) Percutaneous nephrostomy utilizing a pigtail catheter: a new technique. Radiology 132:750

Functional Urography

T. Kröpelin

Albert-Ludwigs-Universität, Zentrum Radiologie, Abteilung Röntgendiagnostik, Sektion Innere Medizin IV, Hermann-Herder-Strasse 6, D-7800 Freiburg/Breisgau

In 1979 urography celebrated its 50th birthday. During this time it has proved its value and has become a standard investigatory procedure of every X-ray department. The prospective study of Mellins et al. [12] showed that even today it has not lost any of its importance and is not performed too often. The fascination of urography has been maintained thanks to the modern, well-tolerated contrast media and the variety of methods developed.

Bolus injection, "undiluted urography":
Standard urography (30 – 60 ml contrast medium)
High-dose urography (>60 ml contrast medium)
- Angiography
- Rapid sequence urography (early serial urography)
- Nephrography (nephrotomography and -zonography)

Drip infusion, "diluted urography":
Commercial preparation
- Nephrography
- Homogeneous demonstration of the urinary tract.

To be able to understand the various urographic methods, it is necessary firstly to consider the *pharmokinetics of the contrast media.* The media considered for urography are eliminated primarily by the kidneys. Using the normal dose of 30 – 60 ml, 10% – 20% is eliminated in the first 10 min, rising to 50% after 1 h and over 90% after 24 h. The renal elimination of the modern contrast media is achieved by glomerular filtration. The extrarenal elimination by liver, small bowel, rectum and salivary glands is normally very small, but rises with decreasing renal function and is dependent on the degree of renal failure [11]. The nephrogenous contrast media reach the glomerula through the preglomerular vessels and the vasa afferentia. After filtration they are excreted into the renal pelvis via the renal tubular system. Where *excess medium* is used, e.g. high-dose urography and angiography, or where a relative excess exists, e.g. *decreased glomerular filtration,* the non-filtrated portion of the medium passes on to the vasa efferentia, is then distributed to the peritubular capillary network and leaves the kidney via the renal vein. After passage through the body, the same material arrives again in the arterial supply, this time in diluted form. This process is repeated until final elimination by the kidney has been achieved (Fig. 1).

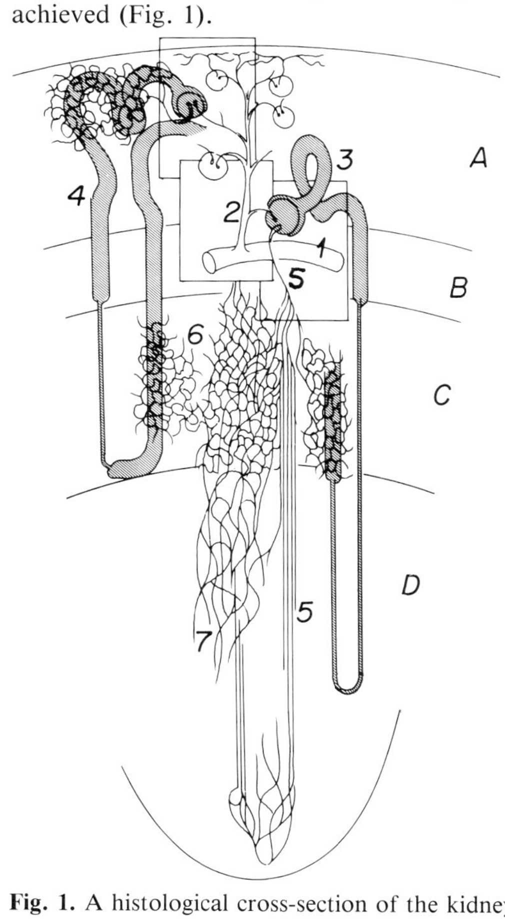

Fig. 1. A histological cross-section of the kidney. *A, B,* cortex; *C, D,* medulla; *D,* medullary pelvic zone; *1, 2,* preglomerular vessels + vasa afferentia; *3, 4,* tubuli (nephrons); *5, 6, 7,* postglomerular vessels + vasa efferentia

Radiology Today 1. Ed. by M. W. Donner and F. H. W. Heuck

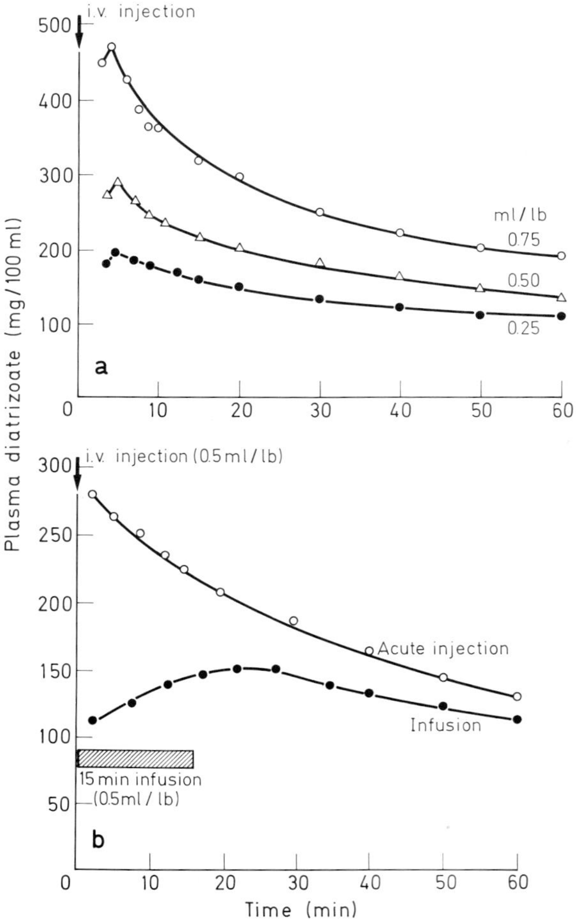

Fig. 2a, b. Bolus injection with **a** varying dose and **b** drip infusion [4]

If X-rays are taken at specific times corresponding to the various phases of contrast medium renal flow and excretion, it is possible to derive detailed functional and morphological diagnostic information about the organ "kidney". This is true for angiography, as well as for urography.

The *intravenously administered contrast medium* which reaches the kidney after passage through the lungs is more diluted than medium which is directly administered intra-arterially under high pressure. As the contrast medium is diluted, there is a tendency which favours glomerular filtration rather than passage through the vasa efferentia.

In *normal renal function,* it is possible to intensify the elimination of the contrast medium and therefore organ opacification by increasing the serum level of the contrast medium.

The increased plasma concentration can be achieved by varying dose or speed of administration (Fig. 2). After *bolus injection,* the serum contrast medium concentration follows a characteristic course. The maximum is reached immediately, the level depending on the dose, but this is followed by a rapid fall over 10 – 15 min, which subsequently levels off. In contrast, the *drip infusion,* with an equivalent contrast medium dose, results in a slow rise in the serum concentration. However, the kidney receives medium over a longer period. The *combination of both methods* is sometimes of value and this will be discussed later.

In *renal failure* the excretion of contrast medium per unit time is reduced and elimination prolonged. The quantity of medium in the primary urine is dependent on:

1. The serum level of the contrast medium;
2. The glomerular filtration rate.

It is therefore possible to derive the following *rule for contrast medium elimination. At all times, the concentration of the glomerular filtrated contrast medium* (= intratubular quantity) *is directly proportional to the serum concentration of the contrast medium and the glomerular filtration rate.* In *normal renal function* it is possible to detect the urographic phases listed in Table 1.

Intravenous angiography has again become a method of interest. It is only possible following a bolus injection of 60 – 100 ml contrast medium within 3 – 5 s and if a circulation time of 9 s up to a maximum of 18 s is taken into account. Using this technique it is possible, for example, to demonstrate a renal artery stenosis. The necessary series of films can be taken on the angiography table or using simultaneous (multilayer) tomography (cf. Fig. 4a) [5, 9, 14, 19].

Table 1. Urographic phases detectable in normal renal function

Urographic phases	Length of administration of CM	Time of film postinjection
Angiography		
Bolus injection	3 – 5 s	9 – 18 s
Nephrography		
– Early (vascular)		
Bolus injection	3 – 15 s	9 – 30 s
– Late (tubular)		
Bolus injection	60 s	2 – 3 min
Drip infusion	5 – 10 min	4 – 8 min
Urinary tract		
Bolus injection	3 s – 2 min	4 – 8 min
Drip infusion	10 min	10 – 15 min

The *early or vascular nephrogram* can be detected in the first 9 – 30 s postinjection. During this time, the major proportion of the contrast medium flows through the preglomerular vessels, the glomerular and later the postglomerular capillaries. The renal cortex and columns are therefore more opacified than the medulla. This can best be visualised using tomography. It is possible to use this method even in renal failure of various causes, as long as an adequate blood supply is still present [1, 2, 3, 7, 8, 17].

The *late, tubular excretion nephrogram* is normally obtained urographically, since slower contrast medium administration is usual. The tubular nephrogram results from the accumulation of the medium in the tubular system and is reached 2 – 3 min following a bolus injection over 60 s, and 4 – 8 min following infusion over 5 – 10 min. In the latter, the demonstration of the kidney over a longer period of time is therefore possible, since the tubules receive significantly more contrast medium over a protracted period. In this case, the intratubular fluid volume can be considerably increased through the intensified osmosis caused by the contrast medium, so that during the infusion urogram, a transitory relative intratubular stasis occurs. This may be desirable in certain parenchymal diseases [15, 16]. In the course of time, the intensity of the nephrogram decreases continuously, following bolus injection more quickly than after drip infusion, whereas the opacification of the renal pelvis increases.

In our experience, it is possible to increase the diagnostic accuracy of urography if contrast medium dose, mode of administration and speed are adapted to the clinical and radiological morphological findings observed.

We begin all our urographies (see Table 2) with a rapid bolus injection in order to obtain information about the renal blood flow. We inject 60 ml contrast medium within 30 – 60 s using a wide lumen butterfly needle and the first film is taken < 1 min postinjection. What follows depends on the findings of the first films (1 – 2). If no pathological findings are detected, the investigation is completed within 12 – 20 min postinjection using three to four films. Should a diminished renal perfusion be observed, a rapid sequence (early serial) urogram is performed.

If the clinical diagnosis is hypertension and renal artery stenosis, an intravenous angiogram with bolus injection of 60 ml contrast medium within 3 – 5 s is performed at the outset. Otherwise, we feel that a rapid sequence urogram with a film series at 1, 2, 4, 12 and 20 min postinjection is adequate to strengthen the clinical diagnosis of a haemodynamically active, unilateral renal artery stenosis. In the first few minutes, a delayed

Table 2. Personal method; excretion urography

1) Basis of diagnosis: plain film ± tomography, zonography
2) Puncture: Butterfly-Needle 19 (1.1 mm)
3) Two ampoules CM in 30 – 60 s (perhaps IV angiogram: 60 ml/3 – 5 s)
4) 1st film (transverse 24/30 cm) 1 – 2 min postinjection (perhaps IV angiogram: 9 – 18 s postinjection)

Decision on further procedure:

Normal nephrogram	Pathological nephrogram		In renal insufficiency[b]
5) 2nd film, 6 min	5) 2nd film, 2 min[a]	– Tumour	5) Infusion urogram; duration, 5 – 10min
6) 3rd film, 12 min	6) 3rd film, 4 min[a]	– Hydronephroses	6) 2nd film, 5 – 20 min[a]
7) (4th upright, film 20 min)	7) 4th film, 12 – 20 min[a]	– Parenchymal lesion	7) 3rd tomogram
	8) (5th upright film, 20 min)	– Anomalies	8) Perhaps late film[a]
			9) (Upright film)

[a] Perhaps tomography, zonography
[b] Serum creatinine > 1.5 ⩽ 6 mg/100 ml
Serum urea < 100 mg/100 ml
() Perhaps upright film

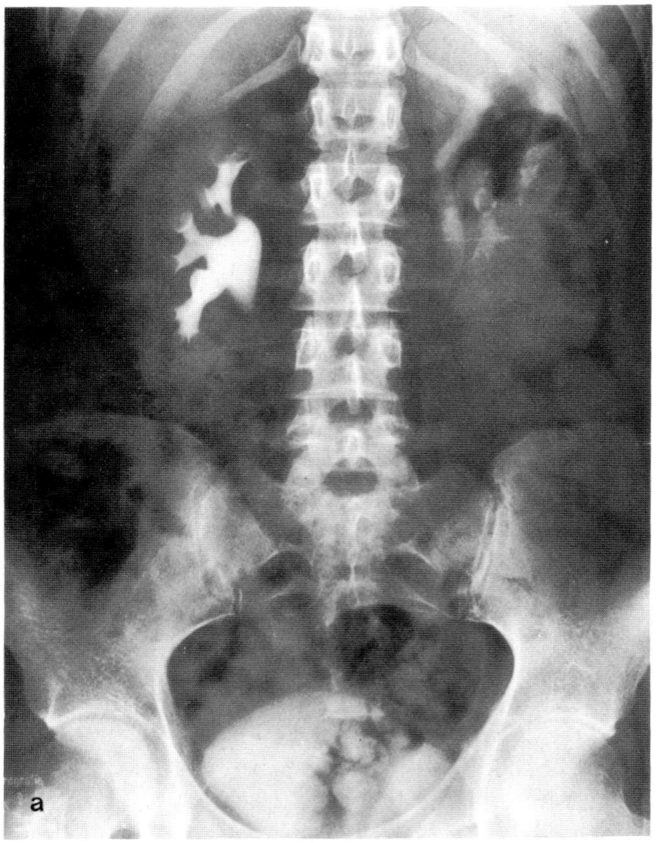

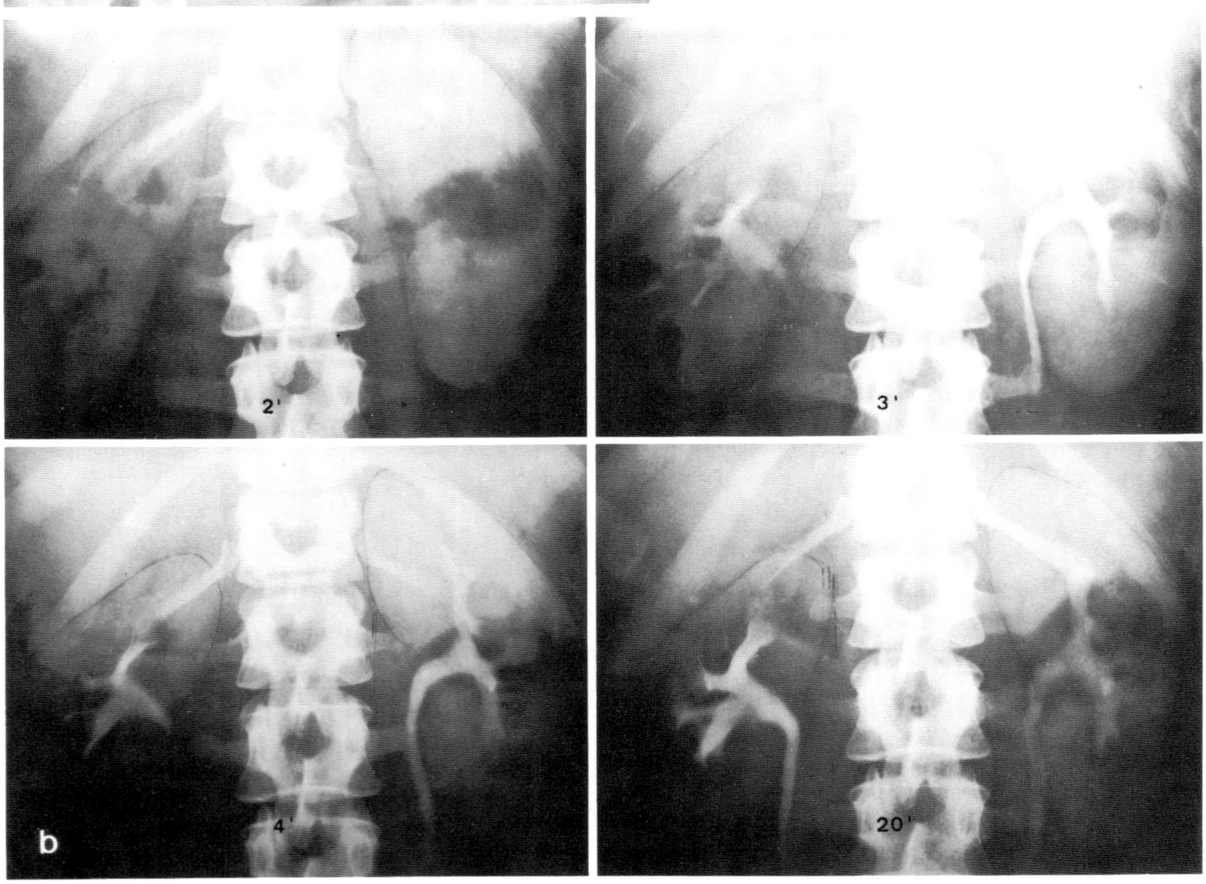

Fig. 3. **a** Standard urography: false diagnosis of right-sided obstruction. **b** Rapid sequence (early serial) urography; the same patient. **c** Angiogram: fibroplastic stenosis of the right renal artery

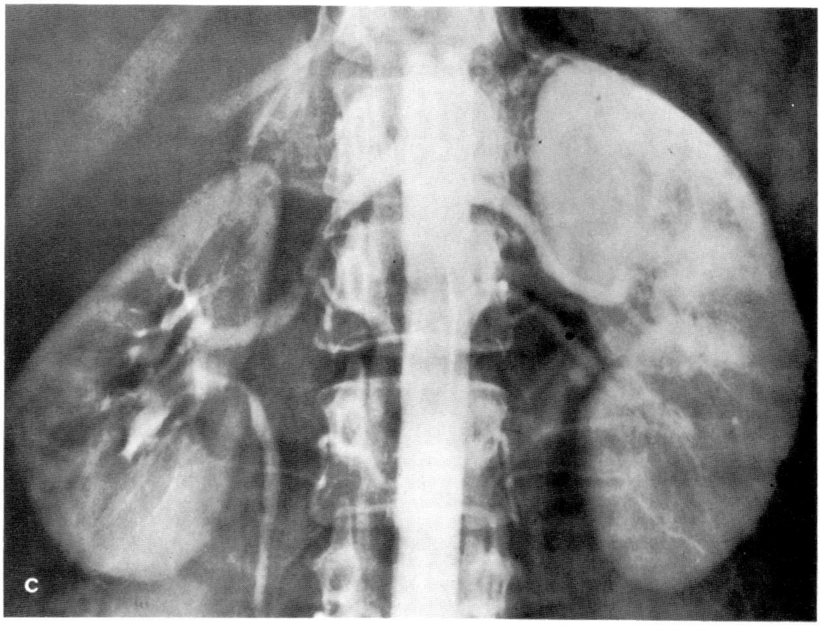

Fig. 3c. Legend see p. 220

nephrogram with delayed filling of the calyces is observed on the side with decreased renal blood flow. Later on, the contrast medium situation is reversed – a hyperconcentration can be seen in the urinary tract of the side with reduced perfusion, whereas the contrast medium has been largely eliminated on the healthy side. The observed differences can be explained as follows. The delayed, weak nephrogram with the slow excretion of the contrast medium into the renal pelvis results from the reduced renal blood flow with subsequent delay and decrease in the glomerular filtration of the medium.

The increased opacification, hyperconcentration of the urinary tract in the late phase, results from:

1. A prolonged filling and persistence of the medium in the renal pelvis;
2. An increased concentration of the excreted contrast medium.

The reduced perfusion of the kidney has the effect that the urine flows more slowly through the tubules. The intact tubule has adequate time to reabsorb water. Therefore, despite the osmotic properties of the contrast medium, in end-effect it is excreted in a more concentrated form. The narrowing of the renal pelvis on the side of the renal artery stenosis represents an adaptation to the reduced urine volume production per unit time. In this case the involved kidney is also often smaller than the normal kidney. The increased opacification of the renal pelvis in the late excretion phase is most often observed in young patients with unilateral fibroplastic renal artery stenosis (Fig. 3); the kidney, however, is not significantly decreased in size. In the case of an arteriosclerotic renal artery stenosis, the increased opacification cannot be detected so readily. The narrowing of the renal pelvis, the decreased size of the kidney and the delayed protracted excretion of contrast medium is more marked. This is most probably due to the secondary arteriolosclerosis with severe tubulus atrophy of *both* kidneys, resulting from long-standing hypertension (Fig. 4, Table 3).

The criteria for a usable or unusable early urogram are listed below.

Usable early serial (rapid sequence) urogram:

1. Delayed nephrogram (1 – 3 min postinjection);
2. Delayed elimination (3 – 6 min postinjection);
3. CM hyperconcentration in late excretory phase (6 – 20 min postinjection);
4. Narrowing of renal pelvis ("spastic");
5. Decreased size of renal shadow < 1.5 cm;

Table 3. Intravenous angiotomography: assessment of renal arteries in 343 patients [9]

	All patients	Patient < 46 yrs	Patient > 45 yrs
Total observed	739 = 100%	325 = 100%	414 = 100%
Complete assessment	83%	91%	77%
Partial assessment	17%	9%	23%

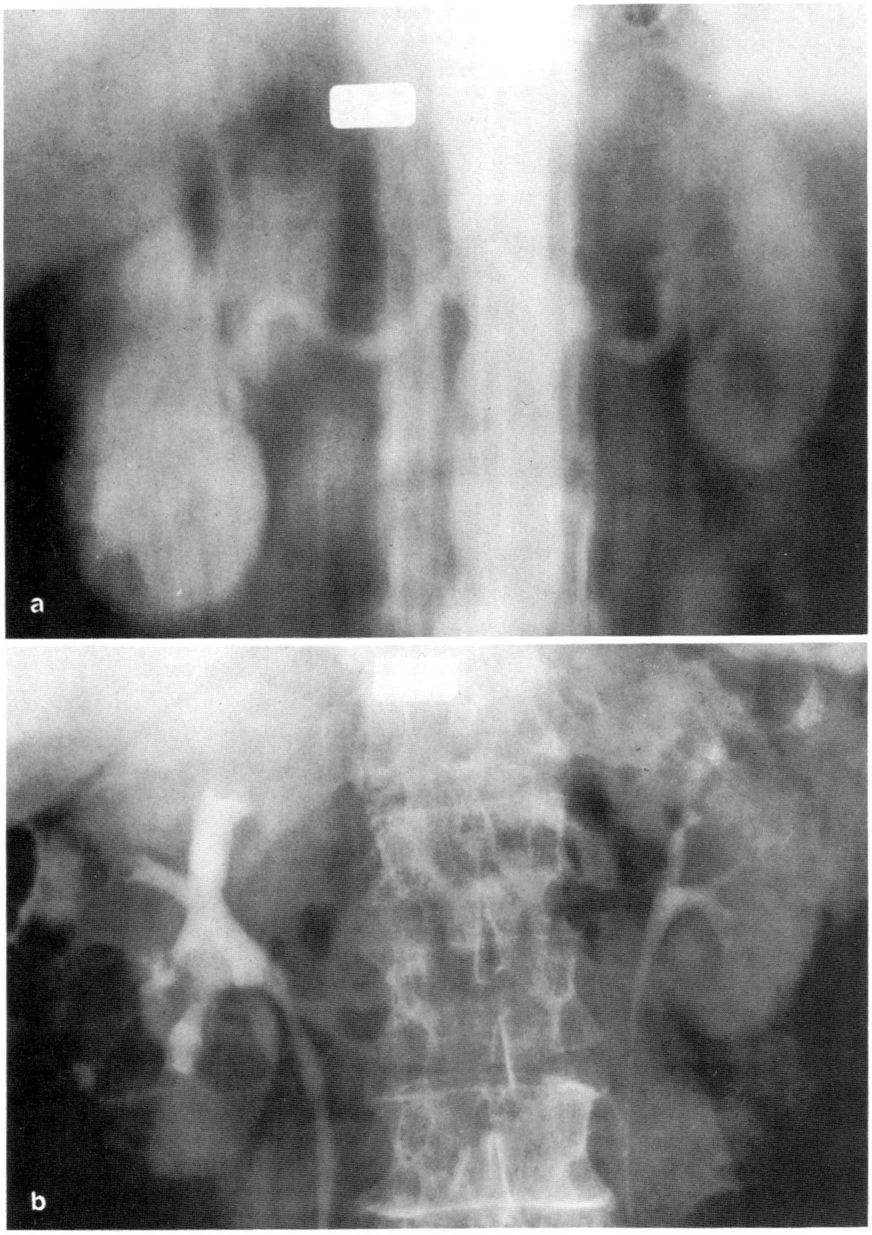

Fig. 4. a Intravenous angiogram – arteriosclerotic stenosis of the left side. **b** The late phase in the same patient

6. Wash-out test: delayed contrast dilution (after early serial urogram: 1 ampoule furosemide IV, 100 – 200 ml 20% mannitol solution).

Unusable early serial (rapid sequence) urogram:
1. No rapid high-dose injection of CM;
2. No serial films;
3. Bilateral (multiple) renal artery stenosis;
4. Contralateral side diseased:
   a) parenchymal
   b) peripheral vessels, e.g. arteriosclerosis
   c) anomalies: hypoplasia, dystopia.

To diagnose a renal artery stenosis on the basis of a rapid sequence urogram, at least three *positive criteria* must be fulfilled. The doubts expressed concerning the value of this method in the diagnosis of hypertension [13, 18] are, in our opinion, not really justified if the above criteria are strictly observed. A combination of intravenous angiography with rapid sequence urography increases the diagnostic sensitivity, so that a renal artery stenosis can be confirmed in the majority of cases.

Nephrography. The rapid bolus injection method for *nephrotomozonography* used alone is only of limited value in differentiating a neoplasm from a cyst. In our experience, a combination of rapid bolus injection and drip infusion provides better diagnostic results. If the following findings are observed in the first two films after the bolus injection we supplement the study with a drip infusion urogram:

1. A tumour of the kidney (neoplasm, cyst etc.);
2. Complete or incomplete, acute or chronic urinary obstruction;
3. Inflammatory, vascular parenchymal lesions;
4. Anomalies of the kidneys and urinary tracts.

It is possible to confirm the presence of a *cyst* more accurately if the initial vascular renal phase after bolus injection and the more marked persisting opacification of the tubular phase of the infusion are compared. *Vascular neoplasms,* such as the hypernephroma, can be well demonstrated in the arterial vascular phase after a bolus injection, but the often demonstrated venous convolutions of A-V fistulas ("contrast medium lagoons") are increasingly better filled by a rapid drip infusion. To improve visualisation, tomography may be necessary.

The combined technique is also better suited for the detection of renal *anomalies.* If renal function is normal, it is possible to demonstrate parenchyma and pelvis equally well over a longer period. The initial perfusion phase, together with the following contrast intensive tubular nephrogram is especially suited for the verification of the diagnosis of horseshoe kidneys and dystopias.

Incomplete urinary obstruction can only be diagnosed with certainty after a forced osmotic diuresis with homogeneous presentation of the urinary tracts. After a single bolus injection no changes may be observed or the site of obstruction may not be properly localised.

The differentiation between *acute and chronic complete urinary obstruction* is also best achieved by a combination of the techniques. In acute obstruction (Fig. 5), the glomerular filtration is still intact and the contrast medium is excreted with the urine into the tubular system. A contrast medium stasis develops as the pressure in the renal pelvis rises to the level of the excretion pressure. Urinary excretion is delayed or ceases. The intact tubulus is still able to reabsorb water and therefore provides room for more glomerular filtrated contrast medium. This results initially in a delayed, later an intensified obstruction nephrogram and a considerably delayed weak opacification of the renal pelvis and ureters [10].

In the case of chronic obstruction (Fig. 6), the intra- and extrarenal contrast medium elimination correlates with the reduced glomerular filtration rate resulting from a pressure atrophy of the renal parenchyma. Using the combined methods described, it may be possible to visualise urographically kidneys which initially appear functionless.

In patients with *renal failure,* it may still be possible to visualise the kidneys. In this case, following a bolus injection of 60 ml contrast medium, a drip infusion with a *diluted solution* is added, the dose being dependent on body weight and degree of renal insufficiency. The procedure is the same as that conducted in all diseases where *dehydration is contra-indicated* because of the danger of aggravation of electrolyte disturbances or the risk of potentiation of the possible toxic effects of the contrast medium, including renal failure, multiple myeloma, hyperuricaemia and diabetes mellitus.

In renal insufficiency, it is possible to achieve satisfactory diagnostic results up to a serum creatinine level of 6 mg/100 ml, if the serum *urea* is less than 100 mg/100 ml. Urea has a *strong osmotic activity.* Even a kidney with a markedly reduced function may still be able to reabsorb sufficient sodium and water if the osmotic urea diuresis is suppressed. By this means, it is possible to achieve an increased concentration of the contrast medium in the urine of the reduced glomerular filtrate. In *severe renal failure* it is therefore necessary to *reduce the serum urea level* by means of dietetic measures or previous dialysis *before urography* is performed. The significance of lowering the serum urea can be well demonstrated in the case of unilateral disease or after renal transplantation. In the latter case, it may be possible to visualise the patients own severely damaged kidneys better than prior to transplantation, at serum creatinine 4 mg/100 ml and urea 160 mg/100 ml (Fig. 7).

By means of urography it is also possible to differentiate prerenal, renal and postrenal causes of *oligo-anuria* [6]. In this case, late films are especially important because of the delayed elimination of the contrast medium.

Where enlarged kidneys with smouth contours are observed, an *acute* illness is most commonly present. In acute *prerenal renal failure,* e.g. the shock kidney, the kidneys are usually clearly enlarged. The nephrogram persists over a number of days, without opacification of the pyelon (Fig. 8).

In contrast, in acute *postrenal* oligo-anuria, the renal pelvis may be detected in the late films,

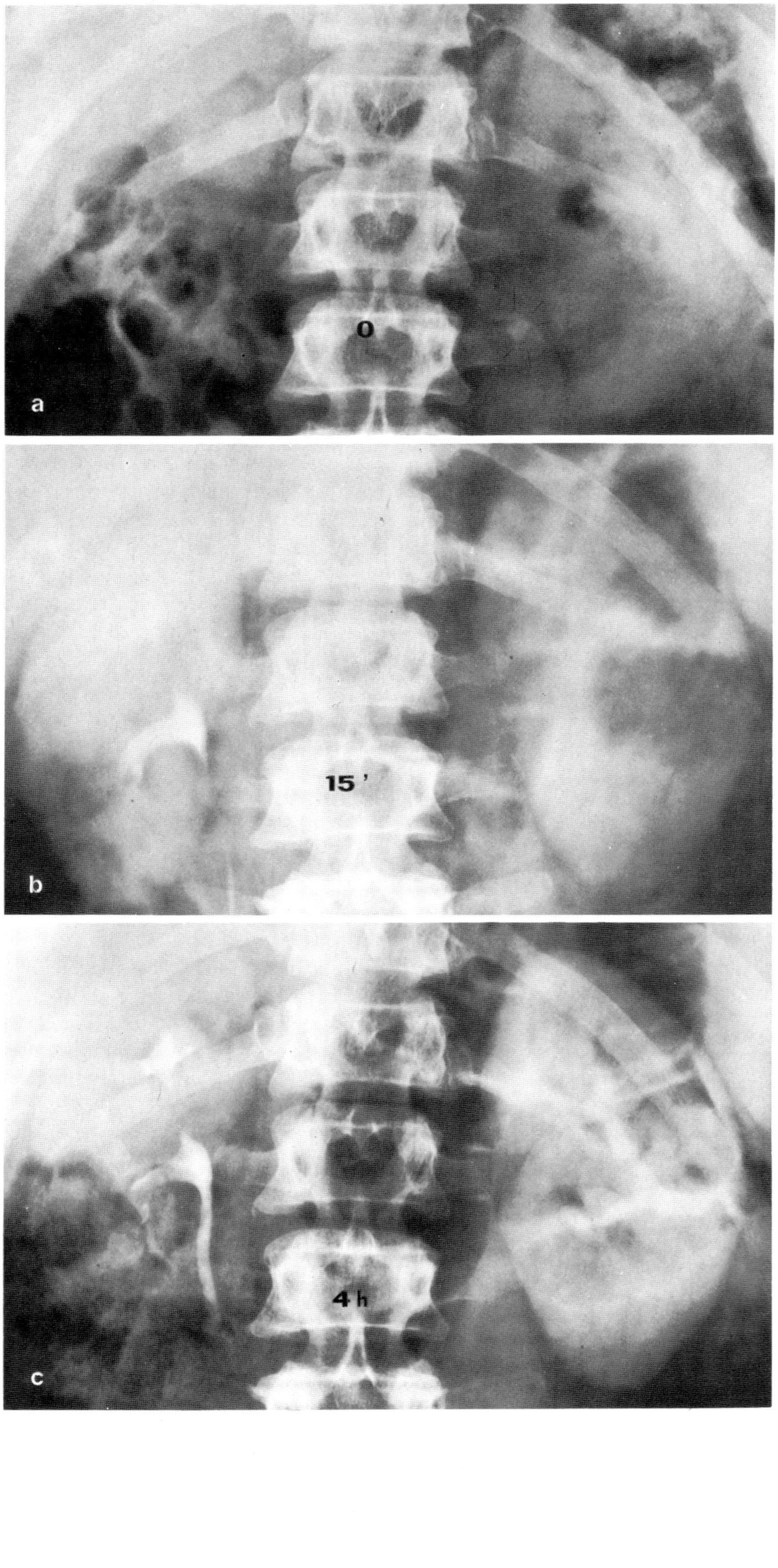

Fig. 5a – c. Left-sided urolithiasis with acute complete obstruction. **a** 0; **b** 15 min; **c** 4 h

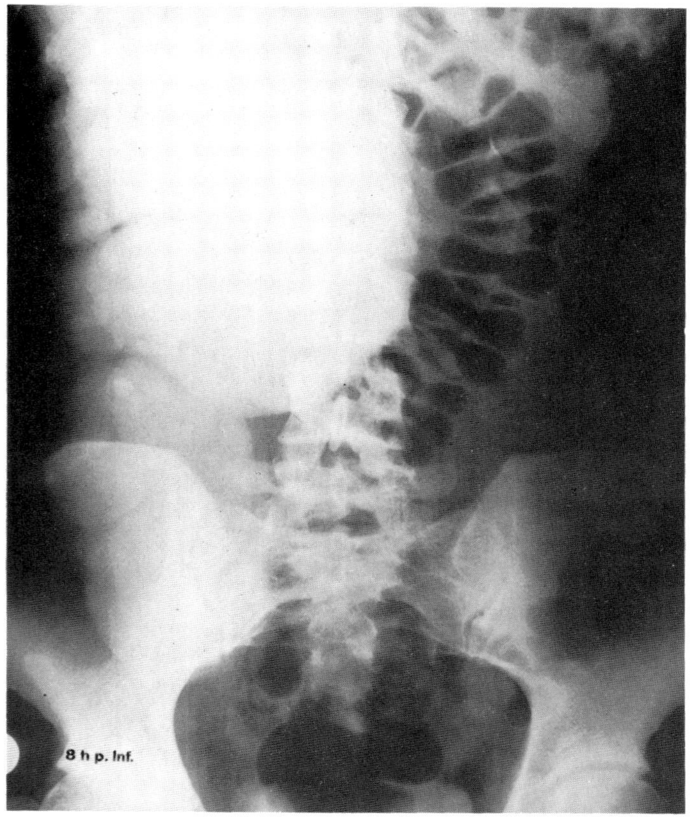

Fig. 6. Severe right-sided chronic hydronephrosis: complete obstruction at pelvico-ureteric junction. *Right,* severe ectasia of pelvis and calyces with displacement of large bowel; *left,* normal-sized kidney, CM practically eliminated

despite the long persistence of an intense nephrogram. The explanation is the same as that already described for the acute unilaterally obstructed kidney. In *renal* diseases of inflammatory origin, e.g. acute glomerulonephritis, the nephrogram is weak and delayed, in the case of vascular disease, weak or absent. In the latter case, the bolus injection nephrotomozonography allows only very weak visualisation of the vascular nephrogram. Also the tubular nephrogram and visualisation of the renal pelvis are inadequate, even in late films [3].

In principle, it is unnecessary to perform urography where chronic terminal renal failure is suspected. Usually visualisation of the kidneys is possible with plain films of the abdomen, using tomography where necessary. If small kidneys are present, symmetrically or asymmetrically, chronic renal disease is present and further urographic studies are not necessary. However, there are borderline cases, e.g. when a gradually progressive renal failure deteriorates acutely or when postrenal obstruction cannot be studied by retrograde pyelography.

However, in our opinion the administration of contrast medium in *oligo-anuria* should be the exception and not the rule! The prolonged circulation of contrast material in the body could easily induce allergic reactions and give rise to toxic accumulation [11]. Because of this, contrast medium investigations in this stage should only be carried out in centres with dialysis facilities. Some authors prefer the "undiluted" bolus injection alone, but we consider this to be inadvisable because of the risk of dehydration. With the combined technique, we obtain more detailed information about the vascular situation (bolus injection) and about any glomerular function (diluted infusion and late film) thanks to the usually delayed nephrogram phase and demonstration of the urinary tract.

Summary

The amount of information which can be obtained from urography depends on the method used. By varying the dose of the contrast medium and mode of application with varying techniques and film sequence, it is possible to perform a detailed diagnostic investigation of the renal artery, parenchyma and urinary tract.

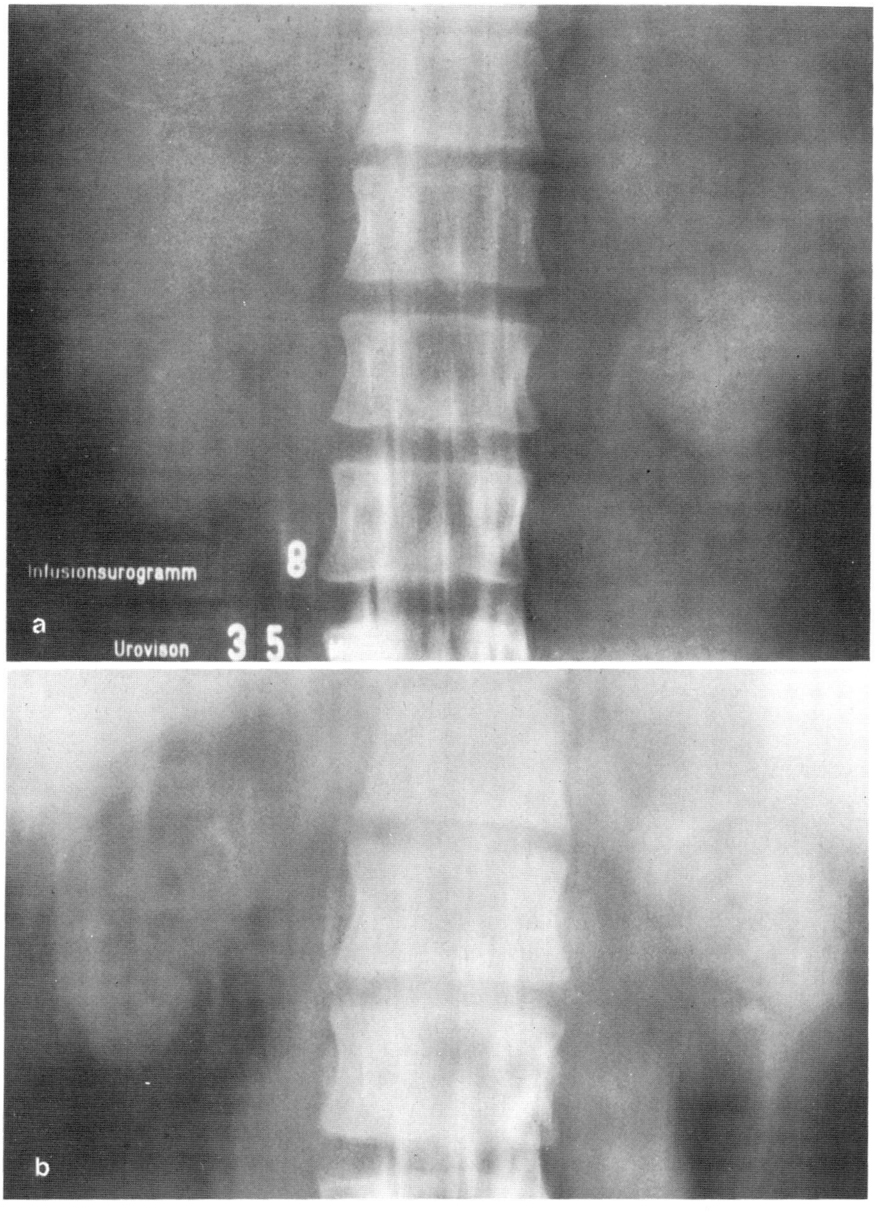

Fig. 7. a 1974: Chronic gomerulonephritis: almost normal-sized kidneys with diminished CM excretion (combined technique, 35 min postinjection. Serum creatinine 4 mg/100 ml; serum urea 160 mg/100 ml. **b** 1979: Demonstration of the patients own "silent" atrophic kidneys following renal transplantation: urea + creatinine normal (35 min postinjection, combined technique). **c** 1979: Same patient with transplanted kidney (35 min postinjection, combined technique)

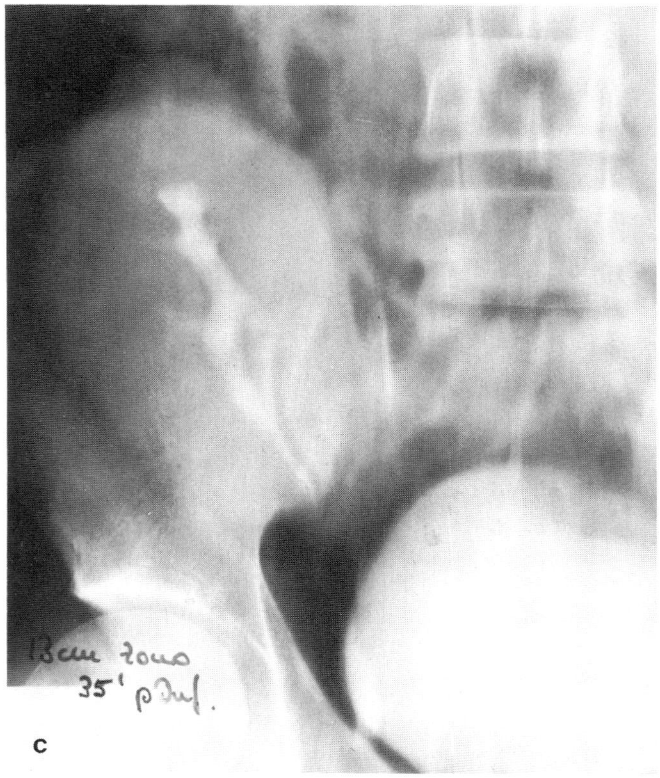

Fig. 7c. Legend see p. 226

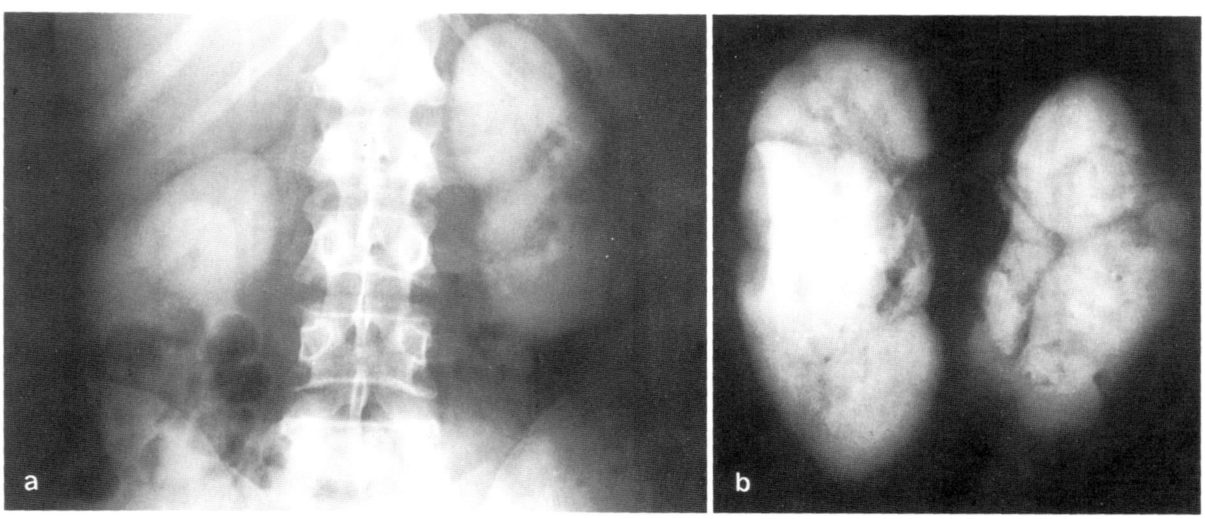

Fig. 8a, b. Persisting nephrogram – acute renal failure (anuria). **a** 3 h postinjection: large kidneys but no opacification of pyelon. **b** 3 days postinjection: post-mortem finding in the same kidneys, persisting nephrogram, no decrease in shadow density despite dialysis

The kinetics of the contrast medium can also be transferred to renal computer tomography, so that a functional morphological analysis and increased diagnostic accuracy are possible.

References

1. Bosniak MA (1974) Nephrotomography: A relatively unappreciated but extremely valuable diagnostic tool. Radiology 113:313 – 321
2. Carlson DH, Simon H (1978) Visualization of vascular structures during routine nephrotomography. J Can Assoc Radiol 29/3:187 – 191
3. Caron-Poitreau C, Vialle M, Friess JJ, Raimbault JP (1978) Apport de la néphrotomographie précoce dans l'insuffisance rénale. J Radiol Electrol Med Nucl 59:175 – 182
4. Cattell WR (1970) Excretory pathways for contrast media. Invest Radiol 5:473 – 475
5. Cecile JP, Guaquiere A, Wallaert C (1976) Intérêt du temps artériel de l'urographie dans le bilan radiologique de l'hypertension artérielle. Ann Radiol (Paris) 19/7:655 – 662
6. Davidson AJ (1977) Radiologic diagnosis of renal parenchymal disease. Saunders, Philadelphia London Toronto
7. Evans JA (1974) Nephrotomography 20 years later. Radiology 113:483 – 484
8. Garc'ia M, Cot X, Rovira JM, Torras A, Teixid'o N, Revert L (1979) Bolus-Nephrotomograf'ia en el diagn'ostico de la hipertensi'on renovascular. Actas Urol Esp 3/3:135 – 138
9. Ingrisch H, Holzgreve H, Sommer B, Westerburg KW, Frey KW (1980) Technik der Nierenarteriendarstellung im Rahmen des Ausscheidungsurogrammes Bolustechnik – Zeitbestimmung – Simultantomographie. ROEFO 132/4:422 – 427
10. Kröpelin T (1980) Röntgendiagnostik der Nephrolithiasis und Nephrokalzinose. Radiologe 20: 300 – 307
11. Kröpelin T, Heuser Y, Gospos C (1978) Kontrastmittelrisiko bei der Ausscheidungsurographie. In: Zeitler E (ed) Kontrastmittelzwischenfälle, Symposium Berlin 1977, German English edn. Schering, Berlin Bergkamen, pp 103 – 115
12. Mellins HZ, McNeil BJ, Abrams HL, van Houten FC, Murphy MA, Korngold E (1979) The selection of patients for excretory urography. Radiology 130:293 – 296
13. Pemsel HK (1979) Nierenarterienstenose: Wertigkeit von Frühurogramm und Isotopennephrogramm. Diagn Intensivther 2:11 – 12
14. Peter JD (1978) Les accidents dus aux produits de contraste utilisés en uro-angiographie. Anesth Analg (Paris) 34/5:1029 – 1037
15. Robbins AH, Rosenfield AT, Pizzolato NF, Irwin GA, Putman CE, Gerzof SG, Ulreich S (1979) Drip infusion urography with meglumine Jodamine. AJR 131/6:1043 – 1046
16. Schuelke J, Freitag J, Mueller R (1979) Die Infusionsnephrotomographie in der urologischen Praxis. Z Aerztl Fortbild (Jena) 73/2:67 – 70
17. Sherwood T, Doyle FH (1974) The I. V. urogram in acute renal failure. Br J Radiol 47:268 – 372
18. Stolle E, Gotzen R, Khalil M (1977) Der Wert des Frühurogramms bei der Abklärung einer arteriellen Hypertonie. Arch Atlas Norm Pathol Anal Roentgenbild 127/3:238 – 242
19. Strub-Mayor F, Jacot C (1978) Urographie avec temps précoces. Schweiz Rundsch Med 67/25: 944 – 948

Radiological Determination of the Renal Circulation

H. K. Deininger

Strahleninstitut der Städtischen Kliniken, Grafenstrasse 9, D-6100 Darmstadt

The known X-ray methods suitable for the examination of the kidneys have been improved continuously and renal contrast media further developed so that they are less toxic. Thus they can be applied faster and at higher doses. As a result of these efforts, contrast enhancement has been improved and details of renal structures are easier to recognize. The progress in the application of contrast media and in the field of technology was decisive for the introduction of new radiological procedures.

These new possibilities of examination of the kidneys allow not only an exact study of the anatomy of the organ but also analysis of physiological and pathophysiological stages of circulation. In this way we get better views of renal function and diseases of the human kidney. The fundamental considerations are based on the known principles of dye dilution techniques. They are transferred to the methodical specialities of an examination using contrast media and X-rays. The roentgenological possibilities and some results of direct measurement of the arterial circulation using water-soluble contrast media were first referred to by Wood and Heuck in 1962 (for complete survey on publications, see [2]).

In the early stages of functional radiological analysis of the circulation two different methods were introduced: densitometric and nuclear medical. These are not competing but complementary procedures. The radio-isotope methods gained wide application in the study of renal circulation, although first attempts at a quantitative measurement of the renal blood flow were not successful. But the radio-isotope renogram is very useful in the diagnosis of a qualitative difference of the kidney circulation. An exact and quantitative measurement of the global renal blood flow can be determined by clearance methods using radiopharmaceuticals. Renoscintigraphy with different, most recent radiopharmaceuticals, a gamma camera and sequential studies allows the imaging of functional and morphological alterations. In this way an anatomical picture of the kidneys as well as a measurement of renal functions can be obtained.

The complementary procedures for the examination of the renal circulation have the drawback of an insufficient time or spatial resolution or both: camera scintigraphy and the isotope renogram are able to record well the periodical flow of radioisotopes within a given time. For both, the resolution of details is less satisfactory. The measurement of the circulation by means of dyestuffs, flow meters and ultrasound will result in quite reliable values of the global circulation of the kidneys. But they permit neither presentation in the form of pictures nor further delineation of the anatomical structures of the kidneys.

Image recording can be done by means of either video tape or cine film. Accordingly, the techniques are called videodensitometry or cinedensitometry. Because angiodensitometry belongs to the group of discontinuous recording techniques, time resolution will be determined by the frame frequency. There is a direct relation between the frame frequency and the exactness of measurement. In the case of very fast events occurring during the measuring of circulation, slow frame frequencies have a poor accuracy. Videodensitometry is limited to a frequency of 25 full frames per second [3, 4, 11].

Normally, a short recording time and the small intervals between each frame can only be attained by cinedensitometry. The flow of the contrasted blood through the kidneys is recorded by means of a high-speed camera which works up to 200 frames per second and exposes a highly sensitive cinema film. The latter must be developed under standardized conditions. It is subsequently projected in the usual way by means of a cinema projector, the picture frequency of which must be precisely adjustable between stand-by and 1 – 25 frames per second [2, 4, 6].

Radiology Today 1. Ed. by M. W. Donner and F. H. W. Heuck

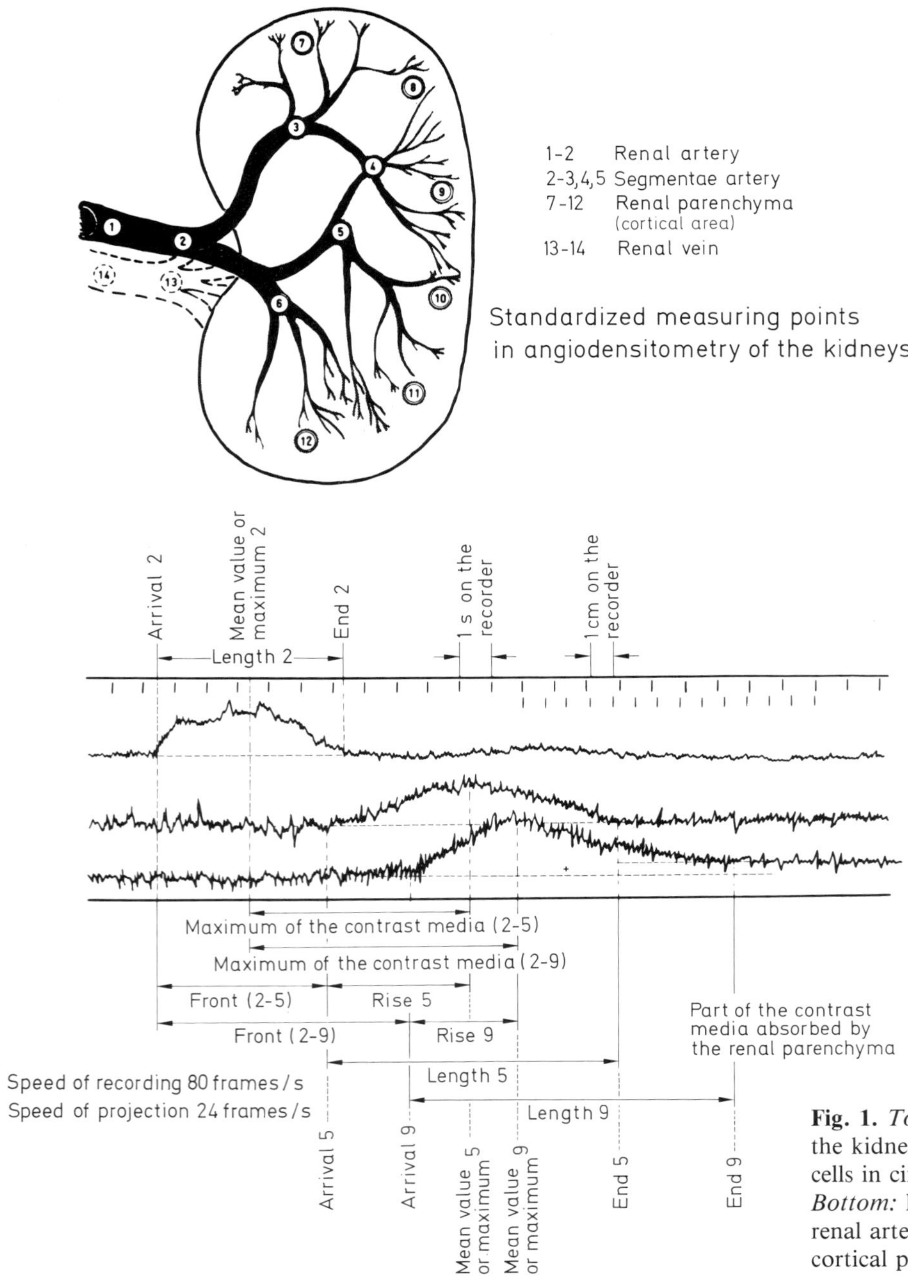

Fig. 1. *Top:* Measuring points over the kidney using photoconductive cells in cinedensitometry.
Bottom: Measuring curves of the renal artery, segmental artery and the cortical parenchyma of the kidney

In cinedensitometry the measurement of density differences as caused by the contrasted blood in the kidneys takes place by means of photoconductive cells (Fig. 1). In spite of their small size, due to which the measuring area becomes as small as a point (1.25 mm in diameter), they respond to even minimal differences in light intensity. The arrangement in pairs of the photoconductive cells in the immediate neighbourhood allows a subtraction of the brightness of background caused by the surrounding tissue from the brightness deviations which are caused when the contrast media flows through the vessels and the tissue of the kidneys. The photo resistors are adjusted by means of a Wheatstone bridge circuit (Fig. 2). If a pair of measuring cells is affected by the same light intensity there is no deviation of tension and thus no deflection on the registering instrument. The method is based on the principle of beam balance, in which an unknown light intensity is compared with a known light intensity.

Due to the above-described facts it is possible to carry out measurements of the systemic circulation and more far-reaching analysis of organic circula-

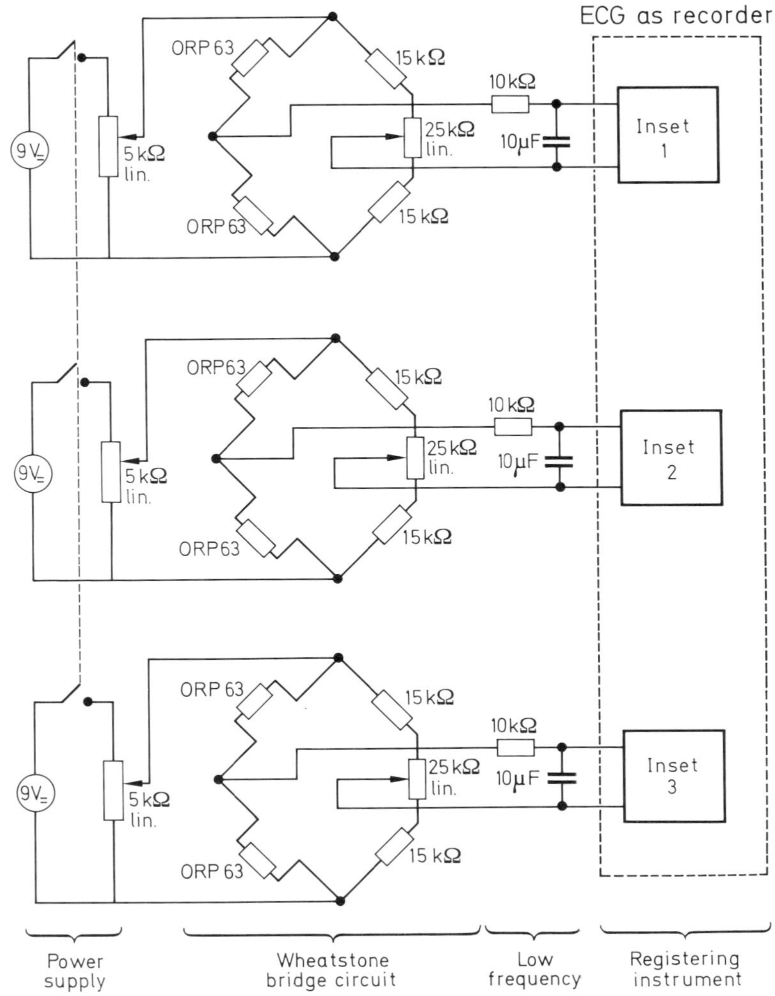

Fig. 2. Circuit diagram demonstrating the use of three pairs of photoconductive cells and one ECG as recorder for densitometric curves

tions in the non-anaesthesized patient under largely physiological conditions. These functional data are providing an important supplement to the conventional angiographical information. No additional stress is involved for the patient, and the additional expenditure is small. By means of examinations carried out on 139 patients, in whom 4400 measurements were taken, it was possible to elaborate standard values for some of the following important parameters of renal circulation [2, 7]:

1. Blood stream in the renal artery (ml/s);
2. Flow in the intrarenal arteries (ml/s);
3. Speeds of flow in the renal artery, segmental arteries and other visible intrarenal arteries (cm/s);
4. Flow times with anatomical definition of the distances of the vessels (s):
   a) Arteriovenous flow time,
   b) renocortical circulation time,
   c) standardized cortical arrival time (s/cm),
   d) intermediate times of intrarenal circulation sections,
   e) renal transit or renopyelal passage time and corticopyelal arrival time,
   f) pulse times (length of the contrast bolus).

Recently, image series of the renal blood flow have been digitized by a system for the real-time processing of video image series [9]. Analogous to videodensitometry, which uses electronic windows for the measuring of the regions of interest, this new technique also records the intrarenal circulation on video tape. In spite of the shorter time resolution in comparison with cinedensitometry, videodensitometry is preferred because its clinical application is more advantageous. For example, storing of data on video tape and the processing of video signals is easier than the handling of a cinema film [8]. Both, cine- and videodensitometry show only a small sector of the picture. They require the setting of multiple and various measuring points or windows to observe the total blood flow through the organ. The technique of a new system for processing the angiogram allows the visualization of all organ phases and thus, the total data of complete angiographic series is available for evaluation.

A system of multiprocessors is used to evaluate the videoangiograms. After digitizing and processing, the results can be obtained as graphs and pictures. By means of a computer the blood flow can be determined in every vessel of the kidney as well as in any point of the renal parenchyma [9, 11].

In densitometry two different methods are usually used to determine the blood flow: Firstly, by measuring time differences of the bolus of the contrast medium for a fixed distance (= 2 measuring points) and measuring the cross-section of the vessel. Secondly, by the integration of the contrast curve, applying the Stewart-Hamilton method to it (= 1 measuring point). A third method involving measurement of the propagation of the bolus in a fixed time interval is only applicable to the angiographic series, which has been digitized by the above-mentioned technique. This method is especially suited for short measuring distances and high velocities, a situation which is typical for blood flow measurements in the human kidney. Corrections for device inaccuracies and background are performed by the multiprocessor system in a relatively simple way [11].

The calculation of the flow by the first-mentioned method requires determination of the front speed and group speed between two measuring points and, furthermore, exact determination of the cross section of the vessel, e.g. by comparison with the catheter tip [2, 10] or with a known vessel radius, or by calculation of the analogous video signal of the profile of the vessel [11].

A similar condition applies in relation to the radius when using the method of Stewart-Hamilton. In addition the concentration of the contrast medium must be measured in absolute units and the vessel must not be ramified between the site of injection and the measuring point.

The third method has the decisive disadvantage that the flow speeds must be calculated by means of the time-concentration curve, which allows steps of only $\geqslant 1/50$ s. Therefore, a high spatial resolution is necessary to measure fast velocities if the measuring distance is short [9, 11].

All parameters and calculations which determine the renal blood flow are influenced by numerous physical and biological factors which cannot be dealt with here [2, 11], e.g. the application of contrast medium, the validity of the laws of absorption, shape and profile of the bolus, the influence of the injection conditions on measurement etc. These factors have to be considered and corrections of the original measurement values must be made to obtain the real and physiological parameters in a renal circulation study.

Independent of the method chosen to determine the specific circulation and optimal signal-noise ratio, the fundamental and most important factor is to obtain correct global or partial results concerning renal circulation and the function of the kidneys [5]. Therefore, we have to gain a high measurement value in relation to interferences, which should be as small as possible. In angiodensitometry they result from the spatial resolution or from small differences of absorption intensity between the vessels and the renal parenchyma in relation to the surrounding tissue during the contrast medium flow through the kidney. They are increased by influences of the photographic material and its processing in cinedensitometry or by many apparatus factors in videodensitometry.

This briefly listing of disadvantageous influences shows that all densitometric methods will be affected by numerous interferences. Besides the problems mentioned there are others which occur during the examination of the blood flow in the kidney and which have not yet been totally resolved [2, 4, 11], i.e. influences of the heart beat, the spatial course of the vessels, the injection of the contrast medium and movements of the patient or the organ.

Up to now the influence of a discontinuous blood flow caused by heart contractions can only be managed partially, either by the use of means obtained from values measured during different contraction phases or by triggering the injection by the ECG signal. Knowledge of the exact site of the vessels requires at least a biplane projection.

The main problem of circulation studies are influences of the blood flow by the injection of the contrast medium, which can cause alterations of the flow, the intravascular pression, the laminar profile of the blood stream, vibrations of the wall of the vessels etc. The site of injection and the kind of catheter (e.g. side holes) are important in order to avoid disturbing the laminar flow. Thus, in routine work it is useful to standardize the injection procedure [2, 11].

By means of cinedensitometry using pairs of photoconductive cells and a Wheatstone bridge circuit, some interferences are already eliminated during the measurement procedure [4, 7]. In this

manner, especially alterations of the light intensity that are influencing the results and are not caused by the contrast medium can be eliminated totally. The measurement values obtained by this technique of cinedensitometry are quite comparable with the results of other methods used in renal circulation studies like radio-isotope clearance, flow meter, etc. [6]. Recently, accuracy of densitometric examinations could be shown by animal experiments and not only by model studies [1].
In our own research group we obtained normal values by examining patients who did not have renal disease but had undergone angiography because they were suffering from another abdominal complaint. It could be shown that some of the normal values measured in these patients are fairly reliable when compared with those of pathological kidneys [2, 3].
The corrected value of the *renal blood volume* was 11.0 ml/s (±7.5 ml/s) when it was calculated from the speed of the contrast media front. The global blood volume determined on the basis of the contrast media front was somewhat lower, as could be expected. A value of 10.6 ml/s (±7.7 ml/s) was measured. It corresponds to a volume per minute of about 600 ml and is thus in harmony with the results of other methods.
According to preliminary studies, a laminar flow with marked flow paraboloid has to be expected in the renal artery. Therefore, it is necessary to distinguish between *front speed and group speed* [2, 11]. The front speed correlates with the minimum circulation time between two measuring points. The group speed is a dimension for the average transport time and thus, in relation to the profile of the laminar flow, it must be somewhat lower than the front speed.
Up to now the phase speed was left unconsidered in renal circulation studies. The problems in connection with measuring speeds of the blood cannot be dealt with here.
On average, 28.2 cm/s (±15.0 cm/s) were found for the front speed and 25.4 cm/s (±15.3 cm/s) for the group speed in the renal artery. The various segmental arteries of the kidney are anatomically extremely different. Therefore, the speeds of intrarenal circulation have a wide scattering field. The mean values for the front speed are about 17 cm/s and for the group speed about 15 cm/s.
From various measurements which are taken, we can then come to conclusions as to the *circulation of the renal parenchyma*. The cortical areas show different distances to the renal hilus. Therefore, it is necessary to find a normalized value with a time dimension related to the dimension of distance: the

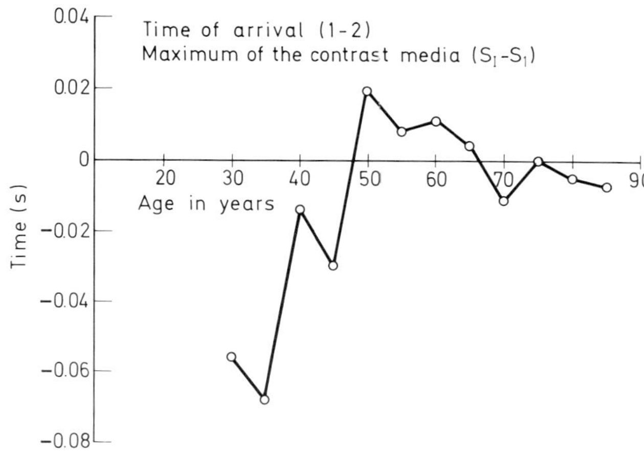

Fig. 3. Correlation between age and cortical circulation of the kidney as measured by a standardized renocortical arrival time. Blood flow in the renal parenchyma is reduced beyond the fifth decade of age

standardized renocortical arrival time (Fig. 3). In healthy persons there are only small differences for the various renal sections. This can be shown very well in digitized angiograms processed by computers [11].
It is of particular importance that it should be possible to compare the circulation of various areas of the renal cortex by means of tissue densitometry. Thus, a small and still localized disturbance of the cortical function can be detected before it becomes evident in the known clinical and radiological methods [3]. The simultaneous recording of the density by curves or by digitized pictures over kidney arteries and the various areas of the renal parenchyma permits precise statements on the blood circulation of the organ [8, 11]. In pathologically changed cortical areas the circulation is reduced, the on-flow of the contrasted blood takes place with delay and the concentration of the contrast medium in the tissue is reduced. These correspond with a diminished local clearance.
Some of the partial functions of renal circulation which can be measured by angiodensitometry were studied in different diseases of the kidneys, e.g. pyelonephritic renal damage, hypernephroid carcinoma (Fig. 4) and renal cysts. Remarkable and characteristic differences could be observed in the various parameters [2, 3, 6].
Thus, circulation measurements are helpful to differentiate between the various a forementioned diseases of the kidneys and to improve its diagnosis in an earlier stage.

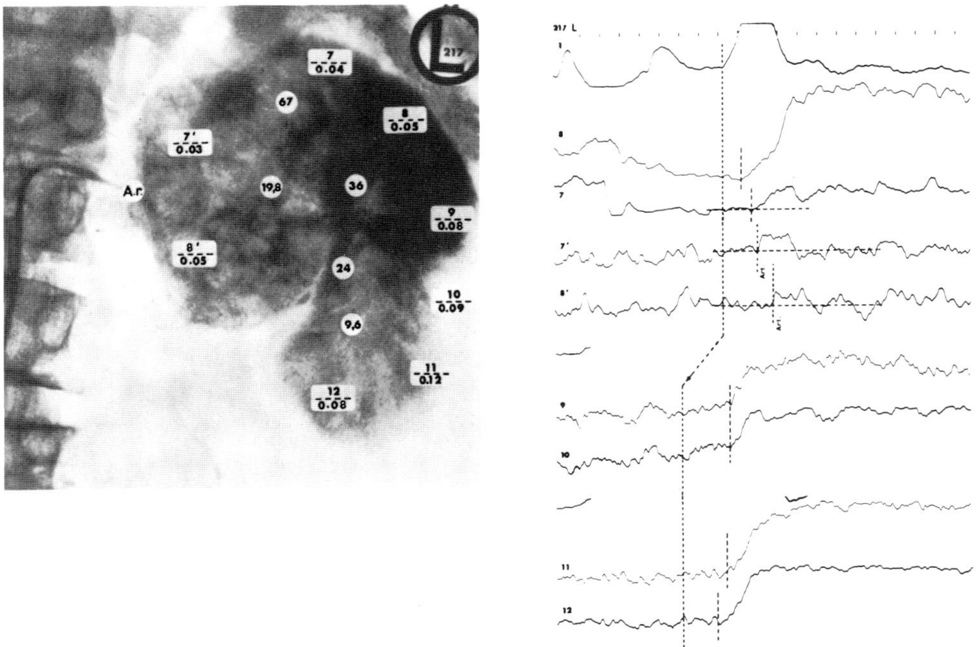

Fig. 4. Hypernephroid carcinoma with significantly changed renal circulation in the lesion as well as in the undestroyed parenchyma of the lower pole of the left kidney

Summary

Angiodensitometry makes possible determination of the specific circulation of the kidneys in the non-anaesthesized patient. Time-to-density curves of the contrast medium injected during the angiographic procedure can be obtained from the individual vessels as well as from the parenchyma. On the other hand, an improved signal-noise ratio can be obtained by means of cinedensitometry.

Due to the formation of a quotient from values measured by a pair of photoconductive cells placed next to each other, interferences can already be eliminated during the measuring procedure.

The digital processing of angiograms also represents an improvement, because it allows higher accuracy and simpler handling. Image series are digitized by a system for the real-time processing of video images. Corrections for device inaccuracies and background are performed by the system. Cine- and videodensitometrical methods have been applied for a long time in the determination of angiograms. Up to now, they have not been used in clinical routine because their handling is difficult. It has been shown that densitometry is especially suited for short measuring distances and high velocities, which is characteristic for blood flow measurements in the kidneys.

In addition, the different methods for measuring renal circulation, the multiple influences and the various interferences have been discussed. Reference values of different circulation functions and renal parameters have been described. In this way, partial functions (e.g. segmental circulation, local cortical circulation, arrival and passage time) can be measured on anatomically defined renal sections beside the global values, which can also be determined by radio-isotope techniques (e.g. total renal blood flow).

References

1. Butt TJ, Jones DR, Wallis AT, Simpson FO Intrarenal haemodynamics in the rat. Paper at the 20th Anniversary International Conference, Biological Engineering Society, London, 23–28 March 1980
2. Deininger HK (1974) Die Angiocinedensitometrie der Nieren. Methodik und Ergebnisse. Kugler, Singen
3. Deininger HK, Heuck F, Vanselow K (1978) Determination of renal circulation by means of angiodensitometry. Contrib Nephrol 11:134

4. Deininger HK, Heuck F, Vanselow K (1978) The determination of the circulation in normal human kidneys by means of angiodensitometry. Ann Radiol (Paris) 21:366
5. Deininger HK, Heuck F, Vanselow K (1979) Densitometric circulation studies of the human kidney. In: ICMBE and ICMP Committee (eds). Digest of XII ICMBE and V ICMP Meeting, ICMBE and ICMP, Jerusalem, p 271
6. Deininger HK, Heuck F, Vanselow K Densitometric circulation studies and measurement of the blood flow of the human kidney. Paper at Bio Eng. 80, London, March 1980
7. Deininger HK, Heuck F, Vanselow K The determination of the renal blood flow in man by means of angiocinedensitometry. Paper at Blood Flow, London, March 1980
8. Höhne KH, Böhm M, Nicolae GC, Pfeiffer G, Sonne B (to be published) Functional imaging – A new tool for X-ray functional diagnostics. Radiology
9. Nicolae GC, Höhne KH (1978) Digital video system for real-time processing of image series. DESV-Report DV-78/02. Deutsches Elektronen Synchroton, Hamburg
10. Piroth HD, Magin E, Georgi M, Marberger M (1977) Ergebnisse der kineangiodensitometrischen Nierendurchblutungsbestimmung. ROEFO 126:126
11. Sonne B, Höhne KH (to be published) Comparison of different methods for measuring blood flow from digital angiograms. Biomed Tech (Berlin)

Radiology of the Adrenals: Overview

M. Georgi, W. Jaschke, E. Böttger, G. Kempmann, and E. Wetzel

Klinikum der Stadt Mannheim, Institut für Klinische Radiologie, Fakultät für Klinische Medizin, Theodor-Kutzer-Ufer, D-6800 Mannheim 1

Radiological diagnostics of the adrenal glands have made substantial progress in recent years, especially due to the introduction of computed tomography (CT). The attempt will be made to evaluate old and new methods of investigation on the basis of recent results communicated in the literature and our own experience. Before going into new techniques such as ultrasound, adrenal radionuclide scanning and computed tomography, older techniques will be subjected to a critical consideration.

Abdominal Plain Film and Excretion Urography

In connection with excretion urography and tomography, adrenal masses can be demonstrated on plain films. Heuck et al. [9] specify the minimum size for this as 2 – 3 cm. Our own experience is consistent with that of Hoefer et al. [10], who specified a threshold value of 2.5 cm for the right side and of over 5 cm for the left side. Otherwise, pathological adrenal processes are only shown up on plain radiographs when they display calcifications giving rise to spontaneous shadows, as after tuberculosis, haemorrhage or in adrenal tumours (Fig. 1).

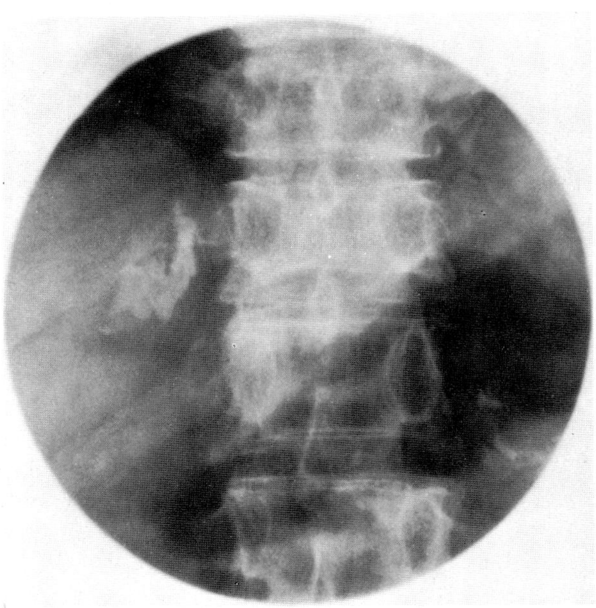

Fig. 1. Plain film of the abdomen: Bilateral adrenal calcifications due to tuberculosis

Retroperitoneal Pneumography

The outer contours of the adrenals can be delineated better after filling the retroperitoneum with gas than on plain radiographs. However, the possibilities of error are great. Whereas visualization of large tumours is unproblematical, there are appreciable difficulties in delineating the normal adrenal with hyperplasia and in differentiating hyperplasia from small tumours. Its accuracy is stated as 56% by McLachlan and Beales [14].
It is to be noted that this technique produces severe subjective discomfort and is not without risks [4]; one can always dispense with it today.

Angiography

Before the introduction of CT, angiography was regarded as the most important radiological technique in the diagnosis of pathological adrenal processes. It is applied as aortography, selective adrenal arteriography or venography.

Aortography

In adrenal diagnostics today, aortography is chiefly performed with the catheter technique. Large or well-vascularized tumours can be demonstrated

Radiology Today 1. Ed. by M. W. Donner and F. H. W. Heuck

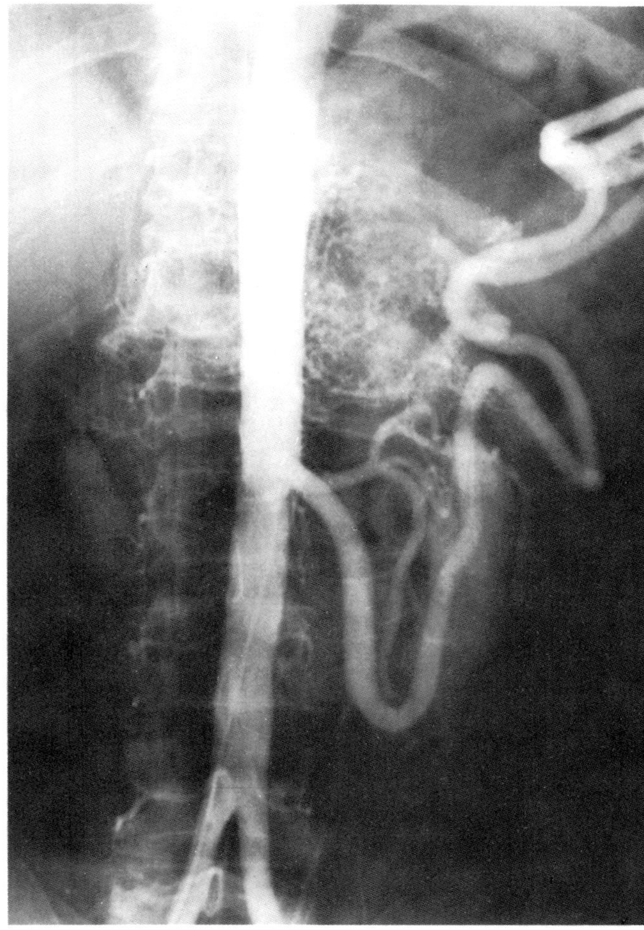

Fig. 2. Aortography: Bilaterally hypervascular, para-aortal tumour at the level of the 11th and 12th thoracic vertebrae. Operation revealed malignant pheochromocytoma

very well (Fig. 2). It is to be noted in the diagnosis of pheochromocytoma that hypertensive crisis can occur during aortography, as in selective adrenal arteriography. This can be avoided by pretreatment with α-blockers.

Selective Adrenal Arteriography

Smaller space-occupying lesions of the adrenal glands or hyperplasia are demonstrated poorly or not at all with aortography. They can be demonstrated without superimposition and with better recognition of details with selective adrenal arteriography (Fig. 3). However, it is difficult and sometimes impossible to show up all supplying vessels due to the triple arterial vascular supply. On the other hand, tumours may also be partly or completely missed. An advantage is the possibility of obtaining information on the origin of masses in the suprarenal space and the growth beyond the organ.

Selective Adrenal Venography

Selective adrenal venography in combination with the collection of blood samples from the adrenal veins and the vena cava systems for homone investigations was regarded up to 2 years ago as the method of choice in the diagnosis of hormonally active adrenal diseases [4, 10].

Hyperplasia of the adrenals as in Cushing's syndrome or in aldosteronism is shown up very well by venography (Fig. 7c).

The possibility of determining the hormone concentration in the adrenal veins separately for each side allows detection of *cortical adenomas* under 1 cm in size, such as sometimes occur in aldosteronism (Fig. 4). According to our own experience *pheochromocytomas* can be demonstrated more reliably and with less risk by means of adrenal venography than with arteriography [2, 5].

The performance of the investigation requires practice. It often succeeds on the right side in only 30% – 90% of cases [17]. The most important

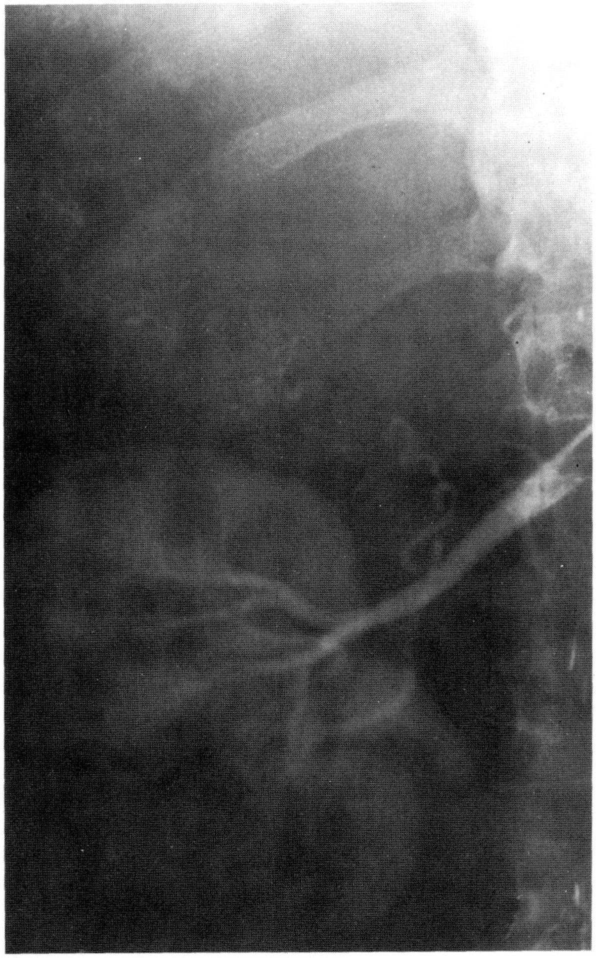

Fig. 3. Adrenal arteriography: Hypervascular tumour of the right adrenal gland. Main blood supply via inferior adrenal artery. Operation revealed adrenal cortical carcinoma

complication of adrenal venography is rupture of the adrenal vein after retrograde injection of contrast medium. If this takes place on both sides, loss of adrenal function has been described [13]. In our own experience, this complication is largely avoidable when thin, non-occluding catheters are used and the highest permissible doses of contrast medium are not exceeded. In normal adrenals these are 1 – 3 ml for the right side and 3 – 5 ml for the left.

Radionuclide Scan

The adrenal scintigraphy with ^{131}I-cholesterol introduced by Beierwaltes and co-workers in 1971 [1] has proved effective in the diagnosis of cortical adenomas and hyperplasia. With the aid of dexamethasone suppression scintigram, 95% of adenomas and 100% of hyperplasias in patients with aldosteronism were detected by Herwig et al. [8]. The recent use of 1-I-methyl-19-norcholesterol made possible a still better radionuclide uptake of the adrenals, so that the periods of examination could also be shortened [19]. The radiation exposure of the adrenals is high, so that younger patients should not be investigated with this technique (Fig. 6a).

Ultrasound

By means of ultrasound, Sample and Sarti [15] were even able to demonstrate a higher accuracy with ultrasound (93%) than with comparative investigations performed with CT (91%). Hofer et al. [10] were able to detect tumours up to 1.5 cm in size in 12 patients investigated by ultrasound. However, they were often shown up larger than they in fact were. These authors nevertheless value ultrasound as a screening method.

Computed Tomography

The introduction of CT is doubtlessly the greatest advance in radiodiagnostics of the adrenals. Information with regard to the normal anatomy of the adrenals is important here. According to Wilms et al. [18] the right adrenal can be shown in 99% of patients; its visualization fails only in thin patients. The left adrenal gland is shown up in 100%.

The results of CT investigations communicated in pathological adrenal processes are based on a relatively small number of cases. The results obtained by different authors already largely agree.

Haertel et al. [7] as well as Karstaedt et al. [12] report on experience in ten and eight *pheochromocytomas* investigated with CT, respectively. These round- to oval-shaped masses display very different densities of 20 – 60 HU; solid masses with 5 – 10 HU were also observed [11]. According to our own experience in four cases, they can almost always be demonstrated, since they are mostly over 2 cm in size (Fig. 5). Smaller, multiple and extra-adrenal pheochromocytomas can give rise to difficulties. They can already be delimited by cava

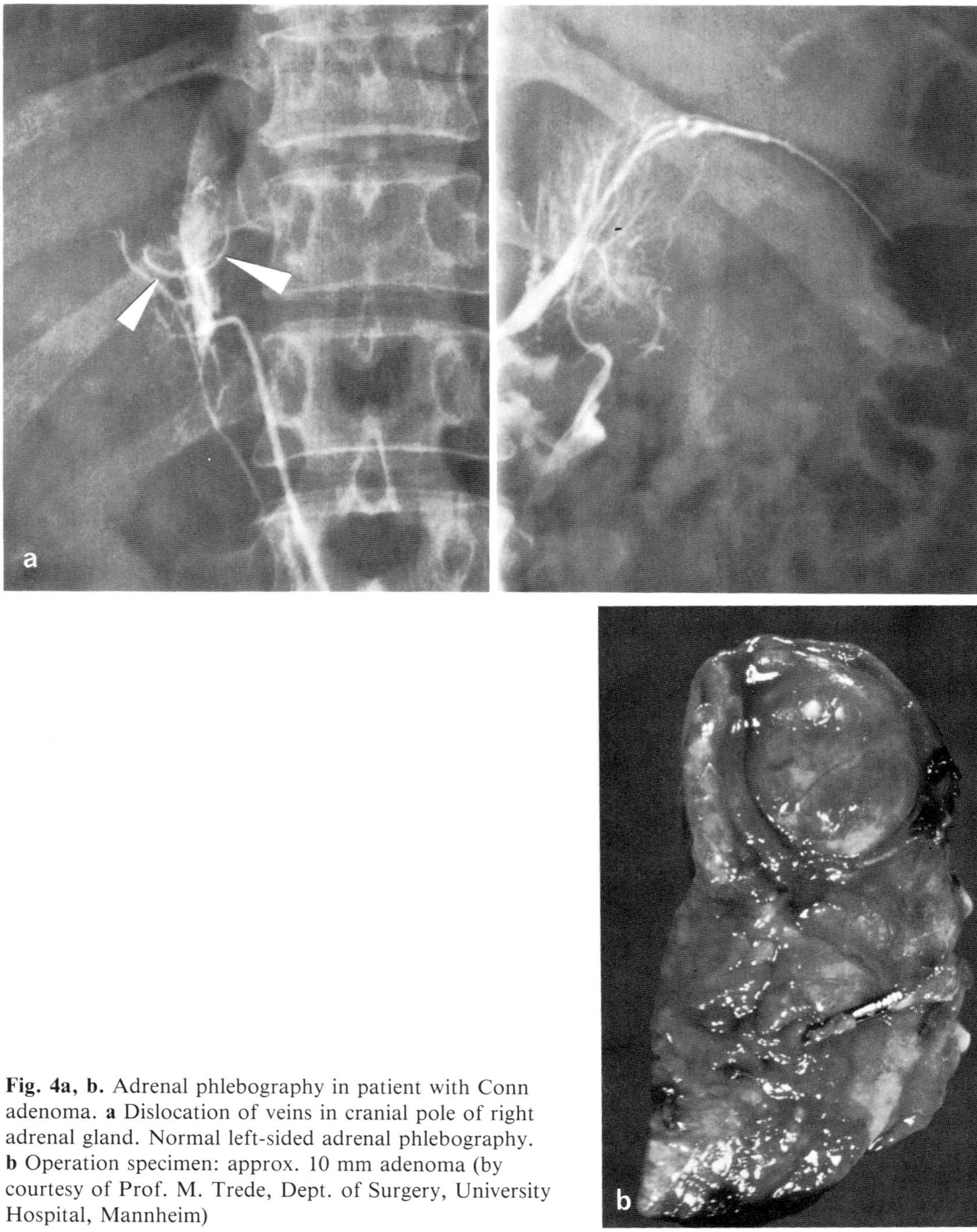

Fig. 4a, b. Adrenal phlebography in patient with Conn adenoma. **a** Dislocation of veins in cranial pole of right adrenal gland. Normal left-sided adrenal phlebography. **b** Operation specimen: approx. 10 mm adenoma (by courtesy of Prof. M. Trede, Dept. of Surgery, University Hospital, Mannheim)

catheterization with hormone investigations in the context of adrenal venography [6].

Adrenal cortical adenomas such as occur in aldosteronism could be demonstrated by Dunnick et al. [3] in seven out of nine cases, by Heuck et al. [9] in three cases and in our own investigations in three out of five cases (Table 1). The tumour is rarely over 2 cm, but not seldom under 1 cm in size (Fig. 6). It displays very low densities and sometimes negative absorption values [6, 16].

Since the tumour may therefore escape CT detection, ^{131}I-adrenal radionuclide scan and adrenal venography with connection of blood for hormone determinations continue to be appropriate as supplementary investigations.

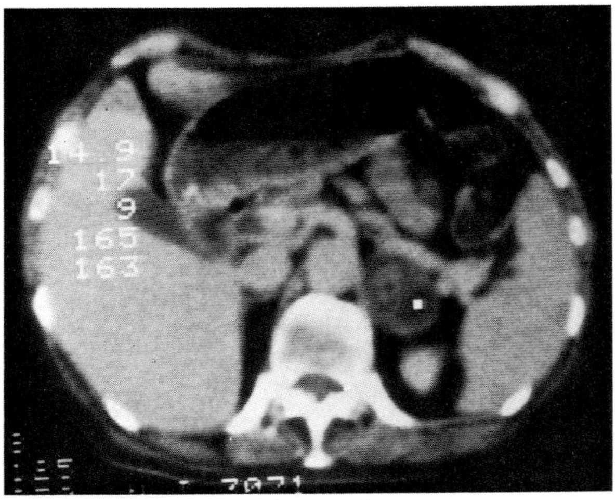

Fig. 5. CT in patient with pheochromocytoma: Demonstration of rounded, hypodense, 2.5 cm tumour

Table 1. Diagnostic methods in patients with adrenal tumours

Case no.	Venous sampling	Angiography		CT	US	Radio-nuclide scan	Surgery	Pathology and final diagnosis
		Veno-gram	Arterio-gram					
1) 53 A (F)	+	+	–	–	–	NP	+	Aldosteronoma
2) 39 A (F)	+	+	NP	–	NP	–*	+	Aldosteronoma
3) 57 A (F)	+	+	NP	–*	NP	–*	+	Aldosteronoma
4) 48 A (F)	+	+	NP	+	NP	+	+	Aldosteronoma
5) 37 A (F)	+	+	NP	+	NP	NP	NP	Aldosteronoma
6) 50 A (M)	–	+	+	+	NP	+	+	Adenoma without function
7) 73 A (F)	–	+	NP	+	–	NP	NP	
8) 34 A (F)	NP	NP	–	+	NP	NP	+	Pheochromocytoma
9) 58 A (F)	NP	NP	NP	+	NP	NP	+	Pheochromocytoma
10) 50 A (M)	+	+	NP	+	NP	–	NP	Pheochromocytoma
11) 25 A (F)	+	–	NP	+	–	NP	+	Pheochromocytoma
12) 45 A (F)	–	–	+	NP	+	+	+	Adrenal cyst

+, Positive for adrenal tumour
–, Negative for adrenal tumour
NP, Not performed
*, Hyperplasia rather than tumour

Cushing's or AGS (adrenogenital syndrome) adenomas give rise to hardly any diagnostic difficulties: they mostly become more than 3 cm in size, and usually display low densities [16]. The relatively rare *myelolipoma* of the adrenal glands is described by Karstaedt et al. [12] in one case as a tumour 4 cm in size of which the density was somewhat higher than that of fat. Demonstration of *adrenal cysts* is also unproblematical; their organ assignment is not always recognized in CT.

Hyperplasia of the adrenals is frequently not detected in CT. Even if they are occasionally shown up very well, assessment of their functional state is not possible (Fig. 7). Besides adrenal scintigraphy, adrenal venography with separate blood sampling from the adrenal vein on each side is able to give more detailed information on hormone production (Table 2). Hyperplasias not visible in CT had been described by Haertel et al. [7] in two out of five cases, and by Dunnick et al. [3] in one out of five cases. Stadler et al. [17] also report one false positive finding.

Primary adrenal carcinomas are mostly shown up as large, in some cases necrotic, tumours displaying marked contrast enhancement. With large size, the organ assignment is ocassionally not possible in CT (Fig. 8). Growth beyond the organ is also not always detected. These questions can be clarified with angiography, which is still indicated before operation.

Adrenal metastases can be detected frequently and well with CT. Further diagnostic methods are unnecessary when the primary tumour is known.
In the view of all authors, the *detection limit of CT* is about 1 cm diameter in the case of circumscribed lesions. CT is unable to give any information on the function of detected lesions when there is no clear clinical or chemical constellation available. Misinterpretations with CT are also possible in

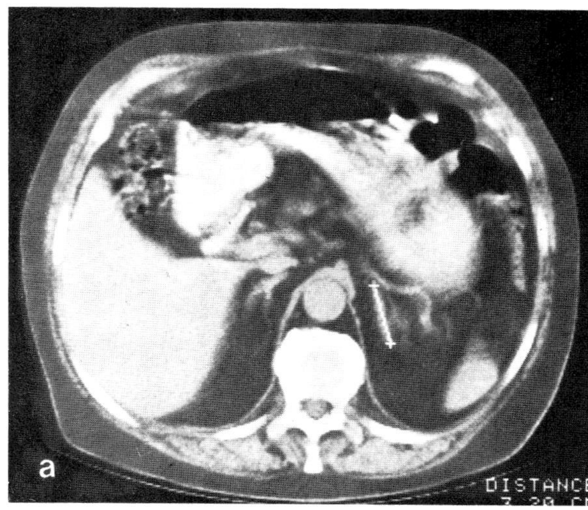

Fig. 7a–c. Hyperplasia of adrenal glands. **a** CT: Enlargement of both adrenal glands. **b** Adrenal phlebography: Hyperplasia of both adrenal glands, more pronounced on left side. **c** Values of cortisol in adrenal veins and in inferior vena cava: Hyperlasia proven at operation. Left-sided adrenalectomy. Regression of Cushing's syndrome following operation

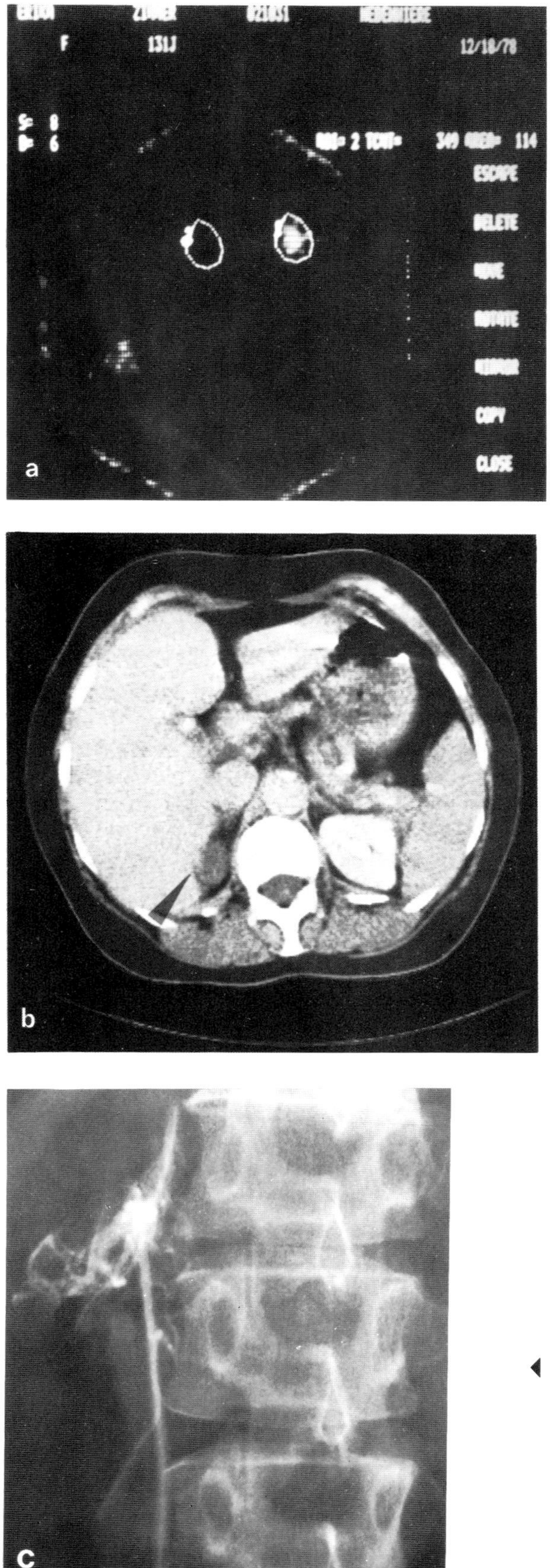

◀ **Fig. 6a–c.** Adrenal scintigraphy, CT and phlebography in patient with Conn adenoma of right adrenal gland. **a** Adrenal scintigraphy following blocking with dexamethasone. Localized, increased activity in right adrenal gland only (examination performed with patient in prone position). **b** CT: demonstration of 2.4 × 1.8 cm right-sided adrenal tumour. **c** Adrenal phlebography: oval, approx. 2.5 × 1.5 cm tumour in right adrenal gland. Operation revealed Conn adenoma

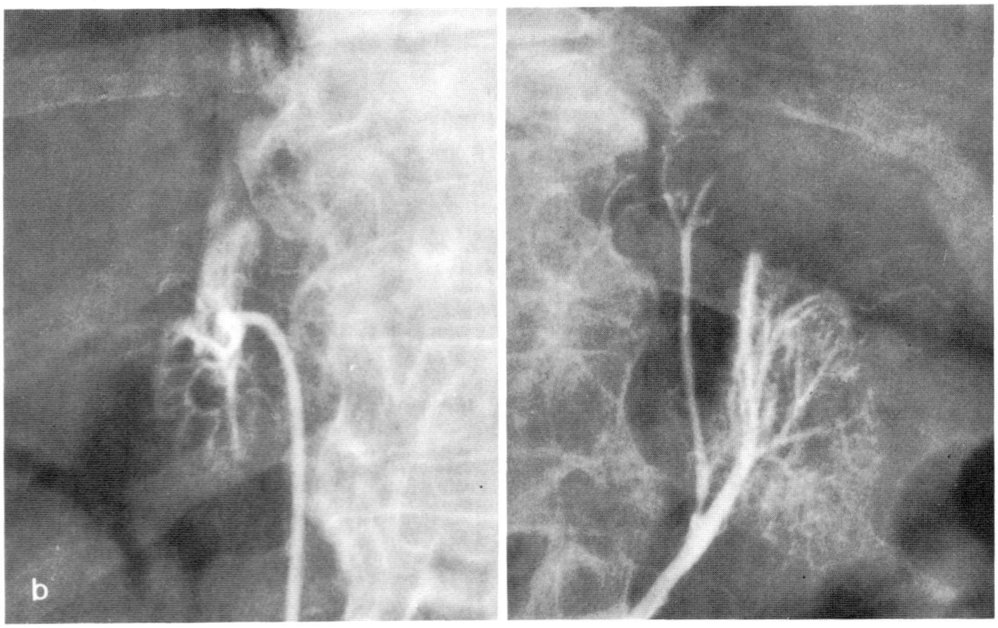

Fig. 7b, c. Legend see p. 241

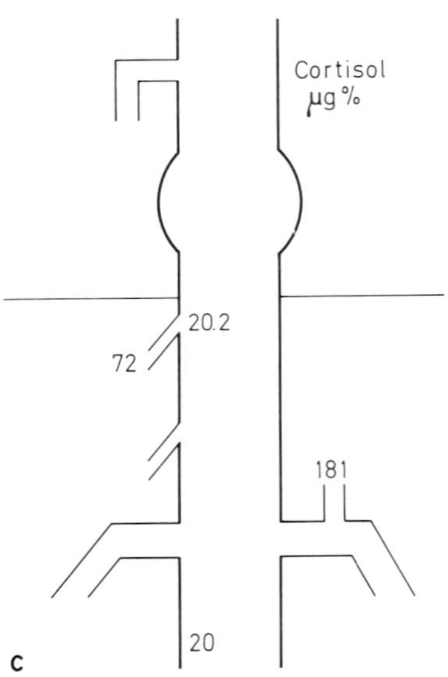

hyperplasia, so that adrenal venography with blood sampling for hormone investigations must also be used. One can agree with the view of Hartel et al. [7] that if clear clinical, chemical and CT results exist, traditional angiographic documentation can be dispensed with.

Summary

New radiological techniques, such as ultrasound, CT and radionuclide scanning, necessitate a new approach to the patient suffering from adrenal disease. Especially CT proved to be extremely

Table 2. Diagnostic methods in patients with adrenal hyperplasia

Case no.	Venous sampling	Angiography		CT	Radio-nuclide scan	Surgery	Pathology and final diagnosis
		Venogram	Arteriogram				
1) 58 A (F)	+	+	NP	+	NP	+	Cushing's syndrome
2) 23 A (M)	+	+	NP	–	NP	NP	Cushing's syndrome
3) 53 A (M)	+	+	NP	+	NP	NP	Cushing's syndrome
4) 48 A (M)	+	+	NP	+	+	+	Aldosteronism
5) 32 A (M)	+	+	NP	+	NP	NP	Aldosteronism
6) 52 A (M)	+	+	–	–	NP	NP	Pheochromocytoma

+, Postive for adrenal hyperplasia
–, Negative for adrenal hyperplasia
NP, Not performed

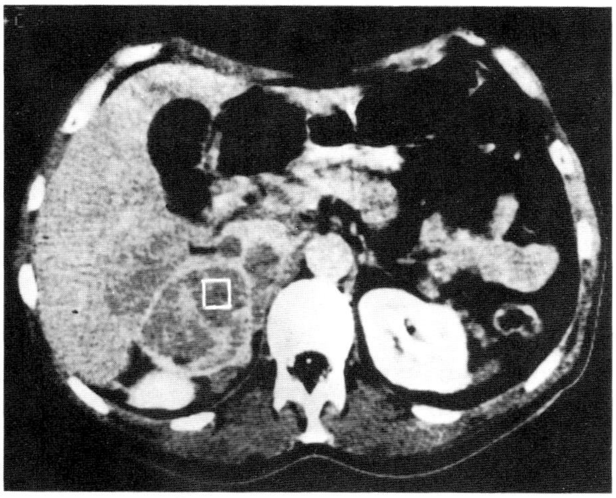

Fig. 8. Primary, adrenal cortical carcinoma: CT demonstrated a large tumour. Suspicion of infiltration of the liver by the tumour. No infiltration found by surgery

sensitive in detecting adrenal abnormalities. Specifying adrenal lesions by CT, however, can be very difficult. Invasive studies, such as arteriography and venography with blood sampling, can add important information in these cases. Plain film radiograph, IVP and ultrasound should still be the first diagnostic tests when looking for adrenal disease.

References

1. Beierwaltes WH, Liebermann LM, Ansari AN (1971) Visualization of human adrenal glands in vivo by scintillation scanning. JAMA 216:275 – 277
2. Cordes U, Georgi M, Günther R, Beyer J (1979) Adrenale und extraadrenale Phäochromozytome – Diagnostik und Lokalisation durch Bestimmung der Plasma-Katecholamine. Dtsch med Wochenschr 104:317 – 323
3. Dunnick NR, Schaner EG, Doppman JL, Strott CA, Gill JR, Javadpour N (1979) Computed tomography in adrenal tumors. AJR 132:43 – 46
4. Georgi M (1979) Röntgendiagnostik der Nebennieren. Roentgenblaetter 32:20 – 29
5. Georgi M, Cordes U, Günther R, Philipp T, Lenner V (1978) Phlebographische Diagnostik des Phäochromozytoms. ROEFO 128:727 – 733
6. Georgi M, Jaschke W, Trede M, v. Mittelstaedt G, Cordes U, Sinterhauf K, Magin E (1980) Erfahrungen mit der Computertomographie und der Nebennierenphlebographie in der Diagnostik hormonaktiver Nebennierenprozesse. Radiologe 20:172 – 180
7. Haertel M, Probst P, Bollmann J, Zingg E, Fuchs WA (1980) Computertomographische Nebennierendiagnostik. ROEFO 132:31 – 36
8. Herwig KR (1979) Primary aldosteronism: Experience with thirthy-eight patients. Surgery 86:470 – 474
9. Heuck F, Buck J, Reiser U (1980) Die gesunde und kranke Nebenniere im Röntgen-Computertomogramm. Radiologe 20:158 – 171
10. Hofer B, Thriller J, Haertel M (1978) Sonographisch-phlebographische Diagnostik der Nebenniere. ROEFO 129:686 – 691
11. Hübener K-H, Grehn S, Schulze K (1980) Indikationen zur computertomographischen Nebennierenuntersuchung; Leistungsfähigkeit, Stellenwert und Differentialdiagnostik. ROEFO 132:37 – 44
12. Karstaedt N, Sagel SS, Stanley RJ, Melson GL, Levitt RG (1978) Computed tomography of the adrenal gland. Radiology 129:723 – 730
13. Korobkin M, White EA, Kressel HY, Moss AA, Montagne J-P (1979) Computed tomography in the diagnosis of adrenal disease. AJR 132:231 – 238
14. McLachlan MSF, Beales JSM (1971) Retroperitoneal pneumography in the investigation of adrenal diseases. Clin Radiol 22:188
15. Sample WF, Sart DA (1978) Computed tomography and Gray scale Ultrasonography of the adrenal gland: A comparative study. Radiology 128: 377 – 383
16. Schaner EG, Dunnick NR, Doppmann JL, Strott CA, Gill JR Jr, Javadpour N (1978) Adrenal cortical tumors with low attenuation coefficients: a pitfall in computed tomography diagnosis. J Comput Assist Tomogr 2:11 – 15
17. Stadler H-W, Grabner W, Fuchs HF (1979) Computertomographische Untersuchung der Nebennieren. Klinikarzt 8:399 – 406
18. Wilms G, Baert A, Marchal G, Goddeeris P (1979) Computed Tomography of the normal adrenal glands: correlative study with autopsy specimes. J Comput Assist Tomogr 3:467 – 469
19. Yun Ryo U, Johnston AS, Kim I, Pinski S (1978) Adrenal scanning and uptake with ^{131}J-6β-Iodomethyl-Norcholesterol. Radiology 128:157 – 161

Direct Magnification and Target CT as Image Optimization Techniques

F. Buchmann

c/o C.H.F. Müller, Unternehmensbereich der Philips GmbH, Alexanderstrasse 1, D-2000 Hamburg 1

CT images are generated by reconstruction of slices from a full set of transverse projections. Both modalities, target scan and direct magnification, are part of the primary data acquisition process which is the pick-up of measurements for the axial transverse projections or profiles of the slice. Target CT results in an image of only a selected area of the body section under examination. Both modalities contribute to the optimization of image quality and show their full effectiveness in a third-generation CT system. This paper has the objective of giving an impression of principle and application range of the target scan modalities of the Philips Tomoscan 300 and similar systems.

Procedures to Provide a Target Image

There are several procedures to provide an image of a region of interest in a CT slice. The best known of these is the simple method of zoom technique: In a reconstructed image the center of a target area is selected by a light pen or another input procedure and all elements of the reconstruction matrix are displayed on 4, 16, or more elements of the display matrix. This results in a linear magnification of two times, four times, or more. As the picture looks coarse if this method is applied, a type of smoothing can be combined with zoom magnification. The procedure allows for more viewing comfort and centration of the details which are important for diagnosis, but it does not enhance image quality or increase information.

As it is an easy image postprocessing method, zoom technique is available on many CT viewing systems and is frequently used.

In CT more primary data are usually collected than displayed on reconstructed picture elements. Therefore in particular cases it is helpful to reconstruct a restricted field only, and in this way to make use of the full reconstruction matrix for a selected area. This technique is called reconstructive zoom. Reconstructive zoom as a primary routine technique is applied in third-generation CT scanners with fixed combination of focal spot – rotation center – detector array. It provides increasing image quality as long as enough detector elements are involved in the data acquisition process.

A particular version of reconstructive zoom is obtained by generating the projections from a full-size image and again reconstructing a region of interest. In this case the procedure serves as a type of interpolation in the visualized field.

Full use of the imaging power of a CT system on a selected field can be made by target reconstruction out of a set of data which was taken directly from the field of interest. If a region of interest out of a full diameter slice is scanned, only so-called truncated profiles, which do not allow for a correct reconstruction of the image, are available. Therefore complements for the truncated profiles have to be found which contain that information needed for correct reconstruction. Several procedures for providing this complementary information have been proposed. In the Tomoscan 300 a somewhat larger area than the target field is scanned for this purpose (Fig. 1).

The Role of Direct Magnification

In the second-generation scanners, which have a translate – rotate geometry, it was easy to concentrate a high number of measurements on a restricted area by just adapting the sampling intervals in the translation parts of the movement. Third-generation scanners also offer a possibility of concentrating their measuring power to an area of

Radiology Today 1. Ed. by M. W. Donner and F. H. W. Heuck

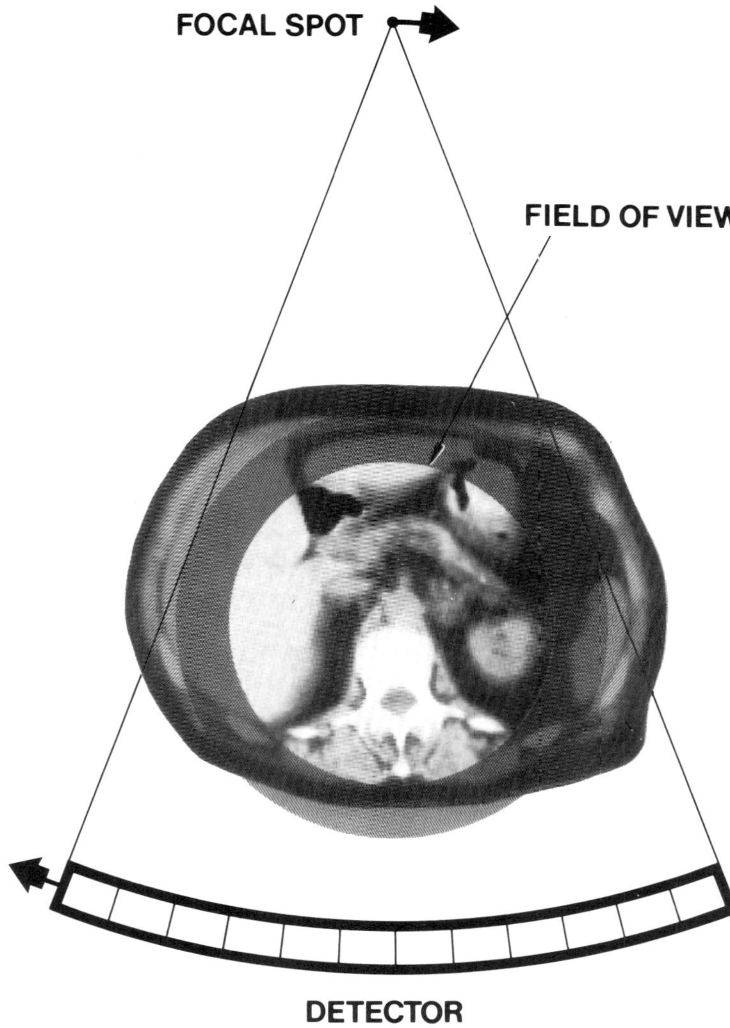

Fig. 1. Target scan implementation by scanning a slightly larger area than the field of interest

particular interest by adapting the magnification factor for the projection of the field of view on the detector array.

Direct magnification technique in CT is implemented by shifting the X-ray source detector combination of a fan scanner toward the rotation center in such a way that in all axial transverse projections of the imaging field a maximum of detector elements is involved for data acquisition (Fig. 2). This means that for all scanned field sizes the full detector array is effective.

By making use of direct magnification the increased number of measurements can be provided for all field sizes and also in target scan operation modes. But this always means that a high number of measurements is available for image formation. The result is optimized image quality.

Conclusions and Applications

If the modalities to provide an image of a selected area are compared, these aspects are obvious: zoom technique allows for more viewing comfort and centration of the diagnostic structures out of a full-size slice. In many cases it is a convenient procedure to produce more instructive multiformat pictures. It also makes interactive measuring procedures easier. However, it does not enhance image quality.

Reconstructive zoom as an interpolation technique helps to overcome restrictions in reconstruction and to display parts of the information transfer channel, which is given in a CT system by concentrating the reconstruction matrix to the area of

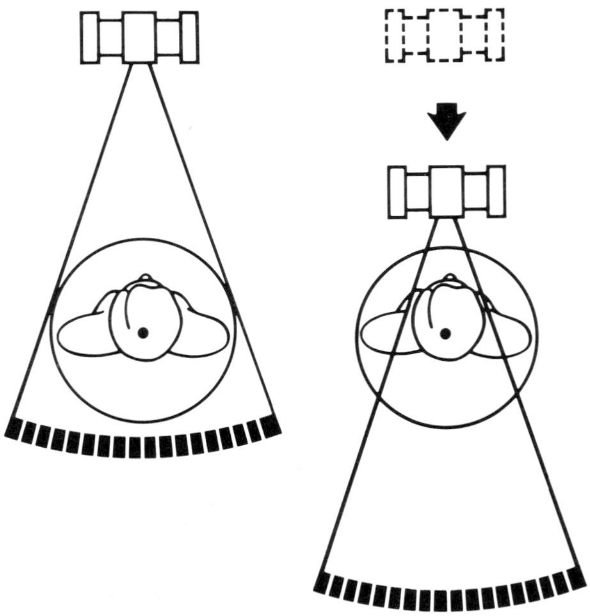

Fig. 2. Direct magnification of the field of view to the full detector array in order to obtain a maximum number of primary measurements

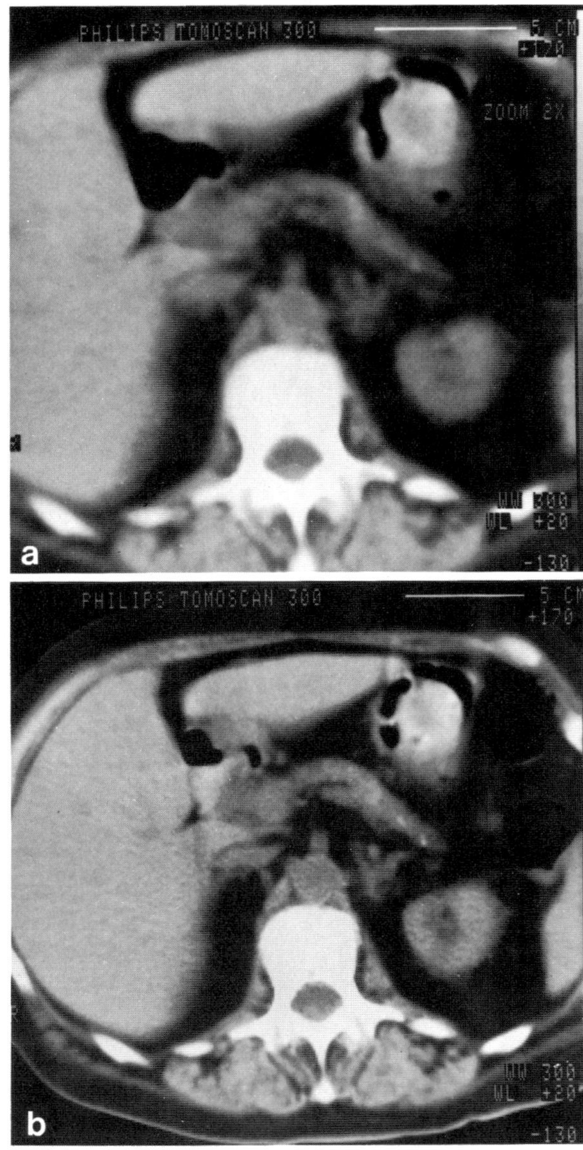

Fig. 3a, b. Example of 2 × zoom **a** from a 400-mm field of view and target scan, **b** with a 240-mm field size

interest. But it is not yet a true target imaging modality.

Target scan procedures include optimization of all parts of the information transfer channel, which can be segmented as follows: data acquisition, reconstruction, display. For data acquisition modified sampling procedures in second-generation systems or variable geometric enlargement of the scanned field in third-generation systems are applicable. The following reconstruction and display processes include the facilities of reconstructive zoom techniques. With the Tomoscan 300 two target scan modes are actually offered. The diameter of the field is either 16 or 24 cm.

There is a wide field of applications for target scan modalities, and this field has just started to be evaluated. Localized objects such as mediastinal structures or the pancreas are already well-known structures for target CT. The larger field is capable of covering even a diameter which is suitable for routine kidney examination or CT of adrenals. Of course, one of the most obvious target scan objects is the spine. Target CT examination in this area, planned by means of scanogram techniques, is supposed to be one of the most powerful means of examination of the near future.

Target CT is expected to be effective in many parts of the total body as it is a procedure that provides the highest resolution mode of the CT system in any part at the expense of a preselectable restriction of field size.

The examples shown in Figs. 3 and 4 demonstrate field size and resolution effect of the target scan modality. They were obtained with Tomoscan 300 equipment and are reproduced with the intention of providing an impulse for the evaluation of the further application range of this modality.

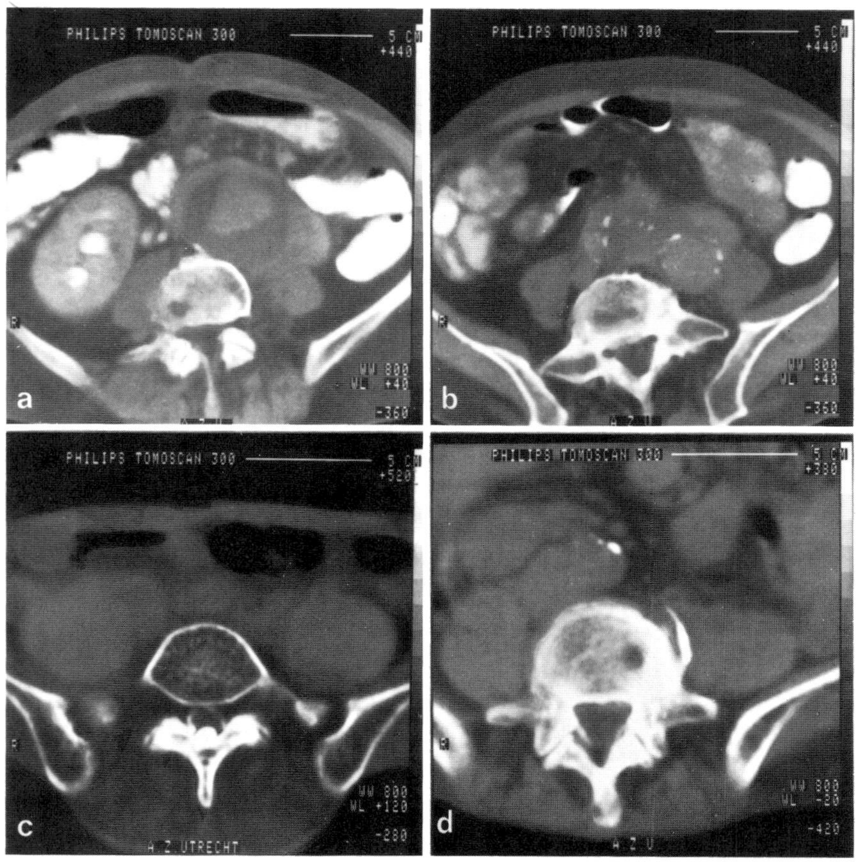

Fig. 4a – d. Four examples of target CT application: **a, b** 240 mm and **c, d** 160 mm fields of view

References

1. Abele M, Erdos J, Chase NE (1978) Artifacts due to non-linear characteristics of X-ray transmission measurements in CT. 64th Scientific Association and Annual Meeting of the Radiological Society of North America, Chicago Illinois, 1978, paper 255
2. Bublitz G, Moeller M (1980) Beispiele für die Erweiterung der diagnostischen Möglichkeiten durch die Ganzkörper-Computertomographie. Roentgenstrahlen 43:16 – 20
3. Buchmann F (1978) CT-Systeme und Anwendungsgesichtspunkte. Medizinal-Markt/Acta Medicotechnica 26:349 – 354
4. Dihlmann W, Gräper P, Buchmann F, Zimmer H (to be published) Target scan in clinical application. Medicamundi 25/3
5. Wagner W (1978) Reconstruction from truncated scan data. (Procedures of MEDITA '78). Sonderheft 1:89 – 96
6. Wijdeveld B (1979) Primäre geometrische Vergrößerung in der Computer-Tomographie. Röntgenstrahlen 41:8 – 13

Computed Tomography in the Urinary Tract, Adrenals, and Pelvis

P. Wozney

General Electric Company, Medical Systems Division, Post Office Box 414, Milwaukee, WI 53201 (USA)

General Electric Medical Systems Division

Computed tomography until recently has principally been of value in imaging anatomy. The diagnosis of pathology has been limited to lesions that alter gross structure. With new advances, however, diagnosis of functional abnormalities may become possible, in addition to an improvement in the resolution of anatomic lesions.

Currently, CT is of great value in identifying pelvic lesions and assessing their importance. Of great value is the staging of urinary bladder carcinoma. By injecting air into the bladder, the tumor is clearly outlined. The degree of involvement of the bladder wall is readily determined on the standard CT scan. If the tumor extends past the bladder wall into the perivesicular fat, total excision is not possible and radio- and chemotherapy is more appropriate than surgery.

A new technical advance called dynamic scanning allows one to evaluate blood flow. This is performed by injecting a contrast bolus in a peripheral vein and obtaining slices rapidly at one location. The scans take 5 s, with an interscan delay of 1, so that five scans are taken in 30 s, or ten a minute. This allows one to see the contrast bolus as it washes in and out of the scan plane.

One straightforward application is the identification of suspicious masses. In one patient with lymphoma, multiple bilateral pelvic masses consistent with enlarged lymph nodes were seen. With the addition of a contrast bolus, they were seen to opacify and wash out rapidly. Their identification as the iliac vessels then became obvious.

Potentially an important use of dynamic scanning is the evaluation of blood flow to the kidney. This would aid in the diagnosis of renovascular hypertension and renal infarcts. Preliminary research has been carried out at Duke University (North Carolina, USA). In these canine studies part of the kidney was infarcted by embolization of the segmental artery. Rapid sequential scans of the area were then taken and evaluated by the computer. By plotting the change in opacity due to contrast from scan to scan, a measurement of blood flow in each part of the kidney section is obtained. Clear differences are apparent when the center of the infarct is compared with the periphery.

Further clinical evaluation in human patients is, of course, necessary. However, these results suggest that dynamic scanning may define decreased blood flow in a patient with unilateral stenosis and may even identify segmental compromise of renal blood flow. This would allow angiography to be more directive, and may eliminate it entirely in those cases where no flow abnormality is identified.

Finally, new reprocessing of computer data allows improvement in image resolution to better than 0.75 mm. This is particularly valuable in diagnosis of small adrenal gland lesions as well as in assessment of the extent of malignancy.

References

Heinz ER, Dubois PT, Drayer BP, Hill R (1980) A Preliminary Investigation of the Role of Dynamic Computed Tomography in Renovascular Hypertension. J Comput Assist Tomogr 4(1):63–66

Radiology Today 1. Ed. by M. W. Donner and F. H. W. Heuck

Computed Tomography of the Pelvis: Overview

A. Breit, U. Rohde, and A. Atzinger

Städtisches Krankenhaus, Radiologische Abteilung, Bischof-Pilgrim-Strasse 1, D-8390 Passau

Two methods have been available for the radiologic diagnosis of pelvic tumors, one noninvasive and one invasive. Besides the information which can be drawn from plain films, by the use of contrast media we can visualize the adjacent organs, such as the ureter, the bladder, the colon, and the ileum. Only with the help of invasive methods such as arteriography and lymphography can tumor masses be demonstrated directly [6, 4]; hysterography might also be used.

Clinical Material and Method

Since 1976, 650 patients with gynecologic tumors have been examined in our department. I would like to distinguish between primary diagnoses obtained by CT, i.e., the examination of untreated tumors, and the diagnosis of recurrent tumors. CT diagnoses in cases after surgery represent a distinct group. Slice thickness amounts to 8 mm without oblique position of the gantry. A cross section thickness of 4 mm is only considered for planning calculations and for sagittal or frontal views. We use contrast media or gas in order to obtain markings of the bladder and ureter. For delineation of the vagina an amber filter or tampon may sometimes be necessary [2].

Anatomy

In order to evaluate the efficiency of our technique as well as of our facilities, in cooperation with Professor Platzer from the Institute of Anatomy, University of Innsbruck, we studied anatomic cross sections of the truncus visualized by CT in 8 mm slices of several males and females [15]. This was made possible because Professor Platzer provided us with almost identical 8 mm thick sections for the CT. With the help of this direct comparison we were able to evaluate the accuracy of the CT very well.

Carcinoma of the Cervix

Primary carcinoma of the cervix is diagnosed by biopsy or curettage. The tumor is clinically classified with the help of palpation. However, in cases with proved carcinomas CT helps to substantiate the results of examination and sometimes to improve them, particularly in cases with infiltrations which could not be delineated cranially or were not palpable at all because of their location (Figs. 1 – 3) [8, 13, 16].

Parametrium

It is important to know that the parametrium consists partly of soft tissue, smooth muscle fibers and dense vein conglomerations which serve to secure

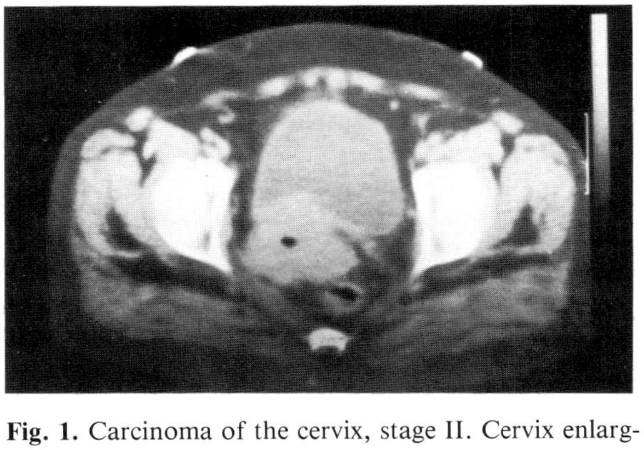

Fig. 1. Carcinoma of the cervix, stage II. Cervix enlarged, visualization of parametric region and rectum

Radiology Today 1. Ed. by M. W. Donner and F. H. W. Heuck

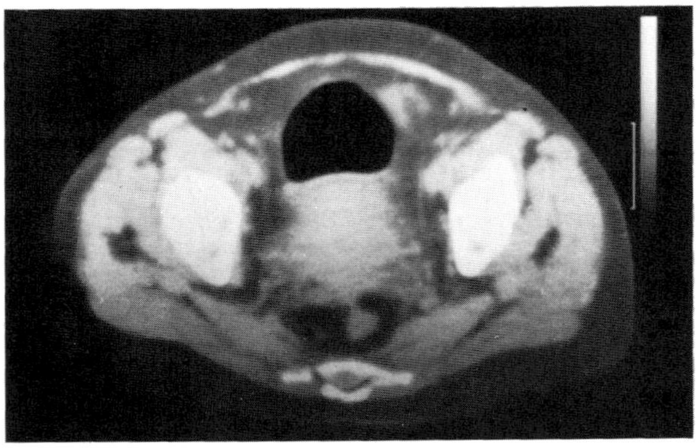

Fig. 2. Infiltration of the parametrium on both sides. Carcinoma of the cervix, stage IIb; bulky structures bilateraly. The infiltration does not reach the pelvic wall

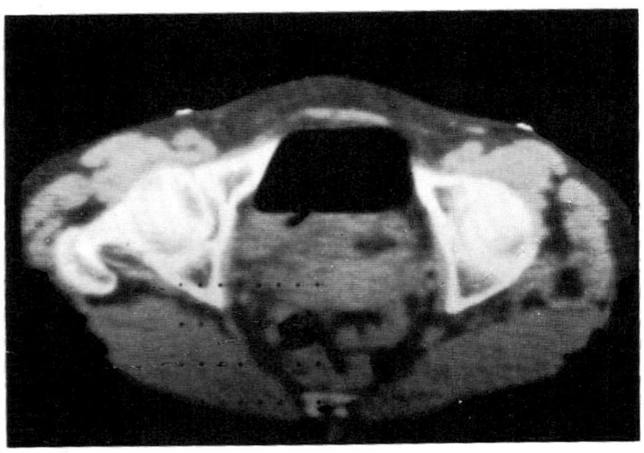

Fig. 3. Infiltration on both sides reaching the pelvic wall; carcinoma of the cervix, stage III

and to suspend the uterus within the frame-work of the pelvis and also to connect the cervix to the adjacent organs [10].

Because of such relevant questions as whether, in carcinoma of the cervix, infiltrations or scar formation has occurred and whether one can distinguish between scar and infiltration and determine the extension to the pelvic wall, it is important to know whether CT examination supplies any additional information to palpation. In our experience CT confirms and corrects the physical examination.

Lymphatic Pathways of Gynecologic Carcinomas

All lymph nodes along the large vessels can serve as regional filter stations for gynecologic tumors. Lymph node metastases are reported in over 18% of patients with stage I carcinoma of the cervix, in over 33% with stage II carcinoma, and in over 52% with stage III carcinoma [17]. On CT scans,

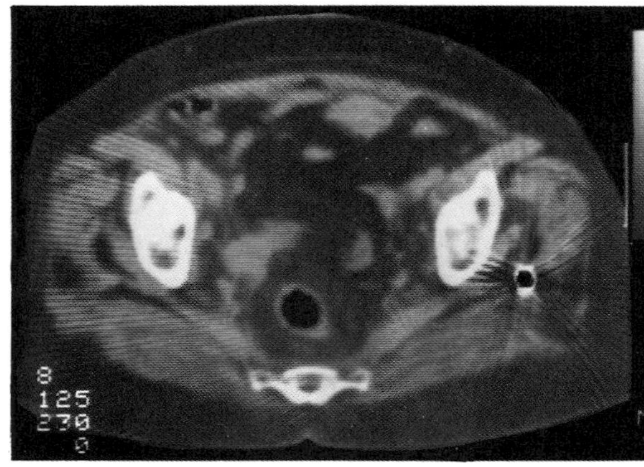

Fig. 4. Lymph nodes enlarged on the pelvic wall

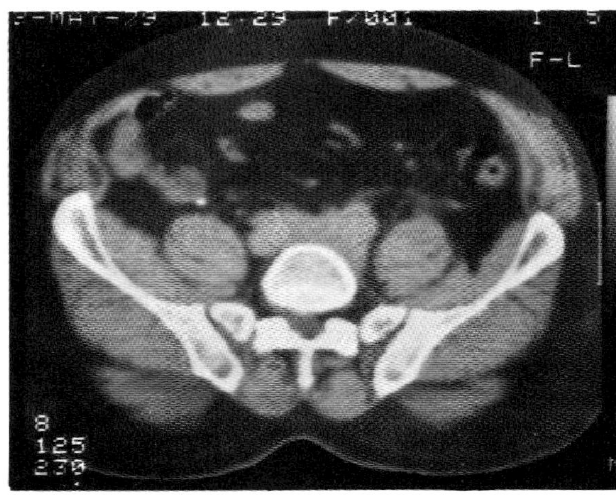

Fig. 5. Lymph node metastases at the bifurcation of the aorta

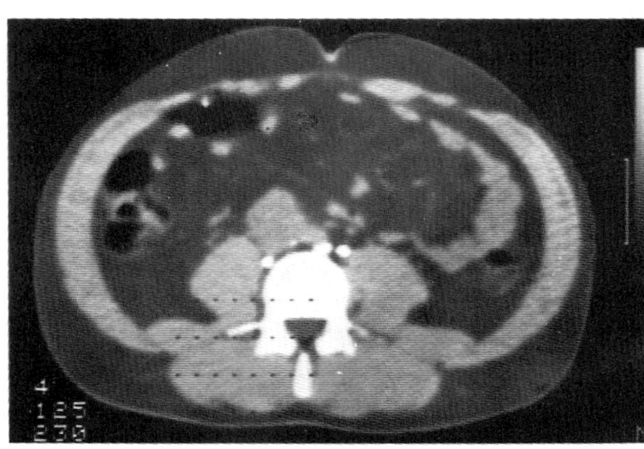

Fig. 6. Lymph node metastasis in the para-aortic region

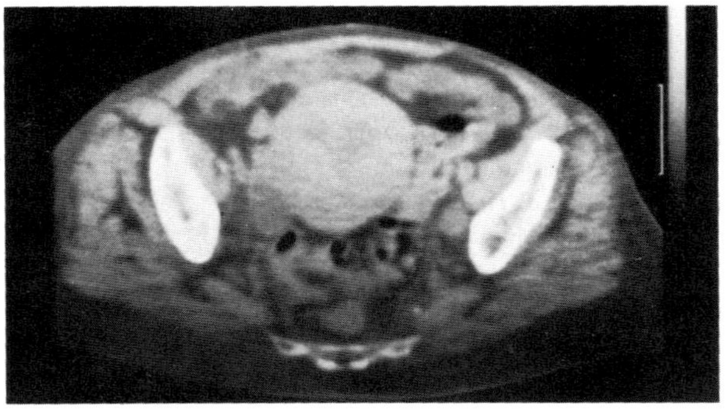

Fig. 7. Carcinoma of the corpus uteri. Carcinoma of the endometrium, stage III; enlarged uterus

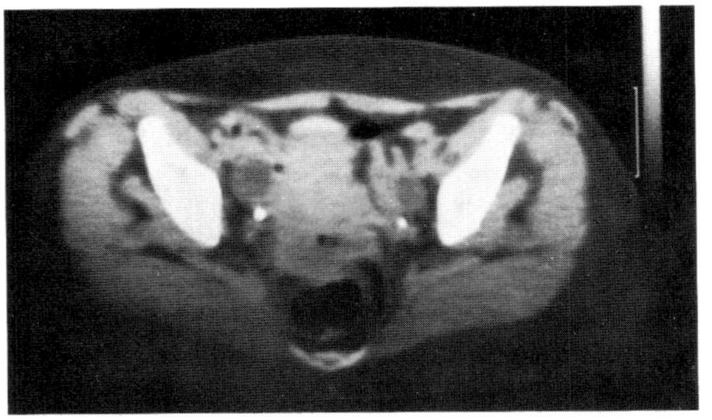

Fig. 8. Small cystic ovaries. Carcinoma of the cervix, necrosis of the enlarged cervix

enlargement of lymph nodes appear as soft tissue masses. Demonstration is dependent on size, number of invaded lymph nodes, and their topographical location.

Enlargement of lymph nodes in the pelvis is only demonstrable from 2 cm upward in size, because if less adipose tissue is present bowels and vessels may be taken as adenopathy. Increase in soft tissue may be seen more easily in the retroperitoneal region filled with fat tissue. Structure of lymph nodes can be determined only by lymphography; on CT, extension of tumor masses into the lymph nodes may be better evaluated. CT is superior to lymphography in demonstrating abnormality in the areas not reached by the contrast material from bipedal lymphography (Figs. 4–6) [5, 7, 9, 11, 12, 14, 21].

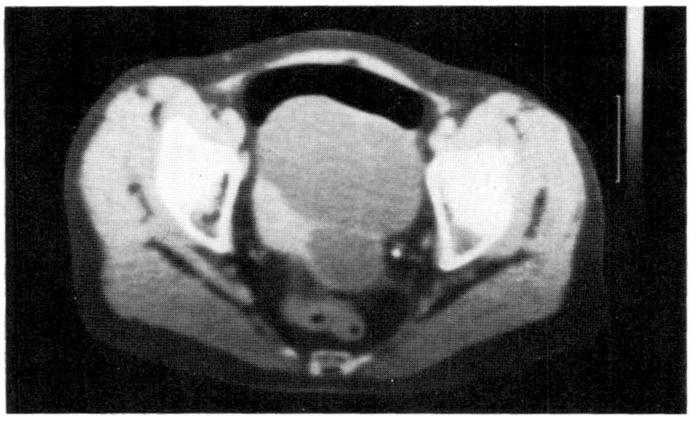

Fig. 9. Ovarian carcinoma. Large cystic and solid masses

Carcinoma of the Endometrium

In cases with primary carcinoma of the endometrium, physical examination with curretage is the most important examination. On CT scans only morphological changes of the uterus can be demonstrated. Stages I and II cannot be verified by CT (Fig. 7) [18].

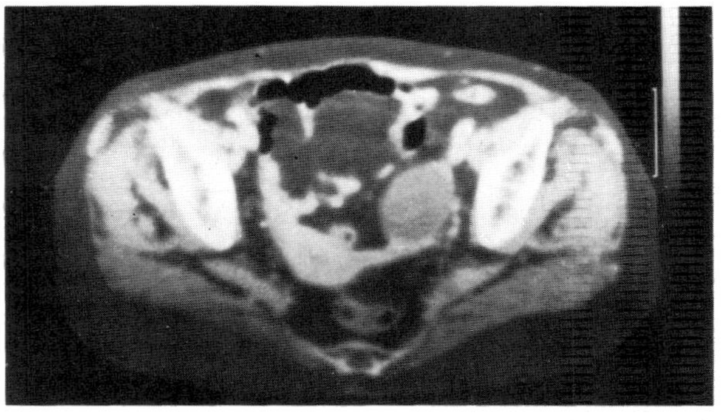

Fig. 10. Ovarian cyst on the left

Carcinomas of the Ovary

Here, we have to distinguish between pre- and postoperative tumors. For the clinical surgeon it is important to know up to which size a tumor can be diagnosed. Localization of the ovaries by CT can be achieved only with filling of the ureter.

Loops of small bowels often overlay the ovarian region. If delineation is needed, filling with Gastrografin is necessary. According to our experience we can conclude that normal ovaries in the premenopause can be visualized. In the postmenopause, however, delineation of the ovaries is much more difficult since the ovaries measure only 1–1.5 cm.

Within the framework of CT diagnosis it is a quite new achievement to visualize even small ovarian tumors.
According to our experience, extension as well as direction of tumor expansion can be delineated with the help of CT [3]. Larger tumors develop upward and the ureter is sometimes displaced. Smooth contours can often be considered as signs of benign lesions. Cystic masses are seen in cases of carcinomas as well as in cases of benign tumors (Figs. 8 – 10).

Recurrences of Gynecologic Carcinomas

Diagnosis of recurrent gynecologic carcinomas presents problems. Palpation is often insufficient to distinguish between fibrosis and recurrence [22]. Pelvic angiographies are positive in only 30% of the studies. Lymphography and transosseous phlebography, both invasive diagnostic methods, often show only indirect signs of tumor growth.

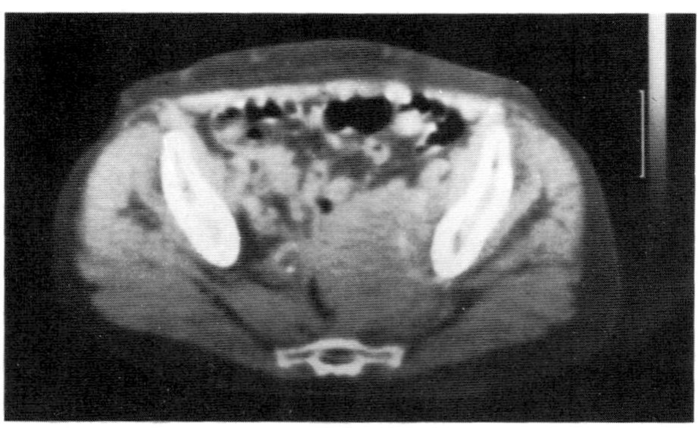

Fig. 11. Bulky lymph node metastases in the iliac region on the left (recurrence)

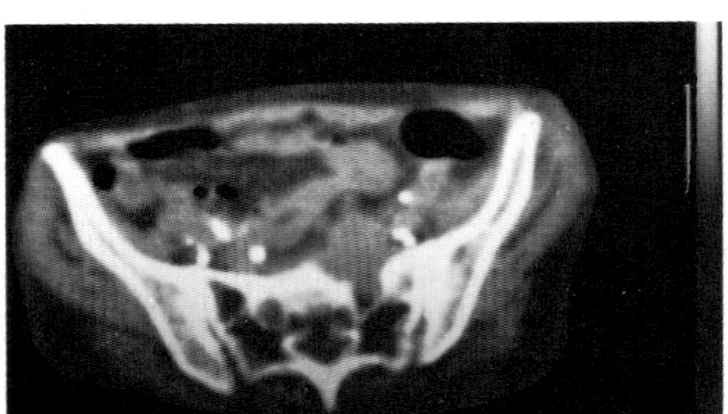

Fig. 12. Lymph node metastases in the ileolumbar region on the left (after lymphography) (recurrence)

The accuracy of CT, i.e., the number of correct positive results, is high in the detection of recurrences to the pelvic wall. Out of 26 lymph node recurrences to the pelvic wall, 25 could be diagnosed on CT [19]. Invasive radiologic procedures should therefore only be applied in cases of negative CT studies. Extensive lumbar lymph node recurrences could be seen more frequently. As a rule, scar tissue proved by palpation and follow-ups cannot be substantiated by CT. In our experience the mistaking of marked fibrosis for a recurrent tumor is quite seldom (Figs. 11, 12).

Possibilities of Angio-CT

Angio-CT in use with faster CT scanners regularly shows an increase in density of the uterus (10 – 20 HE units). The visualization of the pelvic vessels allows a better delineation of the lymph nodes. The technic of bolus injection with CT and timed exposure has recently been developed [20].

Carcinoma of the Rectum

Primary diagnosis of carcinomas of the rectum are made with the help of double contrast enema and endoscopy. CT is only applied to rule out metastases. Recurrence after surgery (rectum amput.) are hard to diagnose by conventional methods. Recurrences with osseous destruction can be detected on conventional tomograms. No better diagnostic means than CT is available in cases with sacral tumoral infiltration [18].
Difficulties exist in differentiation from secondary retroperitoneal fibrosis (Fig. 13).

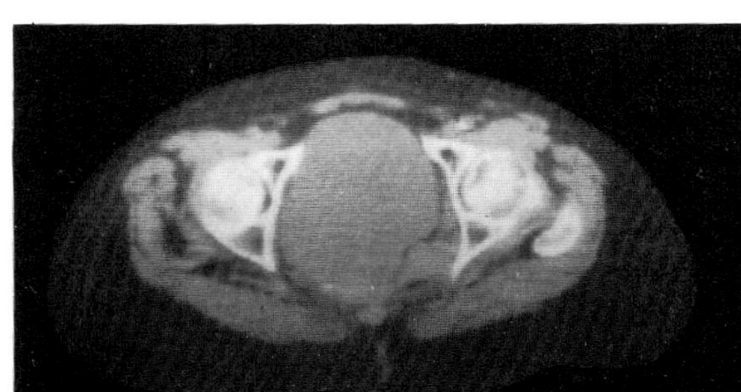

Fig. 13. Recurrent carcinoma of the rectum, *left*

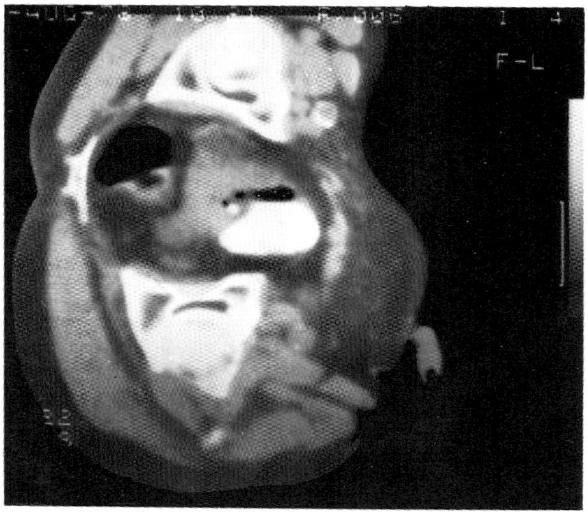

Fig. 14. Carcinoma of the prostate, stage III, infiltration at the level of the seminal vesicles

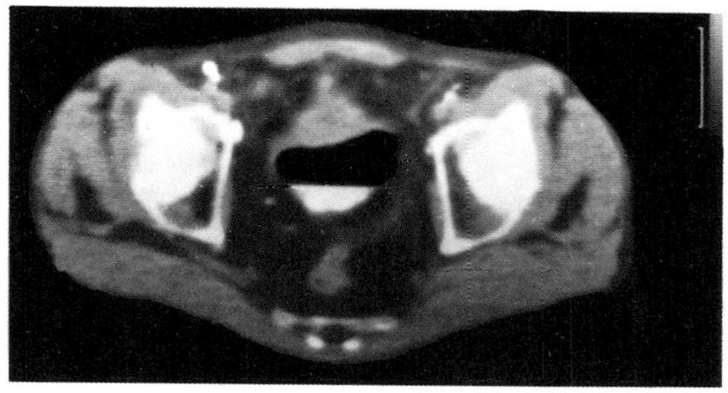

Fig. 15. Carcinoma of the bladder, stage IIIb

Carcinoma of the Prostate

As long as a carcinoma of the prostate has not extended outside the capsule, CT is of no diagnostic value. Obliteration of the seminal vesicle angle is considered an early sign of extracapsular spreading of a carcinoma of the prostate [24]. Diagnostic difficulties may arise if the carcinoma of the prostate extends into the basis of the bladder and surrounding fat is absent (Fig. 14).

Carcinoma of the Bladder

Carcinoma of the bladder is diagnosed with the help of cystoscopy and biopsy. In cases of extravesical extension of the tumor, CT examination has to be preferred to bimanual examination under anesthesia and to the angiological studies. Superficial lesions are not to be differentiated in their stages. Stage IIIb (C) and IV (D) are to distinguish from lower stages. According to the literature, staging was correct in over 80% of the positive findings (Fig. 15) [23, 25].

Lymphatic involvement of carcinomas of the prostate and bladder is frequently observed. The lymphatic pathways run along the external, internal, and common iliac lymph nodes. The accuracy of CT for lymph node metastases has been previously discussed with relation to gynecologic tumors.

Therapy Planning Using CT

At the Department of Radiology in Passau, 1110 patients undergo radiation treatment annually. Therapy planning with CT is carried out in 40% – 50% of these patients. Anatomic cross sections are the basis for computerized isodose mapping. Until a few years ago, the basis for these were anatomic drawings which were projected into the mechanically taken circumference of the patient by optical aids, but there is some inaccuracy in this method.

With the help of CT we get the most exact individual anatomic cross sections of any region. It should be emphasized that it is absolutely necessary to have the same positioning of the patient on the CT and therapy couches. An aid for the positioning of the patient for CT is the topogram. On the anteroposterior topogram the treatment borders and on the lateral topogram especially the position of the patient in regard to the spine can be checked (Fig. 16).

Having found the optimal position, one has to make sure that it can be reproduced on the treatment couch and during the whole course of treat-

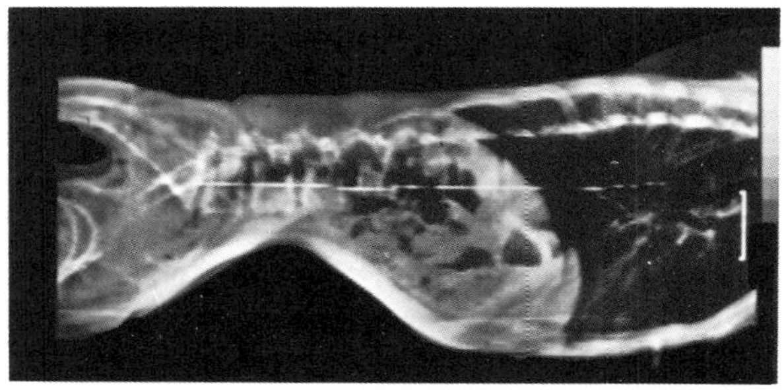

Fig. 16. Lateral topogram showing the position of the spine

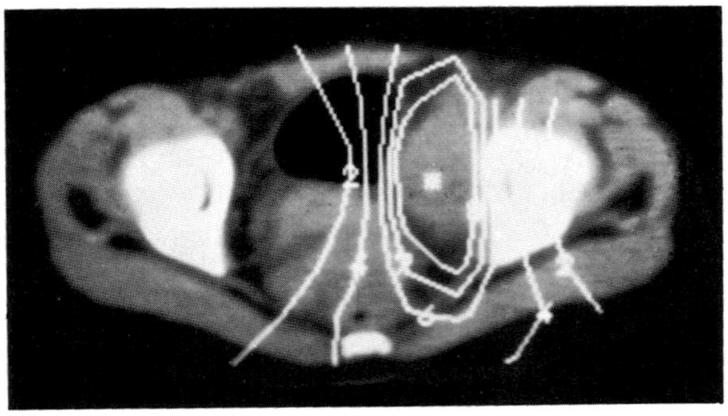

Fig. 17. CT scan with the isodoses overlaid

ment. We therefore had an identical laser installed in the treatment and CT rooms. Having once marked the patient's skin with the help of lateral and medial laser strips, reproduction of the correct position is guaranteed if the therapy laser fits the markings of the skin (made by the CT laser).
In this correct and reproducible position, the CT cross sections for mapping are done. Our therapy planning system and the CT are connected by a floppy disk and therefore isodoses and anatomic cross sections can be overlaid. This overlay can be achieved in any phase of the planning. With this method the complete information of the CT image is available in the background (Fig. 17) [1].
According to our experience and because of the importance of correct and reproducible positioning, it is necessary that the therapist carries out the CT examination himself to avoid errors.

Summary

The application of CT as a staging method for the different carcinomas of the pelvis has been evaluated. Local spreading of carcinomas of the prostate can be evaluated from stage III on. Infiltration of the seminal vesicle angle is suggestive of extracapsular extension of the carcinoma. CT improves staging of the carcinoma of the bladder. CT is superior to conventional methods in the evaluation of perivesical tumor growth. The local spreading can be substantiated in carcinomas of the cervix from stage IIb on, and in carcinomas of the endometrium from stage III on. CT corrects in some cases to a higher stage. To a certain extent, staging and histologic diagnosis of tumors of the ovaries are possible. Lymph node metastases at early stages are better demonstrated by lymphography than CT. CT, however, is the better choice as an initial method in cases of extensive lymph node metastases in advanced stages and in cases with lymph node recurrences to the pelvic wall and lumbar region. Recurrences of carcinomas of the rectum are well diagnosed by CT.
With the help of CT therapy planning is improved.

References

1. Breit A, Atzinger A, Gfirtner H Therapy planning using CT. Honorary Guest Lecture. Meeting of the American Radium Society, April 1980, Philadelphia
2. Breit A, Rohde U (1977) Erste Erfahrungen mit der Computertomographie in der Gynäkologie. Gynäkol Prax 1:661–666
3. Breit A, Rohde U (1980) Primäre CT-Diagnostik gynäkologischer Tumoren. In: Heuck F, Breit A (eds) Röntgendiagnostik des urogenitalen Systems. Weibliches Genital. Springer, Berlin Heidelberg New York (Handbuch der medizinischen Radiologie, vol XIII/2, pp 183–192)
4. Elke M, Lüning M, Richter J, Röder K, Sieber D (1976) Metastasen von Malignomen der männlichen Geschlechtsorgane. In: Lüning M, Wiljasalo M, Weissleder H (eds) Lymphographie bei malignen Tumoren. Thieme, Leipzig
5. Feuerbach St, Rupp N, Rossmann W, Heller HJ, Rothenberger G, Tauber R, Schmidt G (1979) Lymphknotenmetastasen – Diagnose durch Lymphographie und CT. ROEFO 130/3:323–328
6. Fritz H, Köhler K, Platzbecker H (1972) Komplexe angiographische Diagnostik gynäkologischer Tumor-Rezidive-Technik, Indikation, Ergebnisse. ROEFO 117/2
7. Kreel L (1976) The EMI-whole-body-scanner in the demonstration of lymphnode enlargement. Clin Radiol 27:421–429
8. Kreel L (1979) Computed tomography of the abdomen and thorax. In: Sager W-D, Ladurner G (eds) Computertomographie, derzeitige Stellung in Radiologie und Klinik, Symposium Graz 1978. Thieme, Stuttgart
9. Lackner K, Weissbach L, Boldt I, Scherholz K, Brecht G (1979) Computertomographischer Nachweis von Lymphknotenmetastasen bei malignen Hodentumoren. ROEFO 130/6:636–643
10. Langreder W (1955) Das Parametrium. Funktionelle Anatomie der Ligamentzüge sowie ihre Beziehung zur Cervix und Beckenwand besonders während der Schwangerschaft und Geburt. Thieme, Leipzig, p 187
11. Lee JKT, Stanley RJ, Sagel SS, Levitt RG (1978) Accuracy of computed tomography in detecting intraabdominal and pelvic adenopathy in lymphoma. AJR 131:311–315

12. Lee JKT, McClennan BL, Stanley FJ, Sagel SS (1979) Computed tomography in the staging of testicular neoplasms. Radiology 130:387–390
13. Levitt RG, Sagel SS, Stanley RJ (1978) Computed tomography of the pelvis. Semin Roentgenol 13:193–200
14. Marshall WH, Breiman RS, Harell GS, Glatstein E, Kaplan HS (1977) Computed tomography of abdominal para-aortic lymph node disease? Preliminary observations with a six second scanner. AJR 128:759–764
15. Platzer W (1979) Zur Anatomie der Organe des weiblichen Beckens in Berücksichtigung der Computertomographie. In: Olsson O (ed) Handbuch der medizinischen Radiologie, vol XIII/2. Springer, Berlin Heidelberg New York, pp 134–142
16. Redman HC (1977) Computed tomography of the pelvis. Radiol Clin North Am 15:441–448
17. Reiffenstuhl G (1967) Das Lymphknotenproblem beim Carcinoma colli uteri und die Lymphirradiatio pelvis. Urban & Schwarzenberg, Munich Vienna
18. Rohde U, Atzinger A (1980) Computertomographie des Beckens. Roentgenpraxis 33:105–114
19. Rohde U, Breit A (to be published) Computed Tomography, a contribution to the staging of tumors of the minor pelvis with special consideration given to the pathways of metastases. XI Intern. Symposion "Metastatic Tumor Growth", October 22 to 24, 1979 at Düsseldorf. Fischer, Stuttgart
20. Schad N, Schepcke P, Rohde U, Schmidt V, Breit A (to be published) Timing of exposure in Angio-CT. Cardiovascular Radiology
21. Schaner WG, Head GL, Doppman JL, Young RC (1977) Computed tomography in the diagnosis, staging and management of abdominal lymphomas. J Comput Assist Tomogr 1:176–180
22. Scherer U, Lissner J (1980) Röntgen-Ganzkörper-Computer-Tomographie in der Rezidivdiagnostik. In: Heuck F, Breit A (eds) Röntgendiagnostik des urogenitalen Systems. Weibliches Genitale. Springer, Berlin Heidelberg New York (Handbuch der Medizinischen Radiologie, vol XIII/2, pp. 221–229)
23. Seidelmann FE, Cohen WN, Bryan PJ (1977) Computed tomographic staging of bladder neoplasms. Radiol Clin North Am 15/3:419–440
24. Seidelmann FE, Reich NE, Cohen WN, Haaga JR, Bryan PJ, Havrilla TR (1977) Computed tomography of the seminal vesicles and the seminal vesicle angle. Comp Axial Tomogr 1/4:281–285
25. Seidelmann FE, Temes SP, Cohen WN, Bryan PJ, Patil U, Sherry RG (1977) Computed tomography of gas-filled bladder: method of staging bladder neoplasms. Urology 9:337–344

Skeletal Radiology

Bone Diseases: Overview

J. H. Middlemiss

University of Bristol, The Medical School, Department of Radiodiagnosis, University Walk, GB-Bristol BS8 1TD

In considering progress in skeletal radiology one must first consider techniques which have been and are still being developed or which have been rediscovered and applied to new fields. Then one must consider specific fields of skeletal radiology in which these techniques have made a contribution to advancement. Taking another line, one can look for fields of work where new thought has brought about a new concept and altered our direction in such a way that radiology has been able to contribute to the diagnosis, classification and management of disease processes.
First, to consider techniques.

Magnification Techniques

These techniques have been with us for over 30 years. More than 30 years ago the 0.3-mm focal spot X-ray tube was introduced and we were able to take macroradiographs – enlargements up to $1\frac{1}{2}$ × or 2 × the conventional size were possible without unacceptable loss of sharpness. With this type of enlargement the observer did not really see more – he merely saw more easily; it was also simpler to demonstrate lesions to colleagues and classes. An alternative method was by photographic enlargement with the use of fine-grain film using a non-screen technique. The image could then be enlarged photographically. However, film-grain size interfered increasingly with image definition as enlargement was increased, though Meema in Toronto still uses this method successfully. More recently microfocal tubes with an effective tube focal spot size of 20 – 30 μ, produced either by magnetic or electronic focussing of the beam, have been manufactured. By the use of these, remarkable clinical and specimen magnification images can be obtained whereby individual trabeculae can be examined in the clinical state (Fig. 1). By this method metabolic bone diseases, trauma such as hair-line fractures of the scaphoid, arthritides such as rheumatoid arthritis, degenerative processes like Paget's disease and many other disease processes can be studied.

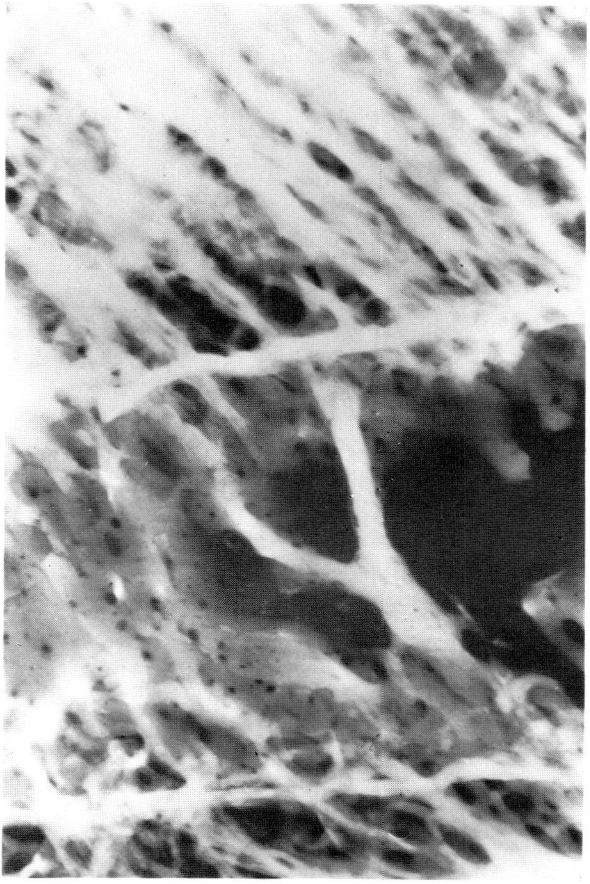

Fig. 1. Macroradiograph showing individual bone trabeculae taken with a 20 μ focal spot

Radiology Today 1. Ed. by M. W. Donner and F. H. W. Heuck

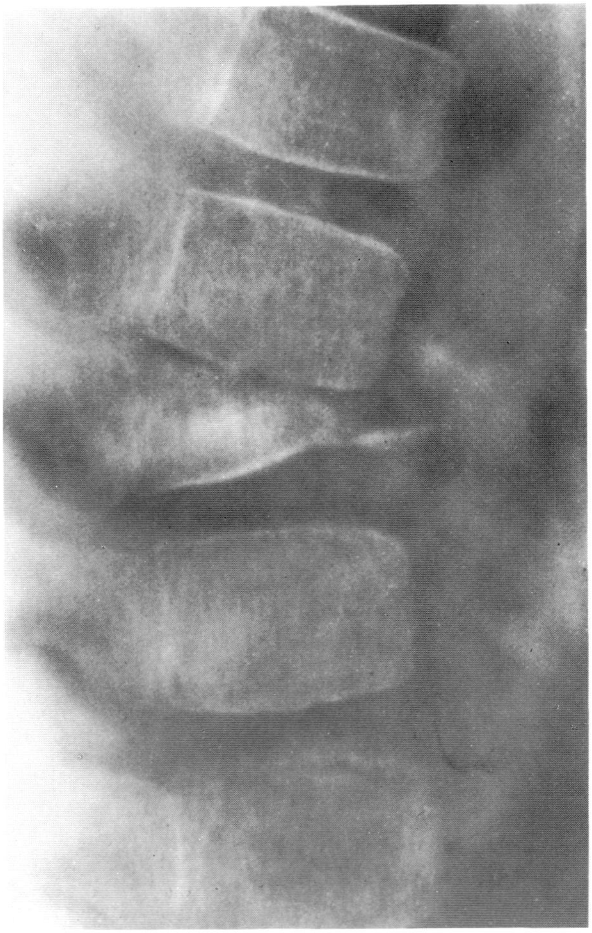

Fig. 2. Conventional tomogram of lateral thoracic spine showing tuberculosis in a child

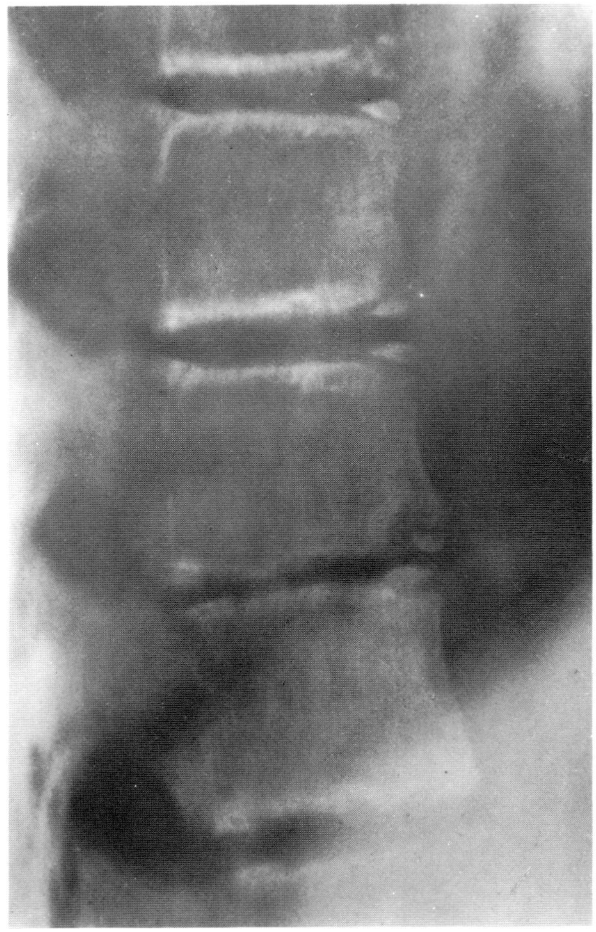

Fig. 3. Conventional tomogram showing Scheuerman's disease in the thoracic spine of a child

Conventional Tomography

As tomographic apparatus has been mechanically improved, so has it developed into a precision technique, useful in its application in the field of bone radiology. This applies particularly in investigations of the spine, where the quality of image obtainable is outstandingly good, allowing detailed study and analysis of a particular bone, section by section, and permitting differentiation in inflammatory processes like tuberculosis (Fig. 2), in degenerative processes like Scheuerman's disease (Fig. 3) and in neoplasm.

Arteriography

Arteriography has never been applied to bone diseases quite to the extent that was originally anticipated, yet in the realm of suspected, or known, bone tumours it can often give useful information (Voegeli 1976). At one time it was hoped that it would contribute materially towards establishing malignancy in a suspected bone tumour. However, inflammatory processes can produce appearances similar to those caused by malignancy. In recognisably malignant bone tumours arteriographic studies can often give useful information regarding the degree of vascularity and will often indicate the optimum site for biopsy.

Computerised Tomography

This new technique is still an expensive one and it is not every department that is able to provide the facility. There is no doubt, however, that it provides us with an added dimension. We are able to observe the relationship of soft tissues to bone, and to see around the contour of long bones and vertebrae in a manner not previously possible. Also it is possible to study the contents of marrow cavities. In his contribution. Dr. Siegelman discusses the applications of CT in the field of bone radiology in some detail.

Now let us look at these techniques and at progress in skeletal radiology in some of the clinical fields of interest to us.

Arthritis

I am not going to consider arthrography as my colleague, Dr. Freiburger, discusses the applications of that technique. Our understanding of some aspects of arthritis has advanced considerably in recent years. For example, histocompatibility antigens are genetically determined antigens on the surfaces of leucocytes. In the case of transplant rejection they are the responsible agent. Many such antigens have now been identified, the better known being designated as "human leukocyte antigen" – HLA. Inheritance of these antigens is genetically determined by several identifiable genes on chromosome 6. Brewerton et al. (1973) reported the high incidence of HLA-B27 in patients with ankylosing spondylitis (Fig. 4). Since then Reiter's disease, psoriatic spondylitis, psoriatic arthritis, the spondylitis accompanying inflammatory bowel disease and salmonella arthritis have also been incriminated.

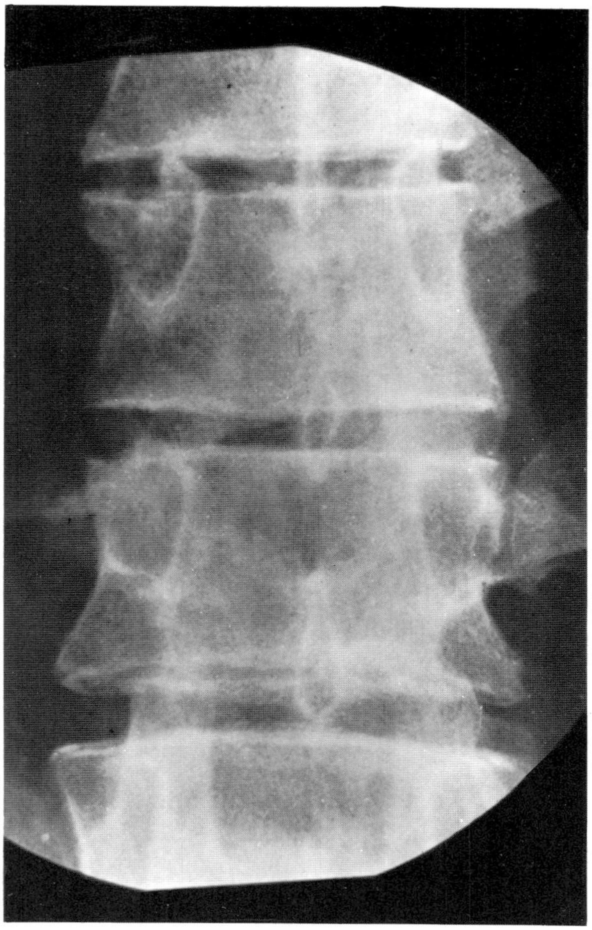

Fig. 4. Example of early ankylosing spondylitis showing marginal erosions of a vertebral body

It is clear that environmental factors are also involved in addition to the genetic factor. It is possible that the HLA gene is linked to another that produces increased susceptibility. Radiologically it may be possible to distinguish these factors.

Bone Tumours

Bone tumours are a relatively uncommon form of neoplasm, and it does not fall to the lot of the general radiologist to see many in the course of his professional life. It is essential therefore that, if advance is to be made, materials and experience should be pooled. It is equally important that we should all use the same terminology so that, when a particular term is used, we all mean the same thing. Thus, classification is important. In Bristol we have a Bone Tumour Registry. The panel consists of orthopaedic surgeons, radiologists, radiotherapists, pathologists and research scientists. During the last 35 years, we have had over 4000 cases referred to us; in most of these cases we reached an agreed diagnosis and classified them accordingly. In 1953 we drew up our classification and this we have modified in a very small way twice since then. It is now used throughout Britain and in some other parts of the world.

Dr. Jacobson discusses in rather more detail some specific bone tumours.

Bone Dysplasias

This is another field in which advance has been made, again on the basis of classification. If dysplasias can be classified and correctly identified, then they can be better studied and followed-up over a period of years, and the eventual outlook can be determined. Correct diagnosis will lead to correct prognosis, and prognosis is what matters to families. Correct counselling can then take place and advice given. We must never forget that as radiologists we are doctors and are concerned with people. In Germany, Spranger has contributed very considerably to this field, while in South Africa both Beighton and Cremin have contributed to it. The Paris classification of Maroteau is the most useful. In Bristol we have a Bone Dysplasia Registry where we collect material, follow up patients over the rest of their lives and investigate and study families. Already in dwarfs prognosis can be reached reasonably accurately on radiological grounds and families counselled and given family planning advice.

Trauma

Finally in the field of trauma radiologists tend to neglet contemplating advance. There is surely much to consider in relation to the possibility of improving techniques in order to further patient care.

References

1. Aho K, Ahvonen P, Alkio P, et al. (1975) HL-A27 in reactive arthritis following infarction. Ann Rheum Dis 34 [Suppl 1]: 29
2. Ansell BM, Kent PA (1977) Radiological changes in juvenile chronic polyarthritis. Skel Radiol 1:129
3. Brewerton DA, James DCO (1975) The histocompatibility antigen (HL-A27) and disease. Semin Arthritis Rheum 4:191
4. Brewerton DA, Caffrey M, Hart FD, et al. (1973) Ankylosing spondylitis and HL-A27. Lancet 1:904
5. Brewerton DA, Caffrey M, Nicholls A, et al. (1973) Reiter's disease and HL-A27. Lancet 2:996
6. Brewer EJ, Bass J, Baum J, et al. (1977) Current proposed revision of JRA criteria. Arthritis Rheum [Suppl 2] 20:195
7. Dahlin DC (1976) Chondrosarcoma and its variants. Bones and joints, IAP monograph 17. Williams & Wilkins, Baltimore, p 300
8. Dahlin DC, Unni KK (1977) Osteosarcoma of bone and its important recognizable varieties. Am J Surg Pathol 1:61
9. Doi K, Genant HK, Rossmann K (1975) Effect of film graininess and geometric unsharpness on image quality in fine-detail skeletal radiography. Invest Radiol 10:35
10. Eastmond CJ, Woodrow JC (1977) The HLA system and the arthropathies associated with psoriasis. Ann Rheum Dis 36:112
11. Fletcher DE, Rowley KA (1950) Radiographic enlargements in diagnostic radiology. Br J Radiol 24:598
12. Genant HK, Doi K, Mall JC (1975) Optical versus radiographic magnification for fine-detail skeletal radiography. Invest Radiol 10:160
13. Genant HK, Doi K, Mall JC, Sickles EA (1977) Direct radiographic magnification for skeletal radiology: an assessment of image quality and clinical application. Radiology 123:47
14. Improved radiological diagnosis of azotemic osteodystrophy (1972) Radiology 102/1:1–10
15. McClusky OE, Lordon RE, Arnett FC Jr (1974) HL-A27 in Reiter's syndrome and psoriatic arthritis: a genetic factor in disease susceptibility and expression. J Rheumatol 1:263
16. Meema HE, Schatz DL (1970) Simple radiologic demonstration of cortical bone loss in thyrotoxicosis. Radiology 97:9
17. Meema HE, Meema S (1972) Comparison of Macroradioscopic and morphometric findings in the hand bones with densitometric findings in the proximal radius in thyrotoxicosis and in renal osteodystrophy. Invest Radiol 7:88
18. Schajowicz F (1977) Juxtacortical chondrosarcoma. J Bone Joint Surg [Br] 59B:473m

Arthrography, a Diagnostic Procedure in Joint Diseases

R. H. Freiberger

Cornell University Medical College, Department of Radiology, 535 East 70th Street, New York, NY 10021 (USA)

Arthrography is by no means a new radiographic procedure, as arthrograms of the knee were reported in 1905, of the hip in 1908, and of the shoulder in 1935, but the procedure has not enjoyed widespread application until recently. Improvements of radiologic equipment has facilitated arthrography and improved the picture quality. Perhaps more importantly there has been an increasing desire by patients, physicians, and surgeons to obtain a diagnosis, preferably by graphic means, before surgical exploration. Knee arthrography is the most widely accepted and is performed most frequently for diagnosis of internal derangement, the depiction of torn menisci and torn cruiciate liagments. It is believed that the menisci do not simply fill an empty space at the margin of the joint, but that they are weight-bearing structures and that the removal of a normal meniscus is detrimental to the patient. Partial meniscectomy, when feasible, is now often performed and in addition to the clinical examination the arthrogram provides the surgeon with more information on which a decision for treatment can be made. The arthrogram has also proved valuable in the diagnosis of cruciate ligament tears, a complex problem with diversity of opinion on treatment. In the shoulder, the most common reason for arthrography is for confirmation of a suspected rotator cuff tear, which can be made with great accuracy. Arthrography is useful in the infant's and the young child's hip joint because it is predominantly cartilaginous and cannot be fully evaluated by conventional roentgen examination. The classic use of arthrography has been the evaluation of congenital hip dislocation and dysplasia and its treatment. Other uses are the preoperative evaluation of Legg-Calvé-Perthes disease and other acquired or congenital growth disturbances to determine congruity of the articular surfaces.

The arthrogram is a valuable adjunct in joint aspiration for suspected infection. It provides proof of intra-articular needle placement in the hip and also at other joints, and in cases of infection it may show capsular ruptures, abscess, and sinus tract formation or provide evidence of destruction of articular cartilages. Arthrograms can show intra-articular masses such as pigmented villonodular synovitis, synovial chondromatosis, or the villous synovitis of a variety of inflammatory diseases. Arthrography has proved to be an accurate, inexpensive, simple, and safe procedure and should be a standard radiographic procedure familiar to all radiologists.

Arthrography of the Knee

Equipment

A fluoroscopic X-ray machine with spot film device and image amplifier and a 0.3 – 0.6 mm focal spot tube for spot filming is required.

Injection equipment and supplies:
One 2-cc Luer-Lok tip glass syringe
One 10-cc Luer-Lok tip glass syringe
One 22-cc Luer-Lok tip glass syringe
One 16 gauge × $1\frac{1}{2}$ in. sterile disposable needle
One 20 gauge × $1\frac{1}{2}$ in. sterile disposable needle
One 19 gauge × $1\frac{1}{2}$ in. sterile disposable needle
One 25 gauge × 5/8 in. sterile disposable needle
Five 4 × 3 in. gauze sponges
One thumb forcep
One medicine glass
One fabric drape with a 2 × 2 in. hole

Additional items available, but not on the sterile set are:
Sterile surgical gloves
A disposable shaver
Povidone iodine solution for skin preparation
1% lidocaine solution
1-cc ampule of 1/1000 epinephrine solution

Radiology Today 1. Ed. by M. W. Donner and F. H. W. Heuck

60% diatrizoate meglumine (Reno-M-60; Squibb) or another meglumine-type contrast agent
Sterile plastic tubing (to permit fluoroscopic monitoring during contrast injection)
10-cc ampules of sterile saline solution without preservative
Sterile 22 gauge spinal needles (for shoulder and hip arthrograms)
Crushable ampules of spirits of ammonia (for patients who feel faint)
An emergency resuscitation set like those on hand for intravenous contrast injections. (Such a set has never been needed in the performance of over 25,000 arthrograms.)

Procedure

The preliminary roentgen examination consists of AP, lateral, tunnel, and tangential views of the patella. The patient is placed supine with a pillow under the knee. The knee is scrubbed with povidone iodine solution and draped. Then 5 cc positive contrast agent is aspirated in the 10-cc syringe and mixed with 0.3 cc of 1/1000 epinephrine solution. Lidocaine local anesthesia is used if deemed necessary. The needle is inserted between the femoral condyle and midpoint of the articular surface of the patella, either from the medial or lateral side. Fluid in the knee must be aspirated as completely as possible. Then, 20 cc room air is injected, followed by the contrast agent – epinephrine mixture, followed by another 20 cc room air; the needle is then withdrawn. The patient is asked to stand and move the knee or the knee is moved passively. A lateral view with the patient sitting is taken for cruciate ligament evaluation. Twelve to eighteen spot films are taken of each meniscus, while distracting the side under examination. Fluoroscopic observation of the overlapping of the condyles helps in obtaining a complete examination from front to back. Lateral views, with forward and downward pressure on the tibia, are made for a second cruciate ligament examination.

Pertinent Anatomy and Arthrographic Findings

The menisci are fibrocartilaginous structures, triangular in cross section, and located at the periphery of the tibial plateau. A moderately loose capsular attachment allows the menisci to slide on the tibial plateau. The medial meniscus is C-shaped and has a complete peripheral capsular attachment. The lateral meniscus is more circular and lacks a complete capsular attachment at the popliteal hiatus, which communicates with the joint cavity. Contrast agent coats all intra-articular surfaces. While contrast agent seen at the periphery of the medial meniscus indicates a tear, contrast agent is normally seen within the popliteal hiatus and the arthrographer must be familiar with the normal appearance of this structure and the more complex attachments of the lateral meniscus. Meniscal tears, seen outlined by contrast agent, are similar

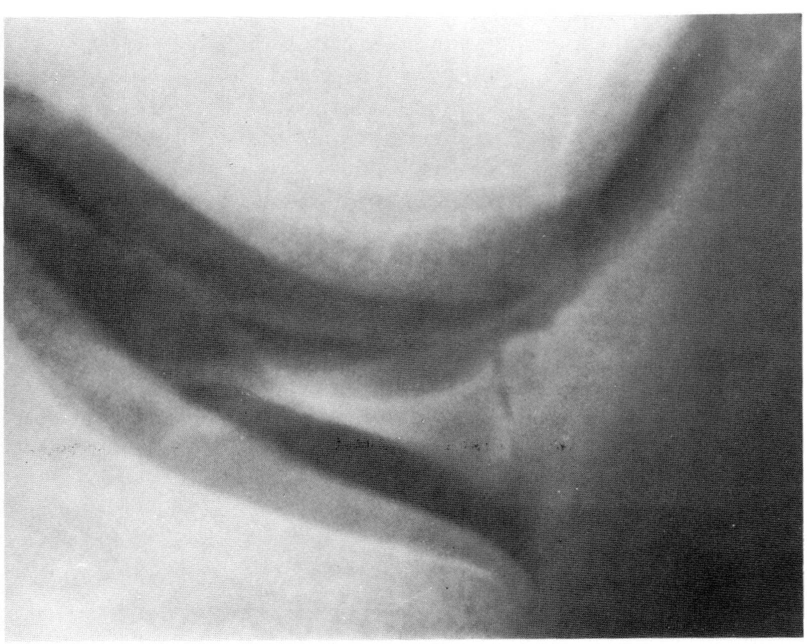

Fig. 1. A vertical tear with minimal displacement of fragments is seen in the anterior horn of the lateral meniscus

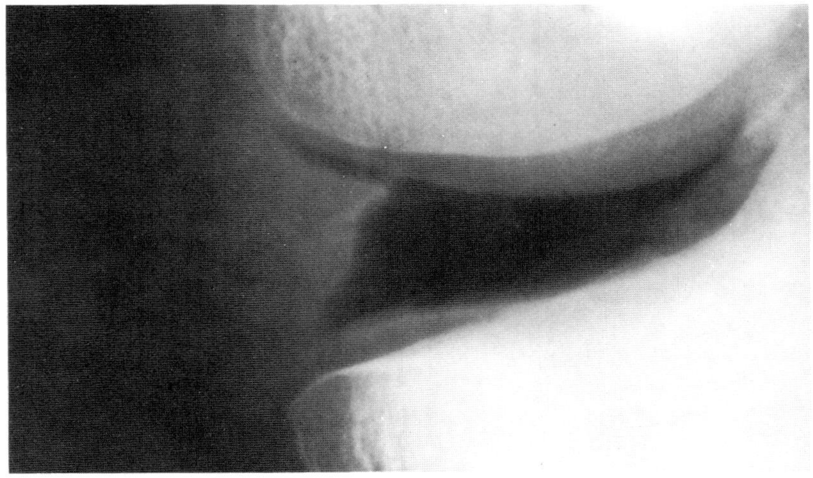

Fig. 2. A displaced tear of the medial meniscus with only the deformed outer fragment visible is shown

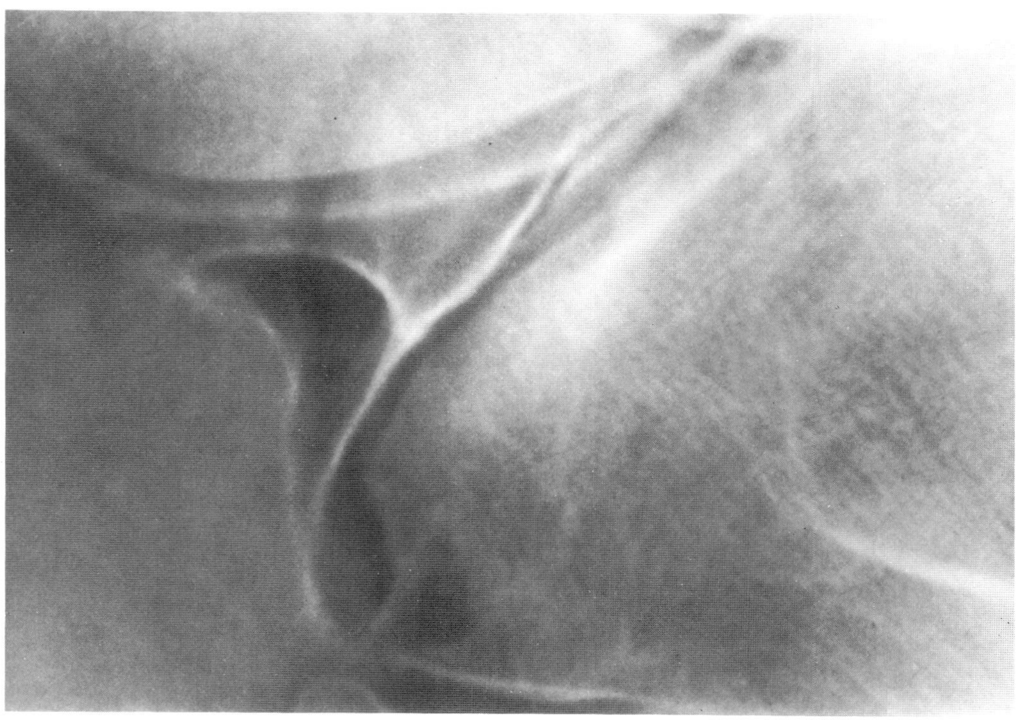

Fig. 3. The complex meniscal attachments of the lateral meniscus at the popliteal hiatus are shown

to fractures and may be simple or comminuted with or without displacement of fragments. Cysts of the menisci, usually located anteriorly in the lateral meniscus, appear as irregular horizontal tears with contrast agent extending beyond the periphery of the meniscus partially opacifying the cyst cavity. Discoid menisci, usually seen laterally, lack a normal wedge shape and are often torn. Tears of the cruciate ligaments are diagnosed by disruption or bowing of their synovial surface. Acute capsular ruptures cause contrast agent leakage from the joint. The arthrogram can also show whether the cartilaginous or bone fragment of osteochondritis dissecans is loose and can outline intra-articular cartilaginous or synovial masses. Examples of arthrographic findings in the knee are given in Figs. 1 – 4.

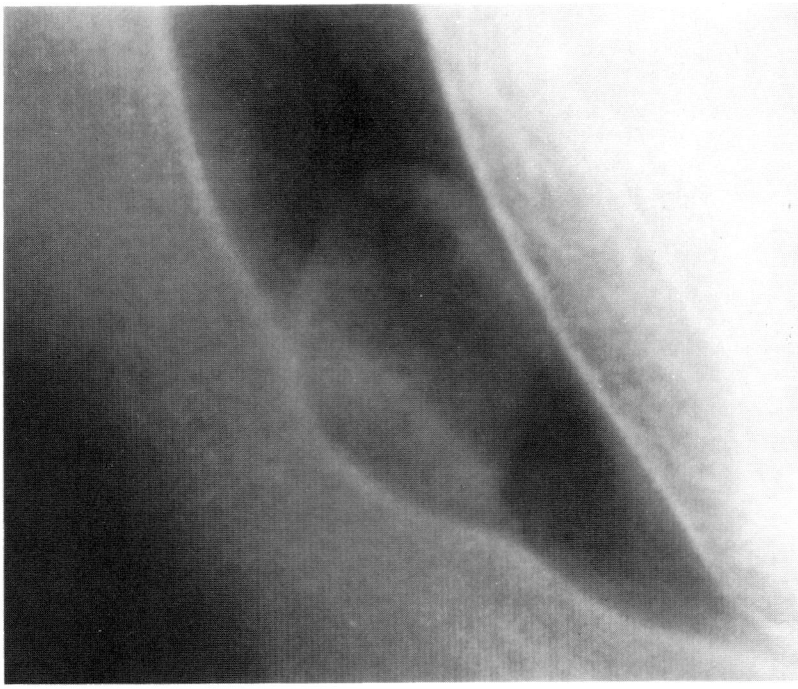

Fig. 4. A nodule of pigmented villonodular synovitis in the suprapatella bursa is shown on the double contrast arthrogram of the knee

Arthrography of the Shoulder

X-ray Equipment

A machine with a overhead X-ray tube and under-table image amplifier is best because there is adequate space above the patient's shoulder and therefore less chance of contaminating sterile equipment than with an overhead fluoroscopic tower.

Injection Equipment

The injection tray described under knee arthrography is used with the addition of a $3\frac{1}{2}$ inch 22 gauge disposable spinal needle. Epinephrine is not used.

Injection Technique

The patient lies supine on an X-ray table with the arm at the side and the thumb up. A spot directly above the junction of the middle and distal third of the glenohumeral joint space is marked on the skin with indelible ink under fluoroscopic guidance. The shoulder is scrubbed and draped in the usual manner and under lidocaine anesthesia a 22 gauge disposable spinal needle is inserted perfectly vertically at the spot marked on the skin and pushed downward until it enters the joint. Entrance of the needle tip into the joint space can be judged by the resistance to the injection of lidocaine and can be verified fluoroscopically by the injection of a few drops of contrast agent, which will immediately leave the needle tip if it is placed intra-articularly. The arthrogram can be performed by single or by double contrast technique. For single contrast technique, approximately 12 cc of a 60% meglumine positive contrast agent is injected and the needle withdrawn. If the patient experiences pain during the injection, this indicates an abnormally tight joint as in pericapsulitis or frozen shoulder syndrome and a lesser quantity of contrast agent is injected. For double contrast arthrography, which is the preferred method at the Hospital for Special Surgery, 3 – 4 cc positive contrast agent is injected, followed by an injection of no more than 10 cc air and the neddle is withdrawn. For positive contrast arthrography, filming can be done in the supine or erect position. The central ray should be angled toward the patient's feet to project the open space between the acromion and humeral head occupied by the rotator cuff to best advantage. In double contrast arthrography most of the roentgenograms are made with the patient in the erect position to provide a double contrast examination of the rotator cuff at the superior aspect of the shoulder joint. Axillary views are taken with the patient prone or supine and the bicipital view is normally taken with the patient in a supine position.

Arthrographic Findings

The diagnosis of complete rotator cuff tear is made by opacification of the subacromial subdeltoid bursa, which is normally separated from the joint by the intact rotator cuff. While the diagnosis of a complete rotator cuff tear can be made with either the single or double contrast method, the size of the tear can only be evaluated by double contrast method. Partial rotator cuff tears show contrast agent within the rotator cuff, but not in the bursa. Articular cartilage abnormalities, particularly those of the glenoid labrum, are best seen with the double contrast study. Synovial abnormalities such as villous synovitis, intra-articular cartilaginous or osseous bodies as well as synovial cysts of the type seen in rheumatoid arthritis can be diagnosed by either method. Pericapsulitis or frozen shoulder is evidenced by an abnormally tight capsular space and leakage of contrast agent from the capsule is common. This leakage occurs at the weakest portion of the capsule at the subscapular bursa and the end of the biceps tendon sleeve. Leakage by itself without a tight capsule, particularly that seen on postexercise films, is not of clinical significance.

Arthrography of the Hip

X-ray Equipment

A machine with an overhead X-ray tube and under-table image amplifier is best because there is adequate space above the patient's hip and therefore less chance of contaminating sterile equipment than with an overhead fluoroscopic tower. However, any image amplified fluoroscopic and radiographic machine is usable.

Injection Equipment

The injection tray described in detail under knee arthrography is used with the addition of a $3\frac{1}{2}$ in. 22 gauge disposable spinal needle for arthrography in the adult or a disposable $1\frac{1}{2}$ in. 22 gauge needle in infants and children. Sterile water or saline solution should be available to dilute a 60% meglumine contrast agent solution to 30% concentration for use in infants and young children. Epinephrine is not used.

Injection Technique

Under fluoroscopic guidance a metal marker is placed over the center or slightly medially on the midportion of the femoral neck and the skin marked with indelible ink. When a metallic prosthesis obscures the marker, a metal ruler or the long arm of a measuring caliper can be used as a guide to place the skin mark. The skin is then scrubbed with povidone iodine solution and draped. There are numerous ways in which a needle can be directed toward the femoral neck. One of the easiest is to puncture the skin laterally and inferiorly of the skin mark and to direct the needle medially and superiorly until its point impinges on the femoral neck. The needle is lateral to the femoral vessels and nerves. When the needle point impinges on the femoral neck, penetration of the hip capsule is achieved more easily by slightly flexing the hip and placing a pillow under the knee. If aspiration is required, it can be performed at this point. When no fluid is obtained, saline solution without preservative is injected, aspirated, and sent for culture. In the infant an injection of 2 cc diluted contrast agent is usually sufficient to obtain a good arthrogram. In the adult approximately 10 cc of 60% meglumine contrast agent is injected. Routinely AP and frog-lateral projections of the hip joint are taken. The number of films and positions of the femur vary with the problem being investigated. When looking for loose bodies or synovial masses tomography is often used.

Arthrographic Findings

The femoral head fits tightly into the acetabulum with only a thin, even layer of contrast agent seen between the articular surfaces. The ligamentum teres femoris is normally not visible. The transverse acetabular ligament causes a smooth filling defect at the inferior aspect of the acetabulum, and the zona orbicularis of the capsule constricts the capsule around the center of the femoral neck. The limbus, which is the cartilaginous extension of the acetabular margin, is larger in children than in adults and can be seen as a sharp triangular radiolucent structure between the femoral head and the capsule.

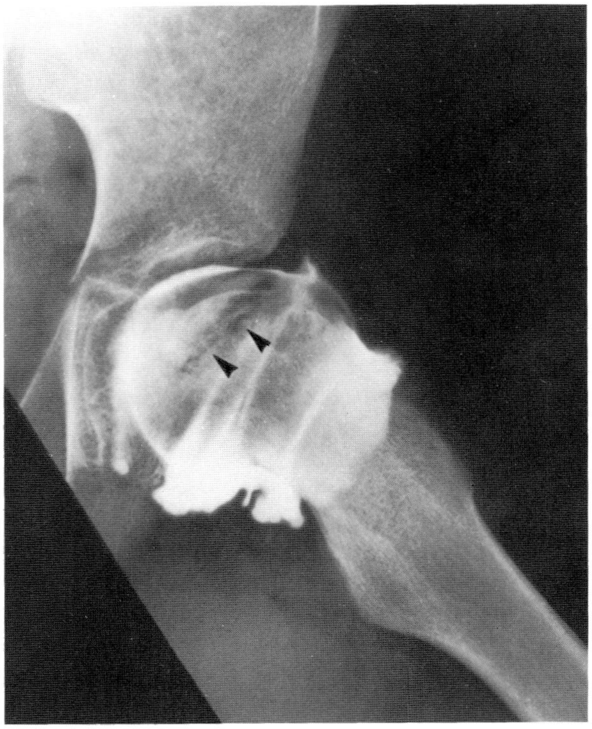

Fig. 5. The incongruity of the joint in the child with Legg-Calve-Perthes disease is shown by puddling of contrast agent between the articular surfaces of the hip joint

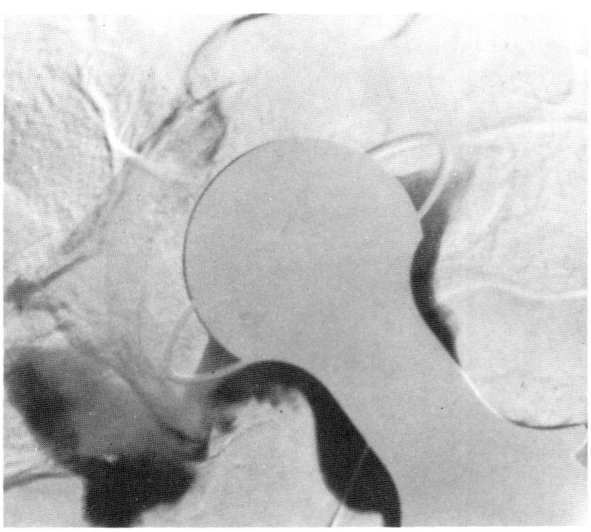

Fig. 6. A subtraction arthrogram of a total hip prosthesis shows loosening of the acetabular component

Incongruity of the joint is evident by puddling of contrast medium between the articular surfaces (Fig. 5). Deformities of the limbus or interposition of the limbus between the acetabulum and femoral head may be seen in congenital hip dislocation. Cartilaginous or synovial intra-articular masses appear as filling defects often best seen by tomography. Occasionally in a patient with chronic arthritis, a communicating distended iliopsoas bursa which clinically mimics a tumor mass can be opacified and correctly diagnosed.

In total hip prostheses, contrast agent filling the bone cement interface confirms loosening of the prosthesis (Fig. 6). However, lack of contrast filling of a widened bone cement interface does not rule out loosening. Only "positive" arthrograms are diagnostic.

References

1. Freiberger RH, Kaye JJ (1971) Arthrography. Appelton-Century Crofts, New York
2. Thinj C (1979) Arthrography of the knee joint. Springer, Berlin Heidelberg New York
3. Dalinka MK (1980) Arthrography. Springer, Berlin Heidelberg New York
4. Haage H (1973) Arthrographie des Handgelenks. Springer, Berlin Heidelberg New York (Sonderdruck aus Handbuch der medizinischen Radiologie, Bd V/2)
5. Haage H (1973) Arthrographie der kleinen Hand- und Fingergelenke. Springer, Berlin Heidelberg New York (Sonderdruck aus Handbuch der medizinischen Radiologie, Bd V/2)
6. Haage H, Fischedick O (1973) Arthrographie des Ellenbogengelenks. Springer, Berlin Heidelberg New York (Sonderdruck aus Handbuch der medizinischen Radiologie, Bd V/2)
7. Fischedick O (1973) Arthrographie des Kniegelenks. Springer, Berlin Heidelberg New York (Handbuch der medizinischen Radiologie, Bd V/2)

Bone Tumors

H. G. Jacobson

Montefiore Hospital and Medical Center, Albert Einstein College of Medicine, Department of Radiology, 111 East 210th Street, Bronx, NY 10467 (USA)

Adamantinoma of Long Bones and Fibrous Dysplasia

This interesting skeletal neoplasm has a predilection for the 4th and 5th decades of life, with an equal male/female incidence. The midshaft of the tibia is affected in at least 95% of cases, but isolated examples of this neoplasm have been encountered in the femur, humerus, radius, and ulna.

Mild pain of long duration and, on occasion, localized soft tissue swelling are generally presenting complaints. Pathological fractures may occur, but are rare.

Pathologically, both epithelial and endothelial origins of the neoplasms are suggested, but it is now the opinion held by Dahlin and others that the lesion is of endothelial origin. The cellular structure varies greatly. Polygonal or spindle-shaped cells with alveolar or tubular arrangement are generally encountered. The cellular pattern may also show considerable collagenization, suggesting sarcoma. Squamous transformation of the tumor cells with definite epithelial pearls may be noted, simulating squamous cell carcinoma. The lesion is generally highly vascular. On occasion, a fibrous tissue element which may suggest fibrous dysplasia is encountered.

The radiological features are generally those of a tibial mid shaft lesion which is mainly lytic and expanding (Fig. 1). The lesion is usually eccentric. It may be multilocular with a wide zone of transition and poor definition of its endosteal margins. Not infrequently, reactive new bone may be present. Satellite translucencies in the tibia are characteristic, removed from the major lesion with apparently normal bone interspersed. Similar satellite lesions may be noted in the fibula.

It must be stressed that cortical fibrous dysplasia may simulate adamantinoma and, in fact, pathologically an erroneous diagnosis of cortical fibrous dysplasia may be entertained because of the considerable overgrowth of fibrous tissue.

Until recently, it was considered that adamantinoma and cortical fibrous dysplasia may coexist

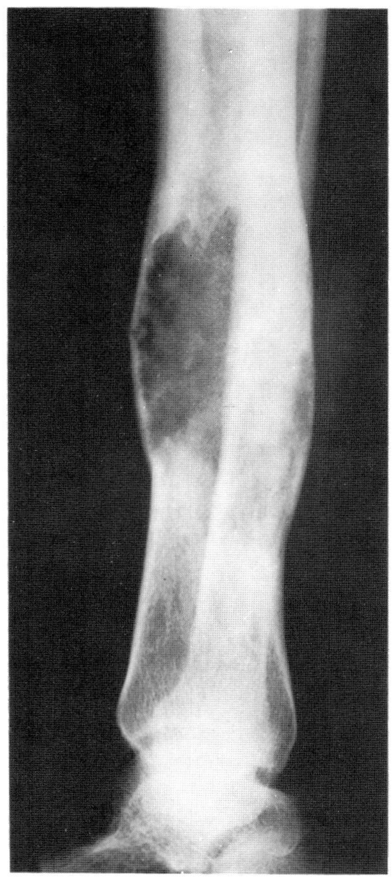

Fig. 1. Adamantinoma of the tibia: A roentgenogram of the lower half of the leg shows an expanding lytic lesion of the tibia below the middle-third with thinning of the cortical margins and some evidence of retained ridges of cortex. The zone of transition around the lesion is relatively narrow, suggest a benign, aggressive lesion. The radiological features are typical; more often adamantinoma involves the middle-third of the tibial shaft

Radiology Today 1. Ed. by M. W. Donner and F. H. W. Heuck

in the same lesion. However, the concept is now held that such cases generally represent adamantinoma with an extensive fibrous tissue matrix, suggesting fibrous dysplasia. Thus the radiological – histological diagnosis of cortical fibrous dysplasia of the tibia in an adult must raise consideration of the possibility of adamantinoma; consequently such cases must be followed carefully. In making the distinction it should also be noted that fibrous dysplasia, which is commonest in children and young adults, has an equal sex incidence, while adamantinoma shows a tendency for a higher female preponderance in a younger age group.

Although adamantinoma is considered a benign neoplasm, a distinct tendency exists for recurrence after local excision and even histologically apparently benign lesions are observed to metastasize after one or two localized resections.

Ossifying Fibroma of Long Bones

This lesion, predominantly involving the tibia (in considering only long bone involvement) has a predilection for the first 2 decades of life and mainly the 1st decade of life. The lesion is slightly more common in females. The child may present with anterior bowing of the tibia, generally with localized pain.

Pathologically, ossifying fibroma of long bones resembles fibrous dysplasia. Osteoblastic and osteoclastic rimming of the bony spicules together with the presence of mature lamellar bone in addition to woven bone is characteristic. The bone spicules are contained in a dense cellular fibrous tissue stroma with no evidence of inflammation or hemosiderin deposits.

Ultrastructural studies with electron microscopy indicate that the osteoblasts rimming the bony spicules and the osteocytes within the bone in ossifying fibroma closely simulate cells described in reactive bone. The osteoblasts are present on the surface of the bony spicules. The cells near the areas of active bone formation have ultrastructural features of both osteoblasts and fibroblasts, suggesting stromal conversion of fibroblasts to osteoblasts. Osteoclasts are also found in apposition to the spicules on ultrastructural studies.

Radiologically, the characteristic features are those of a lesion generally in the middle-third of the tibia characterized by a combination of new bone formation and lytic areas, simulating fibrous dysplasia. Pseudarthrosis may be present. Anterior tibial bowing is common (Fig. 2a, b).

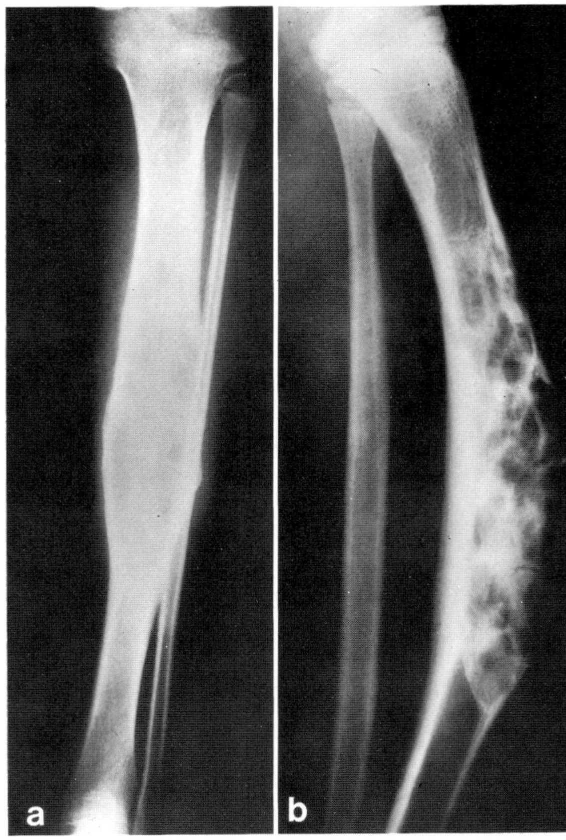

Fig. 2a, b. Ossifying fibroma of the tibia: In these **a** AP and **b** lateral roentgenograms of the leg a large expanding lesion affects the middle-third of the tibial shaft, interspersed with areas of bone sclerosis. The anterior cortical margins are breached by this large expanding lesion. Considerable anterior bowing of the tibial shaft is noted. The findings are characteristic in this child

Calcification, which may be observed in fibrous dysplasia, is generally not part of the radiologic pattern. The lesion may be almost entirely lytic.

Markel is of the opinion that ossifying fibroma and adamantinoma of long bones are related and that lesions resembling fibrous dysplasia in association with adamantinoma of long bones are actually ossifying fibromas.

Ossifying fibroma of the facial bones, e.g., maxilla and mandible, is a well-recognized benign lesion which has the features pathologically of ossifying fibroma of long bones. In the facial bones, the lesion presents as a round or ovoid tumor with the tumor matrix usually of homogeneous density. The tumor is occasionally sclerotic or may be mixed. The histological pattern is similar to ossifying fibroma of the mandible.

Osteoblastoma

This usually benign neoplasm with an osteoid and osseous matrix occurs mainly in the 2nd and 3rd decades of life. It is closely related to osteoid osteoma, both pathologically and often radiologically. Clinically, localized pain and tenderness at the site of the lesion are the usual presenting complaints. The pain is generally less severe than with osteoid osteoma and often is not relieved by aspirin, in contrast to the latter. Neurological deficits and even paraplegia in vertebral lesions may be encountered.

Approximately half the lesions occur in the vertebral column with a predilection for the neural arches, although in contrast to osteoid osteoma, lesions occasionally are observed in the vertebral bodies. The remaining half of the cases have a predilection for the major long bones, although the short tubular bones of the hands and feet, and particularly the hands, are sometimes affected.

Pathologically, the typical lesion is that of a hemorrhagic, irregular, and usually large mass of osteoid and osteoblastic tissue. Numerous giant cells and many thin-walled vascular cavities may be noted. Calcification is not infrequently observed in the lesional tissue. On the one hand a typically occurring benign lesion may be very difficult to distinguish pathologically from osteoid osteoma. On the other extreme, in instances where osteoblastic activity is considerable, an osteosarcoma may be simulated. Not infrequently such an erroneous diagnosis is made. Such lesions Schajowicz has referred to as "aggressive" osteoblastoma and indeed lesions called osteoblastoma have been known to metastasize, suggesting that they were osteosarcoma de novo.

Radiologically, lesions in the axial skeleton tend to be bone forming, although a radiolucent nidus may be observed (Fig. 3). The neural arch is usually affected, although on occasion both the neural arch and the vertebral body may be involved. Rarely, a lesion may only involve the vertebral body.

On rare occasions the lesion in the spine may be completely lytic.

In the appendicular skeleton, the lesions tend to be osteolytic, although lesions present for a long period of time may excite considerable reactive sclerosis. In a long bone, the lesion characteristically consists of a large, irregular translucent center which is as much as 2 – 10 cm in diameter, not infrequently containing an irregular opaque nidus. Lesions in the appendicular skeleton in long and

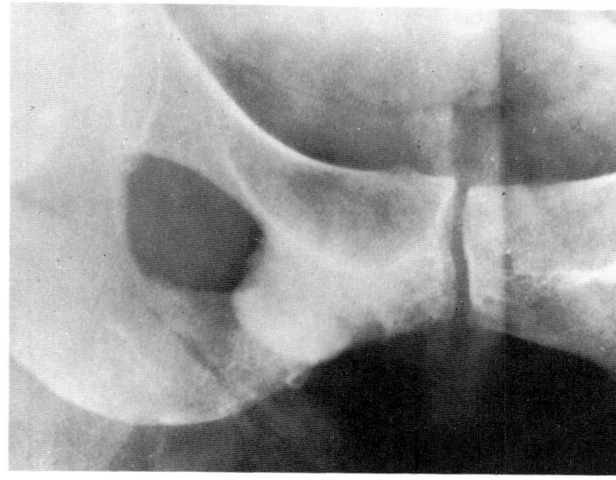

Fig. 3. Osteoblastoma of the pubis: A bony density is noted in the ascending ramus of the pubis with a poorly defined upper border and a fairly well-outlined lower border. Such lesions in flat bones may be grossly lytic. The differential diagnosis between osteoid osteoma and osteoblastoma is difficult at times, both radiologically and histologically

short tubular bones tend to thin, expand, and erode the cortex, sometimes giving an appearance reminiscent of aneurysmal bone cyst or giant cell tumor. The lesions in long bones tend to show interspersed areas of new bone formation and radiolucent zones.

The radiological features in both long bones and vertebral column are often very protean and at times bizarre.

Again, it must be emphasized that the distinction between osteoid osteoma and osteoblastoma may be very difficult radiologically and often pathologically. Thus the term osteoid osteoma – osteoblastoma complex has been coined. Since an occasional osteoblastoma which appears histologically benign may metastasize, and since instances are recorded in which an osteoblastoma apparently has undergone malignant transformation to osteosarcoma, it may be suitable to use the term osteoid osteoma – osteoblastoma – osteosarcoma complex. The concept must again be emphasized that an osteoblastoma which has undergone malignant transformation may have been an osteosarcoma at its inception.

Dedifferentiated Chondrosarcoma

This interesting neoplasm represents a transformation to a highly malignant state of either a benign

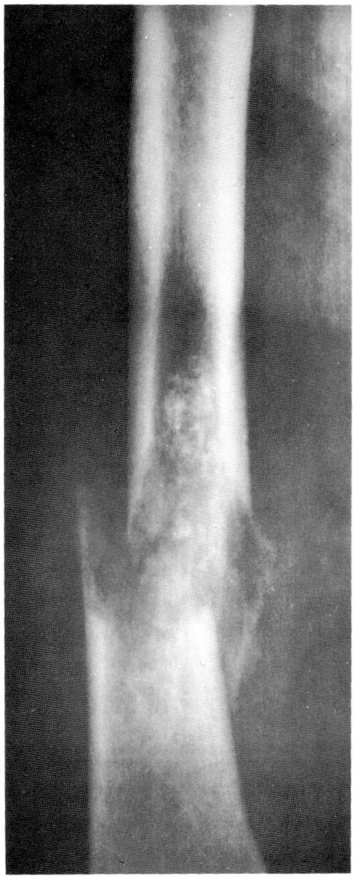

Fig. 4. Dedifferentiated chondrosarcoma of the femur: This AP roentgenogram of the lower two-thirds of the femur shows a pathological fracture through a grossly destructive lesion just below the middle-third of the femur with considerable amorphous collections of calcium within the contour of the lesion. The zone of transition is wide, indicating a malignant lesion. A soft tissue mass appears to be present. The malignant tissue is mainly fibrous histiocytoma – a not uncommon histological determination in dedifferentiated chondrosarcoma. The calcification strongly suggests a preexistent chondromatous lesion

lesion, e.g., osteochondroma, enchondroma (infrequently), or, more commonly, a low-grade chondrosarcoma. Any age group may be affected, but the usual transformation or dedifferentiation occurs in the middle and older age groups. Any bone may be involved, depending on the site of the initial lesion, but the innominate bone and major long bones appear to be more frequently affected. The clinical features are those of pain and swelling at the site of the dedifferentiation.

The histological appearance varies. The portion of dedifferentiation which occurs is most often typical of fibrosarcoma, but osteosarcoma is not infrequently encountered. Classically, the histologic pattern will demonstrate an abrupt transition between the original chondroid lesion and the more malignant dedifferentiated element.

Radiologically, the dedifferentiated chondrosarcoma will show a pattern of classic chondrosarcoma. Calcific foci are generally present within the dedifferentiated lesion. Areas of bone destruction are generally the rule at the site of the dedifferentiation, in contrast to the initial completely or relatively benign appearance of the lesion in comparison with the dedifferentiated area. A typical pattern radiologically is that of an indolent-appearing chondromatous lesion which shows a gross area of bone destruction on one of its borders. On occasion the cortex may be breached at the site of the dedifferentiation and a soft tissue mass may be present (Fig. 4).

The typical dedifferentiated chondrosarcoma is highly malignant, metastasizing early. Death occurs in approximately 90% of cases.

It must be stressed that the cellular pattern may even resemble malignant lymphoma or malignant giant cell tumor of soft parts. Recently instances have been reported by Dorfman of the dedifferentiated lesion being typical of fibrous histiocytoma.

This lesion is of great importance because the risk of a patient developing a dedifferentiated tumor must now be considered when an apparently indolent cartilaginous or osteocartilaginous neoplasm of bone is encountered radiologically. The use of conservative therapy in such instances must now be questioned.

Fibrous Histiocytoma

This neoplasm, which is most often malignant, occurs in a wide age range from the young to the very old, but is most commonly observed in middle age. The lesion may be extraosseous, intraosseous, or both.

Clinically, an occasional lesion may be asymptomatic, but the usual initial complaint is a painful soft tissue mass of long duration. It is of interest that a history of previous trauma is not infrequently elicited. The chest wall, buttocks, and thighs are frequent sites of involvement, particularly in instances of soft tissue tumors (Fig. 5). Such neoplasms have a tendency to invade adjacent tendon sheaths, joint capsules, muscle bundles, and bone.

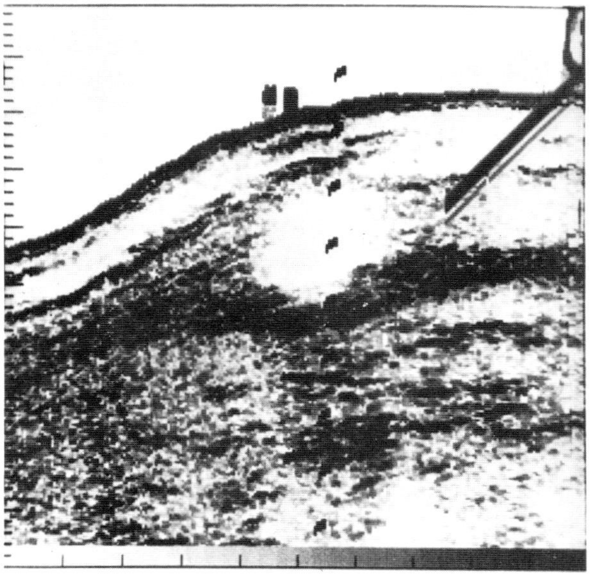

Fig. 5. Malignant fibrous histiocytoma of the abdominal wall: A sonolucent area near the anterior abdominal wall in this ultrasound study represents a malignant fibrous histiocytoma in a 48-year-old woman who was treated for a Stage Ib carcinoma of the cervix 4 years previously. The relationship of this lesion to the radiation therapy was not determined

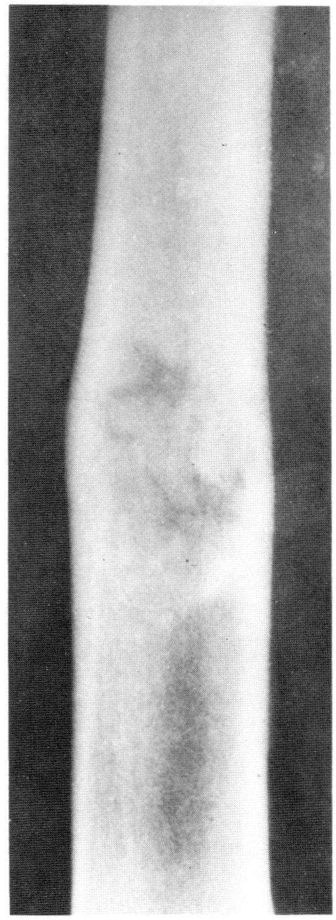

Fig. 6. Fibrous histiocytoma of the femur: A film of the middle two-thirds of the femoral shaft in a 36-year-old woman shows an irregular area of radiolucency with surrounding cortical and subendosteal sclerosis together with periosteal reaction incorporated into the cortex. Poorly marginated central densities are noted within the lytic lesion. The findings are highly suggestive of chondrosarcoma. This appearance in a fibrous histiocytoma is unusual. (By courtesy of Dr. D. J. Stoker, Royal National Orthopaedic Hospital and Institute, London, England)

Primary skeletal lesions are much less common than those affecting soft tissues, although intraosseous lesions may actually extend into the adjacent soft tissues (Fig. 4).

Pathologically, several cell types exist which have been designated as malignant fibrous histiocytoma, malignant histiocytoma, malignant fibroxanthoma, and a much less common type – malignant giant cell tumor. All four types may coexist.

Although varying cell patterns are observed in individual lesions, the typical neoplasm shows pathologically whorls of spindle cells which are reminiscent of fibroblasts. A storiform pattern (radial or pin-wheel appearance) is classic. Spheroid or lobulated pleomorphic cells with multiple nuclei, considerable mitosis, and reticulin fibers are frequently observed. Giant cells are commonly noted and erythrocytes, hemosiderin, and lipids are often incorporated in the individual cells.

The radiologic appearance is generally not specific. With soft tissue neoplasms, the soft tissue mass tends to be well defined and on rare occasions may contain calcium deposits and even osteoid and osseous tissue. Although, multiple bone lesions are observed on occasion, the lesion is usually solitary and is mainly lytic and grossly destructive. The zone of transition tends to be wide and pathological fractures are not infrequently encountered. Periosteal reaction may be present. Lesions of the spine are generally accompanied by a soft tissue paraspinal mass. The typical lesion is often highly reminiscent of fibrosarcoma, particularly in a long bone or innominate bone (Fig. 6).

Metastases after surgical removal to adjacent lymph nodes, lungs, and even other portions of the skeleton occur frequently and often early. In the large series of cases from the Columbia University Presbyterian Hospital Medical Center reported by Feldman and Lattes, approximately 80% of the patients developed a local recurrence after surgery;

72% demonstrated metastases within 1 year after the initial treatment. It must be emphasized that even those lesions designated as benign have a guarded prognosis. In general, therefore, this lesion should be considered malignant.

Hemangiopericytoma

These are uncommonly encountered vascular tumors derived from pericapillary pericytes. A lesion may occur anywhere in the body, but with an apparent predilection for soft tissues of the extremities, retroperitoneal soft tissues, mesentery, omentum, mediastinum, liver, pancreas, and uterus. Skeletal lesions were considered by Stout to be extremely uncommon, but increasing numbers are being encountered.

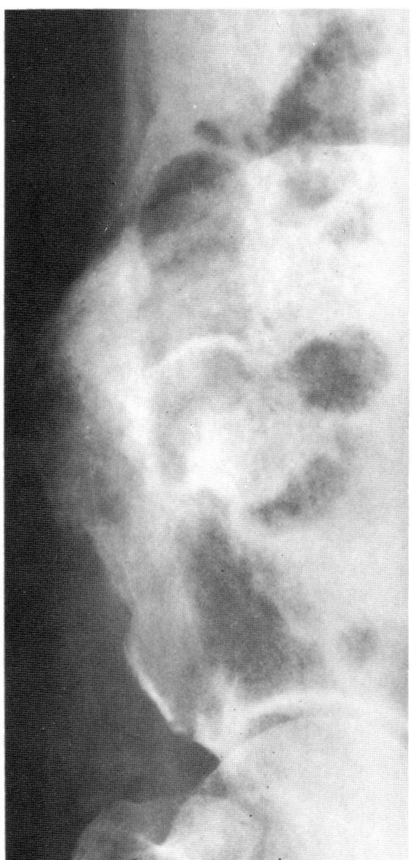

Fig. 7. Hemangiopericytoma in the iliac bone: A large irregular destructive lesion is noted to involve mainly the outer margin of the iliac bone, breaching the cortex at several sites. The zone of transition is wide. Slight reactive sclerosis may be present medially and at the upper margin of the lesion. The findings are indicative of a malignant lesion but are certainly not pathognomonic of the diagnostic entity

Clinically, the usual presenting complaint is localized pain. Although any age group may be affected, this neoplasm is most commonly encountered in young and middle-aged adults. The tumor is usually solitary; any part of the skeleton may be involved but most cases are observed in major long bones, innominate bone, spine, rib, clavicle, and jaw bone.

Pathologically, the characteristic cell is the Zimmerman pericyte, which is observed in the walls of arteries. The cells are elongated, in contrast to the more rounded cell found in a glomus tumor to which the lesion is closely related. The pericytes of Zimmerman are also much more abundant in the histological pattern than the more sparsely arranged cell pattern in glomus tumors.

Radiologically, hemangiopericytoma is virtually always lytic, often grossly destructive, and frequently expanding (Fig. 7). Both benign and malignant forms exist, and great difficulty exists in distinguishing the two. The benign lesion usually shows a narrow zone of transition and other characteristics of a benign neoplasm, but by no means invariably. The pattern often is reminiscent of an aneurysmal bone cyst. On angiography, marked hypervascularity at the site of the lesion is characteristic, but not specific.

In general, the radiological diagnosis can only be suggested by exclusion. A high malignant potential exists and even lesions which were diagnosed as benign histologically may metastasize.

Periosteal Osteosarcoma

This neoplasm represents a very small percentage of primary bone tumors, but it is one of the many types of osteosarcoma which has its own distinctive features.

Clinically, the age range varies widely, but most lesions are encountered in the 2nd decade of life, much like classical osteosarcoma. A slight female preponderance exists. The most common presenting symptoms are pain and localized swelling. The sites of skeletal predilection are the tibia and femur. Although the metaphyses of long bones are most frequently affected, mid-diaphyseal lesions have been encountered.

Pathologically, this lesion is of intermediate malignancy, being more malignant than parosteal osteosarcoma, but less malignant than the classical osteosarcoma. Masses of abnormal appearing cartilage and osteoid are noted to grow from the cortical surface of the affected bone into the adjacent soft tissue. Chondroid areas are noted perpendicular to the cortex with osteoid centrally located, giving a feathery appearance. Lobulated masses which do not actually infiltrate the adjacent soft tissues are typical. The amount and extent of cartilage may vary from large islands of highly malignant cartilage cells to small foci of malignant cartilage. Sheets of anaplastic osteoid-producing spindle cells are typical.

Radiologically, periosteal osteosarcoma is generally limited to the periphery of the cortex of the affected bone. The endosteal surface of the affected bone and the medullary cavity are not affected. Thickening of the cortex with periosteal reaction producing Codman triangles is classic. The typical lesion usually occupies only a relatively small area of the affected long bone. The tumor mass grows into the adjacent soft tissues with varying degrees of calcium deposits and bone noted in the lesion tissue (Fig. 8). Radiating bony spicules perpendicular to the long axis of the involved bone are also frequently noted.

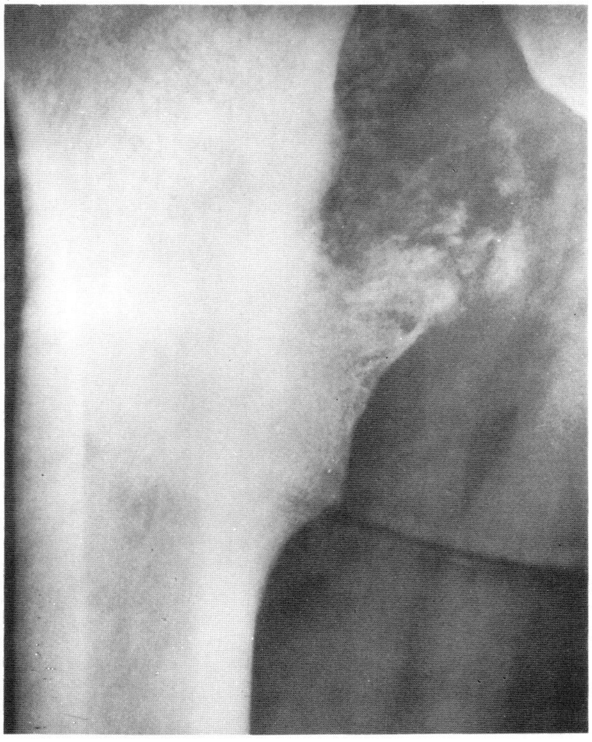

Fig. 8. Periosteal osteosarcoma of the femur: An anteroposterior roentgenogram of the upper portion of the femur shows considerable periosteal new bone adjacent to the lesser trochanter with some compact periosteal reaction along the medial aspect of the femoral shaft just above the lesser trochanter. The periosteal new bone in the soft tissues is irregular and amorphous in appearance. The medial cortical surface appears sclerotic. The findings are typical for this lesion. (By courtesy of Dr. M. Sundaram, St. Louis University Medical Center, St. Louis, MO, United States)

The typical lesion must be distinguished from parosteal osteosarcoma, which tends to occur in slightly older individuals than periosteal osteosarcoma. The duration of symptoms is also shorter in periosteal osteosarcoma than in parosteal osteosarcoma. Parosteal osteosarcoma involves mainly the posterior aspect of the lower end of the femur, in contrast to periosteal osteosarcoma, which most often affects the upper end of the tibia. The histological pattern is different in the two lesions, and the radiological appearance of a parosteal osteosarcoma with a very dense lobulated mass of bone attached to the cortex of the involved bone and encircling the involved shaft is classical. This appearance is completely unlike the typical periosteal osteosarcoma.

The prognosis for periosteal osteosarcoma is intermediate between parosteal osteosarcoma and classical osteosarcoma. In general the prognosis is relatively good.

It should be noted that not infrequently because of the considerable amount of malignant cartilage often encountered in periosteal osteosarcoma, a histological diagnosis of chondrosarcoma may be made. Since the radiological features are relatively typical in periosteal osteosarcoma and completely unlike those encountered in chondrosarcoma, the radiologist has an important responsibility in being aware of both the pathological and radiological appearances of this lesion.

References

1. Baker PL, Dockerty MB, Coventry MB (1954) Adamantinoma (so-called) of the long bones. J Bone Joint Surg [Am] 36:704
2. Byers PD (1968) Solitary benign osteoblastic lesions of bone. Cancer 22:43
3. Cohen DM, Dahlin DC, Pugh DG (1962) Fibrous dysplasia associated with adamantinoma of the long bones. Cancer 15:515
4. Crabbe WA, Wardill JC (1963) Benign osteoblastoma of the spine. Br J Surg 50:571
5. Dahlin DC (1971) Dedifferentiation of low-grade chondrosarcomas. Cancer 28:461

6. Dahlin DC (1977) Case report 27. Periosteal osteosarcoma of the right femur. Skeletal Radiol 1:249 – 252
7. Dahlin DC (1978) Case Report 71. Dedifferentiated chondrosarcoma of the humerus. Skeletal Radiol 3:133 – 136
8. Dunlop J (1973) Primary hemangiopericytoma of bone. Report of two cases. J Bone Joint Surg [Br] 55:854
9. Enzinger FM, Smith BH (1976) Hemangiopericytoma – An analysis of 106 cases. Hum Pathol 7:61
10. Feldman F, Lattes R (1977) Primary malignant fibrous histiocytoma (fibrous xanthoma) of bone. Skeletal Radiol 1:145 – 160
11. Goergen TG, Dickman PS, Resnick D, Saltzstein SL, O'Dell CW, Akeson WH (1977) Long bone ossifying fibromas. Cancer 39:2067 – 2072
12. Kempson RL (1966) Ossifying fibroma of the long bones. A light and electron microscopic study. Arch Pathol 82:218 – 233
13. Lattes R (1973) Case 14, Malignant fibrous histiocytoma – discussion of a case. In: Hartman WM (ed) Proceedings of the 39th annual anatomic pathology slide seminar, american society of clinical pathologists council on anatomic pathology, October 26, 1973. American Society of Clinical Pathologists, pp 75 – 81
14. Lichtenstein L (1956) Benign osteoblastoma: A category of osteoid and bone-forming tumors other than classical osteoid osteoma, which may be mistaken for giant-cell tumor or osteogenic sarcoma. Cancer 9:1044
15. Lichtenstein L (1965) Bone tumors. Mosby, St Louis
16. Markel, SF (1978) Ossifying fibroma of long bone. Its distinction from fibrous dysplasia and its association with adamantinoma of long bone. Am J Clin Pathol 69/1:91 – 97
17. McMaster MJ, Soule EH, Ivins JC (1975) Hemangiopericytoma. A clinicopathologic study and long-term follow-up of 60 patients. Cancer 36:2232 – 2244
18. Mirra JM, Marcove RC (1974) Fibrosarcomatous dedifferentiation of primary and secondary chondrosarcoma: review of five cases. J Bone Joint Surg [Am] 56:285
19. Moon NF (1966) Adamantinoma of the appendicular skeleton. Clin Orthop 43:189
20. Soule EH, Enriquez P (1972) Atypical fibrous histiocytoma, malignant histiocytoma and epithelioid sarcoma. A comparative study of 65 tumors. Cancer 30:128
21. Unni KK, Dahlin DC, Beabout JW (1976) Periosteal osteogenic sarcoma. Cancer 37:2476
22. Unni KK, Dahlin DC, Beabout JW, Ivins JC (1976) Parosteal osteogenic sarcoma. Cancer 37:2466
23. Yaghmai I (1978) Angiographic manifestations of soft tissue and osseous hemangiopericytomas. Radiology 126:653 – 659

Computed Tomography of the Musculoskeletal System

S. S. Siegelman

Johns Hopkins Medical Institutions, Department of Radiology and Radiological Sciences,
601 N. Broadway, Baltimore, MD 21205 (USA)

Introduction

A number of recent reports have indicated that computed tomography (CT) should have a role in the evaluation of patients with musculoskeletal disorders [1 – 12]. We acquired the Pfizer/A.S. & E. Scanner (Model 500) at the Johns Hopkins Hospital in October 1977. In the initial $2\frac{1}{2}$ year period of operation of the unit, we have examined 300 patients with problems related to the bones or soft tissues of the extremities, pelvis, or spine. Although CT has had a much greater impact on evaluation of the chest, pancreas, and retroperitoneum, it does possess a number of features which make it useful for examining the musculoskeletal system. The purpose of this report is to present an overview of the current status of CT of the musculoskeletal system.

General Principles

The key factor which is responsible for the usefulness of CT in evaluating musculoskeletal disorders is that CT provides much greater soft tissue detail than that available from plain roentgenography and standard tomography [2, 3, 4, 8]. An important additional related factor is that CT provides a unique cross-sectional image of the area under study [3, 7, 9, 10]. The combination of these two elements largely accounts for the current contribution of CT to clinical skeletal radiology.

In patients with skeletal lesions detectable by conventional radiography, CT is generally more apt to help plan patient management than to assist in making a specific diagnosis. This is because CT is much more effective in determining the extent of disease, whereas in most cases CT is not superior to standard diagnostic modalities in detecting a lesion or in suggesting a specific histologic diagnosis [2 – 6, 9, 10]. This point was specifically emphasized by Levine et al. who found that in 24 of 29 patients with skeletal tumors, the lesion was located and the correct diagnosis was suggested by plain films and laminography. In the remaining five patients, CT was useful in diagnosis because the lesions were not adequately visualized by conventional radiography [5]. In this same study, CT was deemed useful in patient management in 16 of the 29 patients, generally because it accurately determined the presence or absence of any associated soft tissue component. Thus for patients with bone lesions, CT and standard radiography are complementary: routine methods establish the diagnosis, CT determines the extent of disease.

In our own experience although standard plain roentgenograms are generally adequate for determining the presence of an osseous lesion, CT provides welcome support as a problem-solving device for difficult cases with subtle intraosseous lesions. It is not unusual to encounter a patient with negative plain roentgenograms despite sharply localized pain or a positive radionuclide study. CT almost always settles the issue in such cases. McLeod et al. have also reported success in detecting subtle osseous lesions in the pelvis or spine which were not apparent on routine radiography. These authors also illustrated cases of skeletal metastases in the sacrum and scapula detected by CT alone [6]. A specific role for CT is to evaluate for recurrence of a previously resected osseous lesion [6, 7]. This is illustrated in Fig. 1.

The unique cross-sectional perspective supplied by CT facilitates evaluation of all areas of the skeleton. We have been particularly impressed with the usefulness of CT in the evaluation of the pelvis [7, 8]. In a sense one may conceptionalize that the pelvic area consits of a semicircular bony shell which is lined on its external and internal surfaces by bands of muscle. With standard radiography, the extreme density of the bones interferes

Radiology Today 1. Ed. by M. W. Donner and F. H. W. Heuck

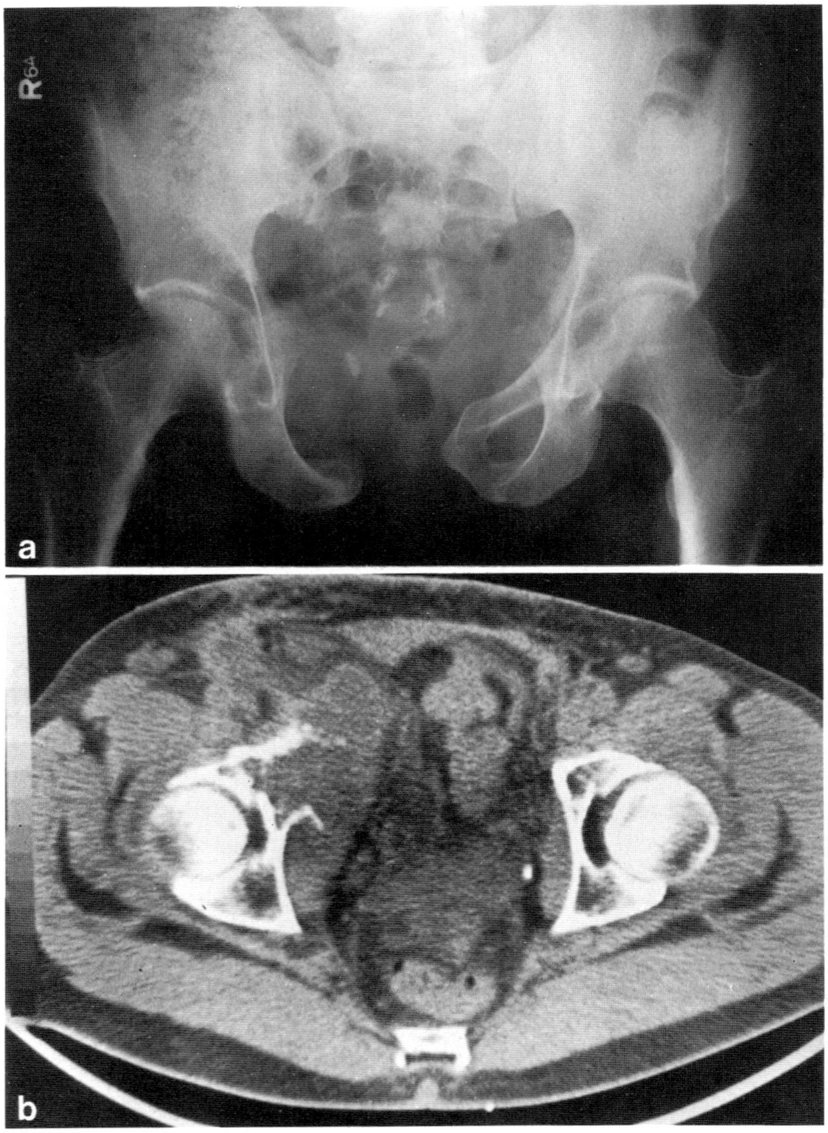

Fig. 1a, b. Recurrent chondrosarcoma. A 49-year-old male with pain in right groin $3\frac{1}{2}$ years following resection of chondrosarcoma of right pubis. **a** Plain pelvic roentgenogram shows questionable soft tissue fullness adjacent to site of previous surgical resection. **b** CT scan demonstrates an expansile osseous mass with contiguous soft tissue component

with visualization of the adjacent soft tissues. In the cross-sectional CT image, bones and soft tissues are clearly separated and may be evaluated independently. It has become necessary for the radiologist to acquire a working knowledge of cross-sectional anatomy [8]. In examining any single section of the pelvis it should be possible to recognize the level as L5, S1, S2, or S3. The radiologist should be capable of tracing on serial sections structures such as the sacroiliac joints, the iliopsoas, obturator, and gluteus muscles, and the iliac arteries and veins.

Although the structure of the extremities is less complex than the pelvis, the cross-sectional image provided by CT can be important. Long bone lesions may be analyzed in terms of cortical and medullary components [3]; and the relationship of soft tissue masses to adjacent vessels and nerves can be assessed [9]. Other areas where cross-sectional images have proved extremely useful are the scapula, the spine, and the sternum with its attachment to the clavicles and ribs.

General Indications

Soft Tissue Mass

Computed tomography is especially suitable for evaluating the patient suspected of harboring a deeply seated isolated soft tissue tumor. Such patients present with some combination of localiz-

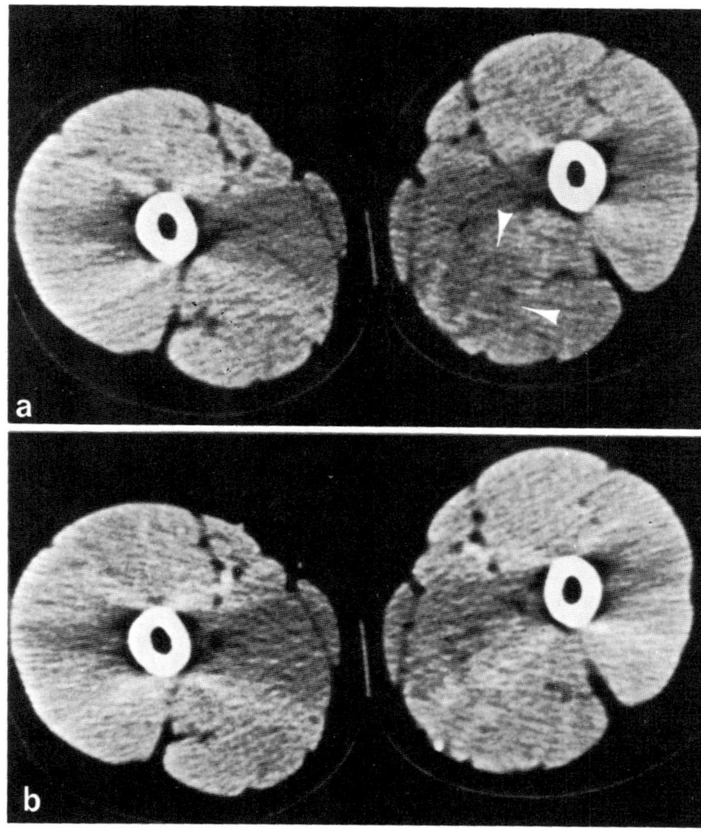

Fig. 2a – d. Infiltrating angiolipoma. A 10-year-old girl noted a dull aching pain in the posteromedial aspect of the thigh. The pain was exacerbated by exercise or prolonged standing. There was considerable relief from rest. Palpation of a soft tissue mass was facilitated during muscle contraction. **a** CT scan unenhanced. Abnormal area of reduced attenuation in posteromedial aspect of thigh (*arrows*). **b** CT scan following the intravenous injection of 50 ml 60% Renografin. The abnormal area has enhanced. **c** Femoral arteriogram, arterial phase shows an abnormal network of fine vessels. **d** Femoral arteriogram, late capillary, early venous phase shows diffuse pooling of contrast in vessels

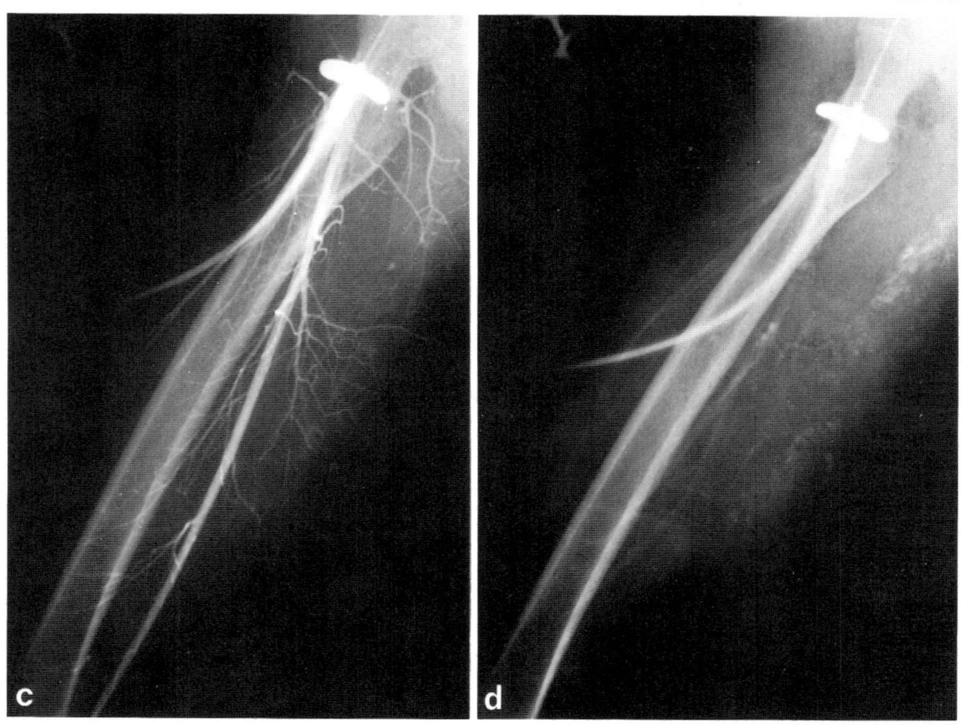

ed pain, tenderness, possible swelling, and a questionably palpable mass usually in the paraspinal region of the thoracolumbar area, the gluteal region, the thigh, or the calf. The typical patient is a 35–45 year old jogger or exercise enthusiast of either sex. Since the pivotal item is whether an actual soft tissue tumor is present a normal CT scan is definitive information. Levine et al. reported six patients with normal CT scans despite serious clinical concern for a soft tissue mass [5]; Wilson et al. had experience of eight similar cases [12]. These latter authors have indicated that the objective determination that no soft tissue tumor is present is one of the most important current contributions from CT. In our own experience, the questionably palpable soft tissue mass in the thigh or calf is often an area of newly acquired muscle hypertrophy, and areas of localized pain are frequently normal appearing muscle groups. The availability of a contralateral extremity to serve as a standard of normal anatomy is most useful in such cases.

Computed tomography has also been employed in the evaluation of the patient with a definite, readily palpable soft tissue mass. In such cases CT will generally not provide a specific diagnosis unless the lesion is a lipoma [5, 9]. The usefulness of CT is in determining the extent of the lesion and the relationship of the mass to the major regional arteries and veins [10, 11].

The optimal examination of a soft tissue mass consists of a baseline study followed by immediate reexamination after intravenous injection of contrast media. Levine et al. found that the use of contrast provided significant additional information in 12 of 30 cases, usually because the lesion was better visualized on the postcontrast studies. In two patients the soft tissue mass was seen only postcontrast [5]. The degree to which a tumor enhances on CT may be correlated with the vascularity of the lesion. Soft tissue masses which enhance to a greater degree than adjacent muscles would generally be associated with tumor vascularity on angiography. The correlation is not absolute since Wilson et al. reported that two soft tissue hemangiomas failed to enhance [12]. Herman and Rose noted that the failure of a lesion to enhance to the same degree as adjacent muscles, "reverse contrast enhancement," usually indicated tumor necrosis [4]. One may anticipate a much lower yield from angiography of soft tissue masses which do not enhance on CT. A soft tissue mass which enhanced following intravenous injection of contrast material is illustrated in Fig. 2. On the unenhanced study (Fig. 2a), the CT number of the lesion was 20 HU, whereas the CT number of adjacent muscle was 50 HU. Following injection of 50 ml 60% Renografin, the CT numbers of the soft tissue lesion and normal muscle were recorded as 70 HU. The mass proved to be an infiltrating angiolipoma, which is a benign unencapsulated soft tissue neoplasm which involves skeletal muscle and adjacent soft tissues [13, 14, 15]. One might anticipate a CT number below zero in a tumor with a large content of fat, but in this instance the extensive pooling of blood within the tumor undoubtedly was responsible for the CT number of 20 HU.

An additional occasional role for CT has been to search for a soft tissue hematoma. The clinical setting is a patient with a recent hip fracture or pelvic fracture who is noted to have sustained a significant fall in blood volume without any palpable mass or clinically apparent site of blood loss. In addition to several large retroperitoneal hematomas, we encountered one patient with a fractured right hip associated with an unsuspected large hematoma in the left gluteal region.

Soft Tissue Component of Skeletal Lesions

Computed tomography is notably useful for the evaluation of soft tissue components of a primary bone lesion [1–12]. Bone lesions frequently include a contiguous extraosseous soft tissue mass which may be difficult to detect by plain radiography. It is particularly difficult to assess the soft tissue component of osseous lesions of the sacrum and pelvis [6, 7]. CT may also be used to evaluate the soft tissues within the medullary cavities of long bones. The intramedullary component of primary bone tumors [1–3], osteomyelitis [4], and malignant lymphoma [6] may be assessed and monitored, if necessary with serial examinations. Evaluation of any juxtaosseous soft tissue masses is particularly important as a guide to radiotherapy treatment planning and as a baseline prior to chemotherapy.

Staging of Tumors

Computed tomography is clearly superior to other currently available imaging modalities in staging of skeletal lesions by determining the precise location, extent, and relationship to surrounding structures. Such information is used in determining the feasibility of resection and in planning the correct surgical approach [9]. For lesions which are not resectable CT serves as a guide for radiotherapy or as a baseline for chemotherapy. Levine et al. found that in the majority of their cases CT was superior to plain films, laminography, radionuclide bone scanning, and angiography in staging of tumors [5]. Wilson et al. found that in 78% of their cases the precise location and extent of a lesion was better defined by CT than by standard imaging procedures [6].

Quantitative Analysis of Bone Mass

Computed tomography has been employed in the analysis of bone mass and bone mineral content [16, 17]. Osteoporosis is a commonly encountered clinical problem and a need exists for a precise, noninvasive method for serial measurement of bone mineral content [18]. Jensen et al. have devised a technique of obtaining objective reproducible measurements of cortical and trabecular bone mass by CT analysis of a cross section of the distal radius [16]. Workers at The University of San Francisco are measuring vertebral mineral content in the first and second lumbar vertebrae by a technique which employs multiple contiguous, nonoverlapping 5 mm thick slices which cover the L1 – L2 region [17]. Longitudinal quantitative studies of cortical and trabecular bone using CT are a promising new tool for evaluating therapeutic programs for postmenopausal osteoporosis and renal osteodystrophy.

Specific Disorders

Special features of CT make it uniquely suitable for the evaluation of the number of clinical disorders. We have studied and obtained critically useful information on at least six patients with osteogenic sarcoma, myeloma, desmoids, and neurofibromatosis. We have had experiences with at least two patients with inflammatory spondylitis, osteoid osteoma. Paget's disease of bone, and intraspinal lipomas. The role of CT in these conditions will be briefly presented.

Osteogenic Sarcoma

Computed tomography has been found to be effective in the evaluation of patients with osteogenic sarcoma [2, 3]. The usefulness of CT in this regard is founded upon CT's unique cross-sectional perspective and superior soft tissue analysis. Knowledge about variation in the degree of malignancy and the spread of osteogenic sarcoma has produced varying plans of treatment [19, 20]. CT defines the epicenter of the lesion and determines if cortex, medullary cavity, or both are involved by tumor. In true parosteal osteogenic sarcoma the medullary cavity is spared [20]. CT discloses if an extraosseous soft tissue mass is present. This information is not routinely self-evident. Using CT, DeSantos et al. found soft tissue masses in three patients with osteogenic sarcoma in whom physical examination and routine radiography did not disclose a soft tissue component [2]. The CT examination is also directed at determining whether the extraosseous component of the lesion consists of irregular tumor infiltration of the periosseous structures or merely a displacement of vital structures by a well-circumscribed mass. Knowledge of the extent of the lesion helps to plan whether the lesion is resectable. Tumors with an extensively infiltrating soft tissue component are not managed by simple en bloc resection.

When less than radical surgery is planned, CT determines the proximal extent of the lesion and assists in planning the level of resection. The normal marrow contents of the medullary canal have a high lipid content and consequently a CT number below 0. Osteoid in the medullary canal may be recognized by its relatively high CT number. Uncalcified osteoid has a CT number of 40 – 80 HU, whereas calcified osteoid ranges from 40 – 400 HU [2]. The extent of tumor spread within the medullary canal is always better seen by CT than by standard tomography.

Myeloma

Myeloma is a disorder produced by a clone of plasma cells with specific immunoglobulin products elaborated by the population of myeloma cells appearing in the serum and urine [21]. The quantity of abnormal immunoglobulin serves as a marker of disease activity which may be monitored by serial examinations. The appearance of an unexplained increase in monoclonal immunoglobulin in the serum or urine indicates an undesirable increase in the tumor cell population. In this situation, if bone marrow aspiration does not reveal a generalized increase in plasma cells, a focal tumor mass is sought. We have used CT in this situation to detect renal, peripancreatic, and retroperitoneal plasmacytomas in addition to large juxtaosseous soft tissue masses.

Desmoid Tumors

Desmoids are benign but aggressive soft tissue tumors which arise from muscles and their enveloping fascia [22]. Lesions are most commonly located in the shoulder area, proximal thigh, and hip regions of young adults [23]. Desmoids are histologically benign with an appearance like dense scar tissues. They do not invade blood vessels and do not metastasize [24]. Despite the innocent microscopic appearance, desmoids are troublesome to manage because the lesions are not encapsulated, they infiltrate widely between muscle fascicles, and they present no clear cleavage plane between tumor and adjacent muscle [22–24]. It may be difficult to remove a desmoid completely by simple surgical excision. An infiltrating desmoid of the shoulder, for example, may entrap the brachial plexus and the axillary artery [23]. Early recurrences following surgery are frequent. Radiation therapy or radical surgery including amputation is frequently employed for recurrent lesions [22–24]. In a series of patients with large desmoids seen at Johns Hopkins Hospital we have used a combination of total excision followed by radiation therapy as the treatment of choice. CT has been a valuable adjunct in the initial evaluation to determine the extent of disease, for radiation therapy treatment planning, and in an assessment for recurrence. A typical case of recurrent desmoid tumor is illustrated in Fig. 3. The use of CT for evaluation of a desmoid of the buttock area has been illustrated by Schumacher et al. [9]. Authors at the same institution have also reported on the use of CT in detecting a recurrent desmoid tumor of the supracapsular region [12].

Neurofibromatosis

The capacity of CT for visualizing both intraosseous and extraosseous soft tissue abnormalities makes it useful in evaluating patients with neurofibromatosis. We have examined a series of patients with various manifestations of neurofibromatosis and have found CT superior to standard roentgenography. Our experience includes cases of dumbbell neurofibromatosis, extensive plexiform

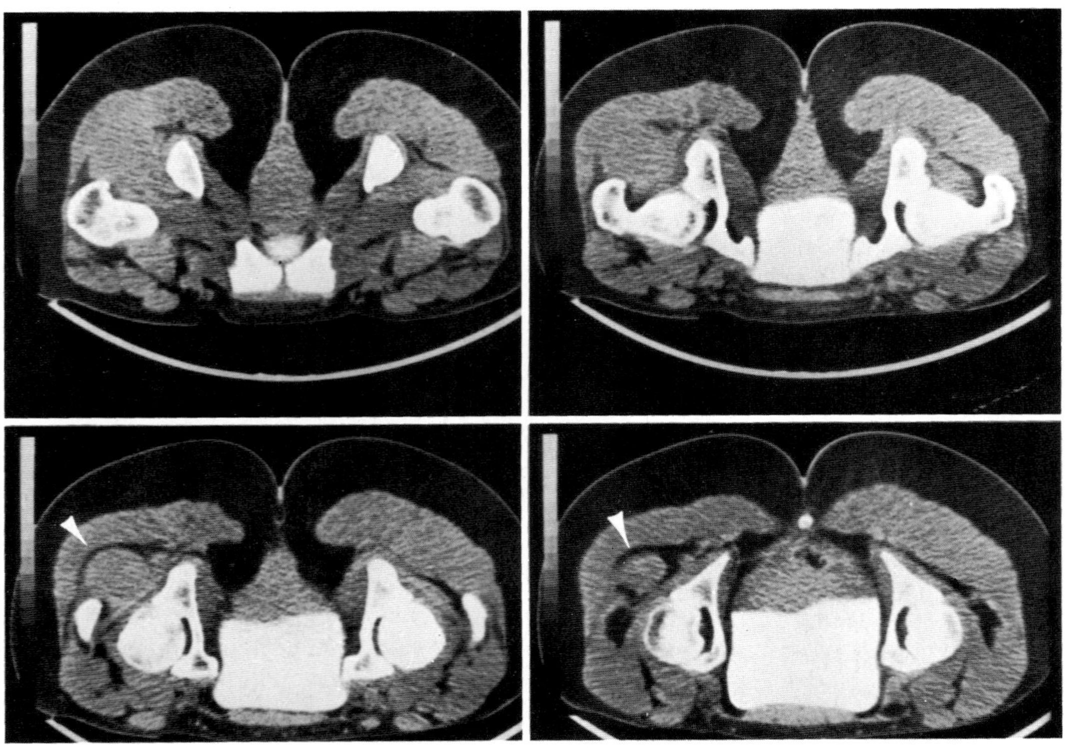

Fig. 3. Recurrent desmoid tumor. A 17-year-old female had a large desmoid tumor resected from the posterior aspect of the left thigh. One year later a questionable fullness of the soft tissues posterolateral to the left hip was detected. No definite mass was palpated. The patient was examined in the prone position. A deeply situated soft tissue mass may be seen on all four CT sections. The mass, which represents recurrent desmoid, is adjacent to the femoral neck (*arrows*). Treatment was excision followed by radiation therapy

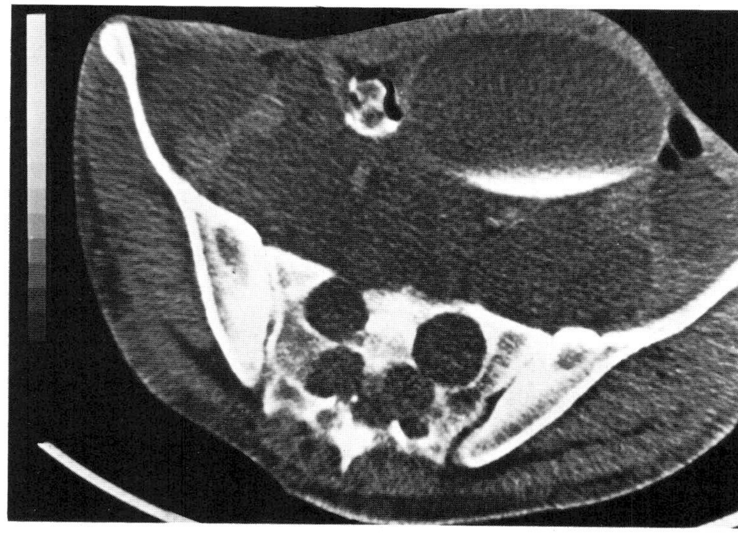

Fig. 4. Neurofibromatosis. A 16-year-old male with known neurofibromatosis. CT scan of pelvis shows enlargement of neural foramina in the sacrum. The bladder, partially filled with contrast material, is noted anteriorly. A series of low density masses in the pelvic soft tissues represent multiple neurofibromata

pelvic neurofibromas, and several patients with juxtaosseous neurofibrosarcoma. A case with intraosseous and extraosseous lesions is illustrated in Fig. 4.

Inflammatory Spondylitis

Inflammatory spondylitis may be diagnosed with confidence when routine roentgenograms show evidence of a narrowed vertebral interspace, destructive lesions in the anterior aspects of adjacent vertebral centra, and a paraspinal soft tissue mass. Occasional cases are encountered in which the osseous findings are less definitive or no soft tissue component is identifiable, or the findings are confusing because the patient has had recent disk surgery. CT is of value in such cases to determine if a soft tissue abscess is present. Schumacher et al. identified such a case in which CT alone detected a soft tissue abscess [9], and we have had experiences with three similar patients.

Osteoid Osteoma

In occasional cases of osteoid osteoma, a small nidus may be obscured by extensive reactive bone destruction. Figure 5 shows a case of pelvic osteoid osteoma in which the nidus was not seen on plain films or standard tomography. The CT number of the nidus was 460 HU and the CT number of the surrounding reactive bone was 1100 HU. The CT number of the nidus was determined by averaging the six voxels in the center of the lesion with the lowest CT numbers. CT was quite useful in this case since the patient's symptoms were not typical and since the radiographic findings were thought to be probably attributable to osteitis condensans ilia. With the patient positioned for optimal visualization of the nidus, a bolus of 50 cc 60% Renografin was given intravenously. Immediately following the injection, the CT number of the nidus increased to 490 HU, and 2 min after the injection the CT number was measured at 620 HU. The lesion was resected and the patient's symptoms disappeared. The use of CT for demonstration of the nidus and osteoid osteoma has also been illustrated by Berger and Kuhn [1] and by Wilson et al. [12].

Paget's Disease

A case which illustrates many of the advantageous features of CT is illustrated in Fig. 6. The patient was a 65-year-old male with known Paget's disease who had unexplained pain, parathesias, and swelling of the right hip and right leg. CT revealed a destructive osseous lesion which had not been seen by routine radiography. The CT examination also detected a large soft tissue mass contiguous with the osseous lesion. A biopsy revealed the malignant fibrous histiocytoma arising within an area of Paget's disease. The CT examination which had demonstrated the extent of the soft tissue mass was used for radiation treatment planning. The patient was treated with radiotherapy and chemotherapy, and he is alive and clinically free of disease 30 months after treatment.

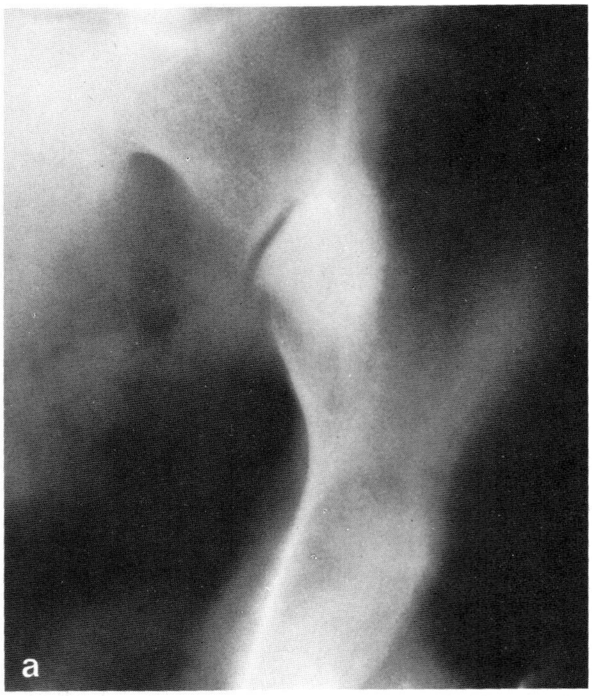

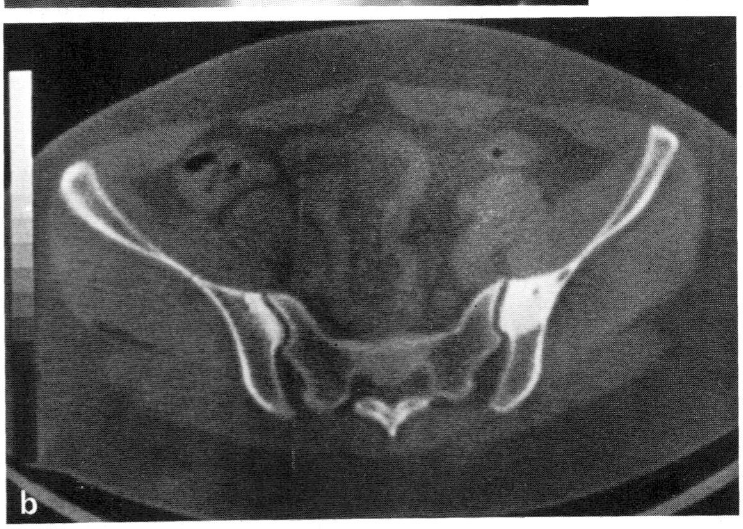

Fig. 5a – d. A 25-year-old female with left-sided low back pain radiating to the left hip. **a** Standard tomogram of the left iliac bone shows zone of dense sclerosis adjacent to the left sacroiliac joint. **b** CT scan (window level, 0: window width, 4000 HU) shows a tiny focus of lesser density (the nidus) in the sclerotic area of the left ilium. **c** CT scan (window level, 1000 HU; window width, 1000 HU) demonstrates the nidus to better advantage. **d** Postoperative CT scan. The patient is now asymptomatic. The lesion has been removed

We have also found CT useful in evaluating several other patients with Paget's disease of the pelvis. Paget's disease can produce circumferential narrowing of the spinal canal leading to spinal cord compression [25]. CT should be useful in such cases to determine the site and the extent of spinal cord compression.

Intraspinal Lipoma

McLeod et al. found CT useful in evaluating patients with widening of the spinal canal and neural arch defects. In addition to the excellent display of the vertebral column and neural arches, CT provides superior visualization of the soft tissue component of any spinal anomaly; hence, the full extent of anterior and posterior meningoceles may be recognized [6]. In some patients with spina bifida and widening of the lumbosacral canal, the associated soft tissue abnormality is a lipoma. Since fat has a CT number of -100 HU, collections of fat may be distinguished from other soft tissue structures. Spina bifida is not uncommonly associated with a subcutaneous lipoma in contiguity with an intradural lipoma [26]. A lipomatous tumor may extend intradurally for a

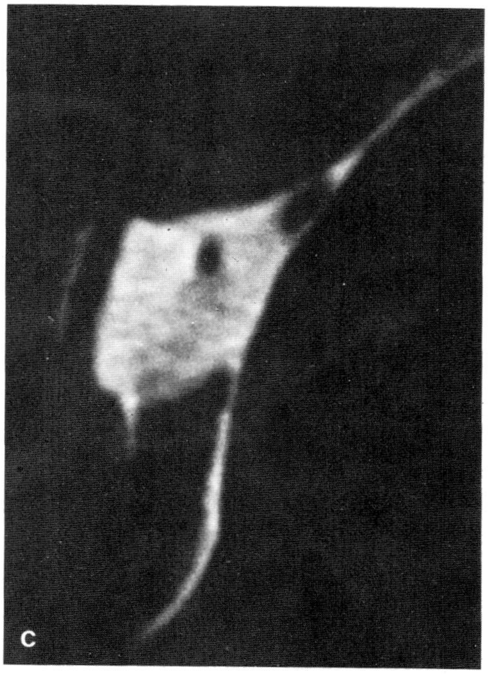

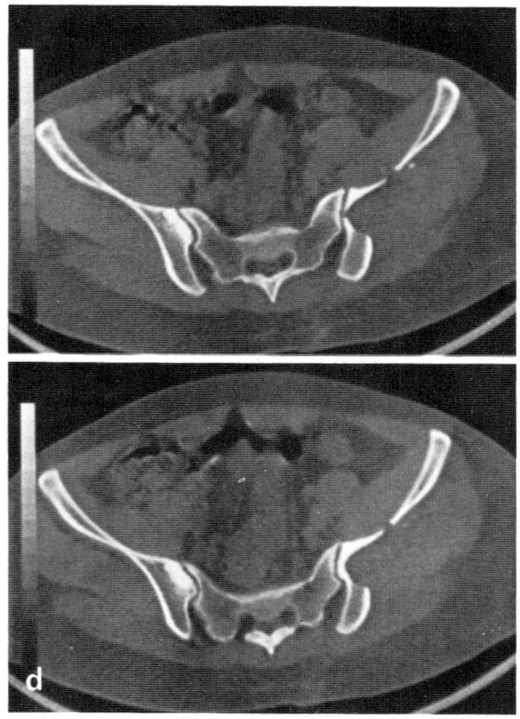

Fig. 5c, d. Legend see p. 284

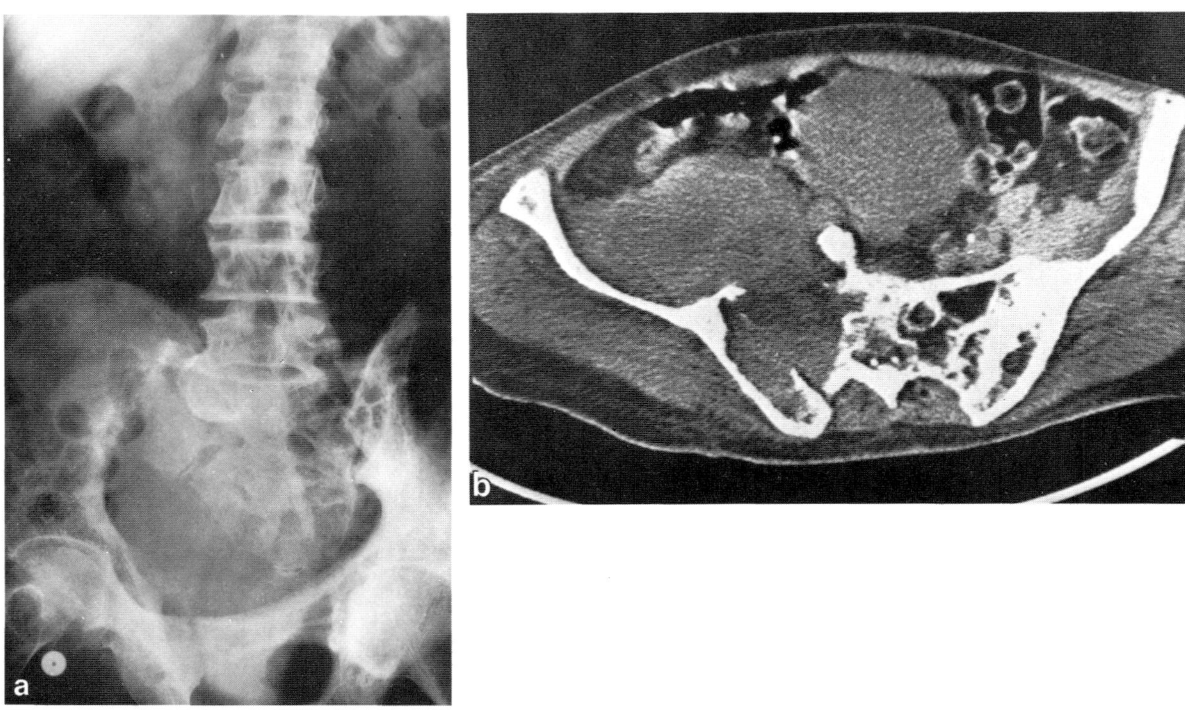

Fig. 6a, b. Malignant fibrous histiocytoma arising in Paget's disease. a Plain film of pelvic and abdomen. Diffuse sclerosis of the pelvis is indicative of Paget's disease. A subtle lytic lesion is present in the sacrum adjacent to the inferior portion of the right SI joint. b CT scan shows destructive lesion in the pelvis with a contiguous large soft tissue mass

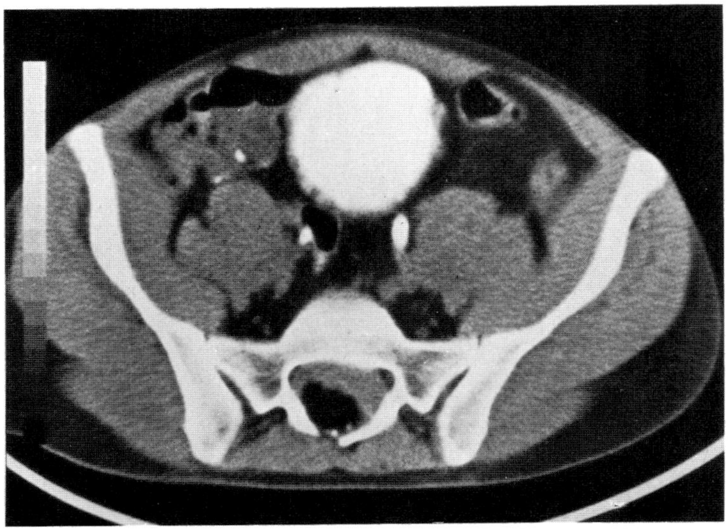

Fig. 7. Intraspinal lipoma. A 27-year-old male with a 15-year history of urinary frequency and urgency and a 6-year history of nocturnal incontinence. Plain roentgenogram showed widening of the canal at the L5 – S1 level. CT scan shows marked widening of the sacral canal. The low density mass within the canal represents a lipoma of the cauda equina

variable distance and may cause compression of the nerves or the cord. This situation may be quite complex in that lipomas and meningoceles may coexist. CT is most useful for evaluating and sorting out the abnormalities in patients with a clinical suspicion of meningocele. CT determines if a soft tissue mass is present, distinguishes between cystic and lipomatous elements, and establishes the intraspinal extension of any component of the disorder. Intradural lipoma is illustrated in Fig. 7.

Conclusion

A list of specific conditions for which CT has proven useful can be readily expanded by the reader. At Johns Hopkins, an additional, important role for CT has been to evaluate for spinal stenosis. This work has been carried out exclusively by our section on Neuroradiology and is not covered in this report. CT is useful as a problem-solving tool when other noninvasive imaging modalities have not provided satisfactory anatomic information on a clinical problem. It is particularly valuable when the perspective provided by a cross-sectional image is needed and when soft tissue details are important.

References

1. Berger PE, Kuhn JP (1978) Computed tomography of tumors of the musculoskeletal system in children. Radiology 127:171 – 175
2. DeSantos LA, Bernardino ME, Murray JA (1979) Computed tomography in the evaluation of osteosarcoma: Experience with 25 cases. AJR 132: 535 – 540
3. Destouet JM, Gilula LA, Murphy WA (1979) Computed tomography of long-bone osteosarcoma. Radiology 131:439 – 445
4. Hermann G, Rose JS (1979) Computed tomography in bone and soft tissue pathology of the extremities. J Comput Assist Tomogr 3:58 – 66
5. Levine E, Lee KR, Neff JR, Markland NF, Robinson RG, Preston DF (1979) Comparison of computed tomography and other imaging modalities in the evaluation of musculoskeletal tumors. Radiology 131:431 – 437
6. McLeod RA, Stephens DH, Beabout JW, Sheedy PF II, Hattery RR (1978) Computed tomography of the skeletal system. Semin Roentgenol 13:235 – 247
7. Naidich DP, Freedman MT, Bowerman JW, Siegelman SS (1978) Computerized tomography in the evaluation of the soft tissue component of bony lesions of the pelvis. Skeletal Radiol 3:144 – 148
8. Naidich DP, Freedman MT, Bowerman JW, Siegelman SS (1980) Ten section approach to computed tomography of the pelvis. Skeletal Radiol 5:213 – 217
9. Schumacher TM, Genant HK, Korobkin M, Bovil EG Jr (1978) Computed tomography. Its use in space-occupying lesions of the musculoskeletal system. J Bone Joint Surg [Am] 60:600 – 607
10. Weinberger G, Levinsohn EM (1978) Computed tomography in the evaluation of sarcomatous tumors of the thigh. AJR 130:115 – 118
11. Weis L, Heelan RT, Watson KC (1978) Computed tomography of orthopedic tumors of the pelvis and lower extremities. Clin Orthop 130:254 – 259
12. Wilson JS, Korobkin M, Genant HK, Bovill EG Jr (1978) Computed tomography of musculoskeletal disorders. AJR 131:55 – 61
13. Finberg HJ, Levin DC (1977) Angiolipoma: A rare benign soft tissue tumor with a malignant arteriographic appearance. AJR 128:697 – 698

14. Gonzalez-Crussi F, Enneking WF, Arean YF (1966) Infiltrating angiolipoma. J Bone Joint Surg [Am] 98:1111 – 1124
15. Lin JJ, Lin F (1974) Two entities in angiolipoma. Cancer 34:720 – 727
16. Jensen PS, Orphanoudakis SC, Rauschkolb EN, Baron R, Lang R, Rasmussen H (1980) Assessment of bone mass in the radius by computed tomography. AJR 134:285 – 292
17. Cann CE, Genant HK, Boyd DP (1979) Precise measurement of vertebral mineral in serial studies using CT. J Comput Assist Tomogr 3:852
18. Siegelman SS (1970) The radiology of osteoporosis. In: Brazel US (ed) Osteoporosis, Chapter 5, pp 68 – 79. Grune & Stratton, New York
19. Rosen G, Murphy ML, Huvos AG, Gutierrez M, Marcove RC (1976) Chemotherapy, en-block resection, and prosthetic bone replacement in the treatment of osteogenic sarcoma. Cancer 37:1 – 11
20. Dahlin DC, Unni KK (1977) Osteosarcoma of bone and its important recognizable varieties. Am J Surg Pathol 1:61 – 72
21. Siegelman SS (1977) Plasma Cell Dyscrasias. In: Jacobson HG, Murray RO (eds) The radiology of skeletal disorders 2nd ed. Churchill, Livingstone, Edinburgh London New York, pp 1923 – 1933
22. Wara WM, Phillips TL, Hill DR, Borill E Jr, Luk KH, Lichter AS, Leibel SA (1977) Desmoid tumors – treatment and prognosis. Radiology 124:225 – 226
23. Enzinger FM, Shiraki M (1967) Musculo-aponeuritic fibromatosis of the shoulder girdle (extra-abdominal desmoid). Cancer 20:1131 – 1140
24. Hill DR, Newman H, Phillips TL (1973) Radiation therapy of desmoid tumors. AJR 117:84 – 89
25. Siegelman SS, Levine S, Wolpin L (1968) Paget's disease with spinal cord compression. Clin Radiol 19:421 – 425
26. Rogers HM, Long DM, Chori SN, French LA (1971) Lipomas of the spinal cord and cauda equina. J Neurosurg 34:349 – 354

Computed Tomography in Bone Imaging

P. Wozney

General Electric Company, Medical Systems Division, Post Office Box 414, Milwaukee, WI 53201 (USA)

General Electric Medical Systems Division

Conventional radiography has imaged bone quite well for over 80 years. Until recently it seemed that computed tomography (CT), although quite valuable in imaging soft tissue, could contribute little to bone radiography. Recent developments, however, indicate that CT has unique value in at least three cases: analysis of bone mineral composition, imaging of minute bony structures, and surgical planning.

Metabolic bone disease, in particular postmenopausal osteoporosis, spurred interest in mineral content. The objective is that by careful measurement the degree of bone resorption can be quantified. This has two benefits. First, absolute measurements would aid in diagnosis. Second, serial measurements over time would allow one to determine if treatment is effective.

The analysis of bone mineral content has been studied extensively at the University of California, San Francisco (USA). Conventional methods, such as radial densitometry, have been disappointing in sensitivity and reproducibility. CT, however, has been shown to be reproducible to within 3% and markedly sensitive.

Prior to CT, the most accessible area for measuring bone mineral content was the peripheral skeleton, principally the radius. However, clinically the earliest and most significant mineral loss occurs in the axial skeleton, in particular the vertebrae.

The UCSF method of quantifying mineral content involves a CT section through the bodies of the first and second lumbar vertebrae. The mineral content of the cancellous portion of the vertebra is determined by comparing the CT number of the bone with external standard solutions of K_2HPO_4 (mineral equivalent), ethanol (fat), glycerol, and water. Long-term precision has been shown to be within 3%. Forty-seven oophorectomized women have been studied using this method. CT was more sensitive in determining bone mineral loss than three other commonly employed methods. When a very high degree of precision is required for diagnosis, dual energy scanning is employed. By measuring the CT number of the bone at 80 and 120 kVp, correction for fat content in the vertebra is possible.

The second major advance in bone CT is in imaging very small bones. Conventional tomograms of such structures as the inner ear are often blurred and difficult to interpret. With new computer postprocessing of the original CT data, resolution better that 0.75 mm is possible. With the addition of an increase in the CT number range from 1000 HU to +3000 HU, detail of the dense temporal bone can be imaged. The clinician can clearly visualize inner ear structures such as the auditory ossicles and assess their involvement in such processes as malignancy and cholesteatomas.

One would think that conventional radiography is quite adequate for evaluating fractures. However, the superposition of structures in projective images is often confusing to the surgeon. Axial CT images are an improvement, but lesions extending perpendicular to the slices are difficult to visualize. A better solution is reformatted images oriented in the natural plane of anatomical structures. This improves the evaluation of joints, particularly the sacroiliac joint, which is often implicated in lower back pain.

However, the surgeon does not operate on a flat picture. His patient exists in three dimensions (3-D). No matter how clever one is at stacking up slices or looking at flat projections, the solid object looks different. Recently 3-D computer reconstructions of facial bones and spines have been produced. Although clinical evaluation has just begun, surgeons have indicated great interest in actually seeing what they will operate on in three dimensions.

Radiology Today 1. Ed. by M. W. Donner and F. H. W. Heuck

References

1. Cann CE, Genant HK (1980) Precise Measurement of Vertebral Mineral Content Using Computed Tomography. J Comput Assist Tomogr
2. Cann CE, Genant HK, Young DR (1980) Comparison of Vertebral and Peripheral Mineral Losses in Dissuse Osteoporosis in Monkeys. Radiology 134:525 – 529
3. Genant HK, Boyd D (1977) Quantitative Bone Mineral Analysis Using Dual Energy Computed Tomography. Invest Radiol
4. Shaffer KA, Haughton VM, Wilson CR (1980) High Resolution Computed Tomography of the Temporal Bone. Radiology 134:409 – 414

Advances in Screens and Film

H. M. Cleare

Eastman Kodak Company, Receiving Department Kodak Park, 66 Eastman Avenue, Rochester, NY 14650 (USA)

Today, there is a new generation of X-ray screens based on modern phosphor technology that has advanced the state of the art of X-ray quantum utilization. This new generation may be more familiar to you by the name "rare earth" screens and is analogous in its impact to that of the cesium iodide input phosphor introduction in image intensifier tubes. Because of their atomic composition, the X-ray absorption of this class of phosphors is particularly high for the energy spectra commonly used in diagnostic radiology.

Also, as a class, they are dense phosphors, permitting screens of high absorption (35% – 60%) to be made without resorting to thick layers wherein light wanders laterally to reduce sharpness. These advantages lead directly to improved quantum utilization. That is, for a given optical image-forming capability (sharpness), screens of this type extract more of the quantum information from the incident X-ray image than do those of the previous generations. In fact, the improvement in quantum utilization can be nearly a factor of two. This leads directly to a number of alternative imaging advantages: improved subject contrast via lower kV, shorter exposure time to arrest motion, the use of smaller focal spots, lower peak capacity generators, less patient exposure, etc.

Yet another advantage of these phosphors is their high X-ray-to-light conversion efficiency, which can be as high as 18% or somewhat greater than half the theoretical maximum of 33%. As a reference, calcium tungstate's conversion efficiency is about 5%. This more than threefold increase in light energy generated can be used either to increase the speed of the screen-film-process combination or to improve the efficiency of silver utilization in the film.

Today's films also are in the process of evolution. Continuing research and development in emulsion technology has led to significant improvements in sensitivity of the photographic grain. These improvements, however, are seldom used to increase film speed. Increased *system* speed by way of increased film sensitivity has the disadvantage that fewer X-rays are used to form the recorded image, a direction found to be unacceptable except in certain specialized instances. Therefore, the innovations in emulsion technology have been used to improve silver utilization: smaller grains with enhanced light sensitivity improve the efficiency of

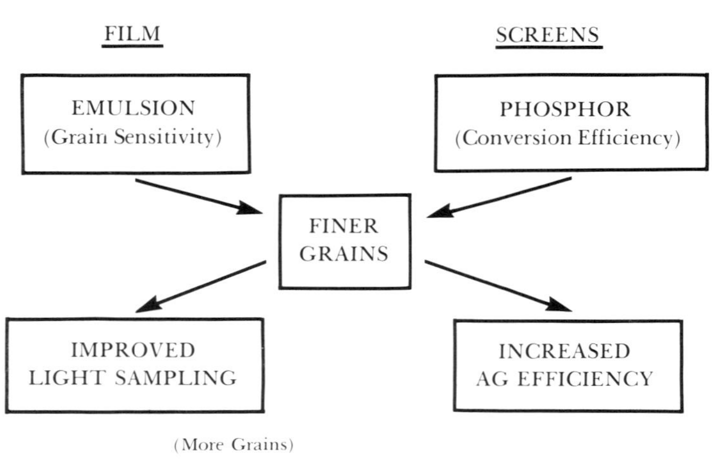

Fig. 1. Advances in technology

Radiology Today 1. Ed. by M. W. Donner and F. H. W. Heuck

the production of photographic film density (less Ag required per unit of density) while leading to an *increase* in the number of image receptor elements (i.e., grains) (see Fig. 1). When these emulsion innovations are coupled with screens of the "new generation" that convert more of the X-ray energy into light, yet further advances in silver efficiency are realized.

I have used the words "image receptor elements" or "photographic grains" to address what in today's electronic terminology would be described much differently. In truth, photographic grains are discrete, solid-state, photon detector/display elements with extremely high gain, typically in the order of 10^8, and with dimensions in the order of 1 μm. Film, then, is a large-scale array of binary, microminiature, solid-state elements with a packing density of about 10^9 per cm^2 (compared to about 10^5 for magnetic-bubble memory elements). In fact, film is a parallel data acquisition device which can be considered a high-capacity, programmable read-only memory (PROM). When used in conjunction with screens, it has a memory capacity of some 10^8 recorded binary bits per 35 × 43 cm sheet (see Fig. 2). Even so, the screen-film image receptor is being challenged on numerous fronts today by *other* electronics/solid-state-based systems such as digital subtraction fluoroscopy via image-intensifier/video technology or CT scan-radiography as well as complementary imaging modalities such as CT, nuclear medicine, ultrasound, and most recently, zeugmatography (NMR imaging). Nevertheless, I am firmly convinced that this century will not see the demise of screen-film radiography, although there will certainly be other electronic/solid-state imaging systems to add to the armamentarium of diagnostic imaging methods.

Grains	■ Binary photon detector elements ■ ~10^8 gain ■ ~1 μm diameter
Film	■ ~10^9 detectors/cm^2 ■ ~10^{12} detectors/35 × 43 cm ■ Parallel data acquisition
Film-Screens	■ Integrated detection/display ■ 10^8 bit "PROM" ■ 90 sec access (5/min)

Fig. 2. Film: A solid-state array device

Mammography

Mammography: Overview*

M. Friedrich

Klinikum Steglitz, Abteilung für Röntgendiagnostik, Hindenburgdamm 30, D-1000 Berlin 45

Over the past 20 years, mammography has evolved as a highly specialized discipline from the field of general radiography. Among the milestones on the way to modern soft tissue radiography were Egan's [5] introduction of the screenless industrial film as an image-recording system and the basic investigations of Gros [15] on the high soft tissue contrast of the characteristic radiation of a molybdenum target. This led to the development of the various well-known mammographic X-ray units in the early 1970s in Europe. Concurrently, in the United States, xeroradiography was inaugurated in the field of mammography by Wolfe. With increasing dose controversy in the United States in the early 1970s, the further development was characterized by a return to the concept of film-screen combinations as an image-recording system in mammography, the first such system being the Lo-Dose I system in 1972 [52]. Since then, the basic concept of conventional mammography has been repeatedly reviewed and is constantly being challenged by various innovations such as:

1. New selective filter techniques (K-edge filtering),
2. "High-resolution" film-screen combinations for mammography,
3. Grid mammography,
4. Microfocal spot mammography,
5. Electron radiography.

This list could easily be extended to include, for example, high-filtration xeroradiography, but I have restricted my choice to those aspects relevant to the European situation.

New Selective Filter Techniques (K-edge Filtering) [8, 17, 23–26, 50, 51]

Shortly after the general introduction of the radiation quality of a molybdenum target, it was recognized that this radiation, under the aspect of contrast vs dose, was optimal only for thin and fatty breasts [26, 32]. With thick and dense breasts there is considerable absorption of the softer molybdenum radiation component and, at the exit side of the object, an unfavorable double-peaked energy distribution of reduced contrast results (Fig. 1). According to some newer calculations,

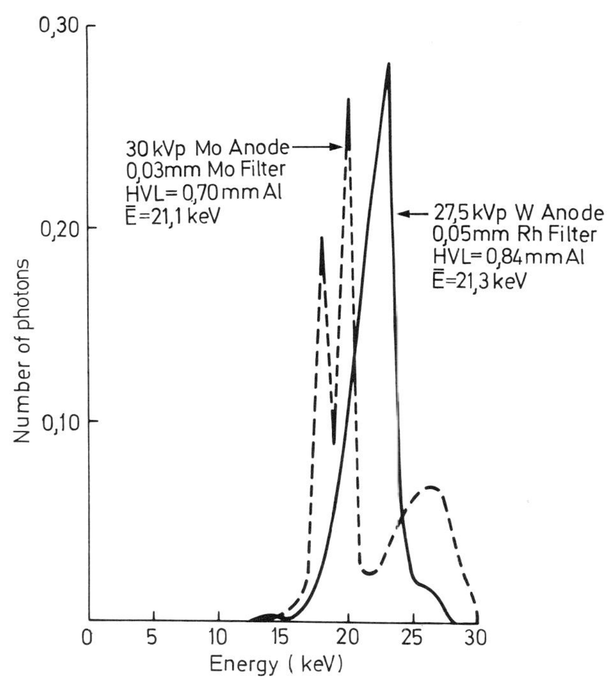

Fig. 1. Dashed line, spectrum from Mo anode tube operated at 30 kVp with 0.03-mm Mo filter. Solid line, spectrum from W anode tube operated at 27.5 kVp with 0.05-mm Rh filter. Both spectra after attenuation by 5-cm lucite phantom [23]

* Paper delivered to the audience of a postgraduate course "Radiology today", Salzburg, June 13th to 15th, 1980

Radiology Today 1. Ed. by M. W. Donner and F. H. W. Heuck

there are two basic guidelines concerning contrast efficiency of mammographic photon energy in relation to dose:

1. The optimal photon energy depends on object thickness. Optimal energy varies between 19 and 25 KeV for object thicknesses between 2.5 and 7.5 cm (Fig. 2).
2. A double-peaked energy distribution behind the object is far less favorable in view of dose than a single-peaked, approximately monochromatic energy band (Fig. 1).

A first suggestion, recommended for thick breasts, was to filter the molybdenum spectrum with 0.5 mm aluminum. Such filters are integrated in most modern mammographic units.

According to recent investigations of Jennings and Fewell [8, 23], through K-edge filtering of the spectrum of a tungsten target, the dose for thick objects can be almost halved with minimal reduction in radiation contrast. For instance, a rhodium-filtered tungsten spectrum shows, after passage through a 5-cm lucite phantom, a single-peaked energy distribution, instead of the unfavorable double-peaked spectrum of the conventional molybdenum anode (Fig. 1). In Table 1 the achievable image contrasts, expressed as a density difference ΔD, are opposed to the necessary average dose for the conventional and new beam qualities. It is apparent that for a 5.0-cm lucite phantom, the average dose with a rhodium-filtered tungsten spectrum is almost halved at more or less the same image contrast as the conventional molybdenum spectrum. There is no need to say that with thin objects (e.g., 2.5-cm lucite phantom) a molybdenum spectrum offers considerably more image contrast than the new filtering techniques.

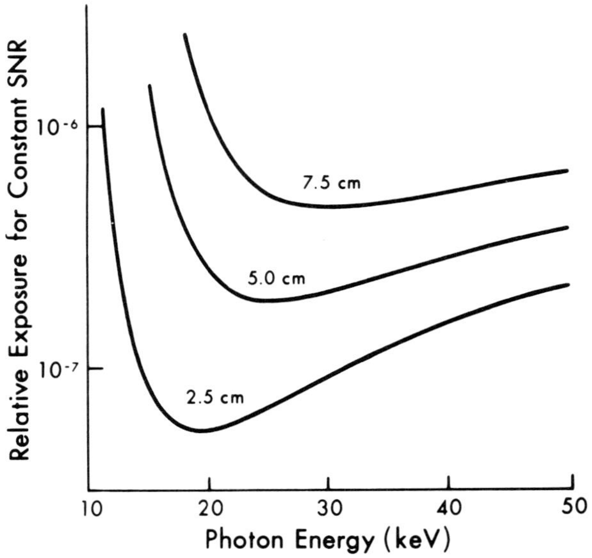

Fig. 2. Photon Energy versus signal to noise ratio for different object thicknesses (Lucite phantom)

Table 1. Relative contrast (density difference, ΔD) of different mammographic radiation qualities vs exposure X_m (mR) for two phantom thicknesses (2.5-cm and 5-cm lucite phantoms) [23]

Data for 2.5 cm lucite phantom

Anode	Filter	kVp	mAs	ΔD	X_m(mR)	X*(mR)
W	0.05 mm Rh	27.5	155	0.32	130	180
W	0.05 mm Pd	30	100	0.29	100	170
Mo	0.03 mm Mo	30	95	0.38	200	200
Mo	0.05 mm Rh	30	110	0.34	185	230
Mo	0.05 mm Pd	30	100	0.32	150	210

Data for 5.0 cm lucite phantom

Anode	Filter	kVp	mAs	ΔD	X_m(mR)	X*(mR)	Average dose (mrad)
W	0.45 mg/cm² Ru	27.5	1100	0.26	560	700	180
W	0.05 mm Rh	27.5	530	0.26	440	550	150
W	0.05 mm Pd	27.5	330	0.22	350	610	130
Mo	0.03 mm Mo	30	400	0.29	1000	1000	270
Mo	0.05 mm Rh	30	430	0.28	720	770	220
Mo	0.05 mm Pd	30	520	0.27	600	700	190
Mo	0.5 mm Al	35	60	0.16	300	990	100

In conclusion, we can say that the development of these new filtering techniques is as yet incomplete, and that it may hold much promise for dose reduction in the near future.

"High-resolution" Film-Screen Systems for Mammography [1, 22, 38, 47, 49]

The principal aims of all commercially available film-screen systems have been the following [52]:

1. High dose reduction factor (about 1/10th),
2. Rapid film processing, and
3. Large exposure latitude to warrant optimal visualization of the skin line and dense parenchymal structures.

Consequently, a film-screen system has been composed of a rapid processing single-coated film and newly developed high-resolution screens [41, 52]. As necessary and valuable as dose reduction in mammography may be, good image quality is just as essential for exact mammographic diagnosis [21, 31]. The significance of fine detail in mammograms [31, 33, 39] can be estimated from the fact that out of the group of 28 occult breast carcinomas [1], which were detected mainly through microcalcifications, in seven cases, i.e., 25%, the diagnosis was made exclusively on the basis of very tiny dustlike microcalcifications of about 200 μm diameter Table 2.

An experimental trial of all commercially available film-screen combinations for mammography, carried out in our clinic, showed that these systems fail to depict small microcalcifications and subtle malignant transformations of interstitial tissue septa with the same clarity as high-resolution screenless film (Fig. 3a, b). The investigations of Haus and co-workers [16] on image degradation by geometric unsharpness, which led to the inauguration of "long-cone" mammography, are not representative insofar as an unusually poor imaging geometry with a rapid processing low-quality screenless film was compared with commercial film-screen combination and long-cone technique.

The major deficiencies of the commercially available single-coated film-screen systems are, in our opinion [14]:

1. Poor image resolution
2. Poor contrast.

1 From the Breast Cancer Screening Program of Hamburg, directed by H. J. Frischbier

Therefore, 5 years ago, we opposed to these systems our own concept of a high-resolution film-screen combination for mammography (Fig. 3c, d), consisting of a panchromatic, double-coated, silver halide-rich, low-granularity industrial film on one of the commerically available high-resolution screens. Especially the panchromatic light-sensitive industrial X-ray films of the Cronex series from the Dupont Company proved successful. According to the practical mammographic situation, two system speeds and qualities are offered: the more sensitive system Cronex 75 with about $\frac{1}{8}$ and Cronex 70 with about $\frac{1}{4}-\frac{1}{5}$ of the dose of industrial film (Fig. 3c, d). In our opinion, the latter system (Cronex 70 on screen, Fig. 5d) offers a generally acceptable image quality, so that we would advocate its general use in mammography. In any case, with this system, the average glandular dose for a 2-view examination would be below 1 rad; with the system Cronex 75 on screen, below 0.5 rad.

In conclusion, we can say that the combination of a light-sensitive panchromatic industrial film on a high-resolution screen is, in the present situation, a good compromise between acceptable image quality and a dose reduction to between $\frac{1}{5}$ and $\frac{1}{8}$ of earlier values. Especially the reduced dose should add to a renewed general acceptance of mammography as a diagnostic and screening tool by the medical profession and public health authorities.

Grid Mammography [3, 4, 9–11, 13, 20, 27, 28, 29, 30, 40, 43, 44]

Two principal modifications of conventional mammographic technique have been developed and tried by various authors during the last 3 years: *grid mammography* [11, 13, 20, 27, 29, 30, 43, 44] and *magnification mammography* [18, 34, 46, 48].

The basic aim of grid mammography is to improve image contrast through elimination of scattered radiation; the goal of magnification mammography is to improve the imaging quality of high-speed film-screen systems for mammography.

The importance and image-degrading influence of scattered radiation in mammography has also been investigated by several authors [3, 9]. The scattered radiation, in mammography usually up to 50% of the image-forming radiation, essentially limits image contrast and the perceptibility of small detail,

Table 2. Size and distribution of microcalcification in 28 clinically occult carcinomas (breast cancer screening program, Hamburg) and "high-resolution" film-screen-system (5c, 5d)

No	Microcalcifications								Soft tissue structure			
	Characteristics of particles							Area of distribution Diameter	Circum-scribed density (cm)	Septa Spiculae Structural disrupture	Detectability with low-dose technique	
	Number (total)	Size			Shape	Density	Particles/ cm^2					
		>500 μ <1 Lp/ mm	500 – 250 μ 1 – 2 Lp/ mm	250 – 160 μ 2 – 3 Lp/ mm	a = amorph r = round i = irregular l = laminal	d = dense w = soft	[N/cm^2]	[cm]				
Σ_{21}^{27}	88 (100%)	13 (14.8%)	34 (36.6%)	41 (48.4%)				1,2 ± 0,8				
Σ_{1}^{27}	697 (100%)	171 (24.5%)	375 (54%)	151 (21.5%)				1,7 ± 1,0				
28	450	20	400	30	i	–	25	8 × 5	–	–	+	
Σ_{1}^{28}	1147 (100%)	191 (16.6%)	775 (67.5%)	181 (15.8%)			19 ± 23		7/28	10/28	21/28	7/28

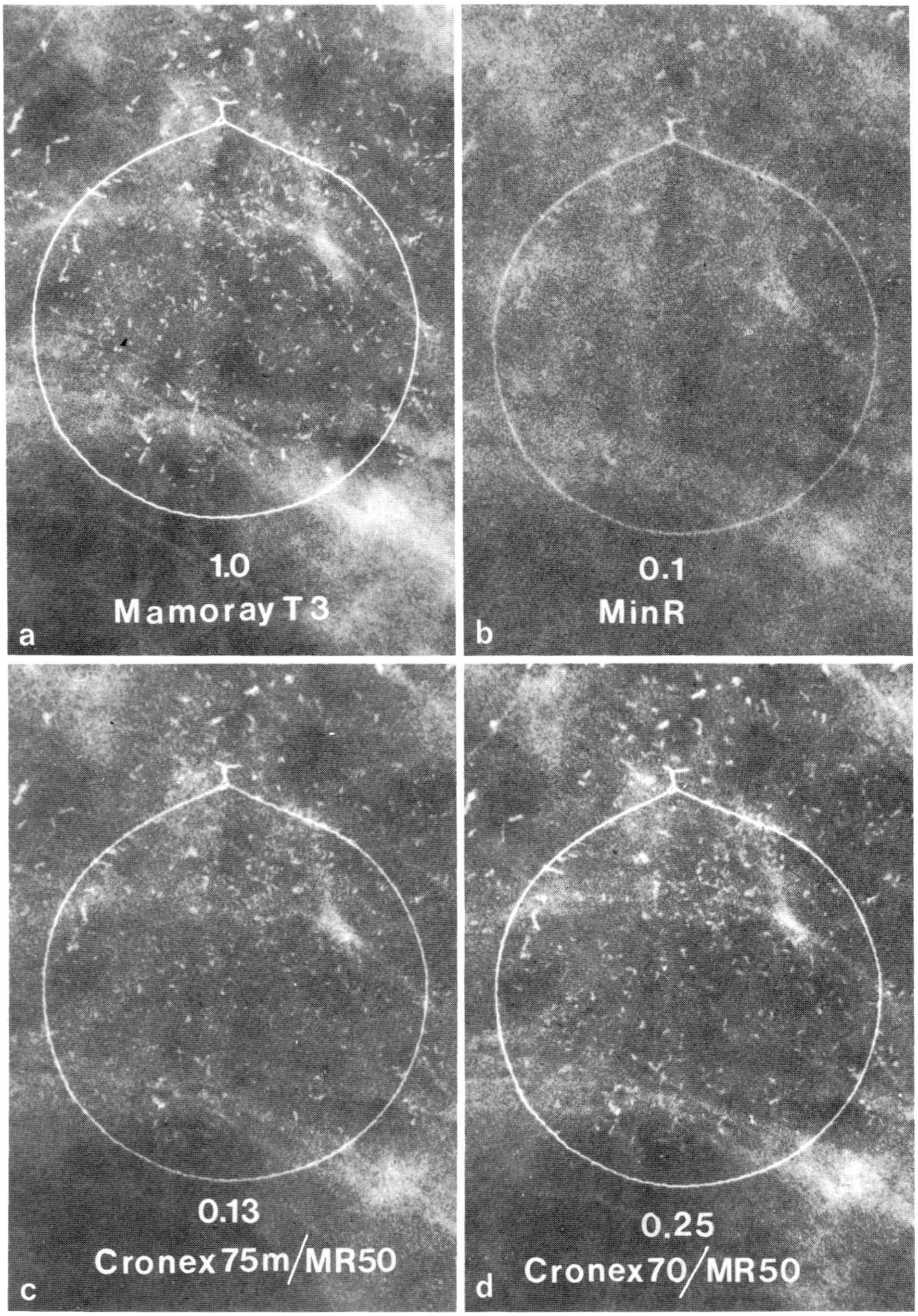

Fig. 3a – d. Detail views (5× magnification) of 80 – 200 micron, microcalcification on screenless film (5a), commercial film-screen-system (5b)

as, for example, microcalcifications and connective tissue septa. Relative scatter strongly depends on the object thickness and can effectively be reduced only by additional technical measures, such as use of a grid or increasing distance between object and film.

The development of grid mammography was carried out essentially during the years 1976 and 1977 in our department [11], the concept is now being adopted by the major European mammography manufacturers. A special soft radiation grid composed of 16 micron thin lead lamellae, a ratio of

1:5, and a high transmission of primary radiation over 90% proved optimal. For practical purposes, the grid mechanism (Fig. 4a, b) has to guarantee the following items:
1. Complete blurring of grid lamellae;
2. Maintenance of good imaging geometry, i.e., small distance between object and film;
3. Unimpaired compression of the breast and visualization down to the prepectoral region; and
4. Unimpaired automatic exposure control.

The technical problems of grid mammography are solved today. Fig. 4 shows the grid mechanism as it has been in daily use in our department for $2\frac{1}{2}$ years. A similar mechanism will be available shortly from all major mammographic manufacturers. The grid is focused at an FFD of 60 cm, thus improving image geometry in grid mammography over the conventional situation. As the mammograms of Fig. 5 show, the main advantages of grid mammography are:
1. Increased general image contrast with an impression of transparency and increased structural content of the image;
2. Better detail rendition, increased visibility of microcalcification; and
3. According to the speed of the image recording system, a dose reduction to $\frac{1}{2}$ or $\frac{1}{4}$ compared to industrial film [40].

The practical value and necessity of grid mammography has been established through clinical series in various hospitals and practices in Europe and the United States [20, 27, 29, 30, 43, 44].

Magnification (Microfocal Spot) Mammography [2, 13, 18, 29, 34, 46, 48]

As an alternate modification of conventional mammographic technique, microfocal spot mammography in conjunction with film-screen systems [18, 48] or Xerox image receptors [18, 46] has been investigated by various groups. Magnification mammography has several technical prerequisites (Fig. 6):
1. A microfocus which should be the same size as the smallest detail to be visualized, in mammography between 100 and 200 μm;
2. An additional mamma supporting tray; and
3. An FFD large enough for effective scatter suppression.

We used an experimental microfocal mammographic unit from Philips, with a molybdenum target and a measured focus of 0.18 × 0.22 mm.

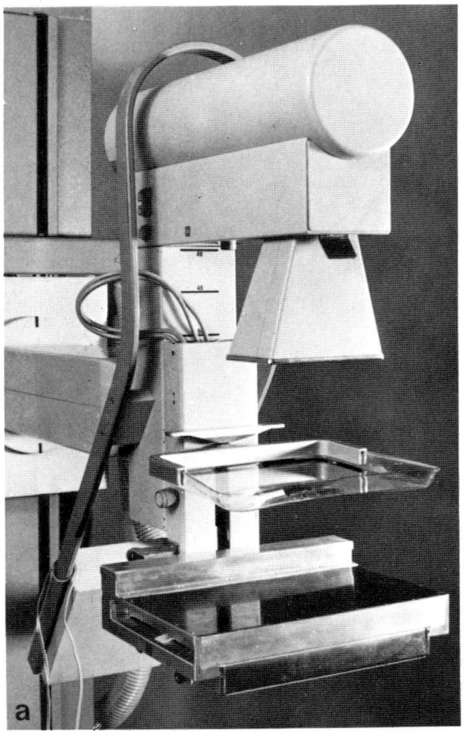

a

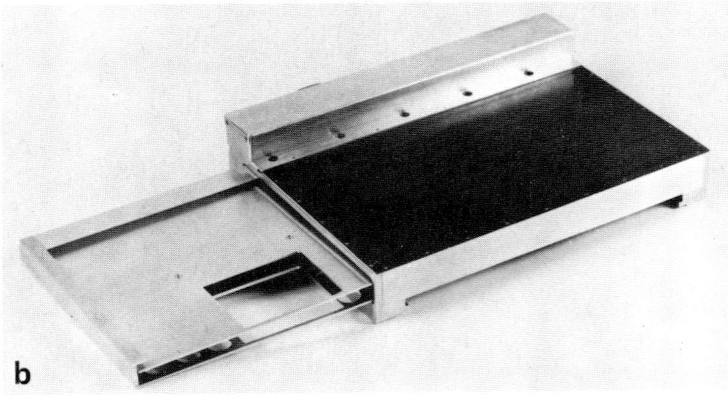

b

Fig. 4a, b. Grid mammography

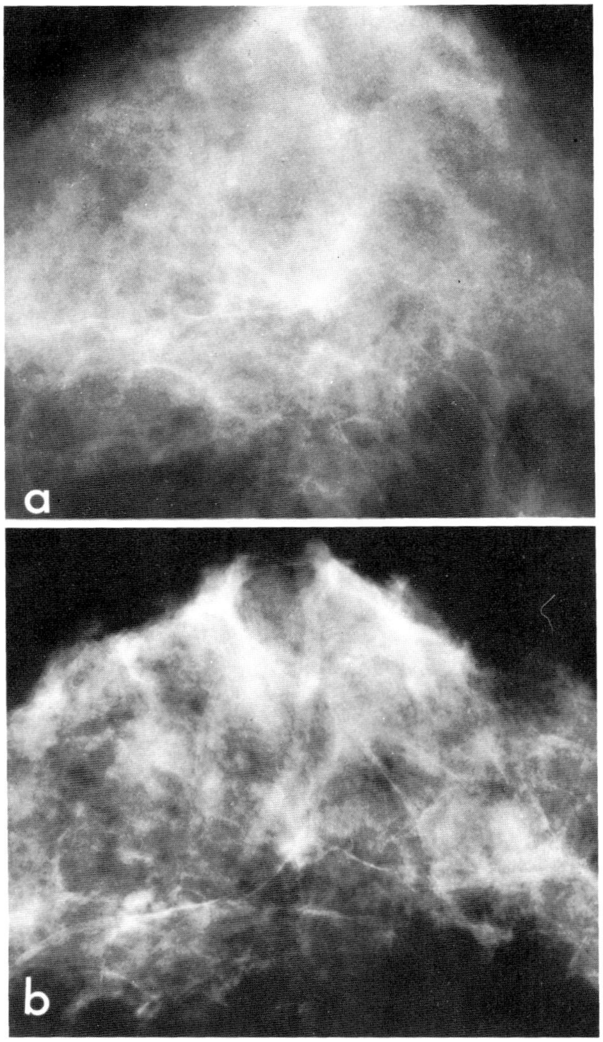

Fig. 5. **a** Conventional mammogram on screenless industrial film; 31 kVp; Mo anode tube; 0.03-mm Mo filter; rel. exposure: 1. **b** Mammogram as in a, with grid, on high-resolution film-screen system (Cronex 75m/MR50); radiation quality as in a; rel. exposure: 0.3

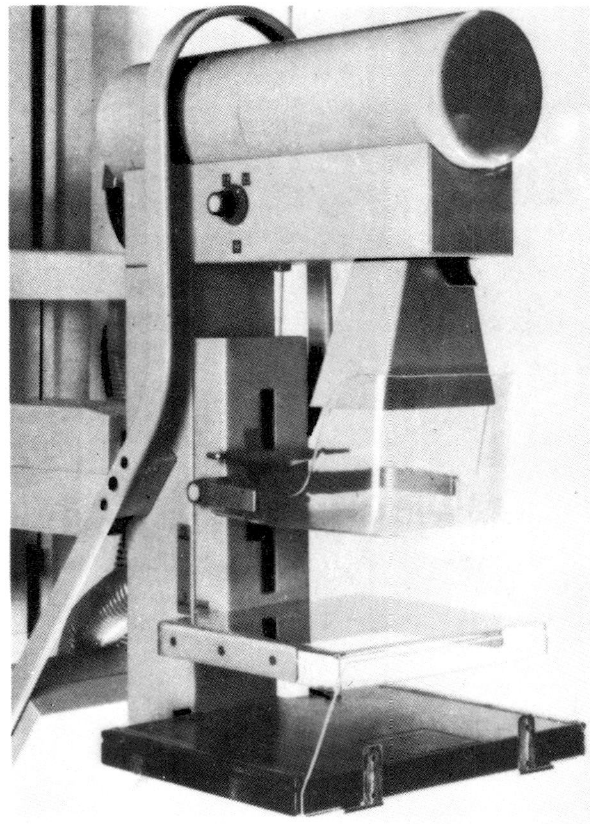

Fig. 6. Experimental microfocal spot mammography unit from Philips/C. H. F. Mueller. Rotating Mo anode; mesured 0.18 × 0.22 mm microfocus

The expected advantages of magnification mammography are:

1. Increased relative sharpness of high-speed film-screen systems through larger projection of details on the image recording system;
2. Reduced effective image noise due to the fact that more statistical imaging elements (e.g., film grains) participate in the visualization of a certain detail; and
3. Reduced scatter by air gap suppression.

As Muntz [37] has shown, scatter suppression through a fixed air gap is proportional to the overall FFD.

The value of magnification mammography is judged differently according to the individual imaging standard in comparison. As can be seen from Fig. 7, a two-fold magnification on a high-speed film-screen system can yield a considerably improved areal resolution and detail rendition, especially with high contrast detail. Also, the effective image noise is greatly diminished. However, this improvement is made at the expense of four times the exposure of the contact image, i.e. the overall speed of the imaging system is considerably slowed down. Because of the higher kV necessary for sufficient emission of the microfocus, the general image contrast is worse in magnification mammography, especially with film-screen systems. Therefore, it remains to be asked whether with a low-speed, high-resolution film-screen system it would not be possible to obtain image results similar to those obtained with the magnification technique.

In a clinical trial on microfocal spot mammography using the RSI-magnification unit, Sickles [46] found that the improved image quality of magnification technique in comparison to film-

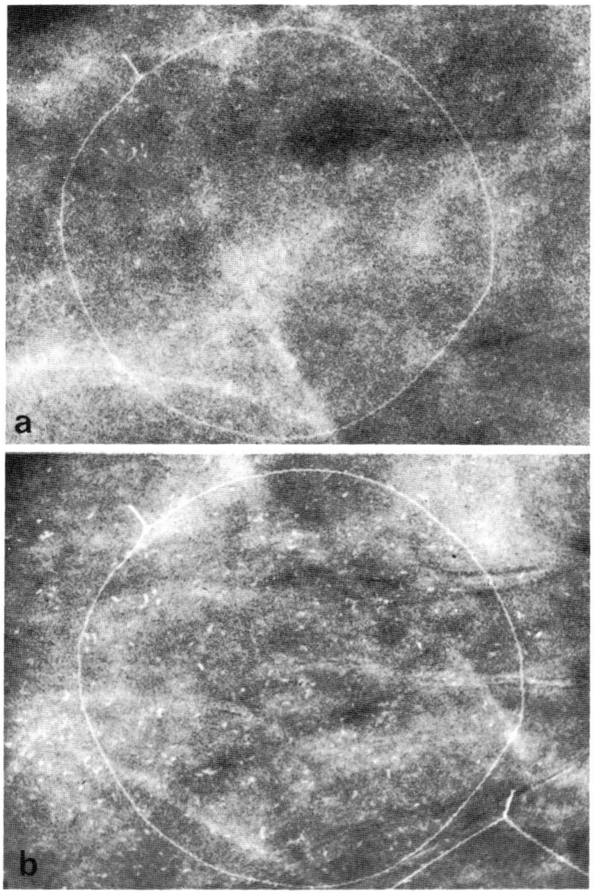

Fig. 7. **a** Microcalcifications on film-screen system (Cronex 75m/MR50); FOD, 3 cm; FFD, 45 cm; contact technique; rel. exposure: 0.13. **b** Microcalcifications as in a, on same film-screen system, with 2 × magnification; improved areal resolution; decreased image noise; rel. exposure: 4 × 0.13 = 0.52

screen mammography resulted in a better diagnostic differentiation between benign and malignant lesions, which remained equivocal to a larger extent with conventional film-screen mammography (Table 3). However, this result confirms our contention about the unsatisfactory imaging properties of high-speed film-screen systems, as well as the diagnostic significance of such inferior image quality. It demonstrates the interference of poor mammographic image quality and diagnostic accuracy.

The advantages and drawbacks of magnification mammography can be summarized in that the value of magnification technique increases in proportion to the deficiencies of the original image-recording system. On an absolute scale it should yield an image quality comparable to high-resolution mammography. However, for practical use it

Table 3. Diagnostic interpretations with pathologic correlation for the 216 biopsy-proved cases

Mammographic diagnosis		
Conventional	Conventional + magnification	Pathologic diagnosis
49 benign	37 benign	35 benign, 2 malignant
	7 equivocal	5 benign, 2 malignant
	5 malignant	5 malignant
145 equivocal	48 benign	48 benign
	56 equivocal	39 benign, 17 malignant
	41 malignant	1 benign, 40 malignant
22 malignant	22 malignant	22 malignant

seems questionable whether the drawbacks of magnification mammography such as larger film formats, more difficult patient positioning, and increased motion blur are compensated by its advantages so as to justify its general use.

Electron Radiography (XERG Mammography, Xonics)

Electron radiography makes use of the electric ions generated during absorption of X-rays in solid, liquid, or gaseous materials. Its proper denomination would be ionography. Its principle has been known and repeatedly investigated in various experimental sets during the last 3 decades [6, 7, 11, 19, 23, 33, 35, 36, 42, 43, 45].

We had the opportunity to do some experimental runs with the XERG system [14], marketed by Xonics, which is a high-pressure gas-ionographic system adapted for mammography. As shown in Fig. 8, a transparent, previously electrically discharged polyester sheet is inserted into a high-pressure ionization imaging chamber. The base and top of the imaging chamber are formed as electrodes for acceleration of the generated ions in the chamber onto the electroneutral polyester sheet. Thus, an electrostatic image is generated, which, after removal from the imaging chamber, can be developed in an electrophoretic liquid toner bath and preserved by polyester lamination. As a result, one gets a transparent negative X-ray image, quite

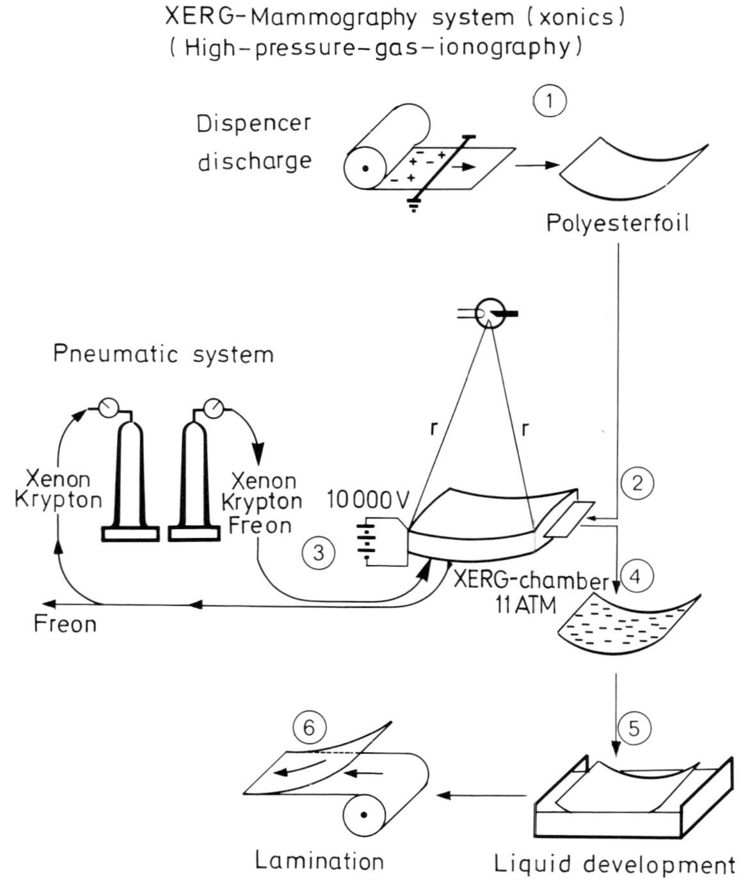

Fig. 8. XERG-mammography system (xonics)

similar to a normal X-ray, but with excellent image contrast and a moderate edge effect (Fig. 9).

The main advantage of this system for mammography is its extreme sensitivity, depending on the electrostatic settings of the machine. As a contact technique, we needed less than $\frac{1}{20}$ of the normal dose of industrial film.

However, besides these advantages of high sensitivity and good image contrast, the system offers only moderate detail rendition because of the limited resolving power of the imaging chamber and a high quantum noise level (Fig. 10). Thus, although various investigators in the United States have found a favorable comparison between XERG mammography and high filtration Xero mammography [41] and comparable quality with film-screen system [18] (Fig. 5b), on the basis of our experience we feel that XERG mammography would not wholly fulfil our European quality standards.

However, in the modification of a 1.5-fold magnification technique, the above-mentioned drawbacks of image noise and limited resolution are easily overcome and an excellent image quality is achieved at $\frac{1}{10}$ the dose of industrial film (Fig. 13b). This quality should be wholly acceptable in Europe too, and seems to be the best compromise between image quality and dose possible with present technology.

Conclusions

1. During recent years, conventional mammography has undergone various technical innovations, the most important being *grid mammography, microfocal spot mammography,* and the use of *high-quality film-screen combinations.*
2. For the near future, the at present still experimental K-edge filtering techniques offer much promise in a further reduction of dose, without compromising image quality.
3. The introduction of a totally new image-recording system, such as XERG electron-radio-

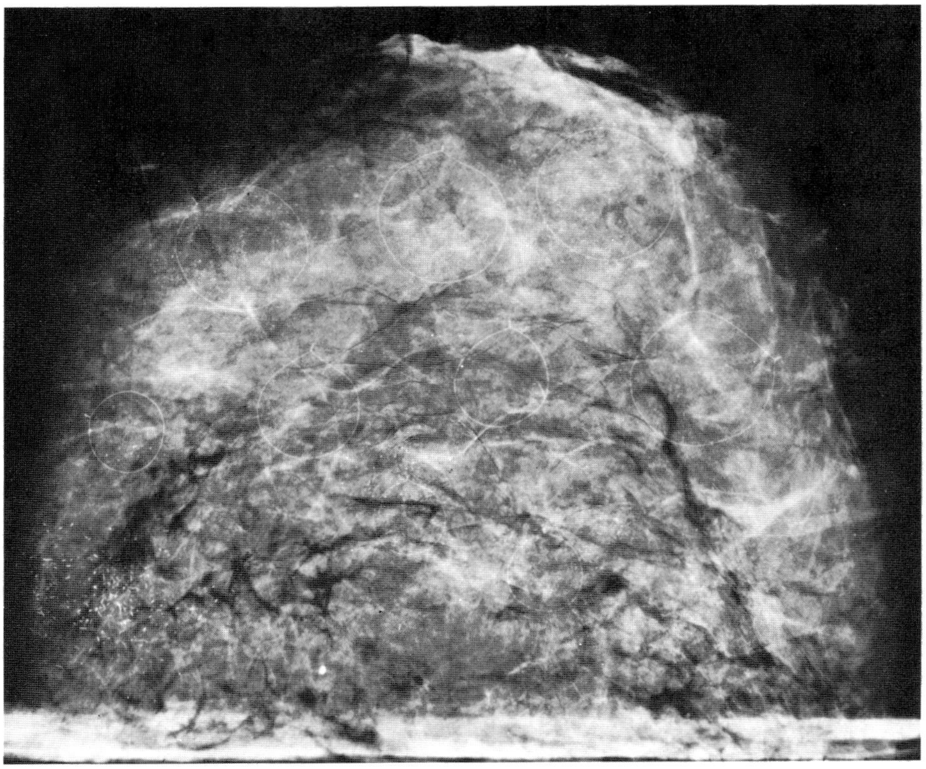

Fig. 9. Electron radiogram (XERG mammogram) of breast phantom; 1.5-fold magnification technique

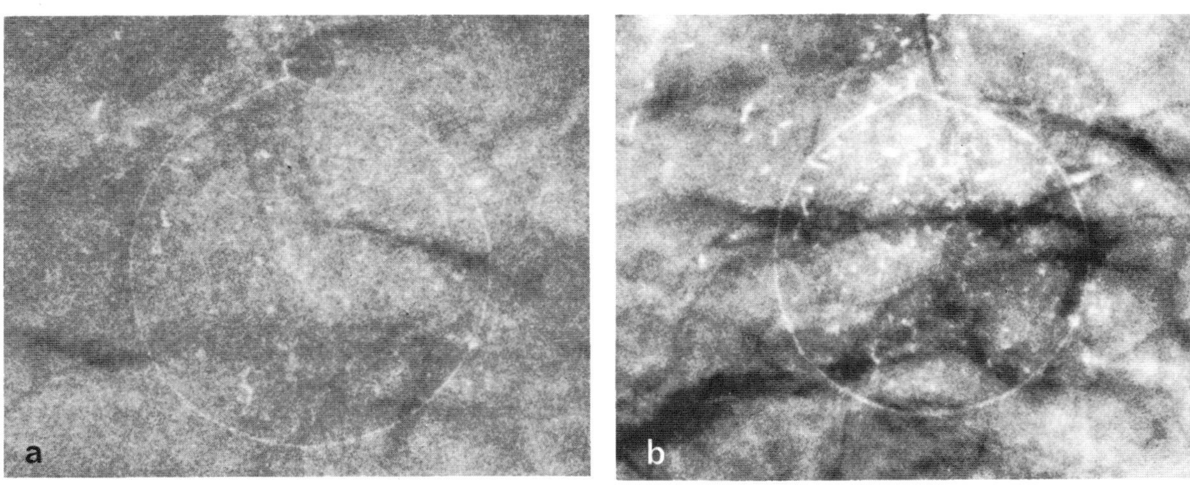

Fig. 10. a Xerg mammogram in contact technique; same detail view as Fig. 5a – d. Rel. exposure: 0.045. **b** Xerg mammogram, 1.5-fold magnification technique; same detail view as Fig. 5a – d. Rel. exposure: 0.1

graphy, opens up a new field of technology for low-dose mammographic imaging, whose future potential cannot yet be wholly estimated.

References

1. Arnold BA, Webster EW, Kalisher L (1978) Evaluation of Mammographic screen-film systems. Radiology 129:179 – 185
2. Arnold BA, Eisenberg H, Bjarngard B (1979) Magnification mammography: a low-dose technique. Radiology 131:743 – 749
3. Barnes GR, Brezovich IA (1978) The intensity of scattered radiation in mammography. Radiology 126:243 – 247
4. Barnes GT, Kleare M, Brezovich IA (1976) Reduction of scatter in diagnostic radiology by means of a scanning multiple slit assembly. Radiology 120:691 – 694
5. Egan RA (1964) Mammography. Thomas, Springfield Illinois
6. Fenster A, Johns HE (1974) Liquid ionography for diagnostic radiology. Med Phys 1/5:262 – 265
7. Fenster A, Plewes D, Johns HE (1974) Efficiency and resolution of ionography in diagnostic radiology. Med Phys 1/1:1 – 10
8. Fewell TR, Shuping RE (1978) A comparison of mammographic X-ray spectra. Radiology 128: 211 – 216
9. Friedrich M (1975) Der Einfluß der Streustrahlung auf die Abbildungsqualität bei der Mammographie. ROEFO 123/6:556 – 566
10. Friedrich M (1977) Bildqualität in der Mammographie, Einfluß der Streustrahlung und der Bildaufzeichnungssysteme. ROEFO 36:4 – 11
11. Friedrich M (1978) Neuere Entwicklungstendenzen der Mammographie-Technik: Die Raster-Mammographie. ROEFO 128/2:207 – 222
12. Friedrich M, Weskamp P (1978) New modalities in mammographic imaging: comparison of grid and magnification techniques. Medicamundi 23/1: 29 – 46
13. Friedrich M, Weskamp P (1979) A comparison of direct film mammography with screen film mammography. In: Logan WW, Muntz EP (eds) Reduced dose mammography. Masson, New York, pp 171 – 193
14. Friedrich M (1979) Ionographie: Mammographie-System der Zukunft? MMW 121/26:870 – 873
15. Gros CM (1967) Méthodologie. J Radiol Electrol Med Nucl 48:638 – 665
16. Haus AG, Doi K, Chiles JT, Rossmann K, Mintzer RA (1975) The effect of geometric and recording system unsharpness in mammography. Invest Radiol 10:43 – 52
17. Haus AG, Metz CE, Chiles JT, Rossmann K (1976) The effect of X-ray spectra from molybdenum and tungsten target tubes on image quality in mammography. Radiology 118:705 – 709
18. Haus AG, Paulus DD, Dodd GD, Cowart RW, Bencomo J (1979) Magnification mammography: Evaluation of screen film and xeroradiographic techniques. Radiology 133:223 – 226
19. Hirschfeld RL (1979) Xerg and low-dose mammography: A comparative clinical study. In: Logan WW, Muntz EP (eds) Reduced dose mammography. Masson, New York, pp 395 – 405
20. Hoeffken W, Jötten G, Richter D (1977) A new method for reducing radiation exposure and improving the image quality in mammography. Medicamundi 22/2:61 – 64
21. Hüppe JR, Schneider H-J (1977) Zur Frage des richtigen Mammographiefilms. Radiologe 17: 195 – 196
22. Jahns RG, Butler PF, McCrohan JL, Thompson WE (1979) The status of film/screen mammography. Radiology 132:197 – 200
23. Jennings RJ, Fewell TR (1979) Filters-photon energy control and patient exposure. In: Logan WW, Muntz EP (eds) Reduced dose mammography. Masson, New York, pp 211 – 222
24. Johns HE, Fenster A, Plewes D, Boag JW, Jeffery PN (1974) Gas ionization methods of electrostatic image formation in radiography. Br J Radiol 47:519 – 529
25. Johnson GA, O'Foghludha F (1978) An experimental "trans-molybdenum" tube for mammography. Radiology 127:511 – 516
26. Kyser K Röntgenspektrometrische und röntgendosimetrische Untersuchungen der Strahlenqualitäten für Weichstrahlaufnahmen. ROEFO 116/6: 818 – 823
27. Lammers W, Kuhn H (1979) Verbesserte Bildqualität in der Mammographie durch Streustrahlenraster. Electromedica 47/1:2 – 10
28. Logan WW, Muntz EP (eds) (1979) Reduced dose mammography. Masson, New York
29. Logan WW, Stanton L (1979) Grid versus magnification use in clinical mammography. In: Logan WW, Muntz EP (eds) Reduced dose mammography. Masson, New York
30. Luska G, Nüsslin F, Wagner HH (1979) Klinische Erfahrungen mit der Raster-Mammographie. ROEFO 131/4:349 – 355
31. Menges V, Wellauer J, Engeler V, Stadelmann R (1973) Korrelation zahlenmäßig erfaßter Mikroverkalkungen auf dem Mammogramm und dadurch diagnostizierter Carcinome und Mastopathietypen. Radiologe 13:468 – 476
32. Mika N, Reiss KH (1968) Optimierung der Röntgenbelichtungstechnik mit Hilfe der Halbleiterspektrometrie. Roentgenpraxis 21:164 – 174
33. Millis RR, Davis R, Stacey AJ (1976) The detection and significance of calcifications in the breast: a radiological and pathological study. Br J Radiol 49: 12 – 26
34. Muntz EP, Logan WW (1979) Focal spot size and scatter suppression in magnification mammography. AJR 133:453 – 459

35. Muntz EP, Welkowsky MS (1977) Characteristics of quantum statistics limited electrostratic imaging in mammography. In: Logan WW (ed) Breast carcinoma: the radiologist's expanded role. Wiley & Sons
36. Muntz EP, Lewis J, Azzarelli T, Welkowsky M, Morsell AL, Kaegi E, Jacobson G (1975) On the characteristics of electron radiographic images in diagnostic radiology. S.P.I.E. 56:208–223
37. Muntz EP, Welkowsky M, Kaegi E, Morsell L, Wilkinson E, Jacobson G (1978) Optimization of electrostatic imaging systems for minimum patient dose or minimum exposure in mammography. Radiology 127:517–523
38. Muntz EP, Wilkinson E, George FW (1980) Mammography at reduced doses: present performance and future possibilities. AJR 134:741–747
39. Murphy WA, DeSchryver-Kecskemeti K (1978) Isolated clustered microcalcifications in the breast: radiologic-pathologic correlation. Radiology 127: 335–341
40. Nüsslin F (1979) Dosismessungen bei der Rastermammographie. ROEFO 130/3:351–355
41. Ostrum BJ, Becker W, Isard HJ (1973) Low-dose mammography. Radiology 109:323–326
42. Porrath SA (1979) Xerg mammography. A review of sixteen months experience plus a comparison with xerography. In: Logan WW, Muntz EP (eds) Reduced dose mammography. Masson, New York
43. Schreer I, Würthner K (1980) Ergebnisse aus dem klinischen Einsatz eines Raster-Mammographie-Gerätes. ROEFO 43:25–27
44. Schreer I, Demelt M, Würthner K (1978) Phantomuntersuchungen und erste klinische Erfahrungen an einem Raster-Mammographiegerät. ROEFO 129: 357–363
45. Seelentag WW (1978) Entwicklungstendenzen in der Ionographie. ROEFO 129:118–125
46. Sickles EA (1979) Microfocal spot magnification mammography using xeroradiographic and screen-film recording systems. Radiology 131:599–607
47. Sickles EA, Genant HK (1979) Controlled single-blind clinical evaluation of low-dose mammographic screen-film systems. Radiology 130:347–351
48. Sickles EA, Doi K, Genant HK (1977) Magnification film mammography: image quality and clinical studies. Radiology 125:69–76
49. Sickles EA, Genant HK, Doi K (1978) Laboratory and controlled clinical evaluations of the image properties of mammographic screen-film systems. J App Phot Eng 4:139–142
50. Siedband MP (1979) System specifications for reduced dose mammography. In: Logan WW, Muntz EP (eds) Reduced dose mammography. Masson, New York
51. Siedband MP, Jennings RJ, Eastgate RJ, Ergun DL (1977) X-ray beam filtration for mammography. S.P.I.E. 127:204–207
52. Weiss JP, Wayrynen RE (1976) Imaging system for low-dose mammography. J App Phot Eng 2:7–10

Bibliography

1. Barth V, Bosnjakovic S, Bach D (1978) Voraussetzungen für ein optimales Mammogramm. Gynäkologe 11:23–28
2. Frischbier HJ, Gregl A, Hoeffken W, Hüppe JR (1977) Vorschläge zur Qualitätsnormierung der Mammographie. Radiologe 17:193–194
3. Hagemann G, Knedel H, Weberling R (1978) Neue Verstärkerfolien in der klinischen Radiologie. III. Mitteilung: Folien-Film-Systeme für die Mammographie. ROEFO 129/2:260–265
4. Hüppe JR, Schneider HJ (1977) Qualitätsprobleme der Mammographie. Vermeidbare Fehler bei Anfertigung und Betrachtung von Mammogrammen. Radiologe 17:197–202
5. John V, Ewen K, Kurz E, Teske HJ (1978) Wertigkeit verschiedener Mammographie-Aufzeichnungssysteme bezogen auf Strahlenexposition und Informationsgehalt. Strahlentherapie 154:101–106
6. Kindl P, Spreizer H, Schneider G (1978) Dosismessungen bei Untersuchungen mit dem Mammomat. Electromedica 1:28–31
7. Kuhn H (1977) Optimierung der Aufnahmebedingungen in der Mammographie. Electromedica 45/2: 31–38
8. Kuhn H, Stahl J (1979) Bildgüte und Dosisbedarf in der Mammographie. Röntgenpraxis 32:18–28
9. Panzer W, Drexler G, Widenmann L, Platz L (1978) Spektren und Dosiswerte in der Mammographie. GSF-Bericht, p 518
10. Paterok EM, Säbel M, Weishaar J, Willgeroth F (1978) Vergleich verschiedener mammographischer Aufnahmetechniken an frisch amputierten Brüsten. ROEFO 129:103–109
11. Richter B, Rausch L (1977) Gegenüberstellung von Risiko, Kosten und Nutzen der Mammographie. Betriebl Strahlenschutz aus ärztl Sicht. Hrsg.: Rausch L u.a., G. Thieme
12. Richter B, Rausch L (1977) Abwägung von Nutzen, Kosten und Risiko bei der Mammographie. In: Messerschmidt O u.a. (ed) Vorsorgemedizin und Strahlenschutz (Risiko) Nutzen-Analyse. G. Thieme, Stuttgart
13. Säbel M, Paterok EM, Weishaar J, Willgeroth F (1977) Untersuchung zur Bildgüte bei der Film- und Xero-Mammographie. 1. Mitteilung: Wiedergabe kleiner Strahlenkontraste. ROEFO 126:529–536
14. Weissleder H, Kiefer H (1977) Mammographie mit minimaler Strahlendosis. ROEFO 126: 520–528
15. Willgeroth F, Paterok EM, Säbel M, Weishaar J (1980) Untersuchungen zur Bildgüte bei der Film- und Xeromammographie. ROEFO 132/4: 433–437
16. Würthner K (1978) Kritische Bemerkungen zu Risikoberechnungen bei der Mammographie. Rö-Bl 31: 318–322

Vacuum and Inflatable Contured Liquid Crystal Flexi-Therm* Contact Thermography

P. H. Meyers

401 Emerald Street, New Orleans, LA 70124 (USA)

Liquid crystal vacuum contoured thermography using Flexi-therm elastomeric film is an inexpensive, noninvasive, nonionizing imaging modality which can be used as the highest risk indicator for breast and other diseases.
Gautherie and Gros [1] state:
Thermography makes a significant contribution to the evaluation of patients suspected of having breast cancer. The obviously abnormal thermogram carries with it a high risk of cancer. This report summarizes the results of patients with questionable or stage THIII thermograms. From approximately 58,000 patients examined between August 1965 and June 1977, most of whom had breast complaints, a group of 1,245 women were diagnosed at initial examination as either normal or benign disease by conventional means, including physical examination, mammography, sonography, and fine needle aspiration or biopsy, when indicated, but nevertheless categorized as stage THIII indicating a questionable thermal anomaly. Within 5 years more than $\frac{1}{3}$ of the group had histologically confirmed cancers. The more rapidly growing lesions with shorter doubling time usually show progressive thermographic abnormalities consistent with the increased metabolic heat production associated with such cancers. Thermography is useful not only as a risk for cancer but also to assess more rapidly growing neoplasms.

Flexi-therm Mark II System

The Flexi-therm Mark II System [2, 3] is a new tool for the clinician: a unique elastomeric thermally sensitive film that can be readily inflated and then contoured to body parts to display the thermal patterns of the body. It produces a crisp, clear, full color thermal pattern and is simple to operate. It can be set up in almost any convenient location, is inexpensive and reliable. It is a safe, nonionizing, noninvasive technique for measuring skin temperatures.
Thermography is the pictorial representation of the heat radiating from the skin. Flexi-therm inflatable system is a new form of contact thermography that involves liquid crystals [4, 5, 6] imbedded in flexible transparent elastomeric sheets which may be contoured to any part of the body. A new physiologic method of performing thermography with these liquid crystal Flexi-therm sheets is presented.
Thermal and vascular pathology is accentuated with rich, high contrast, thermographically calibrated color patterns.
Flexi-therm is a recent development in advanced liquid crystal technology. This technology makes it possible to make thermally sensitive cholesteric crystals and incorporate them into a stable, elastomeric system that can be readily stretched to the contours of the body and maintained in place by an inflatable film mounted in an air-tight Plexiglass box.
Each Flexi-therm film is designed to respond to a selective temperature threshold, enabling the clinican to choose the appropriate range for the individual patient.
The Flexi-therm Mark II System measures skin temperatures in: breast diseases [2, 3, 7], vascular diseases peripheral [7, 8, 9, 10] and cerebral [8, 9, 11, 12], headache [13, 14] rheumatic diseases [1, 5, 16], skin diseases [9, 17] peripheral thermographic manifestations of lumbar disk disease and nerve root injuries with subsequent change in the segmental dermatome heat patterns [18, 8], musculoligamentous injury [9, 18, 19], sports trauma [20], phlebitis [8, 9], and over the thyroid [21], parathyroid [22] and, scrotum [23].

---

* Flexi-Therm Incorporated, 117 Magnolia Avenue, Westbury, NY 11590 (USA)

Radiology Today 1. Ed. by M. W. Donner and F. H. W. Heuck

The Flexi-therm liquid crystal contact thermographic system is applied in the following manner: each Flexi-therm inflatable balloon is designed to respond to a selective temperature range. The Flexi-therm inflatable balloon box is blown up with air and is distended with just five to six compressions of a foot pump which transmits the air through a plastic tube attached to an air valve. To determine the correct Flexi-therm inflatable ballon box. The mid-range box is placed on the contour of the body to be examined. If the colors that appear are in the blue-green range, the Flexi-therm system is in too low a range: use the next higher range. If the colors are tan or brown, use the next lower range. Once the correct Flexi-therm balloon box is selected, one can study the symmetric or asymmetric skin temperature patterns and vascular patterns.

Remember that the Flexi-therm balloon box can be placed anywhere on the skin surface and contoured to the body part of a desired optimal skin temperature reading of that particular body part. The examiner looks through the Plexiglass box to visualize the color response of the skin thermal pattern. The examiner can always cool down the skin surface by a simple spray of alcohol on the skin surface, with cooling afterwards of the skin surface by evaporation or by the use of a hand-held fan.

Skin temperature comparisons can be made, such as comparing the skin surface temperatures of both hands on a single Flexi-therm balloon box. This can be done on any part of the body, such as the toes, ankles, legs, knees, and thighs, simultaneously viewing both extremities and determining if there are asymmetric patterns.

Wexler [18] has demonstrated that thermography provides an objective method of recording the activity of inflammations, tissue trauma, and segmental dermatome irritation. Ring [15, 16] shows that in arthritis repeated thermographic examinations often clearly demonstrate the effect of therapy before it becomes clinically evident.

Ritchie, Lapayowker, and Soulen [19] and others have shown that thermography in peripheral vascular disease such as thrombophlebitis, varicose veins, arteriosclerosis obliterans, and deep vein thromboses show abnormal asymmetric heat patterns. Thermography is specifically useful due to the fact that the thermal patterns associated with these vascular problems can be correlated with the patient's clinical examination and history.

Boyle et al. [11] and Capistrant [12] have shown the usefulness of thermographic facial patterns in occlusive disease of the carotid artery. Boyle and Capistrant have shown that in internal carotid artery stenosis or occlusion, there is decreased blood flow through the ophthalmic artery and through the supraorbital branches of the ophthalmic artery, causing an area of relative coolness of the skin in the supraorbital region of the affected side as compared to the corresponding opposite side.

Arterial insufficiency can be demonstrated by their thermographic patterns in patients with known peripheral vascular disease and following the course of therapy in patients receiving vasodilators and thrombolytic agents. This has been described in papers by Holm et al. [24].

Raskin [9] has shown that thermography can be used to detect positive patch test results as early as 6 h after the application of the allergen to the skin.

Recent papers on the use of thermography for evaluation of the extent of skin cancers, burns, viability of skin grafts, and pressure sores are available [17, 8, 9].

The medical literature shows that thermography of the thyroid [21] can be clinically useful when performed in conjunction with radionuclide scans.

Recent papers by Jones and Hendry [23] show the usefulness of thermographic examination of the scrotum in evaluating varicosities of the scrotum.

Lelik and Kezy [20] show the usefulness of contact thermography in sports medicine; Ching and Wexler [18] demonstrate that thermography is extremely useful in the objective evaluation of acute musculoligamentous injury and have demonstrated peripheral thermographic manifestations of lumbar disk disease, especially when roentgenograms are normal.

Conclusion

The Mark II System is a new, noninvasive, nonionizing, physiologic method of performing thermography; the Flexi-therm TM inflatable medical thermographic system is easy to use, inexpensive, and measures skin temperatures. Numerous recent articles in the medical literature demonstrate how thermography in thermal patterns correlated with the patient's clinical history, physical examination, and other laboratory tests can help in aiding the diagnosis; one can study thermal changes associated with physiologic functions or reactions and obtain the skin thermal effects of pharmacodynamic substances such as vasoactive drugs, cutaneous tests, vasomotor and immunological and hormonal responses.

Mark II System TM is designed to provide you with an instant color photographic record of the patient during the examination.

With specific reference to the breast, vacuum contoured liquid crystal Flexi-therm contact thermography will help you:

1. To identify those high-risk patients who require mammograms for correlation or clarification.
2. To examine younger patients.
3. When you need a deciding factor to initiate a biopsy where palpatory and/or mammographic findings were equivocal.
4. To identify low-risk patients for periodic clinical observation and establish follow-up procedures.
5. As a prepalpation test to attract attention to areas of increased heat emission which may harbor malignant foci.
6. To identify high-risk patients who would require follow-up breast profiles.
7. To identify patients with inflammatory carcinomas which may require special treatment.
8. To follow-up on patients with treated breast cancer to detect new tumor development.

References

1. Gautherie M, Gros C (1980) Breast thermography and cancer risk prediction. Cancer 45:51 – 56
2. Pochaczevsky R, Meyers P (1979) Vacuum contoured, liquid crystal dynamic breast thermoangiography as an aid to mammography in the detection of breast cancer. Clin Radiol 30: 405 – 411
3. Pochaczevsky R, Meyers P (1979) The value of vacuum contoured liquid crystal, dynamic breast thermoangiography. Acta Thermographica 4/1: 8 – 16
4. Fergason J (1968) Liquid crystals in nondestructive testing. Appl Opt 7:1729 – 1737
5. Gautherie M, Quenneville Y, Gros C (1974) Cholesteric thermography. Sheets of liquid crystal. Clinical, pharmacological and physiological applications. Comparison with infra-red thermography. Pathol Biol (Paris) 22:553 – 566
6. Gautherie M, Quenneville Y, Rempp C, Gros C (1975) Valeur informative comparée de la téléthermographie (infrarouge) et de la thermographie de contact (cristéux liquides) en sanologie. J Radiol Electrol Med Nucl 56:316 – 318
7. Nyirjesy I, Abernathy MR, Billingsley FS, Bruns P (1977) Thermography and detection of breast carcinoma; a review and comments. J Reprod Med 18:165 – 175
8. Uematsu S (1976) Medical thermography, theory and clinical applications. Brentwood, Los Angeles
9. Raskin MM, Viamonte M (1977) Clinical thermography. American college of radiology, Chicago, committee on new technology
10. Ritchie WGM, Lapayowker MS, Soulen R (1979) Thermographic diagnosis of deep venous thrombosis: Anatomically based diagnostic criteria. Radiology 132:321 – 329
11. Boyle E, Canosa F, Aparicio A, Bonet E, Owen D, Dash HH (1975) The vertical midsupraorbital pattern in thermographic diagnosis of internal carotid artery disease. Annual Meeting of the American Thermographic Society, Atlanta, September 27 – 28, 1975
12. Capistrant TD, Gumnit RJ (1973) Detecting carotid occlusive disease by thermography. Stroke 4:57 – 64
13. Mumford JM (1979) Thermography and ice cream headache. Acta Thermographica 4/1:33 – 37
14. Lance JW, Anthony M (1971) Thermographic studies in vascular headache. Med J Aust 1:240 – 243
15. Ring EFJ (1975) Thermography and rheumatic diseases. Bibl Radiol 6:97 – 106
16. Collings AJ, Ring EFJ, Bacon PA, Brookshaw J (1976) Thermography and radiology. Complimentary methods for the study of inflammatory diseases. Clin Radiol 27:237 – 243
17. Sowa A (1979) Thermographic estimation of burn depth. Acta Thermographica 4/1
18. Ching C, Wexler C (1978) Peripheral thermographic manifestations of lumbar-disk disease. Appl Radiol: 53 – 58
19. Raskin MA, Martinez-Lopez M, Sheldon JJ (1976) Lumbar thermography in discogenic disease. Radiology 119:149 – 152
20. Lelik F, Kezy G (1979) Contact thermography in sportsmedicine. Acta Thermographica 4/1
21. Moss CE (1977) A review of thyroid thermography. Appl Radiol 6/1
22. Samuels BL (1975) The present status of parathyroid thermography. JAMA 233:907
23. Jones CH, Hendry WF (1979) Thermographic examination of the scrotum. Acta Thermographica 4/1
24. Holm J, Johnsen C, Schersten T (1974) Thermography in vascular surgery. Acta Chir Scand 140: 445 – 448

Noteworthy Aspects of Mammography with and Without Screen Technique

E. Borcke

AGFA-GEVAERT AG Technikum, Anwendungstechnikum Röntgen, Kistlerhofstrasse 75, D-8000 München 70

Noteworthy Aspects of Mammography with and Without Screen Technique

Can the learning process of the choice of optimum density be shortened? Optimum density in the image, which actually renders higher image quality, was only used in mammography many years after the introduction of special films for use without screen. As a transition to screen mammography technique is on its way, the necessary change of the optimum density which is related to it should consequently – and without loss of time – be executed in order not to impair the image quality.
Since the end of the 1950s, the image technique of mammography has been considerably improved by introducing certain film types of the non-destructive testing (NDT) technique (industrial radiography). These films, less sensitive by a factor of approximately 4 as compared with the classic medical film for technique without screens, rendered – by means of the film – more contrast and sharpness for the mammogram and at the same time improved graininess due to more exposure and original lower graininess of the film. These advantages of image quality have only been obtained by means of high dose application.
Even nowadays the films used in mammography technique without screens are often called "material test films," although these film types are of decreasing importance in industrial radiography today. Unfortunately, one had originally only used the film and at the same time not made use of the experience from industrial radiography as to how to handle the film correctly. It even took the pioneers of mammography 1 decade until the optimum density for mammograms was applied.
In recent years there has been a transition from the technique without screens to the screen technique for mammography. To avoid again devoting many years to the learning process of image quality optimum, the following clarification of the best preconditions of both techniques is given. The maximum density is determined by the brightness (physically more exact: luminance) of the viewing box. The generally used luminance in NDT is 40000 cd/m^2 and permits, according to DIN 54116, part 1, the evaluation of density D = 3.6, whereas according to a maximised evaluation feasibility following a physiological point of view, only D = 2.6 would be permissible.
This amazingly low maximum density accounts for the use of special light boxes with a luminance of H_0 = 200000 cd/m^2. These viewing boxes permit D_{max} = 4.3, or with maximum evaluation of D = 3.3. But the "physiological" quality loss is compensated by contrast increase, which is related to this density increase. Therefore, and this only in the case of technique without screens, the higher values can be used as a base.
To avoid glare, the DIN 54111, part 1, requires that for the image part to be evaluated (collimation of the viewing area) the difference of density of various image parts must not surpass ΔD = 1.5.
The average object range O-U in NDT is only O-U = 0.30 (logarithmical unity). But the average object range in mammography is near O-U = 0.75. Whereas the range of an NDT image is easily placed between the densities 2 and 3.5, this is not possible for the object range of mammography. The NDT rules allow quality-reducing exceptions in exposure data in an analogous case of large object range in order to make the image interpretable by the observer. In such cases there is a D_{min} of 1.5 and a contrast decrease of an average of approximately 13% is permissible. This is obtained for NDT with an increase in voltage of approximately 50 kV. The analogous kV increase for mammography would be from 30 to 40 kV referring to soft part structures.
The density range of the mammograms made by NDT rules would be from D = 1.5 to D = 6.17. In other words, the "object" of the female breast cannot be radiographed by the simple rules for

Radiology Today 1. Ed. by M. W. Donner and F. H. W. Heuck

NDT. Are there any such objects in NDT? Yes, but only of iron, and the required solution is a manifold film technique.

In the case of our (average) object range of O-U = 0.75 the material examiner has to use manifold film technique (according to DIN 54111, part 2). He would have to take two films for exposure at same time with a difference in speed of factor 2 and afterward would have to examine the densities from D = 2 to D = 4. He would be forced, though, to use a special viewing box with H_0 = 200000 cd/m^2.

The occasionally used bipack technique in mammography would have its importance, but then the speed of the two films should not be too far apart.

Not only organizational reasons stand in the way of applying the manifold technique in mammography. The spread of occurring object ranges O-U lies between 0.3 and 1.2, with an average of 0.75. Of all mammograms, 12% have an object range of >0.9. Such object ranges cannot be managed as required by the NDT rules with the simple bipack technique.

Thus, when applying the technique without screens in mammography, one is forced to allow reduction of the maximum possible image quality. The used luminance of the viewing box limits D_{max}, and D_{min} results from the mamma type and kV value. Let us assume that there is a viewing box with H_0 = 200000 cd/m^2 available for evaluation, then D_{max} = 4.3 based identical with D_{opt} of an assumed image quality = 100%.

The following D_{min} values and relative image qualities (IQ) result from certain O-Us:

O-U	D_{min}	IQ
0.75	1.1	50%
0.9	0.85	40%
1.2	0.5	20%

The following rule applies if one does not take a strict attitude as regards quality optimization: "Mammograms made without screen should be kept dark". The ever increasingly used screen technique would suffer an image loss if this rule were to be applied here! First observations of people who have changed from technique without screen to screen technique prove this. The density optimization is after all a gradient optimization, and gradient optimizations are quite different with screen technique.

If one takes the typical course of a gradient curve plotted against density for mammography with screen technique for optimization, one gains from the specified O-Us the following D_{max} and D_{min} values for an image quality = 100% for D_{opt} = 1.5:

O-U	D_{max}	D_{min}	$IQ_{D_{max}}/D_{min}$
0.75	2.2	0.9	80%/80%
0.9	2.2	0.6	75%/75%
1.2	2.2	0.5	50%/50%

The similar values of D_{min} of the screen technique and of the technique without screen are striking. As they are not representative for quality maintenance, a control by D_{max} is recommended. A value of D_{max} = 2.5 for all mammograms in screen technique should not be surpassed, if quality loss is to be avoided.

Without looking too closely to the difference of image quality of the non-screen technique versus screen technique, all mammograms with an O-U 0.75 will get a better image quality in lower densities with the screen technique. Together with the big dose advantages, this should be an argument to the advantage of the screen technique in mammography.

Lymphography

Lymphography: Overview

P. E. Peters

Universität Köln, Radiologisches Institut, Josef-Stelzmann-Strasse 9, D-5000 Köln 41

Introduction

At the end of the last meeting of the International Society of Lymphology in fall 1979, Dr. Collard was asked to give a lecture on "new horizons in diagnostic lymphography." He stated: "... lymphography is now falling in agony.

The method which is not without risk, is becoming less and less important since it's diagnostic results, but especially the therapeutic consequences are limited." And he finished his lecture by saying: "Lymphography today is mostly of historical importance" [12]. Is this really true?

There is no doubt that new imaging modalities such as ultrasonography (US) and computerized tomography (CT) are able to show enlarged lymph nodes, even in areas not visualized by conventional pedal lymphography. On the other hand, at present size is the only criterion for malignancy in US as well as in CT, while lymphography also allows the analysis of storage pattern and filling defects in normal-sized lymph nodes due to its higher spatial resolution.

The current status of lymphography, its potential development, and its major drawbacks – as compared to the new noninvasive imaging modalities – will be discussed in the following presentation. The value of US in diseases of the lymphatic system will be discussed and illustrated in more detail by Dr. Beyer in a separate communication. We will take a look into the future, when Dr. Siefert presents the first results of a new lymphographic contrast medium which eventually might improve conventional lymphography as well as CT studies of the lymphatic system.

Computerized Tomography of the Retroperitoneal Lymph System

In the early days of whole body CT, spatial resolution was poor, partly due to motion artifacts. Normal-sized lymph nodes could be recognized only occasionally. Grossly enlarged lymph nodes, however, were easily detected by loss of the paraaortic or paracaval "fat angle" [18]. Involvement of retroaortic lymph nodes produced the so-called floating aorta sign.

The new fast scanning devices possess much better spatial resolution, thus, multiple structures are visualized in the retroperitoneum and the problem of identification of these tiny structures arises.

We have recently completed a prospective study in which every patient scheduled for lymphography underwent CT investigation of the retroperitoneum prior to and after conventional lymphography [32, 37]. Analysis of CT images and lymphograms were performed independently by different radiologists. The aim of this study was (1) to determine the size and the number of apparently normal lymph nodes in prelymphographic CT examinations, (2) to evaluate the gain of information provided by selective radio-opaque marking of lymphatic tissue as compared with the "plain CT examination", and (3) to compare diagnostic accuracy of both imaging modalities.

From this investigation I would like to demonstrate briefly a series of CT images of normal anatomic findings prior to and after lymphography.

In the retrocrural region identification of lymph nodes is fairly easy, provided the patient has enough retroperitoneal fat. Around the aorta we found small lymph nodes, almost never exceeding 6–7 mm in diameter, in 70% of our normal patients. In conventional lymphography they are seldom opacified because of the more distally located chylous cystern through which the oily contrast medium enters the thoracic duct. In the case presented in Fig. 1 two tiny retrocrural lymph nodes are visible after lymphography. Note that they appear to be much larger than in the plain CT images. This is a general observation in postlymphographic CT studies. There are two reasons for the phenomenon:

Radiology Today 1. Ed. by M. W. Donner and F. H. W. Heuck

1) As we know from conventional lymphography, the lymph nodes really increase in volume by about 10% – 15% immediately after lymphography.
2) More importantly, the huge density differences between fat and radiopaque contrast medium create a pseudoenlargement for technical reasons.

Thus, for measurements of lymph node size and number, only plain CT images can be used.

The tiny symmetric structures not opacified in the postlymphographic CT study represent azygos and hemiazygos veins. In addition, one recognizes normal-sized adrenal glands bilaterally. Retropancreatic lymph nodes surrounding the splenic artery and vein can only be identified when they are enlarged.

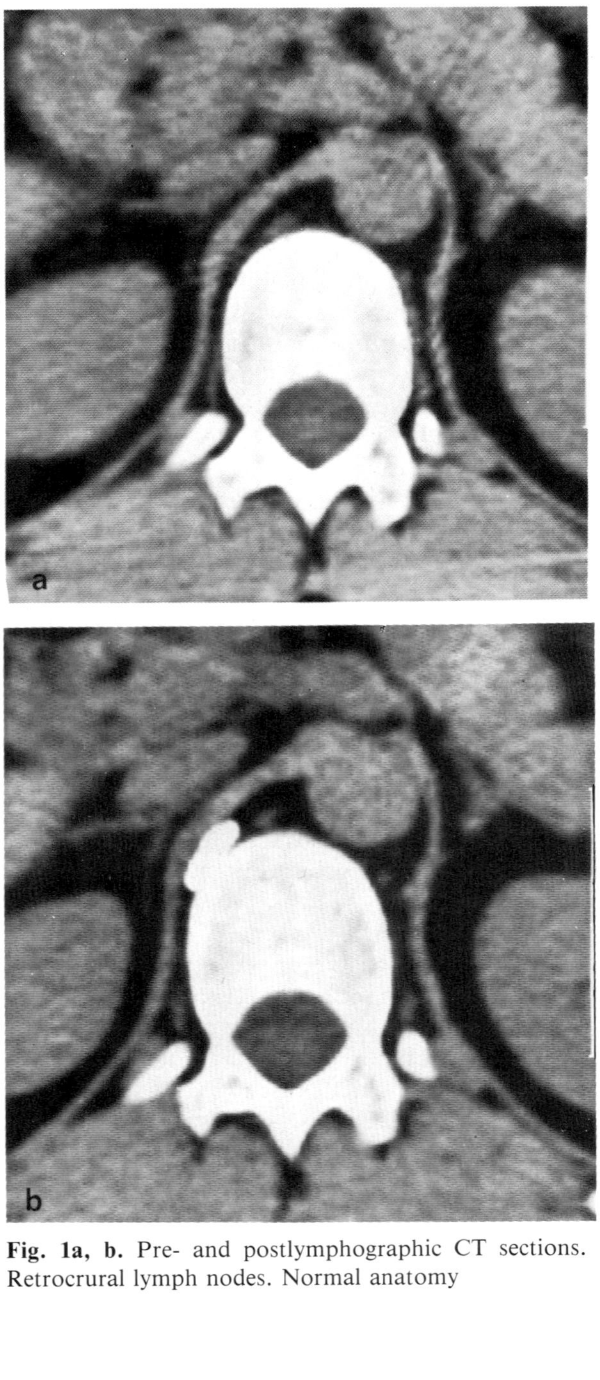

Fig. 1a, b. Pre- and postlymphographic CT sections. Retrocrural lymph nodes. Normal anatomy

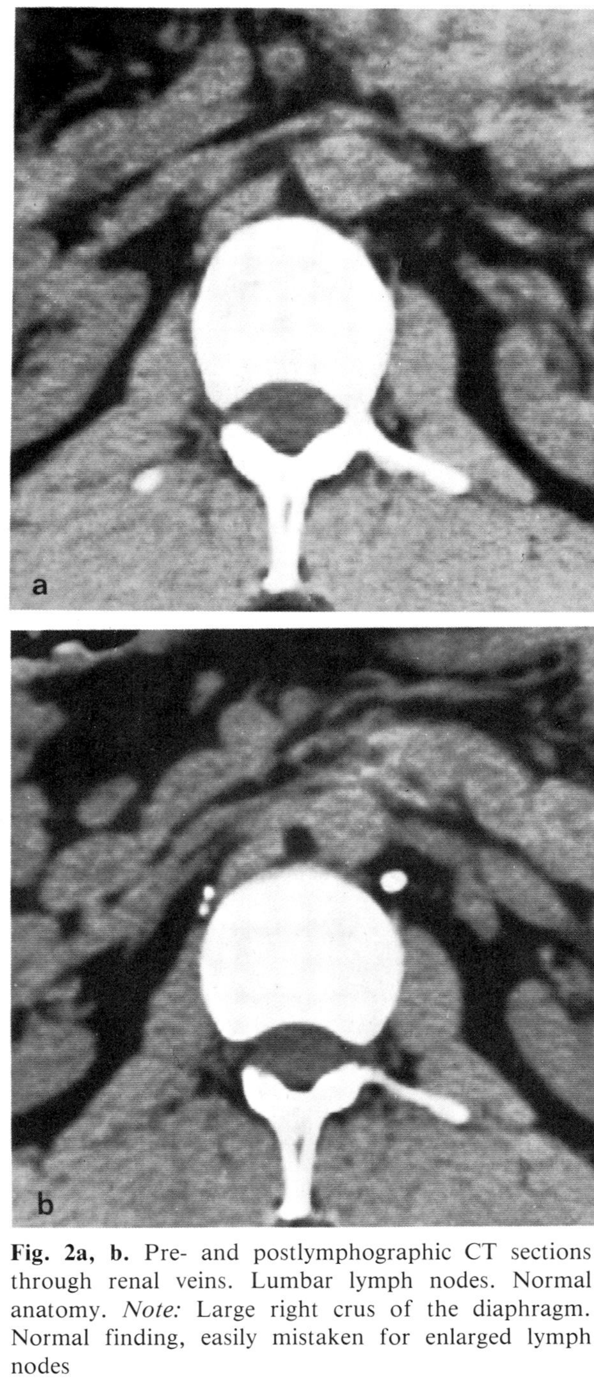

Fig. 2a, b. Pre- and postlymphographic CT sections through renal veins. Lumbar lymph nodes. Normal anatomy. *Note:* Large right crus of the diaphragm. Normal finding, easily mistaken for enlarged lymph nodes

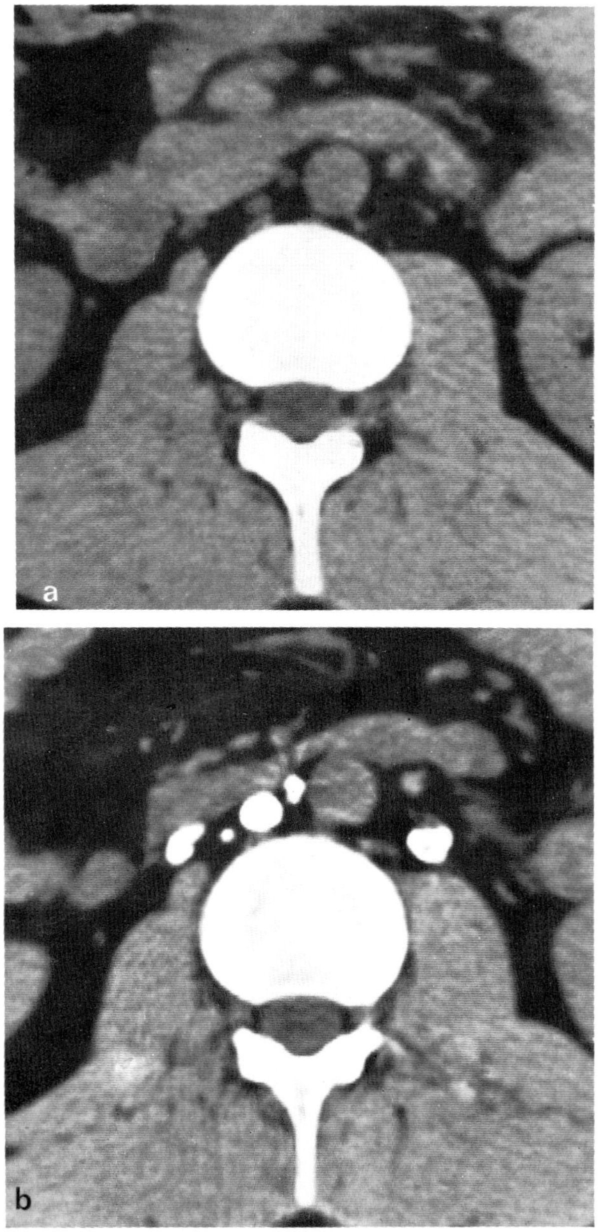

Fig. 3a, b. Pre- and postlymphographic CT sections below renal veins. Demonstration of lumbar lymph nodes in three chains: lnn. lateroaortici, lnn. interaorticocavales, and lnn. retrocavales. Normal anatomy

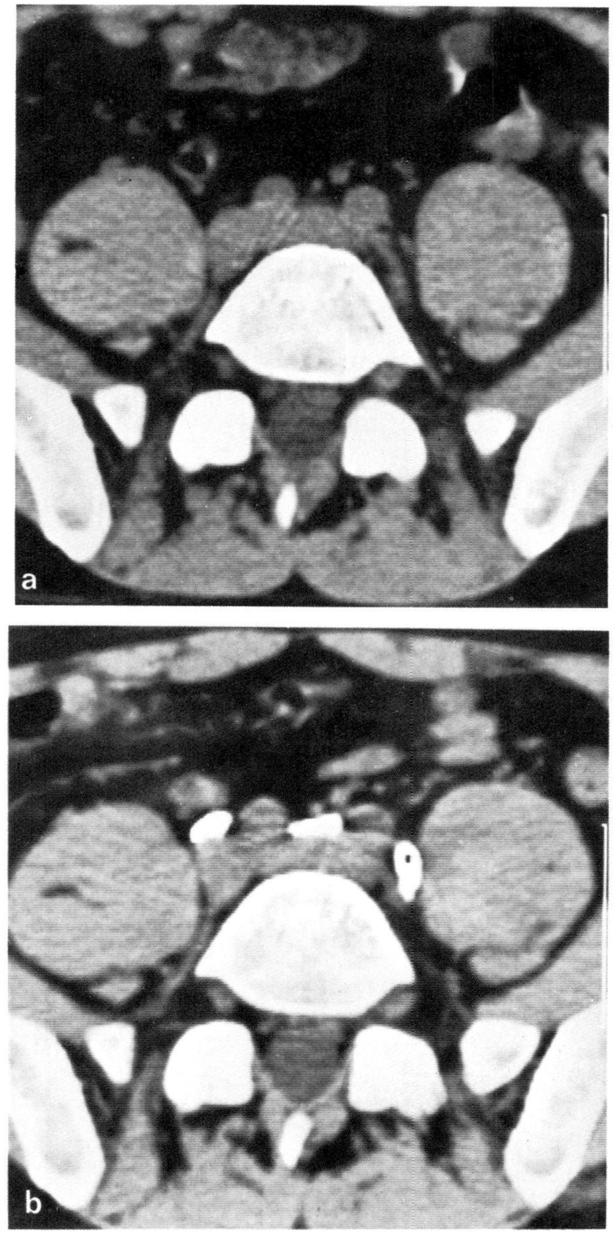

Fig. 4a, b. Pre- and postlymphographic sections just below the aortic bifurcation. Common iliac lymph nodes. Normal anatomy

The next set of figures is a cut through the renal veins. In the prelymphographic CT there is a tiny notch at the dorsal aspect of the right crus of the diaphragm (Fig. 2a) which turns out to represent two very small lymph nodes in the postlymphographic image (Fig. 2b). The right crus of the diaphragm can easily be mistaken for an enlarged lymph node [9].

Infrarenal sections display multiple oval-shaped structures surrounding the aorta and vena cava which seem to be arranged in three longitudinal chains (Fig. 3a, b).

In conventional lymphography, Wiljasalo has always pointed out that normal lymph nodes are elliptic structures while diseased ones undergo "spheric transformation" [43]. In CT cross sections this would indicate that round-shaped lymph nodes might be diseased. So far, we have not seen enough cases to present our own data concerning this assumption. However, differential diagnosis in CT examinations will be very difficult since vascular structures also present as small, round nodules. In our material lymph nodes of normal size tend to appear oval-shaped, sometimes linear, and somewhat less dense than vascular cross sections.

Below the aortic bifurcation identification of normal sized lymph nodes becomes very difficult, and within the pelvic region almost impossible without opacification (Fig. 4a, b).

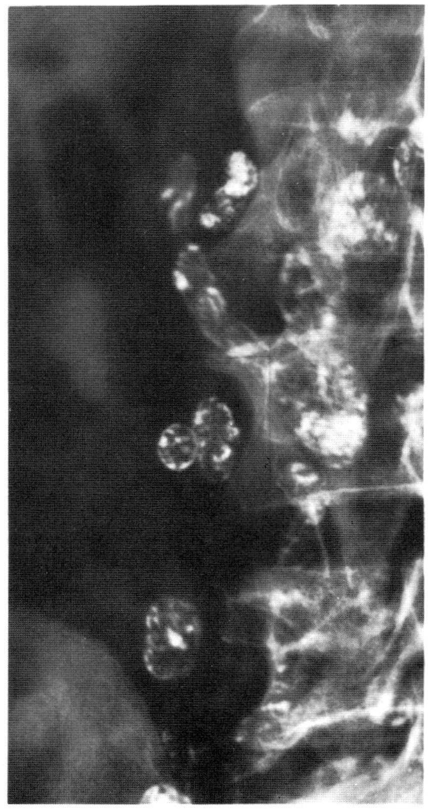

Fig. 5. Lymphography in non-Hodgkin's lymphoma. Grossly pathologic storage pattern and interrupted marginal sinuses in almost normal-sized lymph nodes

Lymphography in Malignant Lymphoma

Extensive histologic-lymphographic correlations have been carried out in patients undergoing staging laparotomy for malignant lymphoma.

In Hodgkin's disease, Castellino and Marglin reported an overall accuracy of 92%, based upon 390 patients. The percentage of true positive findings – sensitivity – was 94%, the percentage of true negative findings – specificity –, 91%. A positive lymphographic interpretation was found to be correct in 79% of the cases, which means 21% false positive readings, as compared to only 2% false negative interpretations [10].

In non-Hodgkin's lymphoma, the same group found an overall accuracy of 88% with 12% false positive and 13% false negative readings (Fig. 5).

There are many other reports on the accuracy of lymphographic staging which do not differ significantly from the above quoted results, so they represent the "state of the art" standard against which other imaging modalities are measured [22].

Comparative studies between lymphography and CT for staging of malignant lymphoma have been published by several authors. Lackner et al. [24] reported an overall accuracy of CT imaging of 86% in the para-aortic and iliac lymph node regions, which was slightly less than the 92% and 93% respectively obtained with lymphography in the same patients (Table 1). Similar results were obtained by Jones et al. [20].

It is interesting to note that by means of US, retroperitoneal periaortic lymph node involvement was correctly predicted in 88% of the cases [5].

While the number of histologically proven cases in CT and ultrasound studies is still much lower than in lymphography, there seems to be general agreement that CT in lymphoma patients shows enlarged lymph nodes in the vast majority of cases in which lymphadenopathy is present. In addition, CT may reveal lymph node disease in areas not visualized in pedal lymphography, e.g., internal iliac, mesenteric, splenic hilar, portal, and retrocrural lymph nodes, and often CT shows more of an individual enlarged lymph node than lymphography does [1, 6, 45, L. Kreel, 1980, personal communication].

CT cannot, however, at present replace staging laparatomy because of its limited ability to detect lymphomatous involvement in liver and spleen [3, 24].

One of the arguments of people endorsing lymphangiography in malignant diseases was the possibility of evaluating response to therapy or relapse of disease by means of a postlymphographic plain abdominal radiograph. Lee et al. [26] recently demonstrated the serious limitations of that ap-

Table 1. Lymphography vs CT in malignant lymphoma staging [24]

	Lymphography (%)	CT (%)
Para-aortic lymph nodes		
Overall accuracy	92	86
Sensitivity	89	80
Specificity	95	93
Iliac lymph nodes		
Overall accuracy	93	86
Sensitivity	90	81
Specificity	97	90

proach. Comparison was made between CT follow-up studies and postlymphographic follow-up plain film, revealing far better results with CT imaging for any time period longer than 1 year after lymphography.

Thus, lymphography, being an invasive procedure which carries a small but definite risk, should be performed only in those patients with suspected infradiaphragmatic disease in which US and/or CT gave negative or equivocal results.

It is conceivable that the concept of staging laparotomy of malignant lymphoma will eventually be changed since fine needle biopsy has proven to be a reliable method in experienced hands [16, 30].

Lymphography in Metastatic Disease

Lymphographic Signs of Malignancy

Lymphographic diagnosis of metastatic involvement is based upon the demonstration of filling and storage defects, obstruction of afferent lymphatics, displacement of adjacent lymphatics, and the visualization of collaterals usually not filled by contrast material [42]. All of these signs can only be detected by means of conventional lymphography.

In US and CT, lymph node enlargement is the only sign of malignancy. Every radiologist knows that there might be lymph node enlargement due to specific or unspecific lymphadenitis, which he will correctly diagnose by analysis of storage pattern and filling phase.

In a recent evaluation of lymphographic accuracy in malignant melanoma we found 90% correct diagnoses in lymph node metastases measuring 10 mm in diameter and more [31]. This is in accordance with Zingg et al.'s [46] proposal to make a positive diagnosis of metastatic involvement only when solitary or multiple well-demarcated filling defects of at least 10 mm in diameter in regional lymph nodes are present. In smaller filling defects the rate of false positive findings is sometimes very high. Fine needle biopsy of small suspicious lesions has been shown to improve diagnostic accuracy in metastatic disease [17, 30].

Lymphography in Tumors of Male Genital Organs

Testicular Tumors. Lymphography in testicular tumors has been performed routinely in many institutions in spite of the fact that application of the contrast medium into lymphatics of the foot does not opacify all regional lymph nodes draining testis, epididymis, and scrotum. Testicular lymphography – as advocated by Chiappa et al. – would demonstrate the first draining nodes, but it has been used only scarcely [11].

The incidence of lymph node metastases in testicular tumors is rather high. Musumeci et al. [34] reported 57% lymph node metastases in 276 teratomas of the testis and 41% lymph node metastases in 266 seminomas. The accuracy of lymphography was found to be 87%. Kademian and Wirtanen reported an overall accuracy of 89% in 45 surgically proven cases [21].

Since testicular tumors most commonly develop metastatic disease in the para-aortic or paracaval lymph nodes, attempts have been made to use US and CT in the evaluation of these regions (Fig. 6).

Burney and Klatte reported an overall accuracy of 75% for US and 76% for CT in testicular carcinoma [8]. Lackner et al. [23] found an overall accuracy of 80% for CT as compared to only 75% for lymphography in 64 surgically proven cases. If these high levels of accuracy can be achieved by noninvasive methods, one should employ either technique as a screening investigation and perform lymphangiography only in those cases in which negative or equivocal results are obtained (Table 2).

On the other hand, if in seminoma patients radiotherapy is scheduled, it is still advisable to perform lymphography for treatment planning. The effect of radiotherapy can easily be monitored by follow-up lymphadenograms. The same holds true for patients suffering from testicular carcinoma, in which case lymphography makes the retroperito-

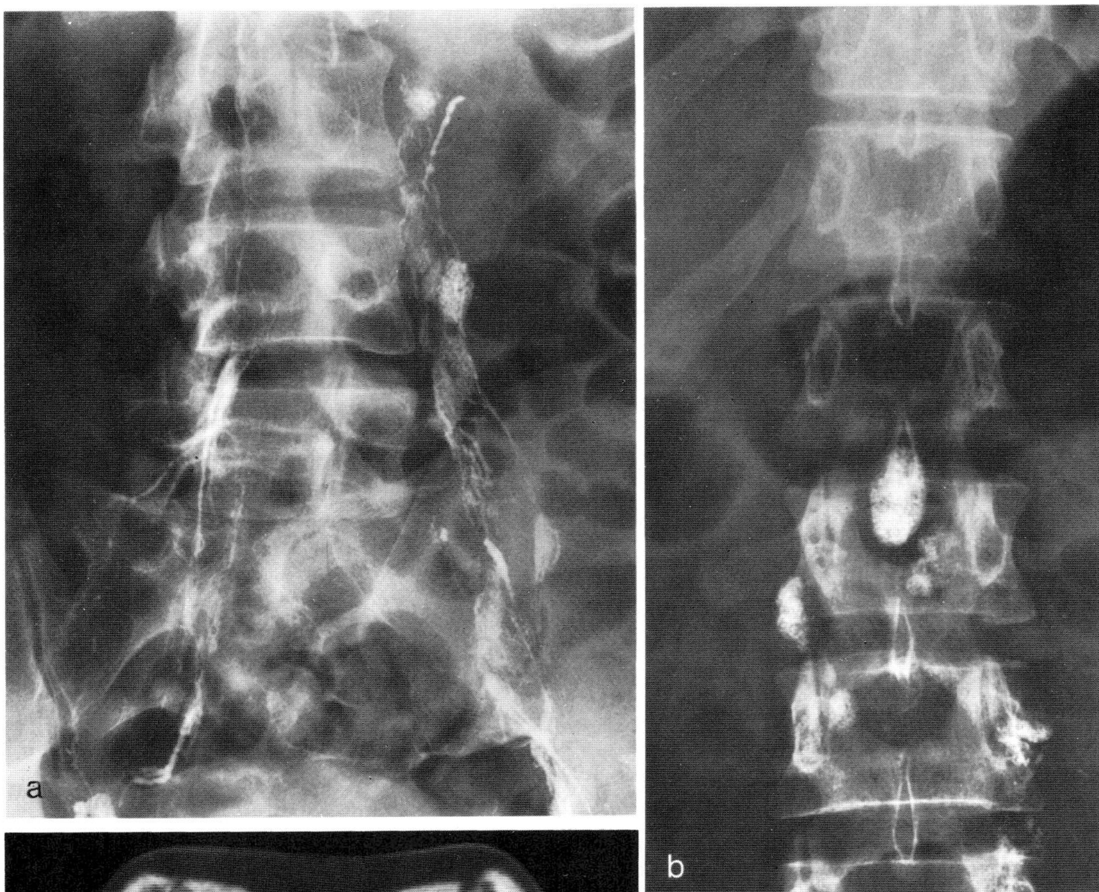

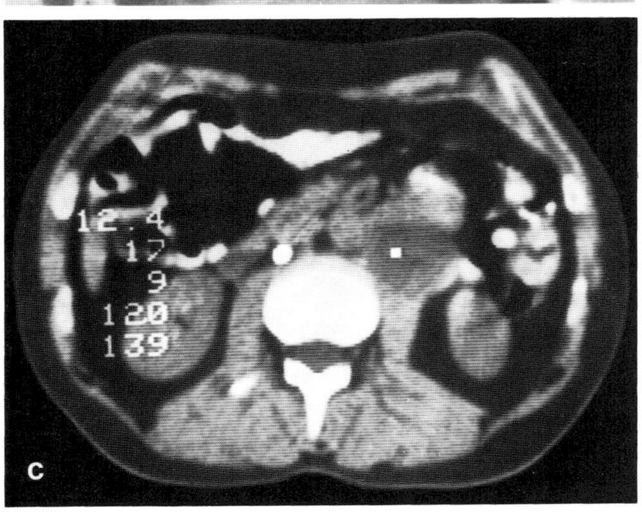

Fig. 6a – c. Metastases of a left testicular carcinoma. **a** Lymphangiogram: Interruption of a left lumbar lymph vessel. **b** Lymphadenogram: Displacement and marginal filling defect in a left lumbar lymph node. **c** CT: Large metastatic mass at the hilum of the left kidney. CT shows the extent of metastatic disease better than lymphography

Table 2. Ultrasonography, CT, and lymphography in testicular carcinoma [8, 21]

	Correct (%)	False + (%)	False – (%)	Equivocal (%)
Ultrasonography	75	2	20	3
CT	76	5	12	7
Lymphography	89	2	9	0

neal lymph nodes visible for radical lymphadenectomy under fluoroscopic control.
In both situations lymphographic diagnosis does not influence the therapeutic regimen, but the visualization of lymph nodes facilitates further treatment.

Carcinoma of the Penis. In carcinoma of the penis the regional lymph nodes are incompletely opacified by foot lymphography. Additional difficulties arise because of unspecific or postoperative reactions of inguinal lymph nodes [42]. Theoretically, penile lymphography would be advantageous but has been performed in only a few centers. The search for retroperitoneal metastases remains the major indication for lymphography. Alternative imaging modalities have not been investigated.

Lymphography in Female Genital Tumors

Carcinoma of the Cervix. Lymphography has long been used as a preoperative routine procedure in stage I and II carcinoma of the cervix although a significant number of primary draining lymph nodes are not visualized by pedal lymphography. Overall accuracy in surgically proven cases has been reported to be as high as 96% [15] and as low as 50% [40]. In a recent study by Musumeci et al. [34], based upon 417 new cases, overall accuracy of lymphography was found to be 86%. Computerized tomography of pelvic malignancies is still in its infancy. Normal-sized lymph nodes are often not well seen, whereas abnormally enlarged pelvic lymph nodes can usually be detected without difficulty. The main advantage of CT seems to be that the rate of false negative studies is very low, thus allowing the use of CT for screening purposes [25].

There has been a lot of controversy about the incidence of lumbar lymph node metastases in cervical cancer. Gerteis observed lumbar lymph node metastases in 12%, with 9% already in stage I disease. This area would, of course, be better suited for either CT or ultrasound investigation. According to Brown et al. [7] lymphographic findings in the para-aortic region are often false positive. They emphasize the need for tissue diagnosis.

Carcinoma of the Corpus Uteri. Lymph node metastases of endometrial carcinoma are found in external iliac nodes and in the lumbar region, and occasionally the spreading occurs via the utero-inguinal ligament to superficial inguinal lymph nodes. However, as in other pelvic malignancies, the primary draining lymph nodes are not opacified by conventional lymphography. The incidence of lymphographically detectable lymph node metastases varies between 17% [33, 34] and 30% [15] with an overall accuracy of 86%.

Lymphography is recommended in operable cases with stage I and II disease. CT of the pelvis shows the extent of the primary tumor and advanced lymph node metastases.

Table 3. Lymphography in gynecologic cancer – incidence of lymph node metastases and diagnostic accuracy [30a, 34]

	n	Incidence of metastases (%)	Diagnostic accuracy (%)
Cervical carcinoma	417	30	86
Endometrial carcinoma	187	17	86
Ovarian carcinoma	225	27	92
Carcinoma of the vulva	86	27	83

Carcinoma of the Ovary. Cancer of the ovary is not only spread by contiguity and intraperitoneal implants but also via the lymphatics. In 225 new cases of ovarian cancer, Musumeci et al. [34] found 27% lymph node metastases with an overall accuracy of 92%. It is of special interest to note that nonepithelial ovarian tumors such as dysgerminomas might have up to 43% lymph node metastases, mainly in the para-aortic region, while ovarian epithelial cancer tends to involve iliac nodes either alone or in combination with para-aortic involvement [33].

Carcinoma of Vulva and Vagina. Metastatic spreading from the cranial portions of the vagina occurs in the same way as for cervical cancer. The lower portion and the vulva drains into superficial inguinal lymph nodes which are inconsistently opacified by foot lymphography but are easy to palpate. The incidence of lymph node metastases in 86 operated cases was 27% with an overall accuracy of 83% [30a] (Table 3).

The presented data indicate that lymphography in tumors of the female genital system has reached an acceptable level of diagnostic accuracy which cannot be much improved by conventional methods. CT offers the advantages of recognition of visceral lymph nodes not opacified lymphographically, but they are difficult to identify without selective marking. The ideal combination would be improved CT with still better spatial resolution and a new contrast agent for easy interstitial application.

Lymphography in Urologic Cancer

Carcinoma of the Bladder. Lymphography in carcinoma of the bladder is positive only in advanced cases, since the paravesical lymph nodes are not opacified by pedal lymphography. In a series of 170 cases the incidence of lymph node metastases seen lymphographically was 32%, with an overall accuracy of 89% [35].

As in other pelvic cancers, CT can outline the extent of the primary tumor and will detect pathologic lymph node enlargement.

Attempts have been made to visualize the regional lymph nodes by injection of oily contrast medium into the submucosal layer of the bladder wall under endoscopic vision. The paravesical lymph nodes could indeed be demonstrated; however, the low local tolerance of the contrast agent prohibited its routine application in humans [4, 19].

Carcinoma of the Prostate. Since the lymphatics of the urinary bladder, prostate, ureter, seminal vesicles, ductus deferens, and rectum form a close mesh, tumors of these organs metastasize in a similar fashion [42]. Positive lymphographic findings in external iliac nodes are mainly seen in T3/T4 stages. Thus, the incidence of positive lymphographic diagnoses varies from author to author according to the distribution of more advanced cases in the particular institution.

In general, lymph node metastases tend to appear earlier and more often than osseous metastases. The combination of both is common – about one-third of patients with positive lymphographic findings also have osseous metastases – while osseous involvement without lymph node disease is rarely observed [29].

Direct intraprostatic injection of Ethiodol has been reported recently. First results in 12 patients revealed good visualization of internal iliac and presacral lymph nodes. There were no serious complications during or after the procedure. Data on accuracy in prostatic cancer are not yet available [39].

Carcinoma of the Kidney. The lymph vessels of the kidneys course toward the renal hilum along the renal vessels and proceed directly to the homolateral lumbar lymph nodes. Since renal carcinomas usually metastasize hematogenously, lymph node involvement is limited to late stages. In large series the incidence of lymph node metastases never exceeded 14% – 20% [27].

Computerized tomography is of utmost importance for staging of renal cell carcinoma and is nowadays performed routinely. The presence of lymph node metastases will be detected in the same examination.

In conclusion, pedal lymphography in urologic cancer (Table 4) is positive only in advanced stages. Since CT is performed routinely in most of these tumors for staging purposes and for treatment planning in radiotherapy, only very few cases with negative or equivocal CT findings will remain for conventional lymphography.

Table 4. Lymphography in urologic cancer – incidence of lymph node metastases and diagnostic accuracy [29, 35]

	n	Incidence of metastases (%)	Diagnostic accuracy (%)
Ca. of the bladder	170	32	89
Renal cell ca.	88	14	100 (n = 13)
Ca. of the prostate	56	29	

Lymphography in Tumors of the Distal Colon and Anus

Only lymph node metastases from tumors of the outer anal region can be detected relatively early by conventional lymphography because of the drainage into superficial inguinal nodes. In all other locations metastatic involvement can be extensive in mesocolic and paracolic nodes without lymphographic abnormalities. Accordingly the incidence of lymph node metastases varies for anatomic reasons. Petrillo et al. [38] observed 31% lymph node metastases in anal cancer but only 12% and 6% in carcinoma of the rectum and sigmoid colon, respectively.

Lymphography in Malignant Melanoma

Patients with malignant melanoma of the lower and upper extremities are subjected to lymphographic investigation in the search for lymphogenous metastases. Since the draining axillary and inguinal lymph nodes are often affected by unspecific or fibrolipomatous reactions, careful lymphographic analysis is necessary. Wiljasalo et al. [44] reported an overall accuracy of 92% in 200 cases with malignant melanoma of the extremities.

Malignant melanoma is known for its early lymphogenous spreading. In patients without palpable lymph node enlargement, Fortner et al. found micrometastases in 38% while performing "prophylactic" lymph node excision [14]. For diagnostic and therapeutic reasons we injected $^{131}J/^{32}P$ labeled contrast medium into lymphatics of the foot. ^{32}Phosphorus emits a high-energy beta radiation which will destroy micrometastases. If the metastatic filling defect exceeds 4 mm in diameter, i.e., more than the medium range of ^{32}P beta radiation, the diseased lymph node must be removed surgically. The results of this ancillary treatment of malignant melanoma of the extremities are encouraging [36].

The role of lymphography in malignant melanoma varies with the treatment concepts from center to center. Those performing prophylactic lymph node excision prefer preoperative lymphography for better demonstration of removed and remaining nodes. The diagnostic information does not influence treatment. The same holds true in centers performing hyperthermic perfusion with cytostatic drugs, which is normally combined with a limited lymphadenectomy.

New imaging modalities are of little importance in malignant melanoma of the extremities as far as lymph node metastases are concerned. Malignant melanoma of the head and neck and of the trunk creates many diagnostic problems since the preferential lymphatic drainage is unknown. Interstitial application of suited radiocolloids can demonstrate the main route of lymphatic drainage, but its spatial resolution does not suffice for recognition of lymph node metastases.

Lymphography in Bone and Soft Tissue Sarcomas

Sarcoma metastases usually are thought to be blood borne, yet Tallroth et al. [41] found a surprisingly high number of lymph node metastases in bone and soft tissue sarcomas. According to their careful analysis the incidence of lymph node metastases varies from 58% in reticulosarcoma of bone to 0% in giant cell tumors. In the group of soft tissue sarcomas the highest incidence of lymph node metastases was seen in rhabdomyosarcoma, the lowest in liposarcoma (Table 5).

Table 5. Lymphography in bone and soft tissue sarcomas – incidence of lymph node metastases and diagnostic accuracy [41]

	n	Incidence of metastases (%)	Diagnostic accuracy (%)
Bone sarcomas	217	21	93
Reticulosarcoma	7/12	58	
Osteosarcoma	16/60	27	
Chondrosarcoma	5/39	13	
Giant cell tumor	0/17	0	
Soft tissue sarcomas	224	28	92
Rhabdomyosarcoma	25/47	53	
Neurogenic sarcoma	8/19	42	
Synovial sarcoma	7/20	35	
Fibrosarcoma	6/45	13	
Liposarcoma	3/37	8	

Lymphography in Fever of Unknown Origin

One of the classic indications for lymphography used to be "fever of unknown origin." The clinicians, having done every laboratory test possible, would refer the patient for lymphography hoping that abdominal lymphoma would be the reason for the fever. In my experience, lymphography very seldom really clarifies fever of unknown origin.

Anfossi and Adami from Italy made different observations: they studied 19 such cases lymphographically and were able to give a reliable diagnosis in 15 out of 19 cases. Interestingly enough, they reported ten cases of retroperitoneal lymph node tuberculosis, which is extremely rare in Germany. In addition, they found four cases of retroperitoneal lymphoma and one case with metastases from an unknown primary tumor [2].

Lymphography in Lymphangiopathies

The original application of lymphography – utilizing water-soluble contrast media – was for studying edematous extremities, and our still limited knowledge of primary and secondary lymphedemas originates from these early studies. Today, the need for lymphographic investigation of lymphangiopathies depends heavily on the therapeutic consequences. Földi – one of the world's leading lymphologists – has taught us that even a minor injury to an edematous extremity may lead to decompensation. This means that lymphography should never be performed just for the sake of a completed patients record or for medical curiosity. If one uses water-soluble contrast media the central portions of the lymphatics cannot be evaluated. If one uses oily contrast media the clinical symptomatology can aggravate due to obstruction of the few draining lymph vessels [13].

In most instances the distribution pattern of subcutaneously injected patent blue violet will allow the diagnosis of a lymphogenic cause of edema by displaying the dermal back-flow sign. The subcutaneous injection of radiocolloid particles – lymph scintigraphy – gives a rough quantitative determination of the degree of lymph flow hindrance.
The current treatment of lymphedema is conservative in spite of the remarkable progress of surgical methods. Lymphography should only be carried out in cases resistant against combined physical – pharmacologic treatment which are considered candidates for plastic and reconstructive surgery such as lymphovenous anastomoses. The only other indication for lymphography in lymphedema is a suspected malignancy in the pelvic or axillary region which cannot be clarified by noninvasive methods. The old medical principle of *nil nocere,* do not harm, should be the guideline for every physician taking care of patients with lymphangiopathies.

New Lymphographic Contrast Media

Coming to the end of this overview, the question arises whether lymphography is, indeed, a slowly or rapidly dying radiologic method which will soon be replaced by better noninvasive techniques? The answer is "yes" and "no".
Conventional lymphography using oily contrast media and direct intralymphatic application can be replaced to the benefit of our patients in many instances by CT and US. Kreel [Kreel L, personal communication] mentioned that in his institution the rate of lymphographies has dropped to about 15% – 20% since introduction of whole body CT.
On the other hand, neither CT nor US nor conventional lymphography can be used to study the lymphatic drainage of tumors in a more selective, individual way. Many attempts have been made to inject Lipiodol directly into the diseased organ in close proximity to the tumor, but the oily contrast medium is not well suited for intraparenchymal, submucosal, or subcutaneous injection. A number of other contrast agents have been developed and investigated in animal experiments. So far, none of these is available for routine application in humans. However, I still hope that there will be a lymphographic renaissance as soon as we have a contrast medium suited for interstitial application.

Conclusions

Lymphography is still the "state of the art" standard against which all other imaging modalities have to be measured.
The advantages of CT and ultrasonography are best proven in the staging of malignant lymphoma and metastases of testicular tumors. In other metastatic diseases, at present, experience with noninvasive techniques is still rather limited. Prospective comparative studies are under way in many institutions, and when we convene again, 2 years from now, we will know more.

References

1. Alcorn FS, Mategrano VC, Petasnick JP, Clark JW (1977) Contributions of computed tomography in the staging and management of malignant lymphoma. Radiology 125:717 – 723
2. Anfossi A, Adami GF (to be published) Remarks on lymphographic and laparotomic findings in patients with fever of unknown origin (FUO). In: Weissleder H, Bartos V, Clodius L, Malek P (eds) Progress in Lymphology, Proceedings of the 7th International Congress of Lymphology, Florence 1979. Avicenum, Czechoslovak Medical Press, Prague
3. Best JJ, Blackledge G, Forbes WS, Todd ID, Eddleston B, Crowther D, Isherwood I (1978) Computed tomography of abdomen in staging and clinical management of lymphoma. Br Med J 2:1675 – 1677
4. Boecker R, Huth F, Juenemann A (1976) Eine neue Methode zur Darstellung der regionalen Lymphknoten der Harnblase. Ein vorläufiger Bericht. Dtsch med Wochenschr 101:1030 – 1031
5. Brascho DJ, Durant JR, Green LE (1977) The accuracy of retroperitoneal ultrasonography in Hodgkin's disease and non-Hodgkin lymphoma. Radiology 125:485 – 487
6. Breiman RS, Castellino RA, Harell GS, Marshall WH, Glatstein E, Kaplan HS (1978) CT-pathologic correlations in Hodgkin's disease and non-Hodgkin's lymphoma. Radiology 126:159 – 166
7. Brown RC, Buchsbaum HJ, Tewfik HH, Platz CE (1979) Accuracy of lymphangiography in the diagnosis of para-aortic lymph node metastasis from carcinoma of the cervix. Obstet Gynecol 54:571 – 575
8. Burney BT, Klatte EC (1979) Ultrasound and computed tomography of the abdomen in the staging and management of testicular carcinoma. Radiology 132:415 – 419
9. Callen PW, Filly RA, Korobkin M (1978) Computed tomographic evaluation of the diaphragmatic crura. Radiology 126:413

10. Castellino RA, Marglin SI (1979) Lymphographic accuracy in consecutive, previously untreated patients with Hodgkin's disease and non-Hodgkin's lymphoma. In: Weissleder H, Bartos V, Clodius L, Malek P (eds) Progress in Lymphology, Proceedings of the 7th International Congress of Lymphology, Florence 1979. Avicenum, Czechoslovak Medical Press, Prague
11. Chiappa S, Uslenghi C, Bonadonna G, Marano P, Ravasi G (1966) Combined testicular and foot lymphangiography in testicular carcinomas. Surg Gynecol Obstet 123:10
12. Collard M (1979) New Horizons in diagnostic lymphography. In: Weissleder H, Bartos V, Clodius L, Malek P (eds) Progress in Lymphology, Proceedings of the 7th International Congress of Lymphology, Florence 1979. Avicenum, Czechoslovak Medical Press, Prague
13. Földi M (1971) Erkrankungen des Lymphsystems. Witzstrock, Baden-Baden, Brussels
14. Fortner JG, Booker RJ, Pack GT (1964) Results of groin dissection for malignant melanoma in 220 patients. Surgery 55:485
15. Gerteis W (1967) The frequency of metastases in carcinoma of the cervix and the corpus. In: Rüttimann A (ed) Progress in lymphology. Thieme, Stuttgart
16. Göthlin J (1976) Post-lymphographic percutaneous fine needle biopsy of lymph nodes guided by fluoroscopy. Radiology 120:205 – 207
17. Göthlin JH, Macintosh PK (1979) Interventional radiology in the assessment of the retroperitoneal lymph nodes. Radiol Clin North Am 17:461 – 473
18. Haaga JR (1979) Vascular fat angle. J Comput Assist Tomogr 3:560
19. Harzmann R, Chiari R, Dhom G, Lehnhardt FH (1978) Indirekte Lymphographie der Harnblase im Tierversuch. Urologe [A] 17:261 – 264
20. Jones SE, Tobias DA, Waldman RS (1978) Computed tomographic scanning in patients with lymphoma. Cancer 41:480 – 486
21. Kademian M, Wirtanen G (1977) Accuracy of bipedal lymphangiography in testicular tumors. Urology 9:218 – 220
22. Kademian M, Wirtanen G (1977) Accuracy of bipedal lymphography in Hodgkin's disease. AJR 129: 1041 – 1042
23. Lackner K, Weissbach L, Boldt I, Scherholz K, Brecht G (1979) Computertomographischer Nachweis von Lymphknotenmetastasen bei malignen Hodentumoren: Vergleich der Ergebnisse von Lymphographie und Computertomographie. ROEFO 130:636 – 643
24. Lackner K, Brecht G, Janson R, Scherholz K, Lützeler A, Thurn P (1980) Wertigkeit der Computertomographie bei der Stadieneinteilung primärer Lymphknotenneoplasien. ROEFO 132: 21 – 30
25. Lee JKT, Stanley RJ, Sagel SS, McClennan BL (1978) Accuracy of CT in detecting intraabdominal and pelvic lymph node metastases from pelvic cancers. AJR 131:675 – 679
26. Lee JKT, Stanley RJ, Sagel SS, Melson GL, Koehler RE (1980) Limitations of the post-lymphangiogram plain abdominal radiograph as an indicator of recurrent lymphoma: comparison to computed tomography. Radiology 134:155 – 158
27. Lüning M, Wiljasalo M, Weissleder H (eds) (1976) Lymphographie bei malignen Tumoren. Thieme, Stuttgart
28. Lüning M, Schulz W, Röder K, Raab K, Rauste J (1977) Wertbestimmung lymphographischer Metastasenkriterien bei malignen Nierentumoren. Radiol Diagn (Berl) 18:315 – 323
29. Lüning M, Plasch J, Schilling H, Schnorr D, Wesirow G, Zyb AF, Jasutkin VV, Cepelenko GV (1977) Lymphographie bei Prostatakarzinomen. 1. Mitteilung. Radiol Diagn (Berl) 18:605 – 615
30. Macintosh PK, Thomson KR, Barbaric ZL (1979) Percutaneous transperitoneal lymph node biopsy as a means of improving lymphographic diagnosis. Radiology 131:647 – 649
30a. Meregaglia D, Kenda R, De Palo G, Musumeci R (to be published) Lymphography in tumors of the vulva. In: Weissleder H, Bartos V, Clodius L, Malek P (eds) Progress in Lymphology, Proceedings of the 7th International Congress of Lymphology, Florence 1979. Avicenum, Czechoslovak Medical Press, Prague
31. Müller RP, Peters PE, Fladerer W (to be published) Diagnostic accuracy in endolymphatic radiotherapy with limited amounts of labelled contrast medium. In: Weissleder H, Bartos V, Clodius L, Malek P (eds) Progress in Lymphology, Proceedings of the 7th International Congress of Lymphology, Florence 1979. Avicenum, Czechoslovak Medical Press, Prague
32. Müller RP, Galanski M, Cramer BM (1980) CT des retroperitonealen Lymphsystems. Lymphatische Systemerkrankungen und Metastasen. 61. Deutscher Röntgenkongreß, Cologne 1980
33. Musumeci R, de Palo GM, Mangioni C, Bolis G, Ratti E (1978) The lymphatic spread of ovarian germinal and stromal tumors. Lymphology 11:22 – 26
34. Musumeci R, de Palo G, Gardani S, Kenda R, Tesoro-Tess G, Volterrani F (to be published) Results of lymphangiography in gynecological cancer. In: Weissleder H, Bartos V, Clodius L, Malek P (eds) Progress in Lymphology, Proceedings of the 7th International Congress of Lymphology, Florence 1979. Avicenum, Czechoslovak Medical Press, Prague
35. Musumeci R, Kenda R, Meregaglia D, Pizzocaro G, Zanini M, Zanoni F (to be published) Results of lymphography in urologic cancer. In: Weissleder H, Bartos V, Clodius L, Malek P (eds) Progress in Lymphology, Proceedings of the 7th International Congress of Lymphology, Florence 1979. Avicenum, Czechoslovak Medical Press, Prague
36. Peters PE, Weissleder H, Kipper S, Ehring F, Makoski HB, Pfannenstiel P, Schnepper E, zum Winkel K (to be published) Intralymphatic isotope therapy – an effective alternative to the "wait-and-

see-policy" in the treatment of stage I malignant melanoma of the lower limb. In: Weissleder H, Bartos V, Clodius L, Malek P (eds) Progress in Lymphology, Proceedings of the 7th International Congress of Lymphology, Florence 1979. Avicenum, Czechoslovak Medical Press, Prague

37. Peters PE, Steinbrich W, Müller RP (1980) CT des retroperitonealen Lymphsystems. Normale Anatomie 61. Dtsch. Röntgenkongreß, Cologne 1980
38. Petrillo R, Doci R, Mauri M, Musumeci R (to be published) Lymphangiography in carcinoma of the sigmoid, rectum and anus. In: Weissleder H, Bartos V, Clodius L, Malek P (eds) Progress in Lymphology, Proceedings of the 7th International Congress of Lymphology, Florence 1979. Avicenum, Czechoslovak Medical Press, Prague
39. Raghavaiah NV, Jordan WP (1979) Prostatic lymphography. J Urol 121:178 – 181
40. Reiffenstuhl G (1967) Das Lymphknotenproblem beim Carcinoma colli uteri und die Lymphirradiatio pelvis. Urban & Schwarzenberg, München
41. Tallroth K, Makai F, Musumeci R (to be published) Lymphography in bone and soft tissue sarcomas. In: Weissleder H, Bartos V, Clodius L, Malek P (eds) Progress in Lymphology, Proceedings of the 7th International Congress of Lymphology, Florence 1979. Avicenum, Czechoslovak Medical Press, Prague
42. Viamonte M, Rüttimann A (1980) Atlas of Lymphography. Thieme, Stuttgart
43. Wiljasalo M, Virtama P, Dean PB (to be published) Spherical form of carcinoma metastases in computerized tomography. In: Weissleder H, Bartos V, Clodius L, Malek P (eds) Progress in Lymphology, Proceedings of the 7th International Congress of Lymphology, Florence 1979. Avicenum, Czechoslovak Medical Press, Prague
44. Wiljasalo S, Lüning M, Raab K (1972) Spezifische röntgenologische Kriterien beim malignen Melanom. Radiol Diagn (Berl) 13:631
45. Zelch MG, Haaga JR (1979) Clinical comparison of computed tomography and lymphangiography for detection of retroperitoneal lymphadenopathy. Radiol Clin North Am 17:157 – 168
46. Zingg EJ, Fuchs WA, Heritier P (1974) Lymphography in carcinoma of the prostate. Br J Urol 46:549 – 554

Real-Time Ultrasonography of the Lymphatic System

D. Beyer

Universität Köln, Radiologisches Institut, Joseph-Stelzmann-Strasse 9, D-5000 Köln 41

Introduction

Since retroperitoneal lymph nodes are frequent sites for spread of a wide variety of malignancies, the detection of the presence and extent of lymph node involvement is of critical importance when evaluating patients with suspected malignant diseases. The question of lymph node enlargement arises most commonly in patients with lymphoma, although the need to identify enlarged lymph nodes in addition to other space-occupying lesions exists in other neoplastic diseases as well.

Accurate anatomic staging is not only important for therapeutic decisions, but often for follow-up studies after chemotherapy as well [1, 4, 10, 14].

There are four major indications for imaging intra- and retroperitoneal lymph nodes by ultrasonography:

1. Evaluation of presence and extent of disease
2. Staging
3. Guide to therapy planning
   a) Prior to fine-needle biopsy
   b) Determination of radiation portals
4. Follow-up examination
   a) Evaluation of completeness of response to therapy
   b) Detection of recurrence of disease

Both ultrasonography (US) and computed tomography (CT) play an important role in this situation and might be able to replace lymphography and intravenous urography in a large number of patients. This report summarizes our findings with real-time US in patients with suspected intra- and retroperitoneal lymphadenopathy, compared with the findings of CT, lymphography, and histology.

Examination Technique

The study of lymph node-bearing areas of the abdomen, retroperitoneum and pelvis does not vary from a routine abdominal real-time study, which is always performed in a systematic fashion. Transverse and sagittal scans of the abdomen are performed in combination with subcostal and lateral views of liver and spleen to assess size and echogenicity as a sign of infiltration or lymphomatous involvement of these organs. Secondary effects such as biliary obstruction from enlarged porta hepatis lymph nodes may be visible as well.

For the pelvic portion of the examination a full urinary bladder is required to permit sufficient visualization of the pelvic walls.

At present we scan with a 2.2 and 3.0 MHz mechanical real-time scanner with a rotating transducer and parabolic mirror in a water bath (rectangular parallel line scan – Vidoson 735 and Vidoson 735 SM). We also use a computer controlled, automatic real-time scanner with compound-scan properties (RA 1 – Siemens).

Results

Normal Anatomy

In the middle and upper abdomen, the inferior vena cava (IVC), the aorta with its branches, and the psoas muscle are the most important retroperitoneal structures to be visualized frequently, usually more completely on sagittal scans.

On the right parasagittal scan the head of the pancreas lying in front of the IVC must be differentiated from enlarged lymph nodes, which usually is not difficult since pancreatic tissue is echogenic while lymphoid tissue is sonolucent because of its acoustically homogeneous texture. Superficially these lymph nodes often resemble fluid-filled abnormalities, but do not show increased through transmission.

Radiology Today 1. Ed. by M. W. Donner and F. H. W. Heuck

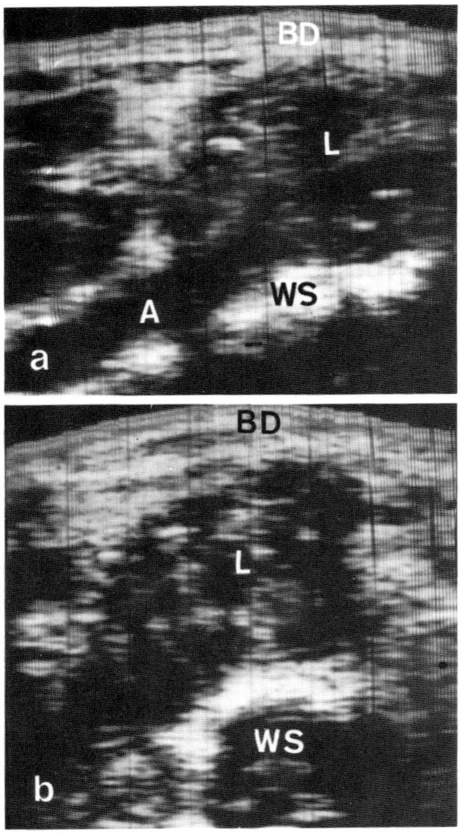

Fig. 1. **a** 30-year-old patient with testicular teratoma. Longitudinal section at the level through the midabdomen demonstrates a big, lobulated, echo-poor mass of lymphoma (*L*) adjacent to the anterior margin of the aorta (*A*). **b** Transverse scan at the level of the midportion of the kidneys demonstrates lack of distinct separation between the aorta and vena cava, indicating para- and preaortic adenopathy (*L*). The prevertebral vessels are totally encased and obscured by the mass ("echo silhouette sign"). *WS,* spine; *BD,* abdominal wall

If these lucent masses change in form and show moving internal echos from peristalsis, they represent bowel loops. In these cases real-time US is extremely helpful and reliable in differentiation.

Pathologic Anatomy

Lymph node enlargements greater than 2–3 cm [2, 15, 16] are shown as one or more sonolucent masses adjacent to the anterior margin of the aorta and IVC and can appear in certain rather classic manifestations, which include:

1. A single, lobulated or confluent mass related to the aorta, IVC, porta hepatis, or mesentery, sausage shaped on corresponding parasagittal scans (Fig. 1a, b).
2. A preaortic, mantle-shaped plate encasing the aorta or IVC, sometimes elevating these structures from the lumbar spine (Fig. 2a–c) ("floating-aorta").
3. Bilateral, symmetrical, preaortic and precaval masses ("dumb-bell appearance") (Fig. 3a, b) and multiple spindle-shaped masses [2, 4, 6, 7, 8, 12, 13, 14].

Nodes involving the root of the mesentery, a fairly frequent occurrence in patients with lymphoma, will show sonolucent, oval-shaped masses with a layered or stratified appearance with plates of echogenic tissue (portions of mesentery) between them, representing lymphoma infiltrating the mesenteric leaves and encasing the superior mesenteric vessels (SMA and SMV) and perivascular fat ("sandwich-sign") [7, 8, 12, 13]. The specificity of

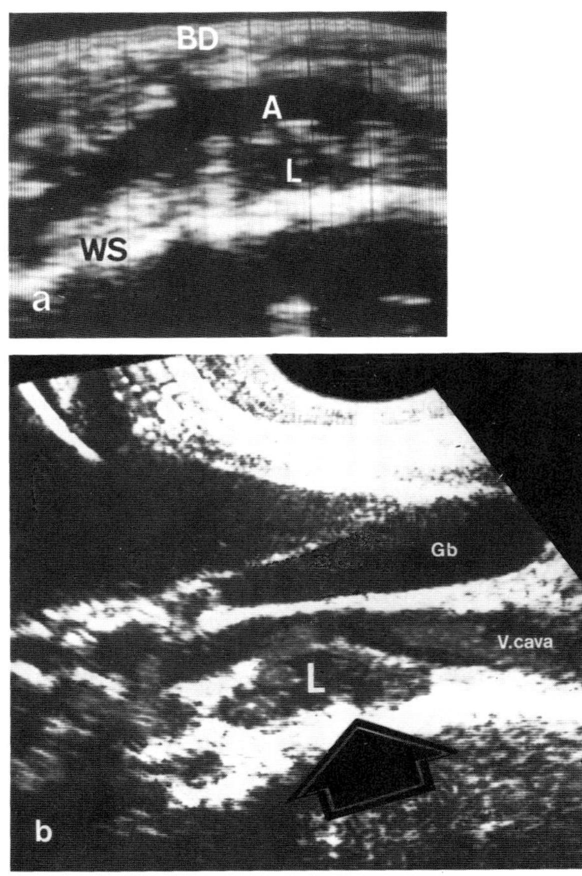

Fig. 2. **a** 21-year-old patient with testicular teratoma. Longitudinal scan of the lower lumbar region involved with lymphoma (*L*). The enlarged lymph nodes separate and elevate the aorta from the spine (*WS*) ("floating aorta"). **b** 39-year-old patient with Hodgkin's disease. Lymphoma (*L*) displacing the inferior vena cava anteriorly from the spine (*WS*)

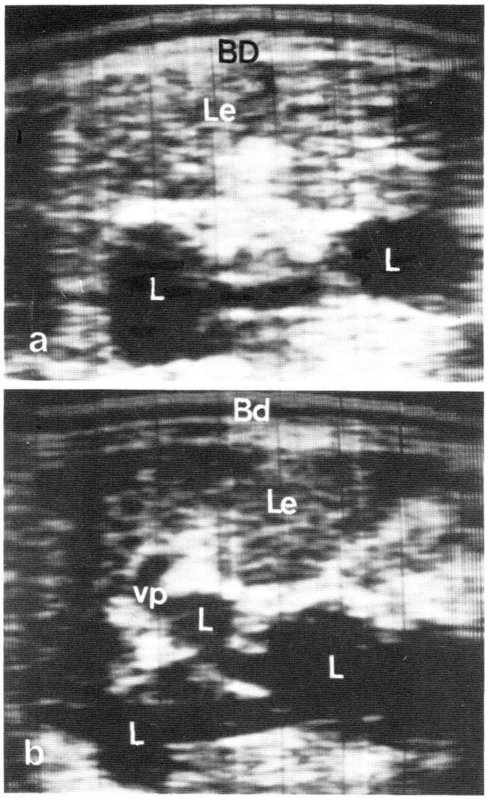

Fig. 3. a 35-year-old patient with non-Hodgkin's lymphoma. Transverse scan shows bilateral, symmetrical, echo-poor pre-aortic and pre-caval masses obscuring vena cava and aorta ("dumb-bell appearance"). (*Le,* liver; *BD,* abdominal wall). **b** Same patient with multiple echo-poor masses (*L*) representing lymphoma in the porta hepatis surrounding the portal vein (*vp*)

this sandwich sign [13] of lymphomatous mesenteric adenopathy is unclear, but no instances of metastatic carcinoma have yet been observed to give this appearance.

Sometimes aorta and IVC are difficult to recognize when they are surrounded by enlarged lymph nodes (Figs. 1a, b, 3a). This "echo-silhouette sign" [7, 8] is caused by the similar density of nodal tissue and the elastic walls of the great vessels most frequently seen in young patients and less commonly in the elderly, where the aortic wall is of harder consistency [12]. Occasionally smaller lymph nodes can be identified by the apparently irregular anterior margin they impose on the aorta.

For identification of these lesions, certain additional features are helpful. The presence of an enlarged spleen or liver sometimes showing a coarse parenchymal texture as a sign of diffuse or nodular infiltration is suggestive of lymphoma as contrasted to other masses [8, 9]. Metastatic disease of the liver can be demonstrated as well.

It is usually more difficult to identify lymph node enlargement on the pelvic sidewalls than para-aortic adenopathy. With more experience and improved equipment we are able to identify lymph nodes larger than 3 cm along the iliac chains anterior to the iliopsoas muscle compartment, but gas in the pelvic colon often prevents adequate evaluation of pelvic lymph nodes.

Diagnostic Accuracy of Ultrasonography in Diseases of the Lymphatic System

During a 12-month period at the University Hospital of Cologne, 160 patients with the diagnosis of Hodgkin's or non-Hodgkin's lymphoma and malignant tumours underwent clinical staging; they compose the case material for this study (Table 1). As a part of this, all 160 patients had a real-time ultrasound examination, and 129 went on to have CT and/or lymphography and staging laparatomy.

The presence or absence of adenopathy was then determined for each of these anatomic regions: porta hepatis; splenic hilum, retropancreatic, celiac and superior mesenteric, right and left para-aortic, right and left renal pedicles, and right and left iliac lymph nodes.

Lymph node groups were interpreted as involved when, in a lymph node group, we were able to demonstrate echo-free or echo-poor masses which could not be accounted for by normal anatomic structures. Also splenic and hepatic size and the echo pattern of these organs were evaluated.

Table 1. Real-time ultrasonography of the lymphatic system (129 patients with malignant lymphoma and metastatic disease)

Result	*n*
Correct positive	61/84
Correct negative	40/45
False negative	23/84
Iliac chains	18
Para-aortic nodes	5
False positive	5/45

Sensitivity of ultrasonography 72.6%
Specificity of ultrasonography 88.8%
Overall accuracy of ultrasonography 78.3%

The sensitivity of a diagnostic procedure is defined as the percentage of tests read as abnormal in diseased patients, and the specificity, as the percentage of tests read as normal in patients without disease. For our group the sensitivity of real-time US was 72.6% for abdominal involvement, the specificity, 88.8% (Table 1). The overall accuracy, defined as the sum of all correct positive and negative results related to the number of all patients studied, was 78.3%. The sensitivity in cases with enlarged abdominal lymph nodes above the pelvis was 91% and the overall accuracy, 90.2%.

Evaluation of the spleen revealed only little correlation between splenic involvement and splenic size, furthermore there were no characteristic changes of the echo pattern as a result of involvement with lymphoma.

The results of our study demonstrate the ability of US to display lymphomatous involvement of many lymph node groups not delineated by lymphography. The demonstration of nodal involvement in these sites merits considerable attention because of revisions in therapy and prognosis which follow.

The main weakness of the method was that in five patients involved and enlarged iliac nodes were missed and that 17 patients had tumor growth in lymph nodes of normal size – demonstrated by lymphography – and consequently were not detectable by US (and CT).

Table 2. Comparison of US, CT, and lymphography: relative advantages in the diagnosis of lymphadenopathy

	US	CT	Lymphography
Average initial investment	+		
Cost of examination	+		
Time for examination (real-time US)	+		
Radiation dose or toxic effect	+		
Invasiveness	+		
Morphological detail			+
Diagnostic accuracy			
Thin patient	(+)		+
Fat patient		(+)	+
Ease of interpretation		+	
Operator dependence		+	
Limitations		+	(+)
Clinician acceptance		(+)	+

Discussion

Both US and CT are increasingly being used to evaluate abdominal and pelvic lymph nodes. Some general statements can be made regarding these now currently used radiologic techniques and lymphography in the evaluation of subdiaphragmatic lymphadenopathies (Table 2).

With current instrumentation US and CT, are of considerable value to those involved in the care of patients with malignant diseases depending upon the detection of neoplastic lymph node enlargement, but unfortunately the appearance of enlarged lymph nodes in US and CT scans is non-specific. Since not every enlarged node contains tumor and conversely, not all tumour-bearing nodes are enlarged, lymphography is still superior in this respect and may still be required after "normal" US and CT results [1, 11]. Lymphography is able to demonstrate the size of lymph nodes, demonstrates their internal structure, detects tumor growth in lymph nodes of normal size, and is able to distinguish the large, but normal reactive lymph node from the large, tumor-containing node [5]. Lymphoid hyperplasia and non-caseating granuloma can give false positive US and CT scans [2].

In contrast to lymphography, both US and CT are capable of showing nodal masses in locations such as the hilum of the liver, in the peripancreatic or retrogastric area or in the mesentery, which are usually not visualized with conventional pedal lymphography [12], but importantly a negative US or CT examination of these regions does not exclude malignant involvement of these lymph nodes. In addition both US and CT often reveal more extensive disease than lymphography.

The resolution of third-generation CT scanners is generally superior to US [3, 11], but patients with thin or normal body habitus are better evaluated by US, because the paucity of retroperitoneal fat makes CT sometimes very difficult to evaluate. However, intestinal gas and obesity are major impediments for US, markedly limiting the ability of this imaging technique to demonstrate mesenteric adenopathy unless they are large enough to displace surrounding air-containing bowel loops. This set of circumstances clearly indicates the complementary nature of these two imaging modalities.

Real-time US is a highly operator-dependent imaging technique; the quality of images and therefore diagnostic information of an examination is closely related to the skill and interest of the operator, while CT mainly requires good interpretation of standard images. Lymphatic can-

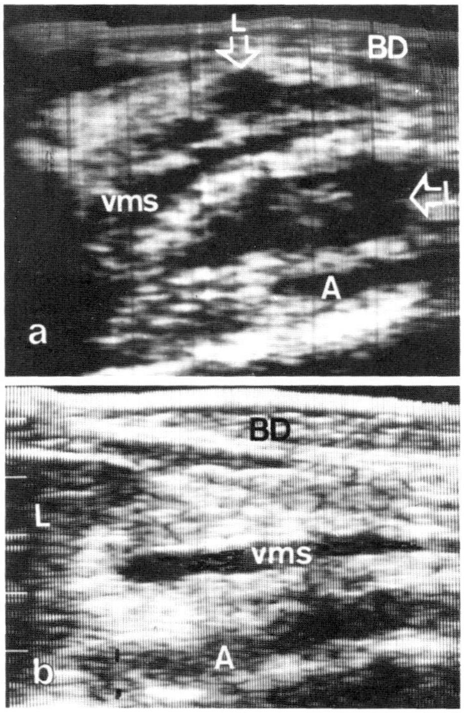

Fig. 4. a 30-year-old patient with malignant lymphoma. Longitudinal scan demonstrates large, sonolucent masses anterior and posterior to the superior mesenteric vein (*vms*) and surrounding central linear areas of increased echogenicity representing fat in the leaves of the mesentery ("sandwich sign"). Behind the masses the aorta is discernible and separate from the mass, indicating that this lymphoma is mesenteric rather than preaortic. **b** Same patient 6 weeks later after cytostatic therapy. Lymphoma is no longer demonstrable. *A,* aorta; *BD,* abdominal wall

nulation and interpretation of lymphangiograms requires high technical skills and advanced training as well.

US is the ideal imaging technique since it is noninvasive and has no known harmful side effects. Both CT and lymphography require radiation, a fact which seems of minor importance in the evaluation of patients with malignant disease which will subsequently undergo radiation or cytostatic therapy. Beyond that lymphography is always invasive and has a small, but definite risk to the patient. CT is usually performed with infusion of water-soluble contrast medium with a remote risk of allergic reaction [5].

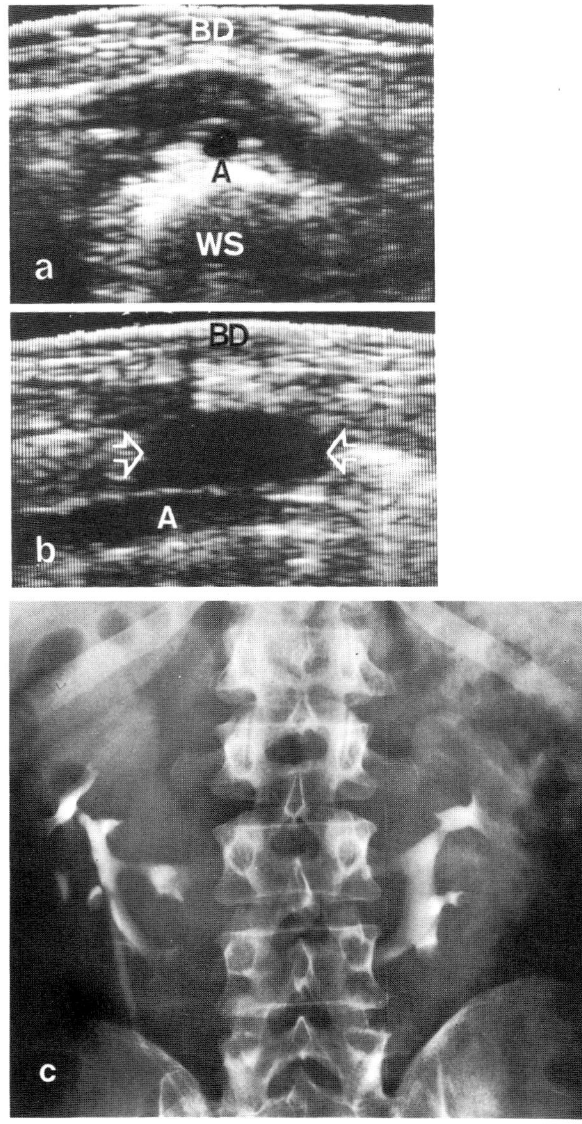

Fig. 5a – c. Pitfall of ultrasonography. 34-year-old patient with non-Hodgkin's lymphoma. **a** Transverse scan demonstrates a large preaortic and precaval, echo-poor mass which is well delineated. **b** Longitudinal scan shows a 6 × 3 cm echo-poor, well-delineated mass anterior to the aorta (*A*). False positive diagnosis: preaortic and precaval adenopathy. **c** Intravenous urogram shows a horseshoe kidney with a large parenchymal bridge anterior to the spine (*WS*). *BD,* abdominal wall

Conclusions

The evaluation of lymphatic disease has been remarkably improved by US and CT, which possess advantages as well as disadvantages. The most apparent disadvantage of both is that they only provide information about lymph node size and relative density whereas lymphography also demonstrates internal lymph node architecture and thus has the potential of displaying abnormalities within normal size lymph nodes.

The obvious advantage of US and CT is their ability to demonstrate many other groups of lymph nodes not opacified by lymphography and the size and internal structure of liver and spleen [1, 11, 14].

Though the interpretation of CT is more reproducible, its resolution is better and there are no limitations by gas-filled bowel, the relative accuracy of US indicates that a patient with suspected lymphadenopathy should have initial evaluation with the quicker and cheaper technique of US as a *baseline study,* especially as liver and spleen can be evaluated simultaneously, particularly using real-time technique.

If US reveals negative findings one should proceed to CT, because our results show a significant number of false negative reports, especially in the pelvis. If CT is also normal, and there is still a high level of clinical suspicion of disease, lymphography is indicated.

If the ultrasonographic study is definitely abnormal, in most instances no further investigation is necessary. In small or equivocal lesions the patient should have CT and both examinations should be interpreted by the same radiologist. If the tests are in agreement, it is likely that this reflects the true pathologic state and obviates the need for pedal lymphography. Contradictory findings indicate an equivocal result and lymphography must be considered.

Follow-up studies in patients with known disease under therapy should be obtained by US with no pain intervention and at reasonable cost. Evaluation to substantiate eradication of metastatic nodes as well as prior to node dissection should be done with both modalities (US and CT). The routine use of lymphography is unnecessary in this patient population [4], but it seems unlikely that US and CT will be able to replace lymphography totally.

By individualizing each case, the radiologist is able to select a proper examination sequence to provide a maximum of diagnostic accuracy and reliability at a minimum of radiation exposure, cost, and annoyance to the patient.

References

1. Alcorn FS, Mategrano VC, Petasnik JP, Clark JW (1977) Contributions of computed tomography in the staging and management of malignant lymphoma. Radiology 125:717–723
2. Brascho DJ, Durant JR, Green LE (1977) The accuracy of retroperitoneal ultrasonography in Hodgkin's disease and non-Hodgkin's lymphoma. Radiology 125:485–487
3. Breimann RS, Castellino RA, Harell GS, Marshall WH, Glatstein E, Kaplan HS (1978) CT-pathologic correlations in Hodgkin's disease and non-Hodgkin's lymphoma. Radiology 126:159–166
4. Burney BT, Klatte EC (1979) Ultrasound and computed tomography of the abdomen and management of testicular carcinoma. Radiology 132:415–419
5. Castellino RA (1979) Abdominal lymphadenopathy – lymphography. In: Moss AA, Goldberg HJ (eds) Computed tomography, ultrasound and X-ray: an integrated approach. Masson, New York Paris Barcelona Milano Mexico City Rio de Janeiro, pp 105–123
6. Filly RA, Marglin S, Castellino RA (1976) The ultrasonographic spectrum of abdominal and pelvic Hodgkin's disease and non-Hodgkin's lymphoma. Cancer 38:2143–2148
7. Freimanis AK (1975) Echographic diagnosis of lesions of the abdominal aorta and lymph nodes. Radiol Clin North Am 13:557–573
8. Freimanis AK (1979) Echography and other diagnostic methods in retroperitoneal node enlargement and other masses. In: Sodee DB (ed) Correlation in diagnostic imaging. Appleton-Century-Crofts, New York, pp 145–152
9. Glees JP, Taylor KJW, Gazet JC, Peckham MJ, McCready VR (1977) Accuracy of grey-scale ultrasonography of liver and spleen in Hodgkin's disease and other lymphomas compared with isotope scans. Clin Radiol 28:233–238
10. Heckemann R, Weichert HC, Röttinger EM, Hossfeld DK (1977) Sonographische Verlaufskontrollen bei retroperitonealen Tumoren unter Chemotherapie. ROEFO 126:236–240
11. Lee JKT, Stanley RJ, Sagel SS, Levitt RG (1978) Accuracy of computed tomography in detecting intraabdominal and pelvic adenopathy in lymphoma. AJR 131:311–315
12. Leopold GR (1978) Ultrasonic evaluation of retropertitoneal lymphadenopathy. In: Korobkin M (ed) Computed tomography, ultrasound and X-ray: an integrated approach. pp 449–455
13. Müller PR, Ferrucci JT Jr, Harbin WP, Kirkpatrick RH, Simeone JF, Wittenberg J (1980) Appearance of lymphomatous involvement of the mesentery by ultrasonography and body computed tomography: the "sandwich sign". Radiology 134:467–473
14. Rochester D, Bowie JD, Kunzmann A, Lester E (1977) Ultrasound in the staging of lymphoma. Radiology 124:483–487
15. Vadrot D, Laval-Jeantet M, Vadrot M, Delmas PE, Bouzac H (1978) L'échotomographie dans l'étude des adénopathies abdominales. Techniques d'examen et séméiologie. J Radiol Electrol Med Nucl 59/6–7:399–406
16. Viamonte M Jr, Rüttimann A (1980) Atlas of lymphography. Thieme, Stuttgart New York

Iotasul, a Water-Soluble Contrast Agent for Direct and Indirect Lymphography: Preclinical Results

H. M. Siefert, H. Miklautz, W. Mützel, C. Schöbel, F. Siegmund, H.-J. Weinmann, and B. I. Wenzel-Hora

Schering AG, Fachbereich Vorklinische Entwicklung, Department Röntgenkontrastmittel, Müllerstrasse 170–178, D-1000 Berlin 65

Iotasul is a non-ionic, dimeric X-ray contrast medium which is distinguished from other representatives of its class of compounds by outstanding physicochemical properties.

If an aqueous formulation of this contrast agent is infused into body fluids such as serum or lymph – in the tests under discussion the iodine content was 275 and 300 mg/ml – it separates into two phases having different degrees of molecular association (see Fig. 1).

The more highly associated phase – it has an apparent molecular weight of >100000 and an iodine content of ~ 465 mg/ml – can be demonstrated by light microscopy in the form of ultrafine droplets or streaks, which sink to the bottom of the test tube. By shaking, this highly associated phase is increasingly disassociated, i.e. it dissolves to a monophasic clear solution.

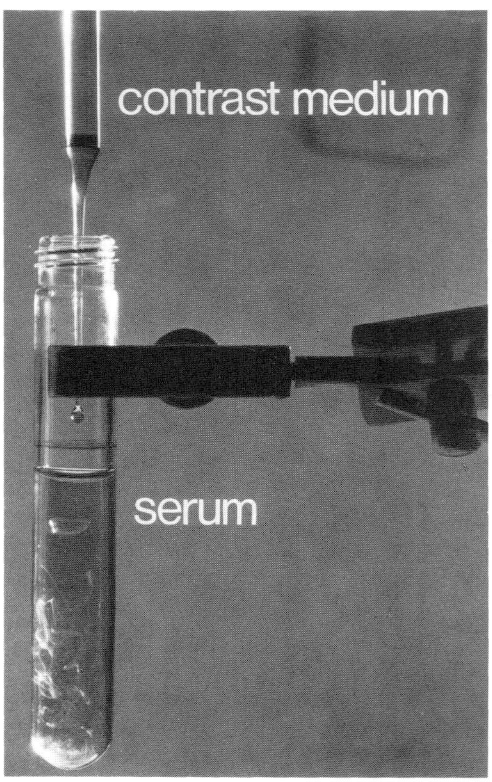

Fig. 1. Physicochemical properties of iotasul

Based on this physicochemical property and the extremely low osmotic pressure of aqueous formulations of iotasul, it is particularly well suited to lymphographic investigations, unlike conventional water-soluble X-ray contrast media.

It shows a strinkingly low tendency to spread through the walls of lymphatic vessels. The continuing flow of lymphatic fluid does not influence contrast quality in any visible way. Thus, retention of the contrast medium in the lymphatic system is sufficient for satisfactory radiographic investigations.

When carrying out direct lymphography in dogs, these properties result in visualization with a quality of contrast and detail at least as good as that obtained after administration of oily contrast media. Information which is usually obtained in two separate stages after instillation of oily contrast media is simultaneously available after intralymphatic infusion of iotasul (Fig. 2a). The course of the thoracic duct up to its entry into the venous system can be visualized homogeneously with this contrast medium (Fig. 2b).

A continuous increase of blood iodine concentration was already demonstrated immediately after commencement of intralymphatic administration of iotasul in the dog. At the end of infusion of the contrast medium, maximum blood iodine concentration was about 0.2 mg/ml (Fig. 3a). This corresponds to about 4% of the dose in total blood volume of the dog. After the end of infusion blood iodine concentration decreased continuously with a biological half-life of about 1 h. This value is consistent with that of conventional X-ray contrast media for urography. After intralymphatic administration in the dog, elimination of iotasul by the renal route is practically complete within 24 h (Fig. 3b). A thin-layer chromatographic analysis of

Radiology Today 1. Ed. by M. W. Donner and F. H. W. Heuck

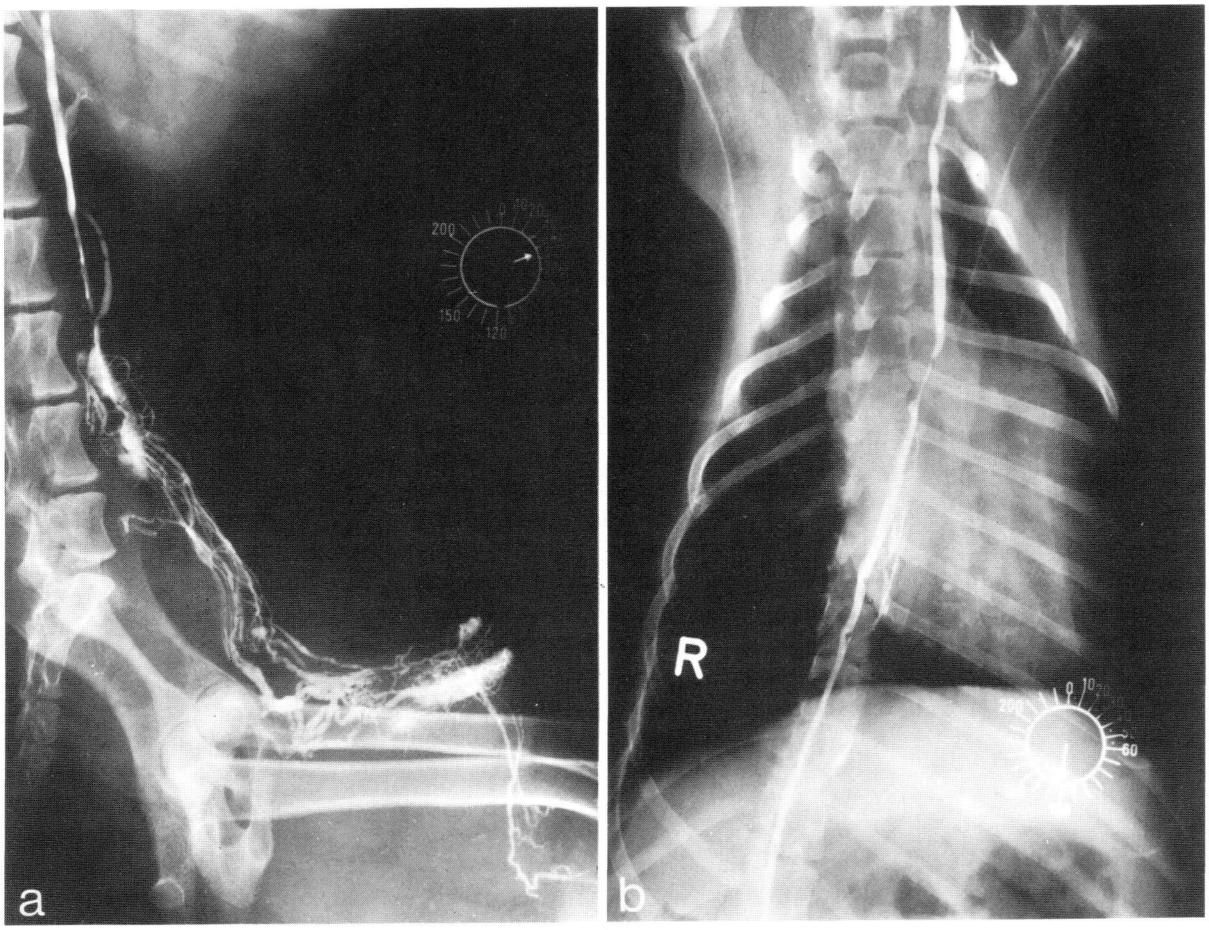

Fig. 2a, b. Direct lymphography in dog after intralymphatic (hind limb) administration of iotasul. **a** Inguinal and iliac lymph nodes with afferent lymph vessels and lumbar trunks. **b** Course of the thoracic duct up to its entry into the venous system

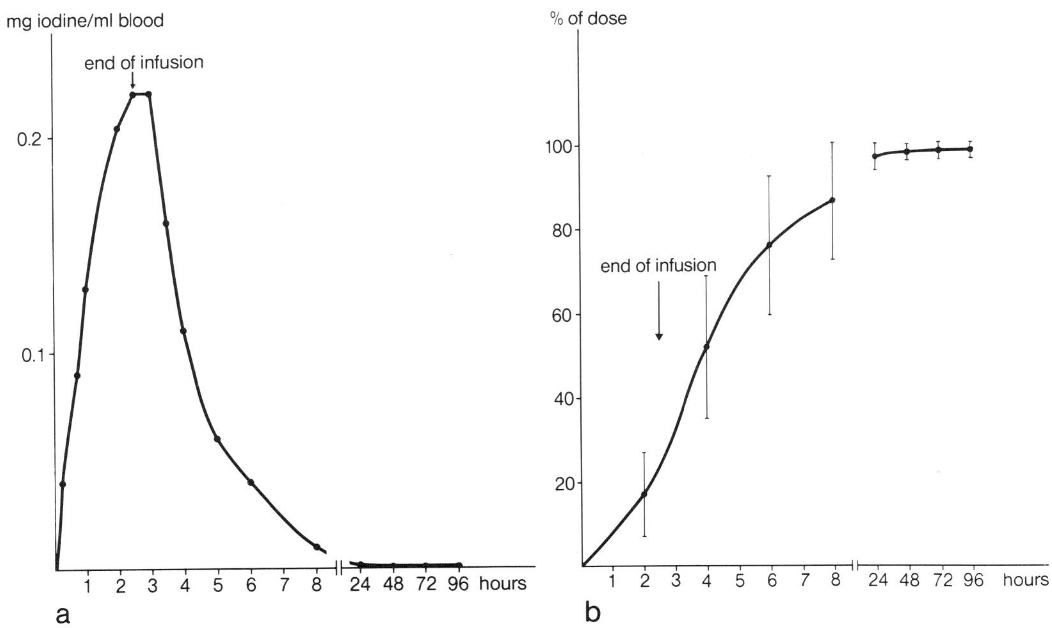

Fig. 3a, b. Pharmacokinetics in dog after intralymphatic (hind limb) administration of iotasul. Dose: 0.3 g iodine/kg body weight. **a** Blood level, mean of five animals. **b** Cumulative renal excretion, mean of five animals

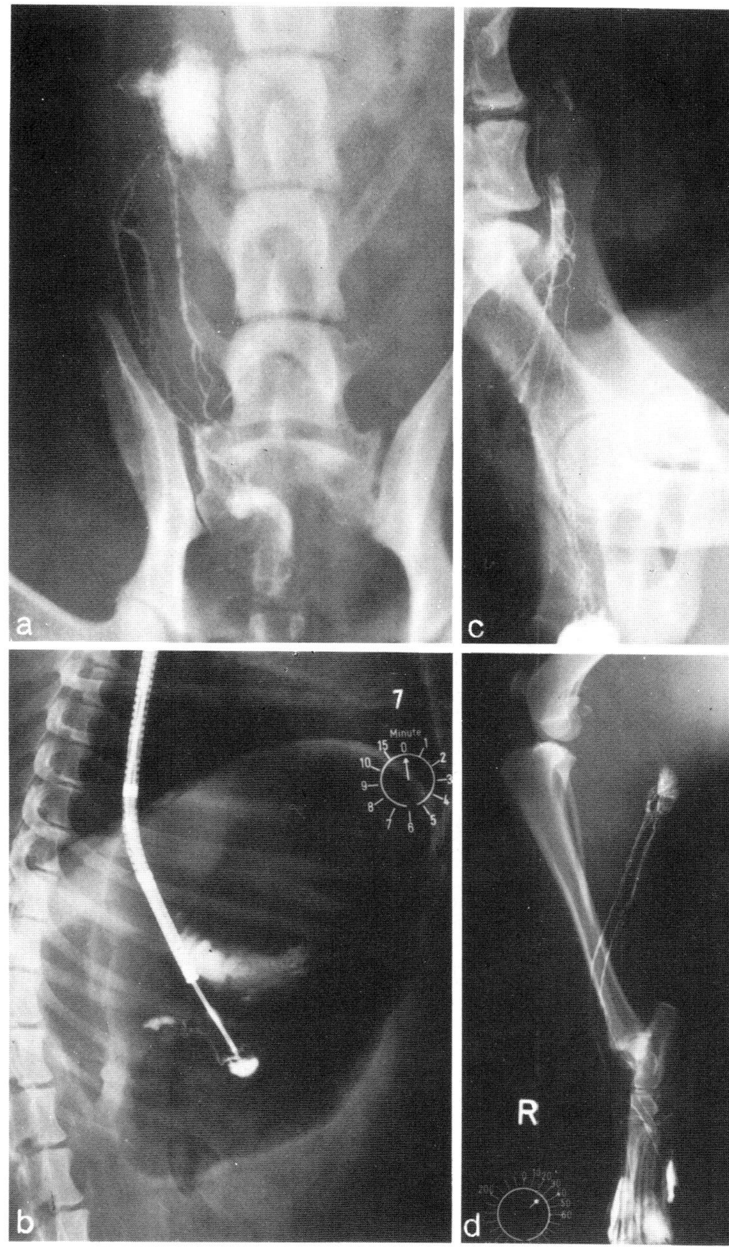

Fig. 4a – d. Indirect lymphography in dog after intraparenchymal, submucosal and intracutaneous administration of iotasul. **a** Superficial inguinal lymph node. **b** Gastric lymph node. **c** Sacral lymph nodes. **d** Popliteal lymph node

dog urine did not reveal any biotransformation of this contrast agent.

Visualization of the lymphatic system comparable to that after intralymphatic infusion of iotasul can also be achieved by injecting the contrast medium into lymph nodes, a procedure which might be termed indirect lymphography. Both after intralymphatic and intranodal administration of the contrast medium the first lymph node group of organs, which is important for early recognition of metastatic involvement, could only very occasionally be visualized. However, by using indirect methods such as intraparenchymal, submucosal, or intracutaneous administration it was possible to visualize the first lymph node stage excellently with iotasul (see Figs. 4, 5). By infusion of greater amounts of contrast medium solution it was also possible to opacify further lymph node stages.

The results of initial toxicological tests in dogs, rats and mice, and observation of more than 300 laboratory animals speak for exceptionally good tolerance of iotasul. The LD_{50} values for this contrast agent might be even higher than those stated in Table 1, especially as no mortality was demonstrated after the highest tested doses. After intralymphatic or intratissue administration of iot-

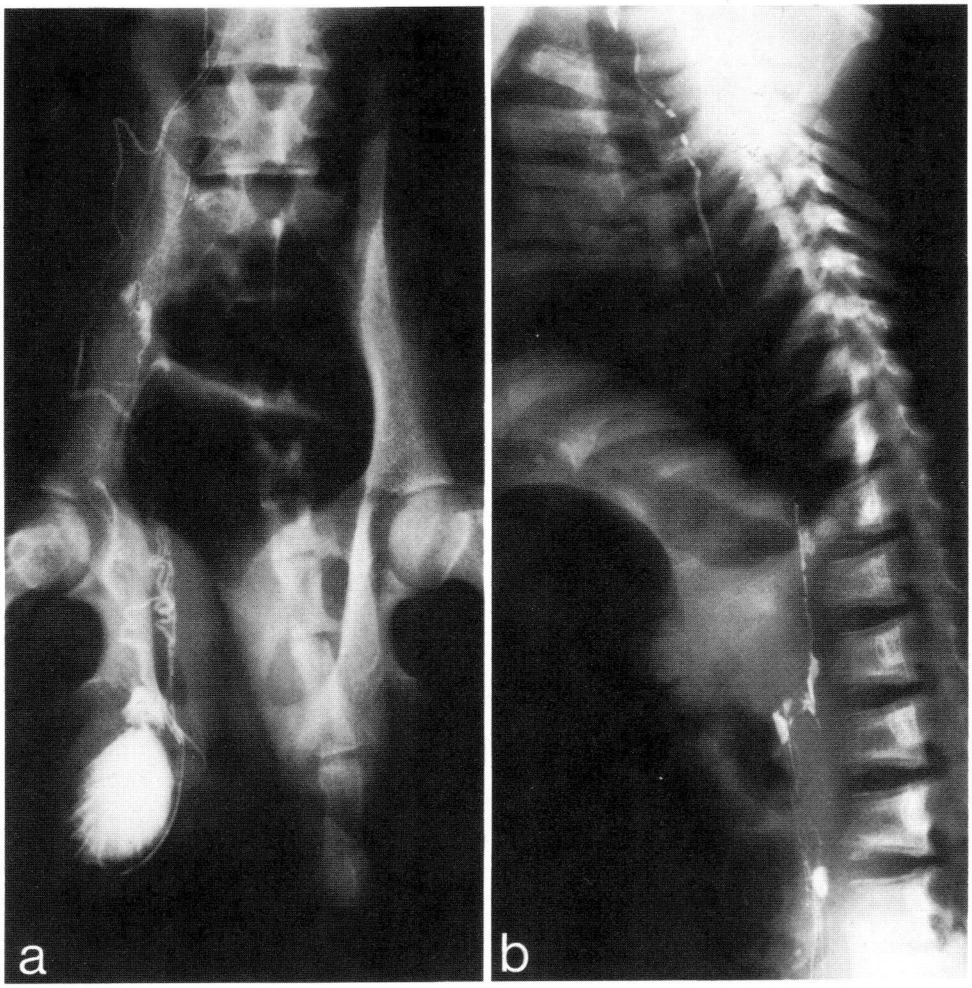

Fig. 5a, b. Indirect lymphography in monkey after intraparenchymal (testicle) administration of iotasul

Table 1. Acute toxicity of iotasul

A	Intraperitoneal administration	
	Species	LD_{50}
	Rat	> 11 g iodine/kg
	Mouse	> 14 g iodine/kg
	Dog	> 10 g iodine/kg
B	Subcutaneous administration	
	Species	LD_{50}
	Rat	> 11 g iodine/kg
	Mouse	> 14 g iodine/kg
C	Intragastral administration	
	Species	LD_{50}
	Rat	> 11 g iodine/kg
	Mouse	> 14 g iodine/kg

asul, no pathological tissue changes were demonstrated in the dog either by light microscopic or electron microscopic methods (Huth, F. and coworkers, unpublished results).
The following clinical advantages in direct lymphography could be attributed to the water-soluble contrast medium iotasul:

1. The ability to recognize details of the lymphatic system is better than after administration of oily X-ray contrast media.
2. The tolerance of iotasul is far better than that of oily contrast media. There is no risk of microembolism in the lungs or pathological alterations in the lymphatic system.
3. Rapid diagnostic procedure; less radiation exposure for the patient.

In addition, iotasul seems to be most suitable for indirect lymphography:

1. An investigation of the lymphatic system is possible without surgery. Local anaesthesia is not necessary. There is less chance of secondary infection or allergy to vital dyes.
2. An investigation of the lymphatic system can be carried out by simplified techniques of administration.
3. Visualization of the first lymph node group of organs permits improved tumour staging.

Ultrasound

Ultrasound: Overview

R. C. Sanders

Johns Hopkins Medical Institutions, Department of Radiology and Radiological Science,
601 N. Broadway, Baltimore, MD 21205 (USA)

Many exciting developments have occurred in the field of ultrasound in the past 2 years.

Kidney

The principal recent advances in the field of renal sonography relate to the detailed elucidation of sonographic renal anatomy and a description of the findings in medical renal disease. Thanks to the painstaking work of Cook et al. [1], who sectioned kidneys in vitro along the axis of a previous ultrasonic scan, it is known that one can identify the renal pyramids and arcuate vessels on a sonogram (Fig. 1). The pyramids appear as a relatively echopenic area compared to the more echogenic cortex. The arcuate vessels are echogenic structures at the apex of the pyramidal zone of sonolucency. In the normal patient the renal parenchyma is less echogenic than the liver, but in medical renal disease the kidney often becomes more echogenic (Fig. 2). Rosenfield et al. [2] have categorized medical renal disease in terms of parenchymal echogenicity. In the earlier stages the renal parenchyma becomes as echogenic as liver parenchyma and at a later, more severe, stage it is more echogenic than the liver and as echogenic as the sinus echoes. Although these changes are common, they do not appear specific, and many renal diseases adopt the same appearance.

The reliability of ultrasound in the assessment of hydronephrosis has been confirmed [3]. In about 15% of cases a false positive sonographic diagnosis of hydronephrosis occurs either in patients with extrarenal pelves or due to the presence of peripelvic cysts or reflux. In less than 1% of patients with renal failure there is a false negative finding. False negative findings which fail to show hydronephrosis occur in patients who have both hydronephrosis and renal calculi; consequently one should be

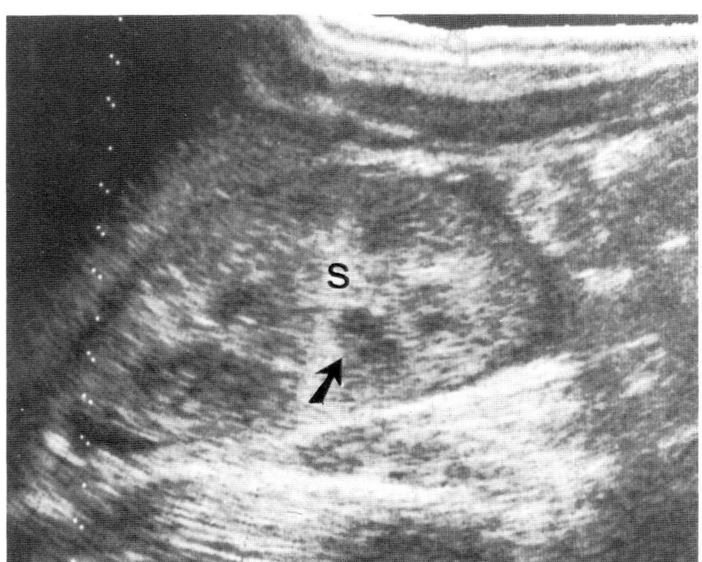

Fig. 1. Longitudinal section. Transplant kidney. Note the relatively insignificant sinus echoes (*S*) and the prominent pyramids (*arrows*). The pyramids are exceptionally large because the patient is suffering from rejection

Radiology Today 1. Ed. by M. W. Donner and F. H. W. Heuck

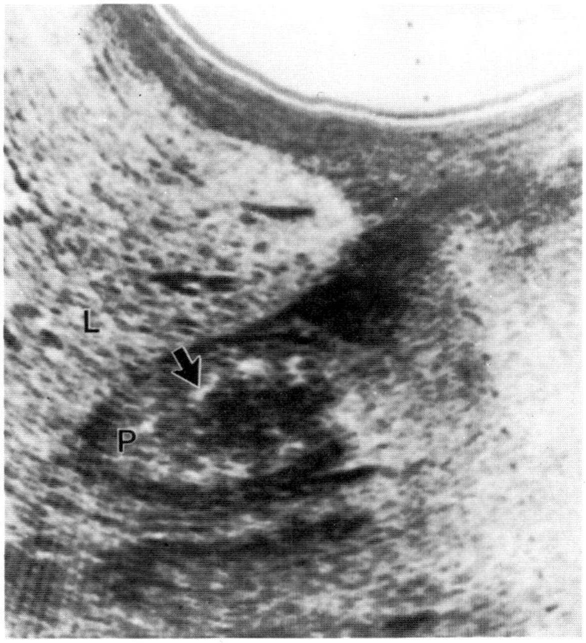

Fig. 2. Supine longitudinal section. Acute glomerulonephritis. Note the increased echogenicity of the renal parenchyma (*P*). This area is more echogenic than the liver (*L*) and almost as echogenic as the renal sinus. The pyramids are sonolucent (*arrow*)

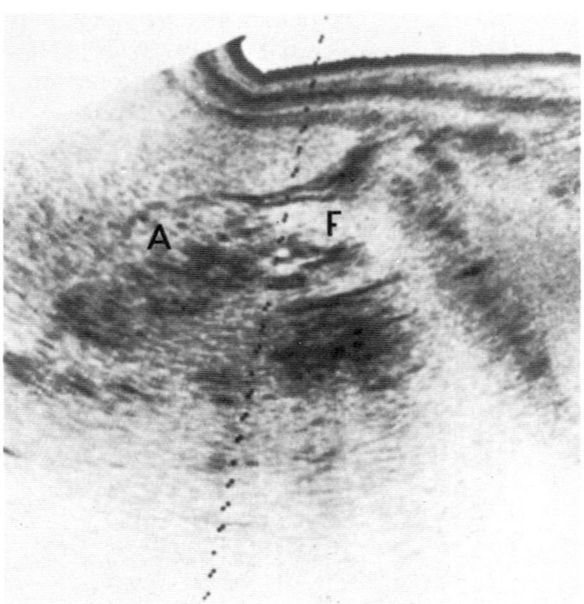

Fig. 3. Longitudinal section. Large angiomyolipoma (*A*) occupying most of the upper pole of the kidney. The normal renal parenchyma (*F*) can be seen at the lower pole

cautious in ruling out hydronephrosis if renal calculi are present.

Further progress has been made in attempts to define typical sonographic patterns for different tumors. So far, angiomyolipomata have always been densely echogenic (Fig. 3) [4, 5]. This appearance coupled with a CT scan showing fat density allows the preoperative diagnosis of this tumors. So far, angiomyolipomata have always echo free when seen within the kidney and Wilms' tumors frequently develop large echo-free spaces which either represent necrosis or fluid [6].

Some experimental work suggesting that rejection, acute tubular necrosis, and renal vein thrombosis can be recognized has been performed in the pig. It is suggested that in rejection, the pyramids become enlarged and more sonolucent and the cortex becomes more echogenic with an overall increase in renal size (Fig. 1) [7, 8]. Changes in renal vein thrombosis are somewhat similar; in acute tubular necrosis it is suggested that the pyramids do not enlarge to the same extent. The problem with these findings is that they require identical ultrasonic technique on consecutive examinations.

Gallbladder

Numerous reports confirm the accuracy of ultrasound in the detection of gallstones and show that the results are similar to those of oral cholecystography. Stones have been seen sonographically, unrecognized on the oral cholecystogram; the reverse has also occurred. Considerable work has been devoted to attempts to discover the significance of gallbladder wall thickening. Gallbladder wall thickening can occur in ascites and hypoalbuminemea and following contraction of the gallbladder with a meal [9]. If gallbladder wall thickening is seen in the absence of these predisposing factors, then the presence of acute cholecystitis can be confirmed [9, 10]. Focal tenderness over the gallbladder (an ultrasonic Murphy's sign) is reputed to be a further ultrasonic method of diagnosing acute cholecystitis. It is not uncommon to see abscess formation alongside the gallbladder in patients with acute cholecystitis [11].

Criteria for the detection of gallstones have been refined. The use of the wrong focal zone and frequency can obscure the acoustic shadowing which is a critical part of the sonographic diagnosis of gallstones [12, 13, 14]. The accuracy of gallstone detection by ultrasound depends on the nature of the ultrasonic findings. If acoustic shadowing is present from a gallstone observed within a fluid-filled gallbladder, one can be 100% certain of the presence of gallstones. If no fluid was present within the gallbladder and the only observation is a dense echo with an acoustic shadow arising within the liver parenchyma, sonographic findings were 96% accurate for gallstone detection. The least accurate sign (about 65%) was the presence of a stone within the gallbladder without evidence of acoustic shadowing but with evidence of movement with different positions [15].

The accuracy of ultrasound in the detection of dilated biliary ducts remains comparable with that of computerized tomography. However, bile duct obstruction located outside of the liver may not be seen with ultrasound if only the extrahepatic biliary tree is dilated. On the other hand, ultrasonic visualization of a dilated duct may precede abnormal liver function tests [16].

Pancreas

Previous attempts to improve the visualization of the pancreas by placing water in the stomach and duodenum have not been very successful. A recent paper [17] using a more meticulous technique showed a vastly increased accuracy when attempts to visualize the pancreatic tail were made. This technique involved the administration of five glasses of water, 1 ml glucagon, and a dose of lipomil. The latter two substances were administered in an attempt to make the pylorous contract and keep the water in the stomach. Erect and semierect views were found to be the most effective in demonstrating the pancreas. An 80% success rate in visualizing the pancreatic tail was claimed.

The accuracy of ultrasound in the detection of neoplastic masses in the pancreas appears to be slightly inferior to that of computerized tomography, though in general the mass displaces associated gas and itself provides an acoustic window [18].

The sonographic appearances of chronic pancreatitis have recently been refined. The pancreas is more echogenic and has irregular margins in pancreatitis [19]. Dense echogenic areas within the pancreas, some associated with acoustic shadowing, develop and represent pancreatic calcification (Fig. 4) [20]. An overall echogenicity can be seen in younger patients with chronic pancreatitis, but in older people this is a common normal finding which may merely represent fatty infiltration. Occasionally a local mass which can be confused with a neoplasm develops due to chronic pancreatitis. Another possible change is shrinkage of the pancreas so that it is barely visible. The normal pancreatic duct has been observed on many occasions, and it is now felt that a width of up 2 mm is a normal variant. Pancreatic duct dilatation can occur when the obstructing pancreatic neoplasm is invisible.

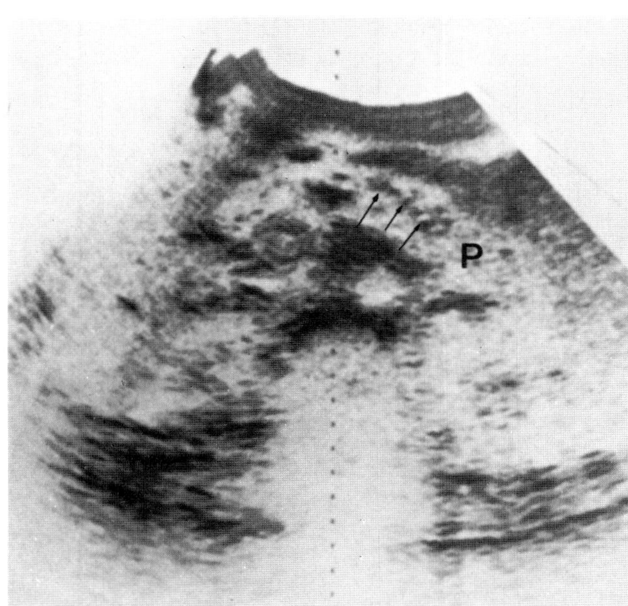

Fig. 4. Transverse section. This patient is suffering from acute on chronic pancreatitis. Within the pancreas (*P*) there are a number of echoes (*arrows*) which are aligned along the course of the pancreatic duct and represent small pancreatic calculi. Note the somewhat irregular border to the pancreas

Liver

Both the detection of liver metastases and the elucidation of diffuse liver disease by ultrasound remain difficult tasks. An attempt to assess the accuracy of ultrasound in diffuse liver disease concluded that a positive diagnosis could be made approximately 80% of the time, but that there was a 20% overcall [21]. The ability to distinguish cirrhosis from fatty liver proved imprecise. The various patterns that hepatoma can adopt have been explored; in general, this is an echogenic neoplasm [22].

Neonatal Heads

An exciting new sonographic field concerned with neonatal heads has developed in the last 1.5 years. Numerous infants are now being saved that weighing less than 1500 g at birth. Within this group there is a significant incidence of germinal matrix hemorrhage with consequent hydrocephalus (Fig. 5). Early detection of hemorrhage and hydrocephalus is important in patient management because the insertion of a shunt may well save the neonatal brain. Portable real-time ultrasound with a mechanical sector scanner proves to be an easy and efficient way of detecting problems in the neonatal brain in the nursery. Even with a sequenced linear array real-time system, adequate images of the lateral ventricles and of intraventricular blood can be obtained [23, 24]. More accurate images of superior quality can be obtained through the anterior fontanelle with a mechanical sector scanner real-time system (Fig. 5) [25]. The detailed structure of the neonatal and fetal brain has been reviewed; what was previously termed the lateral ventricles is in fact the thalamus and basal ganglia. The lateral ventricles lie at a higher level. Both cerebral peduncles and thalami are, for reasons as yet unexplained, relatively echo free. Normal standards have been developed for the upper limits of normal ventricular size in the fetus and in the neonate [26].

Obstetrics

Significant progress has been made in the further definition of fetal anomalies. Examples of omphalocele, gastroschisis, jejunal, and anal atresia, and teratoma have been described in utero (Fig. 6) [27]. Further elucidation of the finding in spina bifida using ultrasound have been described [28]. This remains a difficult diagnosis since in some instances there is no soft tissue component but merely absence of the lamina. A V-shaped indentation with extraspinal tissue usually occurs if spina bifida is present.

Criteria for the detection of limb anomalies have been described by Hobbins. If a real-time system is used to obtain the limb alignment, the detection of unduly short limbs can be made as early as 18 weeks. Examples of achondroplasia, Cornelia de Lange syndrome, and Ellis-van Crefeld and various other dwarf syndromes have been described [29]. Standards for renal size in utero have been delineated [30] and several examples of hydro-

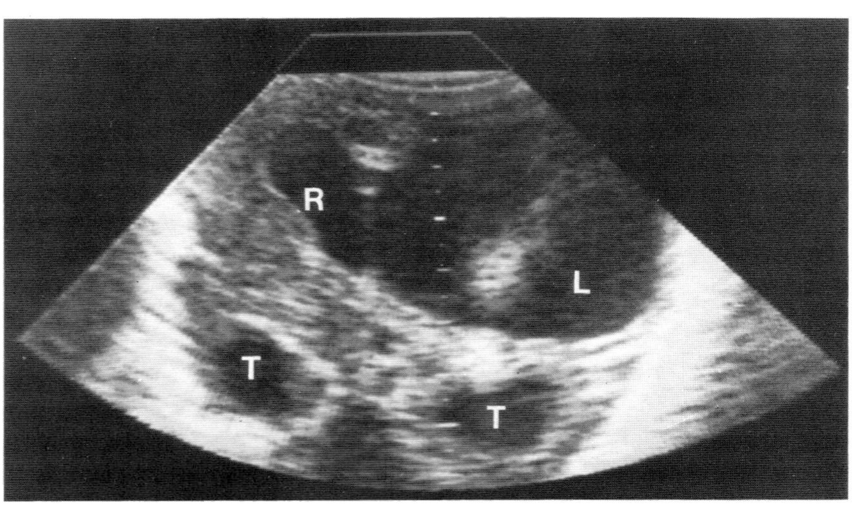

Fig. 5. Transverse section through a neonatal head. Asymmetric hydrocephalus. The left ventricle (*L*) is much larger than the right (*R*). The temporal horns (*T*) can be seen (coronal section)

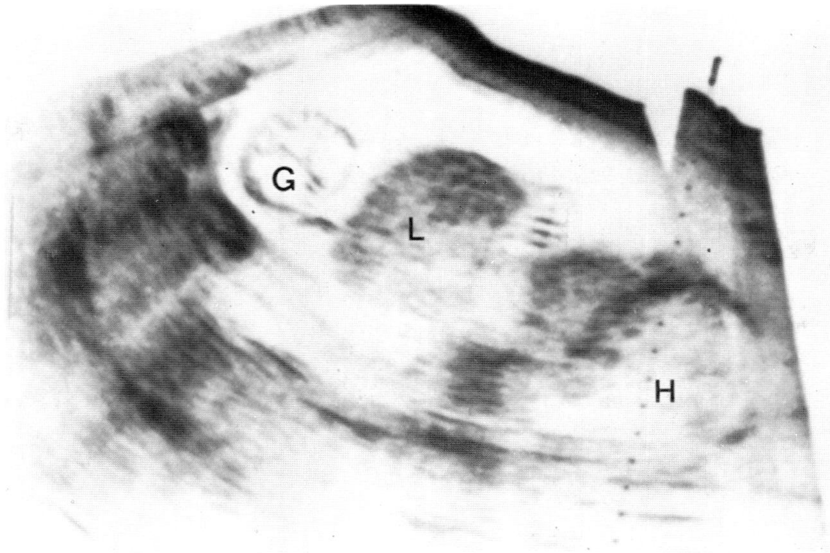

Fig. 6. Longitudinal section through a fetus that has a large ruptured omphalocele. Gut (*G*) and the liver (*L*) can both be seen lying outside the fetal abdomen. The fetal head can just be seen (*H*)

nephrosis, multicystic kidney, and infantile polycystic kidney have been recognized in utero [31].

Measurement data remains the commonest obstetric examination performed in ultrasound departments. Two efforts to combine the various existing scales for biparietal diameter and form a more reliable overall scale have been described [32, 33]. It is now recognized that a great many cases of intrauterine growth retardation (IUGR) cannot be detected using the biparietal diameter alone because the major changes that occur in the fetus are often limited to the trunk. The "total intrauterine volume" has proved of some value in finding fetuses that are at risk for IUGR [34]. In IUGR the placenta, amniotic fluid, and fetus are all unduly small. This measurement, however, is of limited accuracy because it presumes that the shape of the uterus is a prolate elipse, which is often not the case. Further more refined measurement techniques involving the use of the abdominal circumference and the head circumference have proved of value in obtaining information about fetal weight and in showing an abnormal relationship between the head and trunk in IUGR [35].

A problem with the existing ultrasonic literature on placenta previa is that many false positive placenta previa have been reported, although there are few or no false negatives. A major factor in the causation of false positive placenta previa was recently described. It has been shown that with the bladder full, the anterior part of the uterus is compressed against the posterior border, thereby causing an apparent elongation of the region of the cervix and many false positive placenta previa [36,37]. It is now considered essential to perform examinations for placenta previa with the bladder full and empty. This finding has made it unclear whether the phenomenon of "migration" of the placenta was a real one or whether it reflected a technical artifact.

Examinations for fetal movement have long been performed on the Continent. This area has been neglected in the United States; however, with the introduction of sequenced linear array real-time systems, much work has been devoted to the assessment of fetal movements and to the further discovery of the significance of fetal breathing. It has been shown that many of the observations made in the past with A-mode were inaccurate. It is now recognized that fetal breathing occurs at intervals throughout the day, though it is less frequent at night, and that it should be present at least once or twice over a period of 45 min. Decreased fetal limb movements have long been known to have prognostic significance. The clinical value of the examination of fetal breathing and fetal movement has been defined by Manning and Platt [38], who have devised a "biophysical profile" based on the number of movements seen, the presence of fetal breathing, the quality of fetal movement, and the "nonstress" test. An abnormally low "score" has proved to be of more accuracy in the discovery of fetuses at risk for problems at delivery than the "nonstress" test alone.

An important practical observation was made by the group at Yale [39] who showed that the changes that occur in the placenta toward the end of pregnancy are associated with fetal lung matu-

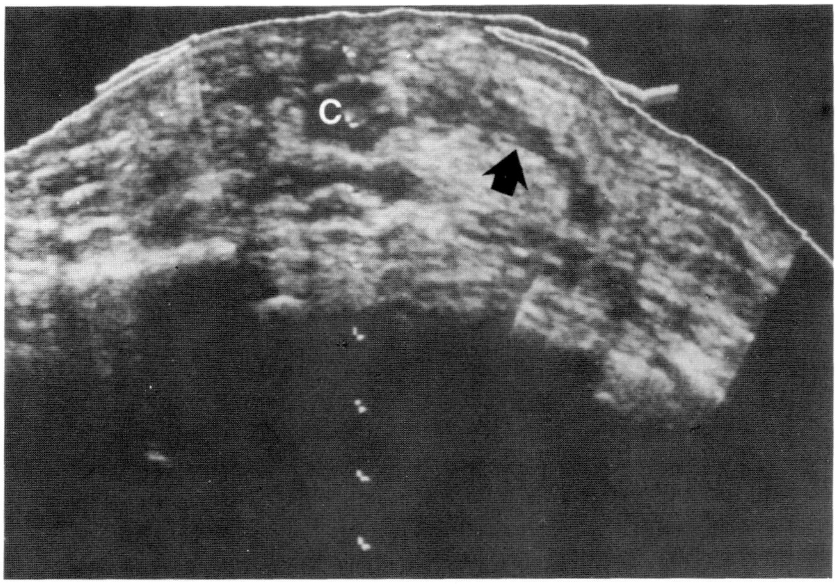

Fig. 7. Section through the breast of a patient with a duct carcinoma (*C*). Note the enlarged duct (*arrows*) leading up to this mass

rity. Grannum et al. divided the changes into four groups and found that there was a 100% correlation between changes in the severest group and fetal lung maturity [39]. The changes they observed were differentiation of the base plate, the development of internal echoes within the placenta, and the formation of circles thought to be due to bleeding into cotyledons. They also found that if these changes developed prior to 36 weeks, there was a strong chance that the fetus would have intrauterine growth retardation.

Breast

Considerable efforts have been devoted to discovering whether or not ultrasound can be used as a screening tool for the location of breast masses. It has been found to be almost as accurate as mammography in the characterization of breast masses into cystic, solid benign, and malignant lesions (Fig. 7) [40, 41]. Its value as a screening procedure remains more controversial. In my view it is of value in the young glandular breast where mammography is difficult. In the older, fatter breast, mammography remains a superior modality.

Carotids

Much attention has been focused on investigating the carotid artery to discover the presence of plaques. Although it is possible to visualize plaques in the carotid artery with static, real-time or with "small parts" scanners, it is as yet uncertain whether it is possible to see excavated plaques [42]. (Small parts scanners are systems optimized for visualization of the 4 cm under the skin using high-frequency transducers.) The clinical significance of the ultrasonic findings of a plaque in the carotid artery are unclear, although it is apparent that atheroma and calcified plaques are seen quite often. Doppler, on the other hand, has been shown to be a reasonably good way of quantitating the reduction in flow that occurs with plaque formation. Ultrasonic instruments which incorporate both small parts scanning and Doppler have been developed and are currently being assessed. So far their track record from the point of view of reliability has been poor; however, the small parts scanners that have been used to examine the carotid artery have very high resolution and have proved to be of value in other areas where superficial organs are examined, such as in the testicles and thyroid and in pediatric age group patients.

References

1. Cook JH, Rosenfield AT, Taylor KJ (1977) Ultrasonic demonstration of intrarenal anatomy. AJR 129:831–835

2. Rosenfield AT, Taylor KJ, Crade M, DeGraaf CS (1978) Anatomy and pathology of the kidney by gray scale ultrasound. Radiology 128:737–744
3. Ellenbogen PH, Scheible W, Talner LB, Leopold GR (1978) Sensitivity of gray scale ultrasound in detecting urinary tract obstruction. AJR 130: 731–733
4. Bush WH, Freeney PC, Orme BM (1979) Angiomyolipoma. Urology 24/5:531–535
5. Lee TG, Henderson SC, Freeney PC, Raskin MM, Benson EP, Pearse HD (1978) Ultrasound findings of renal angiomyolipoma. JCU 6/3:150–155
6. Sanders RC (1981) Renal masses. Clinics in ultrasound 6.68–89
7. Hricak H, Toledo-Pereyra LH, Eyler WR, Madrazo BL, Aammit M (1979) The role of ultrasound in the diagnosis of kidney allograft rejection. Radiology 132:667–672
8. Maklad NF, Wright CH, Rosenthal SJ (1979) Gray scale ultrasonic appearances of renal transplant rejection. Radiology 131:711–717
9. Sanders RC (1980) The significance of gallbladder wall thickening. JCU 8:143–146
10. Handler SJ (1979) Ultrasound of gallbladder wall thickening and its relation to cholecystitis. AJR 132:581–585
11. Kane RA (1980) Ultrasonographic diagnosis of gangrenous cholecystitis and empyema of the gallbladder. Radiology 134:191–194
12. Jaffe CC, Taylor KJ (1979) The clinical impact of ultrasonic beam focusing patterns. Radiology 131: 469–472
13. Taylor KJ, Jacobson P, Jaffe CC (1979) Lack of an acoustic shadow on scans of gallstones: a possible artifact. Radiology 131:463–464
14. Filly RA, Moss A, Way LW (1979) In vitro investigation of gallstone shadowing with ultrasound tomography. JCU 7:255–262
15. Crade M, Taylor KJ, Rosenfield AT, De Graaff CS, Minihan P (1978) Surgical and pathologic correlation of cholecystosonography and cholecystography. AJR 131:227–229
16. Zeman R, Taylor KJ, Burrell MI, Gold J (1980) Ultrasound demonstration of anicteric dilatation of the biliary tree. Radiology 134:689–692
17. MacMahon H, Bowie JD, Beezhold C (1979) Erect scanning of pancreas using a gastric window. AJR 132:587–591
18. Hessel S, Siegelman S, Sanders RC, McNeil B, Finberg H (to be published) A prospective comparison of CT and ultrasound in the pancreas. Radiology
19. Lees WR, Vallon AG, Denyer ME, Vahl SP, Cotton PB (1979) Prospective study of ultrasonography in chronic pancreatic disease. Br Med J 1:162–164
20. Weinstein BJ, Weinstein DP, Brodmerkel GJ (1980) Ultrasonography of pancreatic lithiasis. Radiology 134:185–189
21. Joseph AE, Dewbury KC, McGuire PG (1979) Ultrasound in the detection of chronic liver disease (the "bright liver"). Br J Radiol 52:184–188
22. Broderick TW, Gosink B, Menuck L, Harris R, Wilcox J (1980) Echographic and radionuclide detection of hepatoma. Radiology 135:149–151
23. Johnson ML, Mack LA, Rumack CM, Frost M, Rashbaum C (1979) B-mode echoencephalography in the normal and high-risk infant. AJR 133:375–381
24. Pape KE, Gusick G, Houang MT, Blackwell RJ, Sherwood A, Thorburn RJ, Reynolds EO (1979) Ultrasound detection of brain damage in preterm infants. Lancet II:1261–1264
25. Babcock DS, Han BK, LeQuesne GW (1980) B-mode gray scale ultrasound of the head in the newborn and young infant. AJR 134:457–468
26. Denkaus H, Winsberg F (1979) Ultrasonic measurement of the fetal ventricular system. Radiology 131:781–787
27. Lee T (1980) The principles and practice of ultrasonography in obstetrics and gynecology. In: Sanders R, James E (eds) Prenatal fetal thoraco-abdominal ultrasonography. Appleton-Century-Crofts, New York, pp 179–190
28. Little DJ, Campbell S (1980) The diagnosis of spina bifida and intracranial anomalies. In: Sanders R, James E (eds) The principles and practice of ultrasonography in obstetrics and gynecology. Appleton-Centrury-Crofts, New York, pp 179–190
29. Hobbins JC (1980) The diagnosis of skeletal dysplasias with ultrasound. In: Sanders R, James E (eds) The principles and practice of ultrasonography in obstetrics and gynecology. Appleton-Century-Crofts, New York, pp 191–203
30. Grannum P, Bracken M, Silverman R, Hobbins JC (1980) Assessment of fetal kidney size in normal gestation by comparison of ratio of kidney circumference to abdominal circumference. Am J Obstet Gynecol 249–254
31. Cooperberg PL (1980) Abnormalities of the fetal genitourinary tract. In: Sanders R, James E (eds) The principles and practice of ultrasonography in obstetrics and gynecology. Appleton-Century-Crofts, New York, pp 161–168
32. Kurtz AB, Dershaw DD, Rubin CS, Cole-Beuglet, Wapner RJ, Goldberg BB (1980) Analysis of biparietal diameter as an accurate indicator of gestational age. J Clin Ultrasound 8:319–326
33. Wiener SN, Flynn MJ, Kennedy AW, Bonk F (1977) A composite curve of ultrasonic biparietal diameters for estimating gestational age. Radiology 122: 781–786
34. Gohari P, Berkowitz RL, Hobbins JC (1977) Prediction of intrauterine growth retardation by determination of total intrauterine volume. Am J Obstet Gynecol 73–78
35. Sanders RC (1980) The role of ultrasound in the evaluation of intrauterine growth retardation. In: Sanders R, James E (eds) The principles and practice of ultrasound in obstetrics and gynecology. Appleton-Century-Crofts, New York, pp 139–148
36. Bowie JD, Rochester D, Cadkin AV, Cooke WT, Kunzmann A (1978) Accuracy of placental localiza-

tion by ultrasound. Radiology 128:177 – 180
37. Zemlyn S (1978) The effect of the urinary bladder in obstetrical sonography. Radiology 128:169 – 175
38. Platt LD, Manning FA, Lemay M, Sipos L (1978) Human fetal breathing: relationship to fetal condition. Am J Obstet Gynecol 132/5:514 – 518
39. Grannum PA, Berkowitz RL, Hobbins JC (1980) The ultrasonic changes in the maturing placenta and their relation to fetal pulmonic maturity. Am J Obstet Gynecol 915 – 922
40. Cole-Beuglet C, Goldberg BB, Rubin CS, Kurtz AB, Feig S, Patchefsky A, Soriano R, Ezo M, Lehman D (1980) B-scan diagnostic criteria of benign-appearing solid breast masses correlated with pathology, including analysis of the fibrosis tissue content in fifty cases. AIUM symposium 1980, Montreal
41. Zusmer NR, Gilson AJ, Janowitz WR, Smoak WM, Leborgne J, Fleming RM, Dick D (1980) Early experience with an automated scanner in the detection of benign and malignant breast disease. AIUM symposium 1980, Montreal
42. Cooperberg PL, Robertson WD, Fry P, Sweeney V (1979) High resolution real-time ultrasound of the carotid bifurcation. JCU 7:13 – 17

CT Versus Ultrasound

R. C. Sanders

Johns Hopkins Medical Institutions, Department of Radiology and Radiological Science,
601 N. Broadway, Baltimore, MD 21205 (USA)

The conference commenced with a review of the relative value of ultrasound and CT in abdominal diagnosis. The two systems have significant differences: Ultrasound is portable, able to show movements in real-time, quick, relatively cheap both to perform and to buy, and has no radiation risk. CT, on the other hand, gives a total abdominal cross section without aberrations due to gas or bone, though only in a transverse plane; whereas ultrasound gives oblique and longitudinal sections. Superficially, ultrasound offers a very high resolution, but at depth CT appears to be slightly better at resolving small structures. CT is able to examine large, fat, gassy people who are unsuitable for ultrasound. Thin people and small children may be best shown with ultrasound. Additional information about structures other than the one that is being examined is obtainable with both techniques, but more often with CT. Since a total cross section is obtained, CT has significantly better physician acceptance even though the same information may be displayed.

Because of the real-time features and the absence of radiation risk, ultrasound is the preferred technique in obstetrics, small infants, and cardiology. There can be no dispute that CT is the preferable system in the chest and brain because the air and bone that surrounds that anatomy prevents ultrasonic transmission. Only in small children up to about the age of 2 years can ultrasound image the brain in a two-dimensional fashion.

It was concluded that certain other organs in the abdomen are best imaged with ultrasound. The partial volume effect seen with stones in the gallbladder with CT means that the accuracy in the detection of gallstones is much greater with ultrasound. The real-time feature makes the aorta readily examinable with ultrasound. Superficial structures such as the testicles and the thyroid are close to the transducer so high-quality images are obtained with ultrasound. CT, mainly because of the variable presence of gas, is the preferred technique in the examination of the pancreas, nodes, and renal masses. Adrenals are exquisitely defined by CT and difficult to examine with ultrasound. Radiotherapy planning is simpler with CT than ultrasound.

In certain areas it is not yet clear which modality is preferable, but since ultrasound is significantly cheaper and quicker, it appears to be the appropriate first modality. Such areas include liver masses, the evaluation of dilated bile duct, the bladder, prostrate, and gynecologic lesions.

The engineering aspects of CT and ultrasound were then discussed. Significant improvements in CT can be expected not only in image quality but also in the speed with which the examination can be performed. Several images a minute are readily obtainable with some as yet not commercially released instruments, and it will be possible to perform rapid serial views of the heart. Image reconstruction over a few seconds is becoming commonplace. Ultrasound also does not appear to have reached the limits of development; increasingly powerful transducers are being developed so higher frequencies can be used for routine work with a subsequent increased resolution. The phased array systems, which require considerable computer expertise, are considered to have not yet reached their full potential.

A discussion then took place concerning the different practice in Europe and the United States in the way in which ultrasound is performed. In Europe all examinations are performed by physicians and real-time is the main modality used. In the United States the bulk of the examinations are performed by technologists under the supervision of a radiologist, with real-time being used as an aid to a static scanner. This difference in practice is partly related to the economics. Since physicians are paid much more than technologists, but instrumentation is relatively easy to obtain in the United States, it is an economic proposition to have several technologists working for one physician. In

Radiology Today 1. Ed. by M. W. Donner and F. H. W. Heuck

Europe ultrasound instruments are difficult to obtain, but physicians are not in short supply. The legal aspects of documenting what is seen loom large in the United States because litigation is common. It is not as important to document findings in Germany, and the impression of the physician at the time of the examination is helpful in patient management because one can observe the movements of different organs and pinpoint the site of pain. It was agreed, however, that the contribution of real-time is increasing rapidly and that image quality with real-time is approaching that obtained with a static scanner. A static scanner has one significant advantage – the entire mass or structure being examined can be imaged and documented in one view.

Sonography Versus CT

R. Hauke

Firma CGR Koch & Sterzel, Kruppstrasse 82–96, D-4300 Essen 1

It is a well-known fact that ultrasound is able to detect small density variations much more better than CT does. Measurements recently published [1] prove that qualitatively. It is due to this ability, together with noninvasive and real-time features, that ultrasound came to be used in many fields of medical diagnosis. However, one domain seems to remain where purely CT is used: brain imaging. Due to the rapid development of CT in neurologic applications and the good pictures obtained therewith, in most cases the clinician uses only CT for diagnosis.

In this paper some emphasis is laid on using modern sonography equipment too, at least for newborns and infants up to 2 years old, and some specialized techniques for adult brain imaging with ultrasound are described.

A review of the evaluation of echoencephalography was recently published by de Vlieger [2]. Figure 1 shows a comparison between compound scan (A) and multielement scan (B) in a hydrocephalic child. These pictures are very hard to interpret, only the midline being visualized. Somewhat better pictures were obtained by Johnson [Johnson ML, personal communication] (Fig. 2). As comparison with CT shows, the intracranial hemorrhage is clearly shown with both methods. Using the most modern and commercialized linear array scanners, the image quality in newborns and infants (up to 2 years old) may be further improved. The images obtained by H. C. Rücker [Rücker, personal communication] are presented in Figs. 3–5, in connection with which the help of Einighammer [Einighammer HJ, personal communication] is appreciated.

These images include so much detail and information that there is no need to use CT imaging with regard to most clinical problems. With the real-time capability of ultrasound there is no need to sedate children.

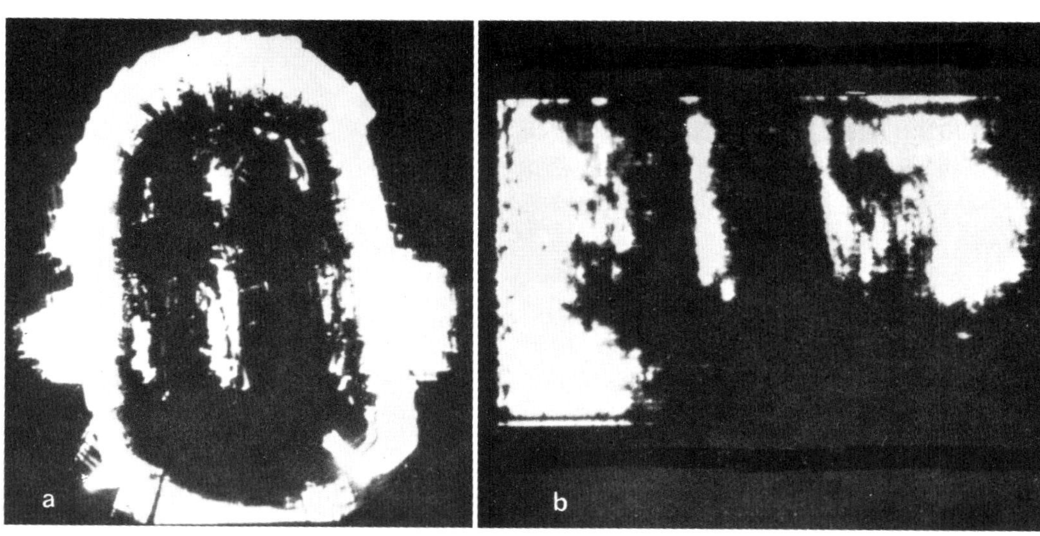

Fig. 1. Comparison of two-dimensional echoencephalograms **a** with mechanical compound scanning and **b** with multielement array in hydrocephalic child (horizontal cross-section)

Radiology Today 1. Ed. by M. W. Donner and F. H. W. Heuck

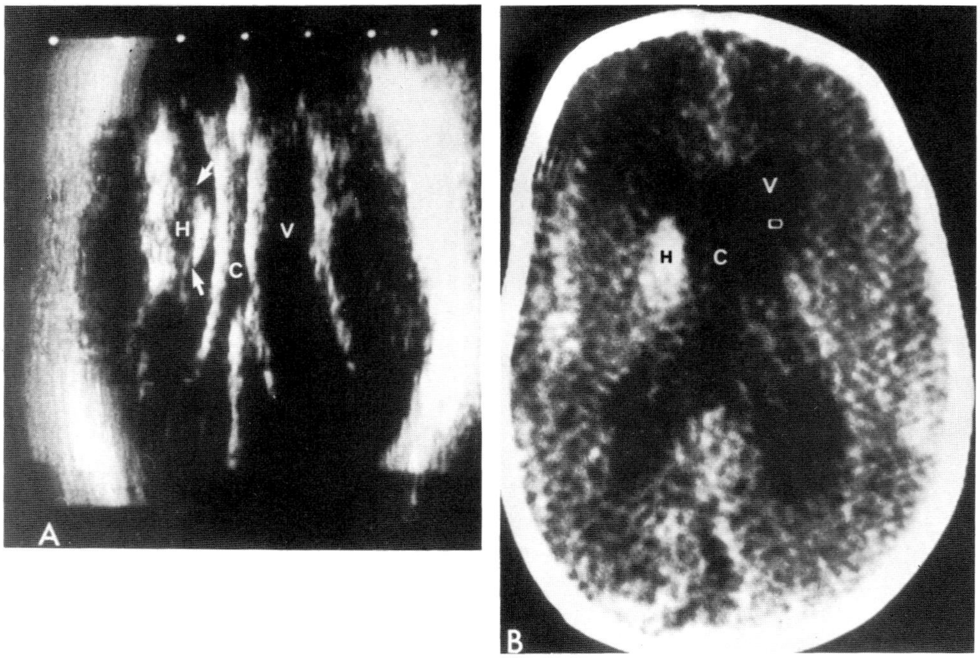

Fig. 2A, B. Intracerebral hemorrhage (ICH). **A** Axial ultrasound and **B** CT scans of a 31-week-old, 1220 g premature infant through the bodies of the lateral ventricles (*V*) with subependymal hemorrhage (*H*). The hematoma bulges into the right lateral ventricle (*arrows*). A cavum vergae (*C*) is noted between the mildly dilated lateral ventricles

As a new feature compared with CT, the intracranial pulsations are also well visualized. Absence of pulsation is a strong indication of vascular occlusions. The problem of examining adult brains stems from the high absorption of the skull bone and the possible image artifact caused by the bone itself. As shown in earlier papers by Freund [3], there is one method which overcomes these problems, i.e., a phased-array system. It is well known that the skull is very thin at the temporal bone as compared to other parts of the skull. Looking through this acoustic window with an electronic sector scan allows production of sector images of the adult brain; in 89% of cases the important structures, such as midline, side ventricles, temporal horns, etc. are well visualized together with the intracranial pulsations. This idea was pursued by several other authors, e.g., Thurstone and von Ramm [4], who discussed in great detail the bone influence and also gave some compensation methods.

The following conclusions can be drawn:

1. Brain imaging in newborns and infants up to 2 years of age should in most cases be done with ultrasound, offering the following advantages:
   a) Good resolution in soft tissue,
   b) Harmless application,
   c) Real-time (intracranial pulsations),
   d) There is no need for sedation of children since image reconstruction is done in several milliseconds.
2. Compared to CT ultrasound has a better price/performance ratio, for ultrasound in medical application is considered a screening method.

References

1. Filly RA (1980) Radiology 134:167 – 171
2. De Vlieger M (1980) JCU 8/1
3. Freund (1973) Neurology (Minneap) 23/11
4. Thurstone, v. Ramm, AIUM-meeting, 1977 Dallas
5. Becher S (to be published) Atlas der Anatomie des Menschen, 16th edn, part 3. Urban & Schwarzenberg, Munich

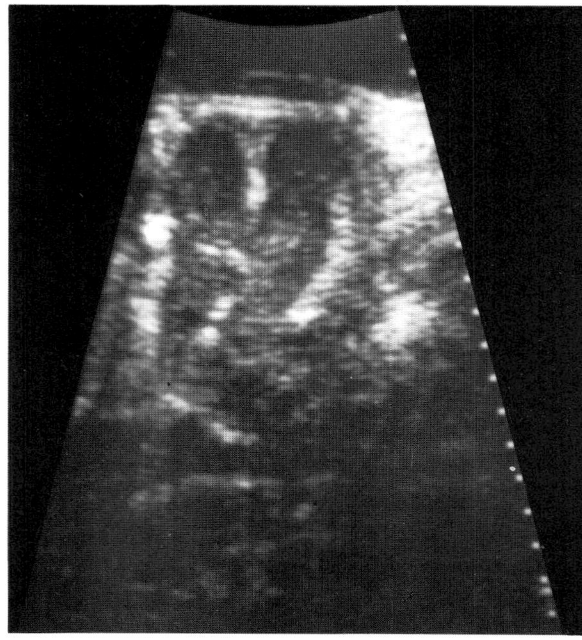

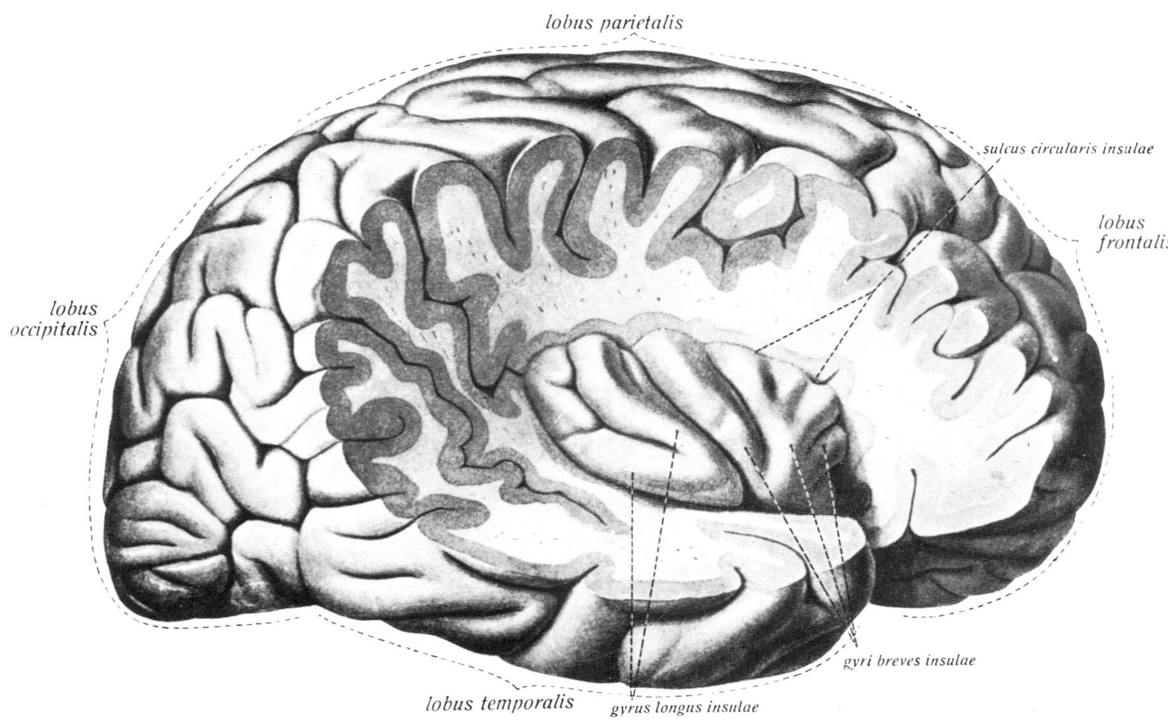

Fig. 3. *Top:* Imaging through fontanella with 8 MHz in 3-month-old child. Marker spacing is 2 mm. Two gyri with sulcus are clearly shown. Pulsations of arteries are seen. *Bottom:* Anatomic cross-section corresponding to above view [5]

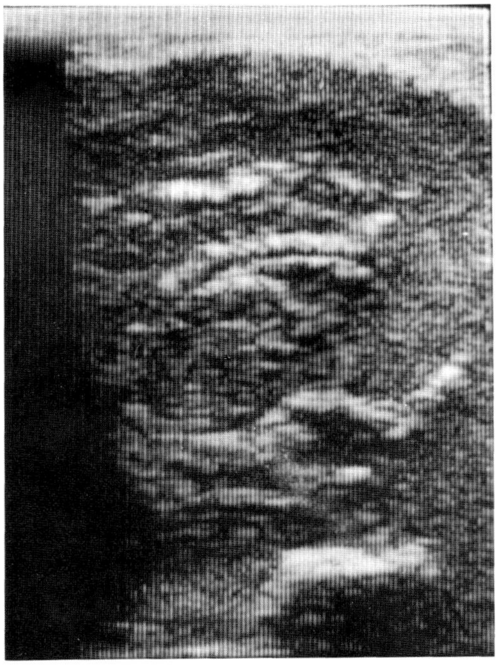

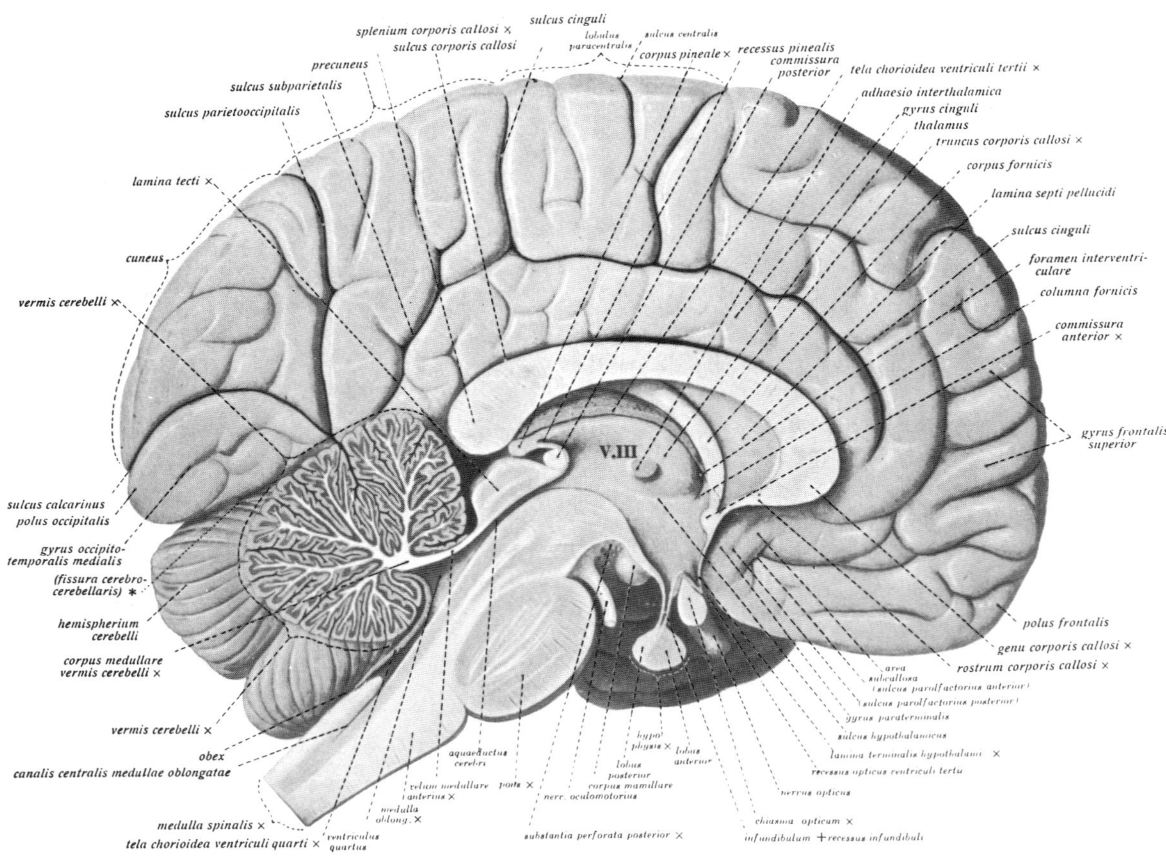

Fig. 4. *Top:* With 2.4 MHz one may see from top to bottom in a 3-month-old child: sulcus cingulis, gyrus cinguli, arteria cerebri anterior (longitudinal, pulsating), corpus callosum, base of the skull. *Bottom:* Corresponding anatomic cross section [5]

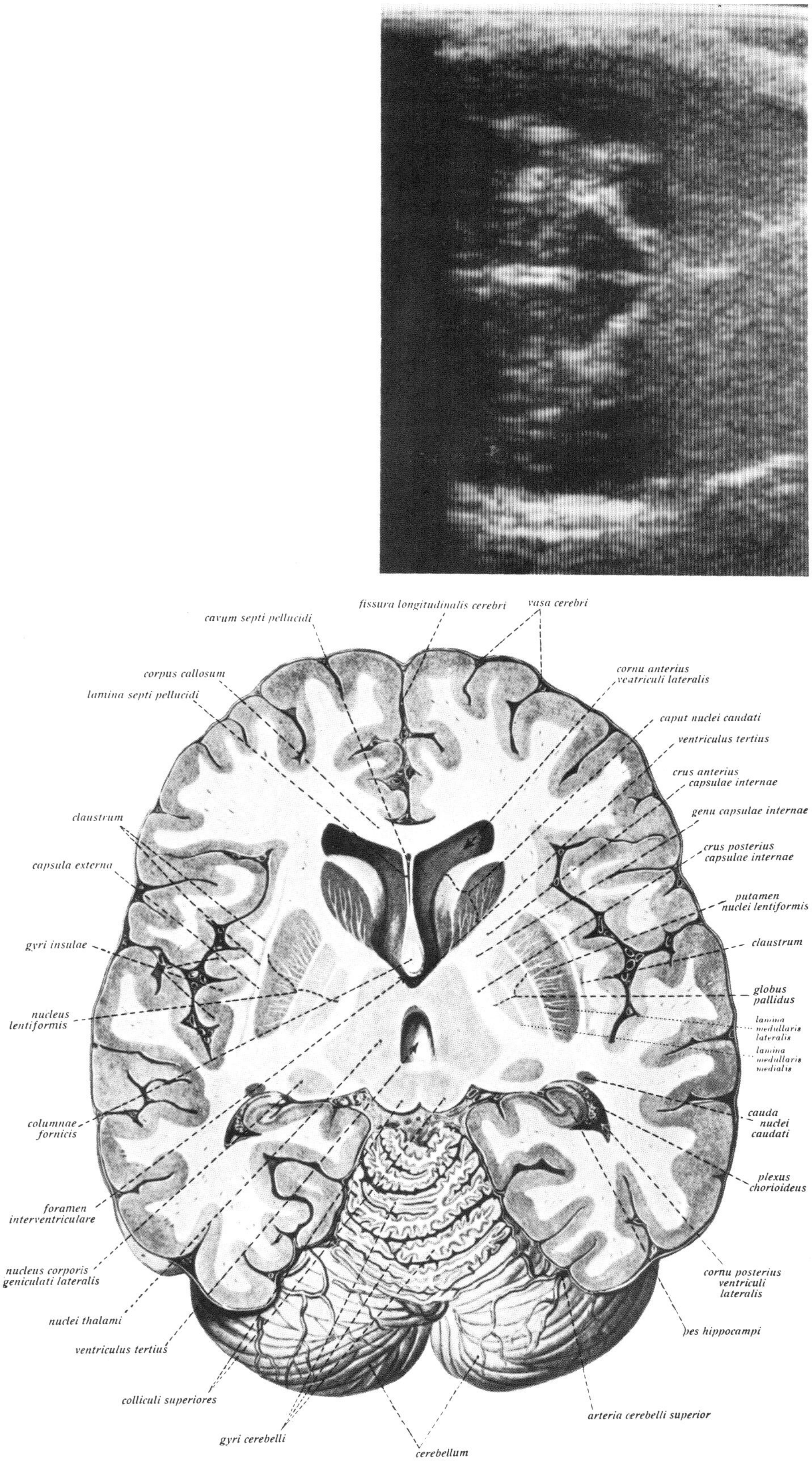

Fig. 5. *Top:* With 2.4 MHz the following may be seen in a 3-month-old child: bone, cortex, cornu anterius ventriculi lateralis, septum pelliculum, nucleus lentiformis. *Bottom:* Corresponding anatomic cross section [5]

ENT Radiology

The Ear: Conventional Tomography Versus Computed Tomography: Overview

A. Bollaert, F. Hotton, E. De Smedt, and D. Baleriaux

Hôpital Universitaire Saint-Pierre, Service de Radiodiagnostic, Rue Haute 322, B-1000 Bruxelles

Introduction

The temporal bone represents an extremely rich neurosensorial region. Its internal structure is very complex, and many of its elements measure only 1 mm or slightly more. Radiologists have been interested in it for a long time and have been trying to visualise and identify its different components using various techniques.

The temporal bone plays an important role in the process of hearing and in the maintenance of balance. The facial nerve (with its three parts) goes through it, as does the carotid artery.

Nevertheless, as Jacqueline Vignaud said in Brussels in 1977, "le temporal s'est laissé peu à peu déflorer dans ses régions les plus secrètes": radiology now permits a detailed analysis of the temporal bone.

Technical and Historical Survey

In the early stages of technical development only plain films were available: Remember the special projections as described by Stenvers, Schuller, Chaussé and others. Next, the principle of intracranial centering was developed by G. L. Dulac. The craniograph permits easier investigation of the ear structures which can be studied with a tangent beam. These conventional projections are now defined by the angulation of their central X-ray beam with regard to the sagittal and the orbitomeatal planes. After this global approach, Ziedses des Plantes decided to make sections of the temporal bone in order to isolate plane by plane the different components of the image. Tomography was born.

The 1950s and 1960s saw the advant of body section radiography, first with linear and later with multidirectional sweepings (spiral and hypocycloidal).

These techniques gave us the opportunity to progress quickly in the study of the normal and pathological radio-anatomy of the ear – important contributions in this field were made by Cova, Mundnich and Frey, Fischgold, Juster, Laval-Jantet, Valvassori, Rabischong and Vignaud.

The 1970s saw the arrival of the CAT scan, which makes possible study of the distribution of the

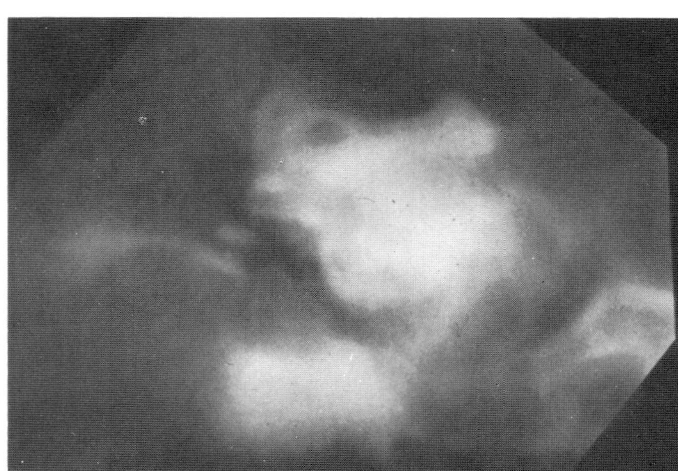

Fig. 1. Normal petrous bone. Stapes and incus. Guillen section. Hypocycloïdal sweeping

Radiology Today 1. Ed. by M. W Donner and F. H. W. Heuck

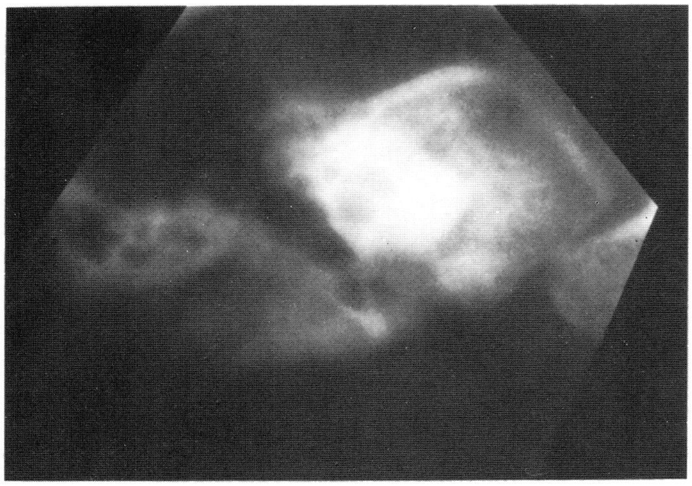

Fig. 2. Normal petrous bone. Cochlear and facial nerves. Guillen section. Hypocycloïdal sweeping

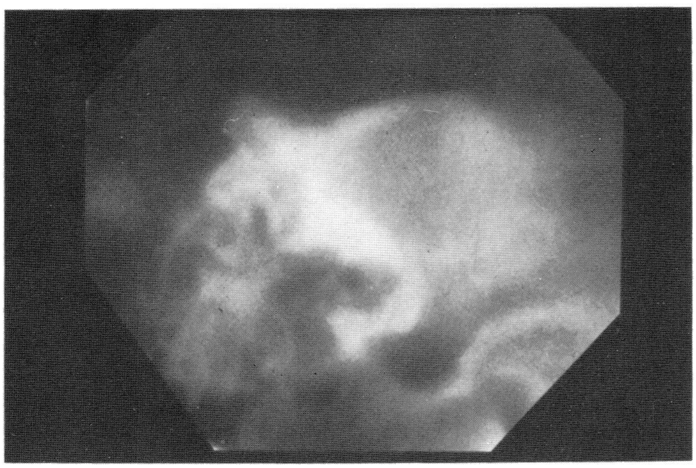

Fig. 3. Modification of the size of the internal auditory canal by neuroma. Frontal section. Hypocycloïdal sweeping

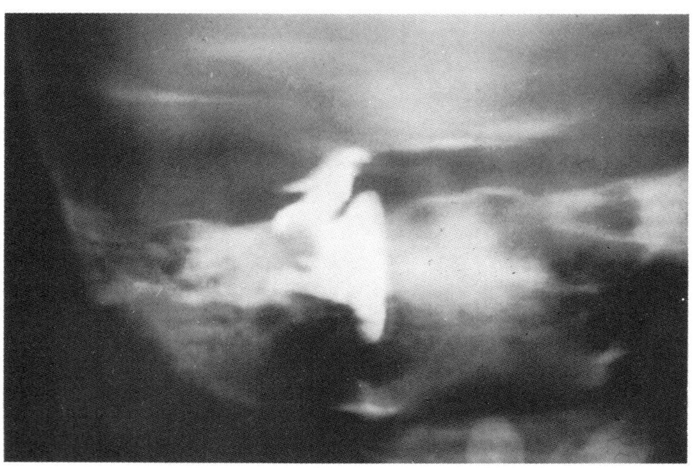

Fig. 4. Same patient as in Fig. 3 Linear sweeping. Intracisternal Lipiodol delimiting the tumor

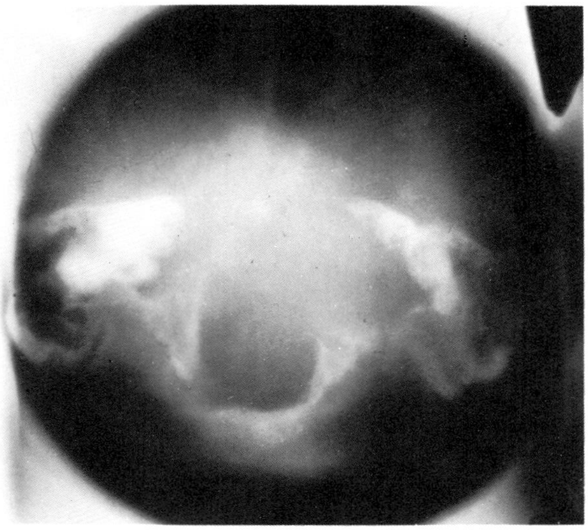

Fig. 5. Right acoustic neuroma. Spiral sweeping; semiaxial section

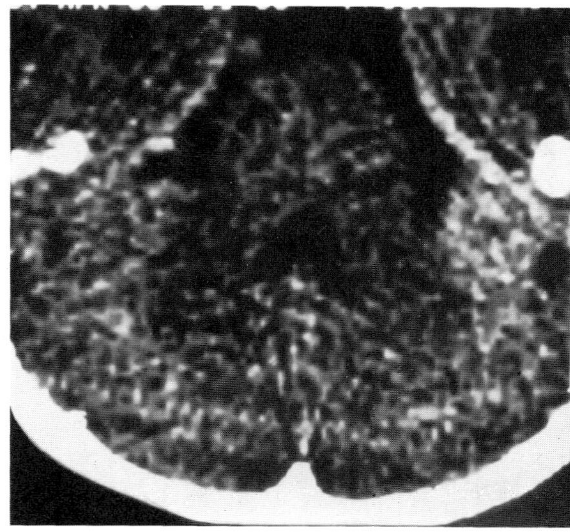

Fig. 7. Hyperdensity without contrast in the right pontocerebellar angle. The circumpeduncular cistern is enlarged. Obtained with Somaton Siemens

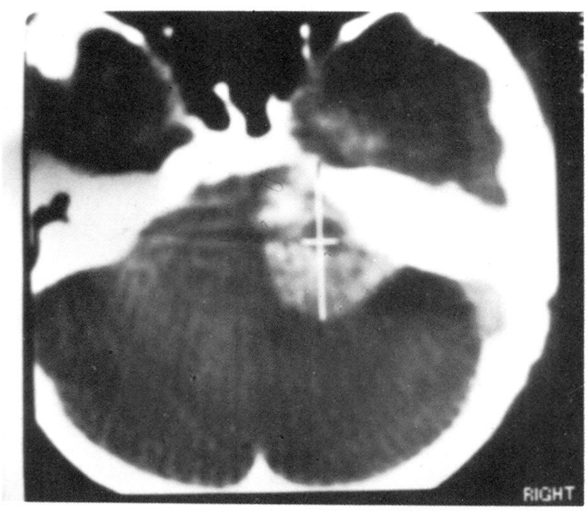

Fig. 6. Same patient as Fig. 5. CAT Scan with contrast. The tumor is centered on the internal auditory canal. Obtained with Varian

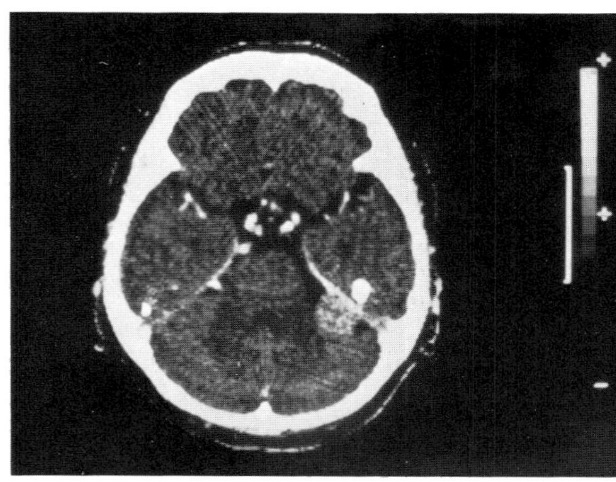

Fig. 8. Same patient as in Fig. 7 with contrast. Homogeneous enhancement of the tumor. Centered on the internal auditory canal. Obtained with Somaton Siemens

tissular densities in a given section. At first this was mainly a complementary examination and was especially used to determine the intracerebral extent of inflammatory and tumoral lesions of the ear. CAT led us to change our methods of exploration in various pathological conditions, of which acoustic neuroma is the best and the most typical example. Indeed, the exploration scheme in the beginning of the 1970s began with conventional radiography, to be followed by tomography. If acoustic neuroma was suspected, arteriography and encephalography were performed. For neuroma located in the internal auditory canal, opaque cisternography was used.

Thanks to the improvement of image quality, the CAT scan can now often replace conventional tomography in the evaluation of the internal auditory canals when looking for acoustic neuroma. Moreover, CAT scan can directly show the tumoral mass, especially after contrast enhancement. When combined with air cisternography, very small extracanalar or even intracanalar neuromas can be detected.

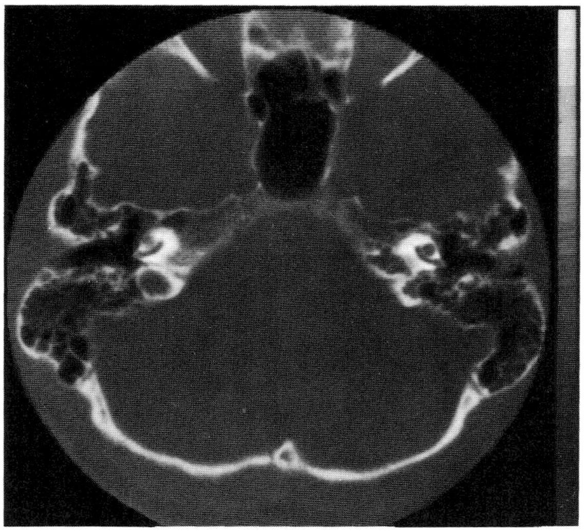

Fig. 9. Horizontal slice showing both petrous bones, at the level of the cochleas. Note also the excellent visualisation of the sphenoid sinus. Obtained with Elscint 705

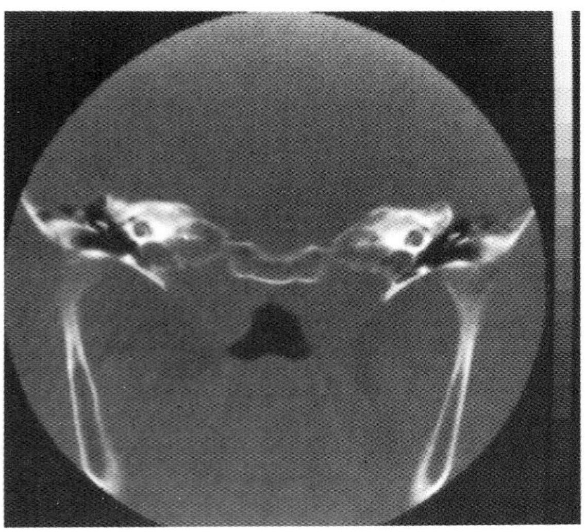

Fig. 10. Normal frontal section showing both petrous bones and the basal part of the sphenoid bone. The slice passes through both cochleas. The first part of the facial nerves is seen at both sides, above the cochleas. Note the ossicles in the tympanic cavities and the demonstration of the mandibles and the cavum. Obtained with Elscint 705

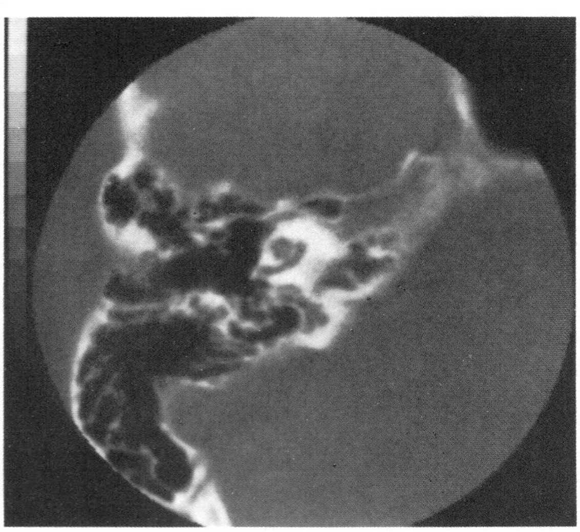

Fig. 11. Same patient as in Figs. 9 and 12. Normal horizontal slice at the level of the cochlea. Part of the handle of the malleus is seen in the tympanic cavity. Mastoid air cells are clearly demonstrated. Obtained with Elscint 705

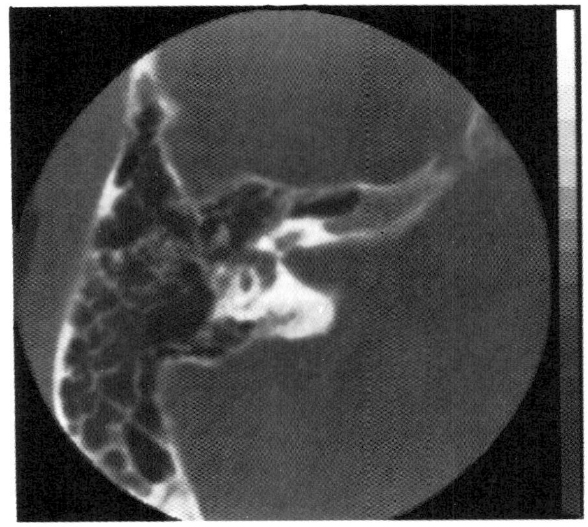

Fig. 12. Same patient as in Figs. 9 and 11. Normal horizontal section passing through a short and wide internal auditory canal (normal anatomical variant). Parts of the cochlea, the vestibulum and the semicircular canals are seen. The auditory ossicles are recognised in the tympanic cavity. Note the clear demonstration of the different mastoid air cells. The larger air cell directly anterior to the lateral sinus corresponds to the mastoid antrum. Obtained with Elscint 705

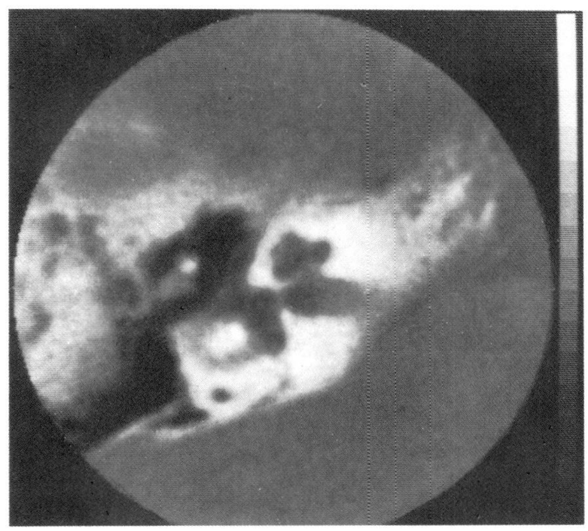

Fig. 13. Horizontal section. The auditory ossicles (head of malleus, body and short process of the incus and part of the long process of the incus) are clearly demonstrated in the tympanic cavity. Note also cochlea, vestibulum, external and posterior semicircular canals and part of the vestibular aqueduct. Obtained with Elscint 705

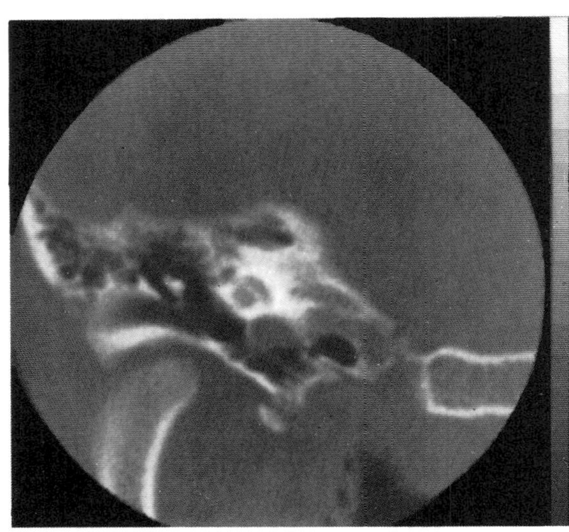

Fig. 14. Frontal section showing part of the external auditory canal and of the temporomandibular joint. The auditory ossicles are seen medial to the lateral wall of the epitympanic recess. The first part of the facial nerve is recognised above the cochlea; under the cochlea, the carotid canal is seen. Note the air density in the tympanic cavity and in the mastoid air cells. Obtained with Elscint 705

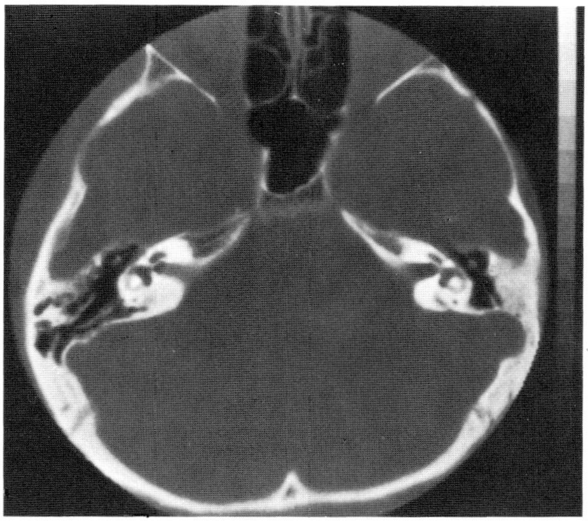

Fig. 15. Horizontal section. Normal pneumatisation at the right side, compared to sclerosis of the mastoid at the left. No other anomalies were found in this patient. Obtained with Elscint 705

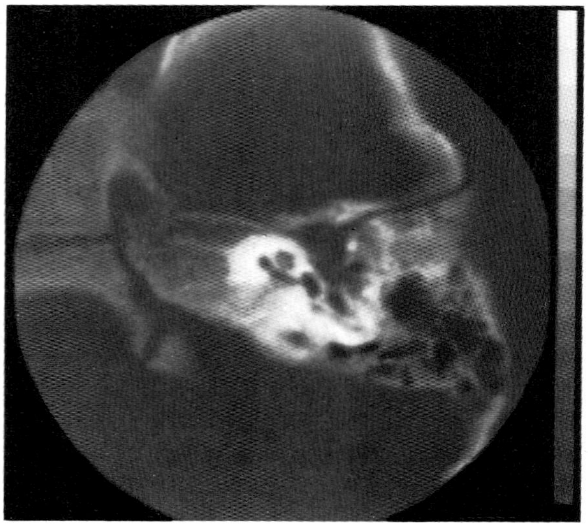

Fig. 16. Severe head trauma in a 5-year-old boy. This horizontal CT section shows a fracture line running from the protympanum laterally, above the level of the external auditory canal and slightly anterior to it. Clouding of the tympanic cavity because of bleeding (haemotympanum). Obtained with Elscint 705

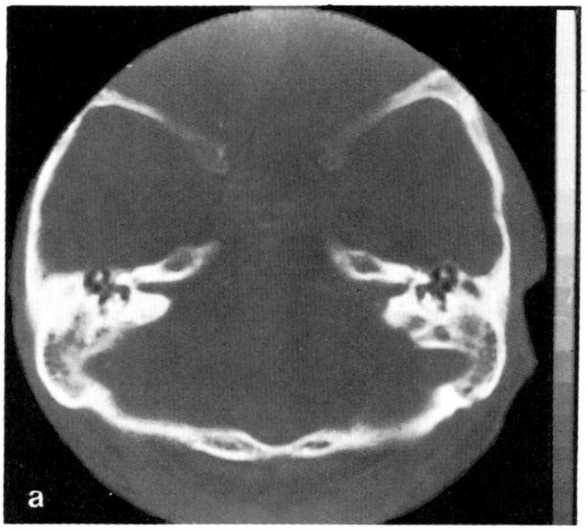

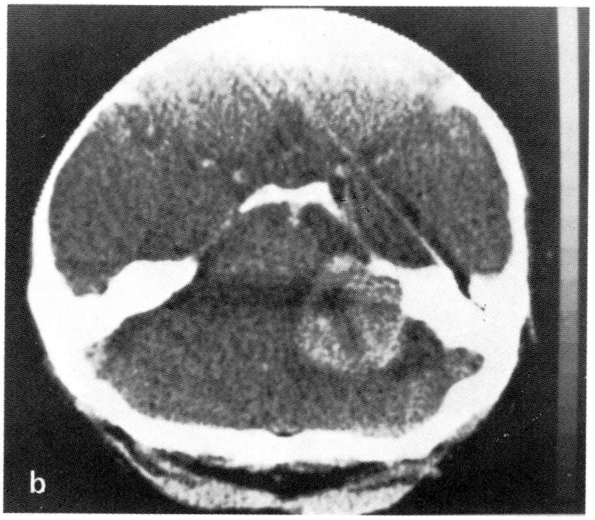

Fig. 17a, b. Large acoustic neuroma. **a** Widening of the internal meatus on the left, with shortening and destruction of the posterior wall and erosion of the anterior wall. **b** A huge acoustic neuroma is clearly visible after contrast enhancement. Both figures were obtained with Elscint 705

Discussion

High resolution computed tomography (CT) permits visualization of structures smaller than 1 mm. Thanks to this excellent geometrical resolution and thanks also to its excellent density resolution, which is far superior to that of conventional tomography, CT can now be used for the detailed examination of the petrous bone. Its important role in the diagnosis of acoustic neuroma has been emphasised, but CT also provides excellent results in many other pathological conditions.

In chronic inflammatory disease, it is possible to find by CAT the elementary lesions that are demonstrated by conventional tomography. Opacification of the tympanic cavity and of the antrum are easily recognised. Localised opacities are even better evaluated. Erosion and destruction of the ossicular chain and its components can be shown.

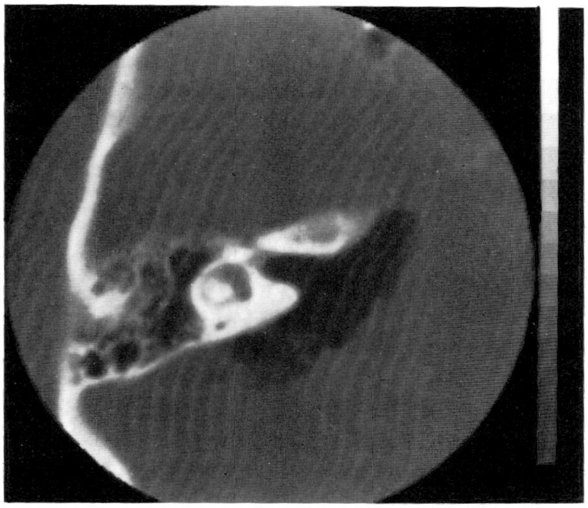

Fig. 18. Cisternography and canalography after lumbar injection of 7 cc air. The air occupies the cerebellopontine cistern and penetrates freely into the internal auditory canal, indicating absence of acoustic neuroma. Also, clear demonstration of the vestibulum, the external semicircular canal and the vertical portion of the posterior semicircular canal, cut perpendicularly. Obtained with Elscint 705

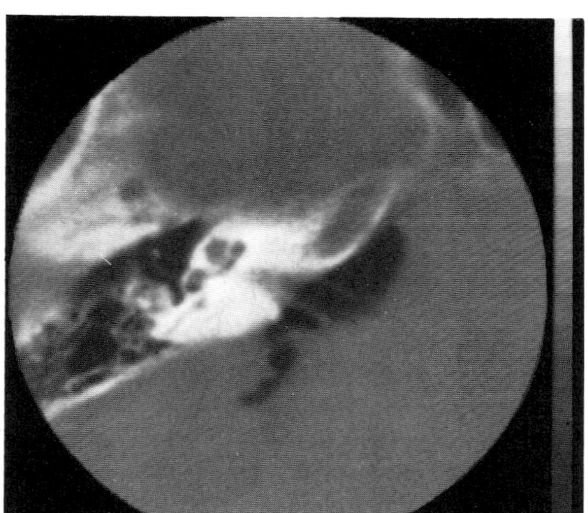

Fig. 19. Air cisternography. The seventh and eight cranial nerves are visualised in the cerebellopontine cistern, as they are running towards the internal auditory meatus. Obtained with Elscint 705

In traumatology, it is possible to demonstrate fracture lines and blood in air-containing cavities. Luxation of the ossicles can be recognised. As all parts of the ear may be visualised, it is possible with CAT to obtain a complete evaluation of malformations. The limits of tumoral lesions can be determined in soft tissue as well as in bony structures. Air cisternography of the cerebellopontine angle allows visualisation of the seventh and eight nerves and earlier diagnosis of small acoustic neuromas.

Finally, we think that with further improvement of CAT technology and with more widespread availability of CAT facilities, high resolution CAT will gradually replace conventional tomography in the diagnosis of various temporal bone diseases.

References

1. Bollaert A, Hotton F, Kleiner S, Courtoy M, Appel L (1972) Étude tomographique des malformations congénitales de l'oreille. Ann Radiol 15 (11/12): 907 – 914
2. Chiesa A, d'Attoma N (1979) Guida anatomo clinica alla radiologica del tamporale. Cortina, Verona
3. De Smedt E, Potvliege R, Pimontel Appel B, Claus E, Vignaud J (1980) High resolution CT scan of the temporal bone. A preliminary report. J Belge Radiol 63:205 – 212
4. Hotton F (1973) Etude des affections congénitales et acquises de l'oreille par la tomographie en balayage hypocycloïdal. Mémoire de licence spéciale en radiologie. Brussels
5. Kritcheff I, Pinto R, Bergeron RT, Cohen N (1980) The diagnosis of small acoustic neuromas by air CT. Cisternography and canalography. Springer, Berlin Heidelberg New York
6. Rabischong P, Vignaud J, Paleirax P, Lamoth AP (1979) Tomographie et anatomie de l'oreille. CGR, Paris New York
7. Valvarossi GE, Buckingham RA (1975) Tomography and cross sections of the ear. Thieme, Stuttgart
8. Vignaud J, Baleriaux D, Aubin ML, Jeanmart L (1980) CT scan diagnosis of lesions causing an angle or internal auditory canal syndrome. J Belge Radiol 63:295 – 311

High Resolution Computed Tomography in the Staging of Carcinoma of the Larynx: Overview

S. S. Sagel, J. F. Auf der Heide, D. J. Aronberg, R. J. Stanley, and C. R. Archer

Washington University, School of Medicine, The Edward Mallinckrodt Institute of Radiology, 510 South Kingshighway, St. Louis, MO 63110 (USA)

Abstract

The normal anatomy of the larynx as displayed on computed tomography is illustrated. Pathologic alterations in patients with carcinoma of the larynx are depicted and discussed.
Computed tomography is recommended as the initial radiologic procedure when additional diagnostic information is required to supplement the findings of laryngoscopy; it will help to determine whether conservative surgery as opposed to total laryngectomy is possible.

Introduction

Laryngeal carcinomas are detected by indirect and direct laryngoscopy, but the limitations of clinical methods to determine the exact anatomic location, size, and extent of such tumors are well recognized. Only the mucosal surfaces are seen, and deep spread must be inferred from increased bulk or altered physiology. Neoplastic invasion of the paralaryngeal and pre-epiglottic space or adjacent supporting cartilaginous structures may be difficult or impossible to ascertain, even with deep biopsy, and the base of the epiglottis and subglottic space often are poorly seen. In the past, when the only alternatives for treatment of carcinoma of the larynx were total laryngectomy or radiation therapy delivered through relatively large ports, correct delineation of the extent of tumor was less important. With the development of conservation surgery designed to preserve a useful voice and food swallowing function, precise delineation of tumor has become imperative for proper operative planning.
The usefulness of radiologic examination, especially laryngography, to provide supplementary information to the clinical examination, has been known for many years. Nevertheless, certain areas – such as the paraglottic soft tissues and laryngeal cartilages – may still be difficult to assess. With the recent introduction of computed tomography (CT), a noninvasive imaging technique capable of a unique three-dimensional anatomic display of the larynx has been provided [1 – 5]. This report details our experience with rapid (3-s scan time) thin section (5 mm) CT of the larynx.

Technique

Since significant anatomic relationships change within millimeters, and because respiratory motion may cause the entire larynx to move 1 cm or more, thinly collimated sections obtained with rapid scanning times are necessary for optimal portrayal of laryngeal anatomy and tumor extent. A rotary motion, stationary detector array computed tomographic scanner (EMI 7070) is used in our medical center. The scanner is operated at 120 kVp, between 20 and 60 mA, with a 3-s scan time. The neck is extended with the patient supine to make the larynx as parallel to the table top as possible. Contiguous 5-mm thick sections are obtained over the entire laryngeal area (from the base of the tongue above the hyoid bone down to the upper trachea). Approximately 14 slices are required to cover the area of interest. Most scans are performed during quiet inspiration. The patient is cautioned against swallowing, moving, or talking. Scanning is occasionally performed during a modified Valsalva (to balloon out the pyriform sinuses) or reverse "e" (to fill out the ventricles and aid separation of the true from the false vocal cords) maneuver when clarification about these areas is required.

Radiology Today 1. Ed. by M. W. Donner and F. H. W. Heuck

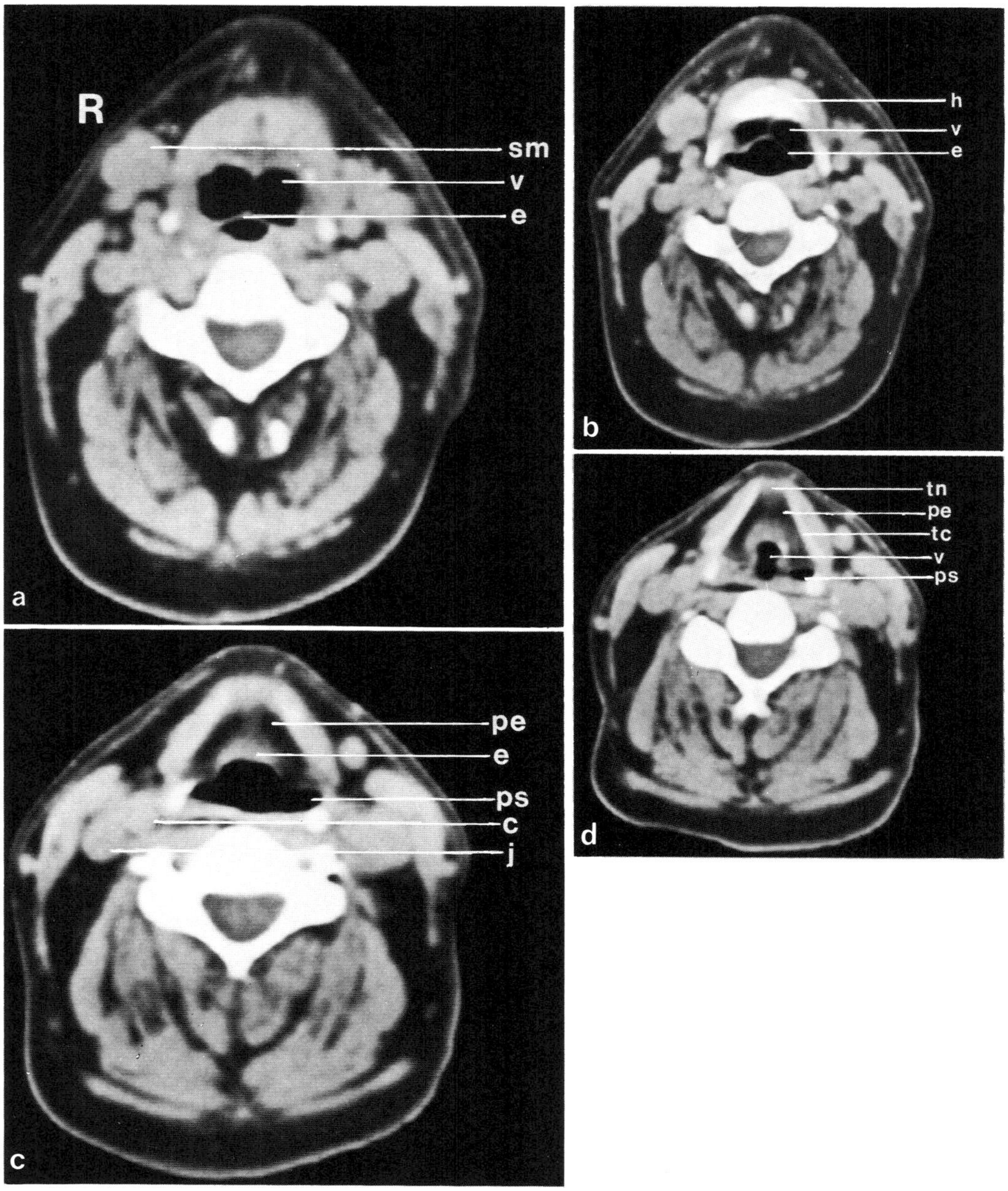

Fig. 1a – e. Normal laryngeal anatomy. **a** Above the level of the hyoid bone, the thin epiglottis (*e*) is seen posterior to the air-filled valleculae (*v*). Just posterolateral are the cornua of the hyoid bone. The inferior portion of the right submandibular gland (*sm*) is present. This structure often is asymmetric and should not be confused with enlarged lymph nodes. (Note that by convention all CT scans of the body are viewed as if from below, with the patients right side (*R*) on the viewers left). **b** Proceeding inferiorly, at the level of the hyoid bone (*h*), the valleculae (*v*) have become slightly asymmetric, a normal variation. The thin epiglottis (*e*), is profiled by surrounding air. **c** Anterior to the midportion of the soft tissue density epiglottis (*e*), the fat containing pre-epiglottic space (*pe*) is seen. This space is contiguous laterally with the paralaryngeal space, posterior to which is the piriform sinus (*ps*). Posterolateral lie the carotid artery (*c*) and internal jugular vein (*j*). **d** At the level of the superior portion of the thyroid cartilage, a space is present anteriorly, the thyroid notch (*tn*), between the paired thyroid laminae (*tc*). The fat containing pre-epiglottic space (*pe*) again is seen. The inferior portion of only the left piriform sinus (*ps*), lateral to the vestibule (*v*), is seen; such mild asymmetry in caudal extension is relatively common. **e** At the level of the true vocal cords (*tvc*), the thyroid laminae (*tc*) fuse anteriorly. The soft tissue space behind the thyroid cartilage, the anterior commissure (*ac*), at the glottic level should be less than 2 mm in thickness. Likewise, only a minimal soft tissue density should be seen at the posterior commissure (*pc*) extending between the arytenoid cartilages

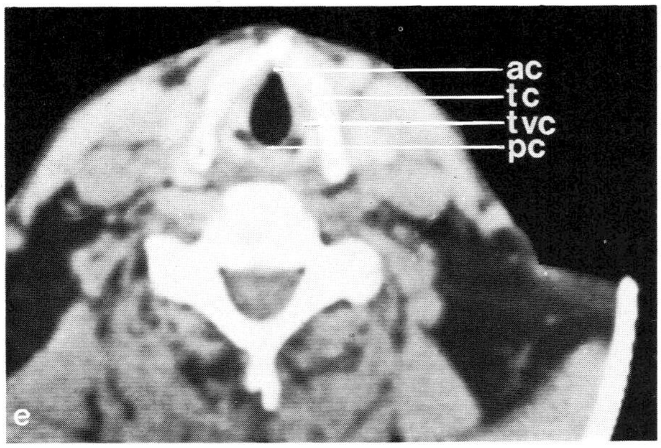

Fig. 1e. Legend see p. 367

Normal Anatomy

The larynx is a fibromuscular organ supported by a group of cartilaginous structures [6]. Certain features of the normal cross-sectional anatomy of the larynx as displayed on the CT scans could cause confusion in interpretation. These anatomic variations will be stressed (Fig. 1).

The *thyroid cartilage* is composed of paired laminae which are fused anteriorly to form the laryngeal prominence. Above the prominence is the suprathyroid notch, where the laminae do not meet in the midline; this normal defect should not be mistaken for cartilaginous destruction (Fig. 1d). There is no consistency in the density or contour of the laminae, which may be variably composed of calcified or noncalcified hyaline cartilage or bone (with even a marrow cavity). The process of calcification and ossification often is irregular, resulting in short segmental interruptions along both the outer and inner margins of the laminae that may simulate cancer invasion. Localized tubercles may form along the margins. The superior and inferior cornua are extensions of the posterior border of the laminae; the inferior cornua articulate with the posterolateral margins of the cricoid cartilage.

The *cricoid cartilage* is the most inferior of the supporting laryngeal cartilages and is a signet-ring shaped structure with a broad posterior quadrate lamina measuring 2 – 3 cm in vertical height and a much narrower anterior arch. Like the thyroid laminae, the posterior ring often has a mixed composition of cartilage and bone. A dense cortical bony rim with a relatively low density center due to a medullary space is the most common occurrence.

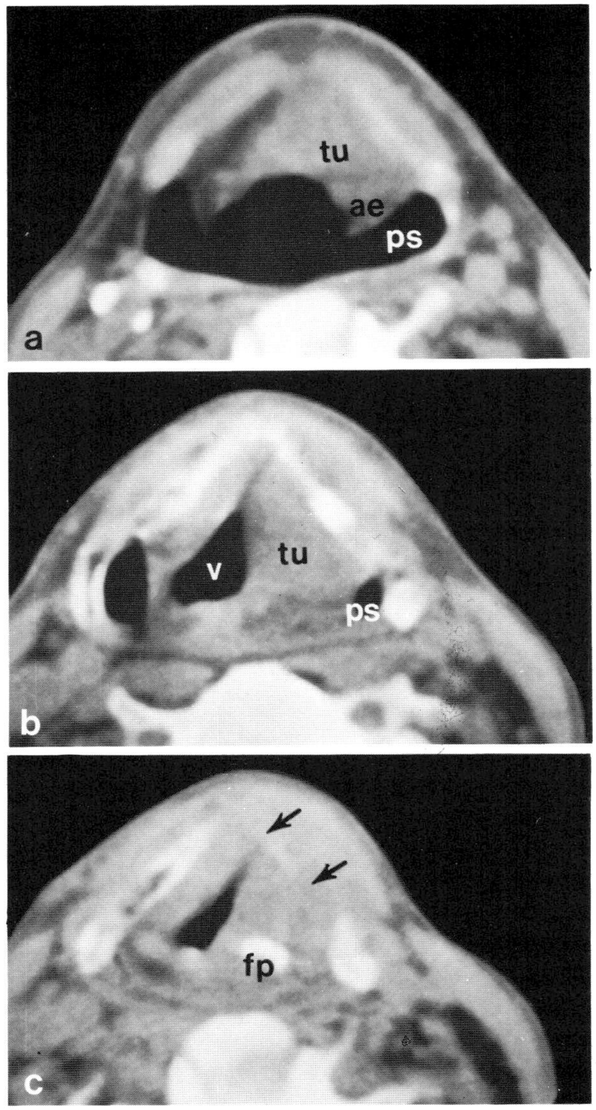

Fig. 2a – c. Transglottic carcinoma. **a** A bulky tumor (*tu*) infiltrates the left pre-epiglottic space and extends deep into the left aryepiglottic fold (*ae*). The superior portion of the left piriform sinus (*ps*) is normal. **b** 1 cm inferiorly, the tumor (*tu*) extending into the aryepiglottic fold compresses and displaces both the laryngeal vestibule (*v*) and the left pyriform sinus (*ps*). **c** 1 cm inferiorly, at the level of the muscular (foot) process of the left arytenoid (*fp*), the vestibule is markedly narrowed by the tumor. Destruction of the left thyroid ala (*arrows*) is present, with the tumor appearing to infiltrate into the subcutaneous tissues. These latter findings were not appreciated on clinical examination. The initial surgical incision disclosed tumor growing through the left thyroid lamina and a total laryngectomy was performed

In the area of the cricoid ring, which demarcates the subglottic space, the mucosa normally is closely adherent to the surface of the cartilage.

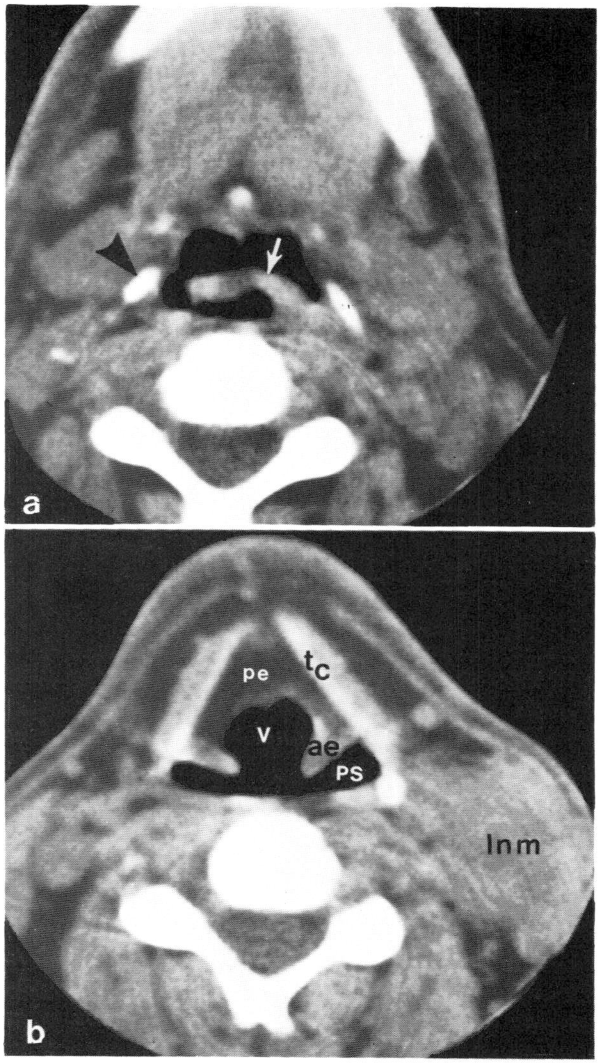

Fig. 3a, b. Epiglottic carcinoma with metastases. **a** Carcinoma producing moderate thickening of the epiglottis (*arrow*) at the level of the cornua of the hyoid bone (*arrowhead*). **b** 1.5 cm inferiorly, the infrahyoid portion of the epiglottis, the pre-epiglottic space (*pe*) and the aryepiglottic folds (*ae*) are free of gross tumor infiltration. The vestibule (*v*) and piriform sinuses (*ps*) are normal, and the superior portions of the thyroid laminae (*tc*) are intact. Despite the relatively small size of the primary tumor, lymph node metastases (*lnm*), clinically palpable, are seen surrounding and obscuring the left carotid artery and internal jugular vein

The *arytenoid cartilages* are paired structures lying superior and slightly lateral to the middle of the upper border of the posterior cricoid lamina; they are roughly pyramidal in shape. The sharp anteriorly projecting vocal process extends from the base of the arytenoid cartilages and attaches to the true vocal cord, while the laterally projecting muscular or foot process spans a height from the base to the level of the false cord or laryngeal ventricle (Fig. 2c). These cartilages usually are homogeneously dense, although apparent inequality in size is not infrequent due to some differences in bony or cartilaginous composition.

The *epiglottis* is a thin band-like structure whose superior margin extends above the hyoid bone and whose apex or inferior margin, the petiole, ends immediately superior to the anterior attachment of the true vocal cords to the thyroid cartilage.

The *paralaryngeal space* is a mixture of fibrous and fatty tissue deep to the endolarynx, bounded laterally by the thyroid laminae. At the level of the true cords it is a very thin space, but it markedly widens superiorly. Anterolaterally the paralaryngeal space is contiguous with pre-epiglottic space. The normal fat content in this space, present in virtually every adult patient; causes a definite decreased density on the CT scans in comparison to the paralaryngeal musculature or neoplastic tissue (Figs. 1c, d, 3b).

The *vestibule* is the portion of the laryngeal airway above the false cords, it is wide superiorly and narrower in its lower portion, with the anterior wall wider than posteriorly (Figs. 3-B and 4-B).

Piriform sinuses are bilateral air-distended structures which bulge into the paralaryngeal space; they are separated from air in the laryngeal vestibule by the aryepiglottic folds (Figs. 2a, 3b, 4a, b). Asymmetry in size and caudal extent (Fig. 1c, d) is not unusual.

True vocal cords are bilateral soft tissue density structures which are normally seen in an abducted position during quiet inspiration. Posteriorly, at their widest horizontal portion, the true cord measures about 9 mm in thickness (Fig. 1e). In this region between the vocal processes of the arytenoids lies the posterior commissure; only a minimal mucosal soft tissue density should be seen in this area when the cords are abducted. The true cord tapers to a thickness of about 2 mm anteriorly where it meets the contralateral cord to form the anterior commissure just behind the thyroid cartilage attachment. Again, only a very small amount of mucosal tissue should be seen behind the midline thyroid cartilage at the level of the true vocal cords. In contradistinction, the false cords are seen as a thicker band of density crossing the midline anteriorly. Only in approximately one-third of patients can the laryngeal ventricle be seen on the cross-sectional images separating the true and false cords.

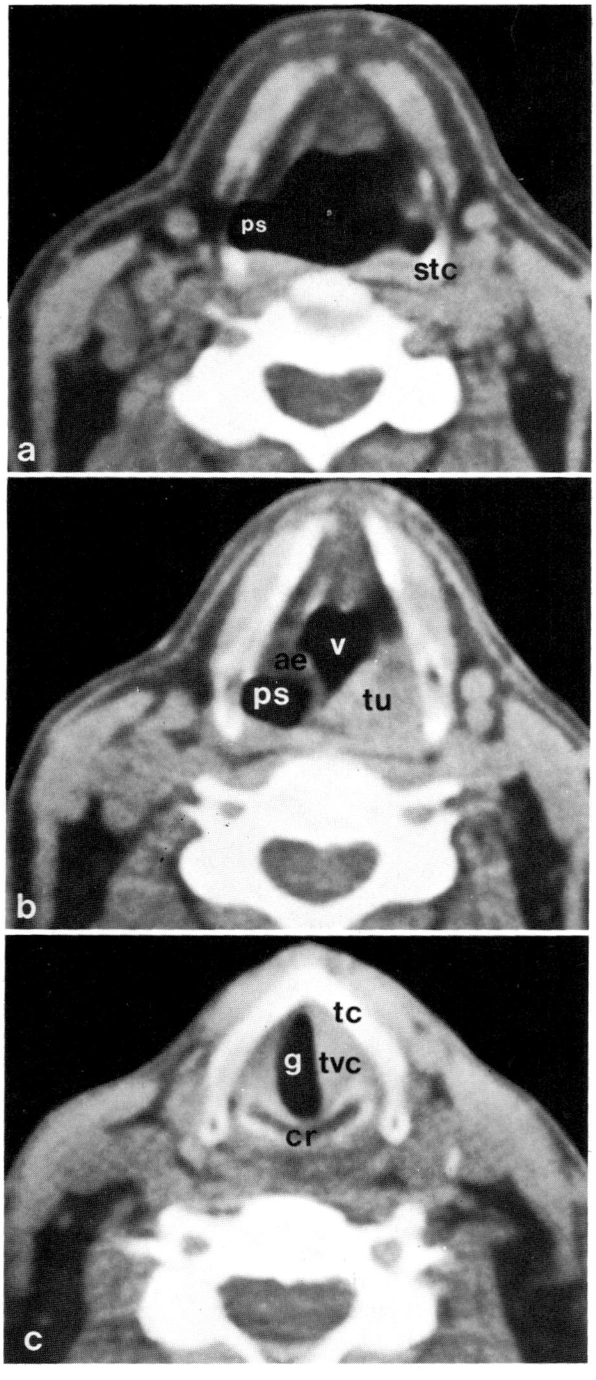

Fig. 4a–c. Piriform sinus carcinoma. **a** The superior portion of the left piriform sinus is narrowed by tumor in comparison to the normal right side (*ps*) at the level of the superior cornua of the thyroid cartilage (*stc*). **b** The middle and inferior portions of the left piriform sinus are totally obliterated by tumor (*tu*). The vestibule (*v*), right aryepiglottic fold (*ae*), and right pyriform sinus (*ps*) are normal. **c** At the level of the glottis (*g*), a paralyzed left true vocal cord (*tvc*) is seen in the midline. The thyroid (*tc*) and cricoid (*cr*) cartilages are intact

Vascular Structures. The carotid artery lies posterolateral to the thyroid cartilages; just posterolateral to the carotids lie the jugular veins which typically are larger and usually asymmetric (Fig. 1c). Identification of the major arteries and veins may be improved by contrast enhancement.

Pathology

Neoplasm is identifiable on CT either because it contains tissue of greater density than the normal laryngeal soft tissues and/or because it distorts, displaces, or destroys normal anatomic structures. CT is especially valuable in assessing the paralaryngeal and pre-epiglottic spaces, areas that should be considered a continuum and that serve as a pathway for the superior, anterior, and inferior spread of supraglottic neoplasm. Deeply infiltrating tumor usually obliterates the normal low density fat content of these spaces (Fig. 2). Such early extension of epiglottic carcinoma to the pre-epiglottic space is difficult to assess clinically or by laryngography.

Computed tomography presents accurate estimation of the posteroinferior spread of tumor (Figs. 3, 4). Spread between thyroid and arytenoid cartilages, or insinuation of tumor between the inferior cornua of the thyroid cartilage and the cricoid cartilage, a not infrequent finding in piriform sinus lesions, is well demonstrated (Fig. 5). Spread deep to the anterior or posterior commissure is reliably

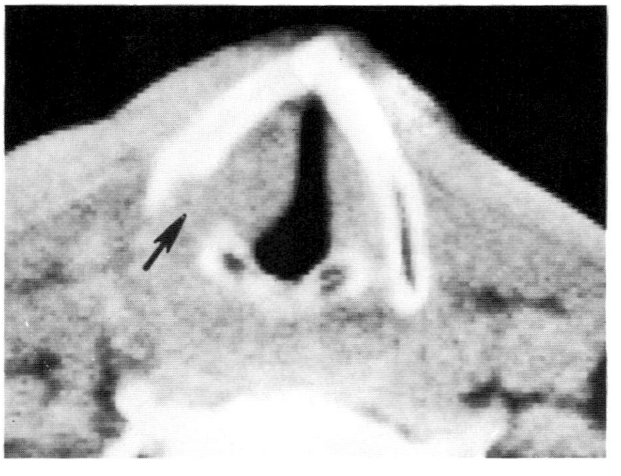

Fig. 5. Inferior extension of a right piriform sinus carcinoma producing destruction of the posterior portion of the right thyroid lamina and widening of the thyrocricoid joint (*arrow*). A paralyzed right true vocal cord is seen extending to the midline

detected on CT (Figs. 6, 7). Such determination can be very difficult on laryngography with bulky tumors. The relationship between any subglottic tumor and the cricoid cartilage, well demonstrated by CT (Fig. 8), is critical information for the surgeon to know, and is more important than some arbitrary measurement of the extent of tumor downward from the inferior margin of the true vocal cords. The cricoid cartilage provides major support for the larynx and only a minimal portion of the superior margin can be sacrificed in conservation therapy if the patient is to retain a viable airway, voice, and "sphincter" to prevent aspiration.

The cross-sectional area of the airway lumen, especially when it is irregular, can be very difficult to estimate on conventional radiography. CT scans accurately depict the airway size.

Computed tomography is an excellent method for detecting cartilaginous invasion, although definite pitfalls and limitations exist. Especially in the thyroid cartilage, because of the normally irregular and nonuniform patterns of calcification and ossification, only moderate to far advanced involvement can be confidently identified. Care must be exercised in diagnosing neoplastic invasion of the cartilaginous structures and not confusing irregularity due to foci of noncalcified cartilage, since conservative surgery would be contraindicated. Even the proximity of tumor to the cartilage can be misleading (Fig. 7a), and it is best with suspected early involvement to tell the surgeon that the findings are equivocal and that inspection and possible biopsy of the cartilages should precede commitment to radicle surgery. Despite the problems encountered, we have still found CT to be the best radiologic technique, superior to soft tissue radiography (including xeroradiography), in determining cartilaginous invasion (Figs. 2d, 7b). Clinical appreciation of such involvement comes only very late when fixation is present.

Rarely, if ever, does CT identify enlarged lymph nodes that cannot be palpated (Fig. 3b). On rare occasion, in patients with substantial body fat, CT may be useful in identifying tumor extension or metastatic lymphadenopathy obliterating the normal low density cleavage plane around the carotid artery and jugular vein; in these circumstances, surgical salvage becomes unlikely.

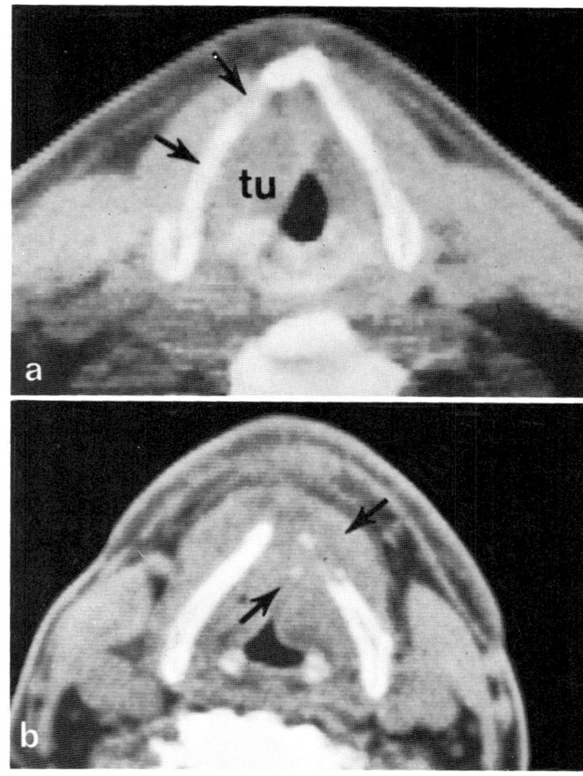

Fig. 7. a A bulky carcinoma (*tu*) of the right true vocal cord is seen with involvement of the anterior commissure (cf. Fig. 6). Adjacent to the tumor, irregularity and marginal defects in the ossification of the right thyroid lamina (*arrows*) is present. This finding was considered very suspicious for tumor invasion of the cartilage. Histologic examination disclosed that the tumor stopped at the margin of the cartilage without invasion; the CT appearance was produced by incomplete ossification and bone marrow production in the right thyroid lamina. **b** In another patient with a carcinoma involving the anterior commissure, destruction and fragmentation of the left thyroid ala are present (*arrows*)

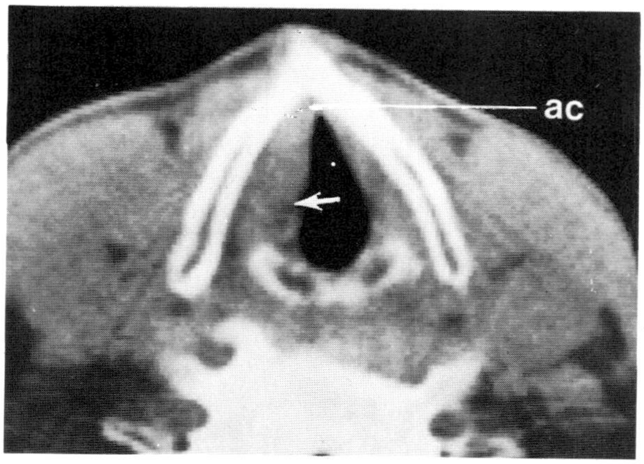

Fig. 6. Carcinoma producing marked thickening of the right true vocal cord (*arrow*). The tumor extends to the anterior commissure (*ac*), but does not cross the midline

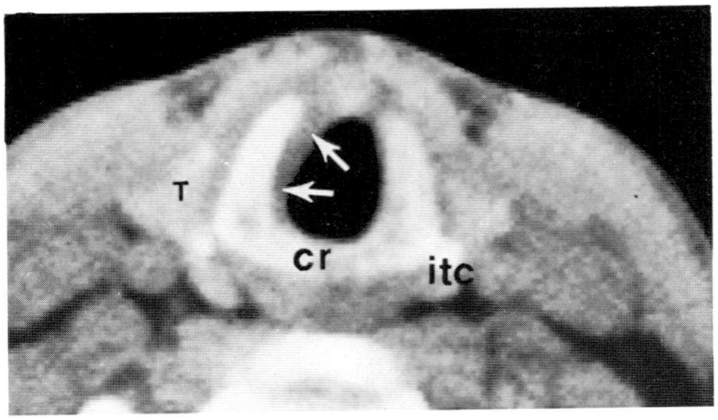

Fig. 8. Substantial subglottic extension of a right true vocal cord carcinoma, contraindicating conservation surgery, is manifested as soft tissue thickening (*arrows*) medial to the right lateral arch of the cricoid cartilage (*cr*) at the level of the inferior cornua of the thyroid cartilage (*itc*). The thyroid gland (*T*) is delineated incidently as a structure of increased density due to its normal high content of iodine

Limitations of CT

A major weakness of CT is its inability to define consistently a transition zone from the false to the true vocal cords. The ventricle is seen in only about 30% of patients. Spread of tumors from the false to the true cords, or vice versa, can be very difficult to determine on CT. Future ready availability of coronal and sagittal reconstruction may diminish this problem.

The status of the piriform sinus is not always clear on the inspiratory phase CT images. Repeating the scans during a modified Valsalva maneuver may fill these structures and improve the evaluation of this region.

Minor mucosal abnormalities will not be imaged with CT, but this is generally of no clinical importance since such irregularities can be depicted by endoscopy. Motion, also, is much better evaluated by clinical examination, since CT is essentially an anatomic study.

Computed tomography only identifies changes in tissue density and fascial planes, and does not permit a histologic diagnosis. Consequently, fibrosis or edema in adjacent tissues can simulate malignant extension on CT. Because of this, CT study should be performed prior to any biopsy or at least 48 h after such a procedure.

Comparison with Laryngography

Computed tomography is cost-competitive (actually slightly less expensive at our hospital) with laryngography. It can be performed with no appreciable discomfort or morbidity to the patient. Laryngography is an invasive procedure carrying some risk, albeit small, particularly in massive tumors. Premedication and substantial cooperation are required for that examination. Most important, we have found equal or superior clinically relevant information provided by CT in over 90% of cases studied by both modalities [7]. CT has a clear superiority in assessing the laryngeal cartilages and deep extension, and should be the initial radiologic procedure, and usually the only one, when such an examination is required. The indications for its use are similar to those established for laryngography, and patients with far advanced or very early lesions usually do not require the procedure.

Computed tomography displays the larynx in a three-dimensional format allowing direct demonstration of tumor in both the larynx and paralaryngeal soft tissues, as well as the cartilages. In contradistinction, laryngography suggests extension of tumor involvement more by inference than by direct determination, except at the mucosal interface.

Discussion

Conservation surgery may successfully manage tumors restricted to the supraglottic compartments; once the neoplasm extends beyond these boundaries or deeply into the paralaryngeal tissues, to involve, for example, the apex of the piriform sinus or the laryngeal cartilages, total laryngectomy is usually indicated.

Computed tomography is a quick (usually requiring less than 20 min to complete) and noninvasive (no discomfort or risk to the patient) method of examining the larynx. CT provides information that adds to or reinforces the clinical examination. Deep extension of neoplasm is well depicted, and the supporting cartilages and subglottic area can be assessed. It is complementary to, rather than a substitute for, laryngoscopy. CT is most valuable when additional data is required to make a decision as to whether conservative surgery as opposed to more radical operation or irradiation is indicated.

Computed tomography is playing an increasingly important role in the management of the patient with carcinoma of the larynx at our medical center. Technologic improvements (thin collimation, rapid scan time) permitting detailed studies during suspended respiration or during physiologic maneuvers is now routinely possible. The study can be accomplished in virtually every cooperative adult. Not only can the structures deep to the mucosal surface of the laryngeal cartilages be accurately evaluated, but subglottic extension of tumor and the cross-sectional size of the airway can be depicted.

Acknowledgement. Reproduced in part with permission from Laryngoscope 91:292–300, 1981

References

1. Mancuso AA, Calcaterra TC, Hanafee WN (1978) Computed tomography of the larynx. Radiol Clin North Am 16:195–208
2. Archer CR, Yeager VL, Friedman WH, Katosontonis GP (1978) Computed tomography of the larynx. J Comput Assist Tomogr 2:404–411
3. Archer CR, Friedman WH, Yeager VL, Katosontonis GP (1978) Evaluation of laryngeal cancer by computed tomography. J Comput Assist Tomogr 2:618–624
4. Mancuso AA, Hanafee WN (1979) A comparative evaluation of computed tomography and laryngography. Radiology 133:131–138
5. Archer CR, Yeager VL (1979) Evaluation of laryngeal cartilages by computed tomography. J Comput Assist Tomogr 3:604–611
6. Cunningham's Manual of Practical Anatomy (revised by Romanes GJ) (1967) vol 3: Head and neck. Oxford University Press, London, pp 168–178
7. Archer CR, Sagel SS, Yeager VL, Martin S, Friedman WH (1981) Comparative accuracy of computed tomography and laryngography in the staging of carcinoma of the larynx. Am J Roentgenol 136:571–575

Neuroradiology

Cerebral Computed Tomography: Overview*

S. Wende

Neurochirurgische Universitätsklinik, Abteilung für Neuroradiologie, Langenbeckstrasse 1, D-6500 Mainz

Introduction

We have examined 3500 patients suffering from cerebral tumor by means of CT, and the results concerning the value of CT have not changed as compared to those of our investigations made on more than 2000 cerebral tumors and published some years ago (see Table 1). The accuracy of localization is still about 98%. In approximately 70% of cases the nature of the tumor can also be exactly diagnosed.

Technical advances in CT have led to better resolution, which allows improved detail recognizability, particularly for structures in the region of the base of the skull.

The reduction of the duration of examination enables more investigations to be made within the same period of time. This short period of examination is of special relevance for uncooperative patients and infants. Anesthesia – which has previously been necessary – can now be omitted and no longer causes any risk.

The reduction of the scan time with special programs has one more advantage: The static examination becomes dynamic: Both the cerebral blood flow and the contrast enhancement in cerebral tissue can be measured in certain intervals. Nowadays it is possible to produce 16 scans in series within 3 s of scan time. These rapid examinations make possible differentiation between the arterial and venous phases as well as the phase of diffuse contrast enhancement. This is of special relevance for patients with cerebral infarct: prognostic assessment can now be made.

Distinct increase in density in a hypodense region during the arterial phase indicates hyperperfusion – a reactive hyperemia. If further measurements do not exhibit any later contrast enhancement in this area, a disturbance of the blood-brain barrier does not come under consideration. Thus, the prognosis is to be considered favorable. The region of infarct will regress and so will the neurologic symptoms.

If, however, during the arterial phase, there are high density values in the vicinity of the pathologic area, indicating vasoparalysis – a luxury perfusion – and if contrast enhancement in the damaged cerebral region occurs after the phase of blood circulation, a distinct blood-brain barrier disturbance exists. This signifies the destruction of the damaged cerebral tissue with permanent neurologic deficiency.

In Germany these investigations have particularly been carried out by the team of Traupe, Cologne, and in the United States by Heinz and co-workers.

The Sortland Technique

In my opinion, the greatest progress in CT diagnosis in recent years was achieved through the Sortland technique for the demonstration of cerebellopontine angle tumors. In 1978 Sortland reported a new technique of examination for the demonstration of small tumors in the cerebellopontine angle region. By means of gas cisternography in combination with CT, Sortland was able to demonstrate the cerebellopontine angle cistern and the internal auditory canal, and thus small intracanalicular tumors. At the Department of Neuroradiology in Mainz, Sortland's technique of investigation has been applied since January 1979 to 98 patients with suspected cerebellopontine angle tumor because of otologic symptoms.

Some information about the technique: In order to exclude larger space-occupying processes in the

* The paper on "Progress of cerebral computed tomography" begins with a statistical cooperative study by the University Hospitals Berlin, Mainz und Munich

Radiology Today 1. Ed. by M. W. Donner and F. H. W. Heuck

Table 1. CAT of 2015 brain tumors

Type of neoplasm	n	Tumor not detected in the plain scan	Post contrast scan			Perifocal edema
			n	pos.	neg.	%
Astrocytoma grade I	104	–	94	–	94	1.9
Astrocytoma grade II	100	4	90	77	13	64
Glioblastoma	375	13	360	354	6	88.5
Oligodendroglioma	93	–	83	32	51	37.6
Pilocytic astrocytoma	45	3	39	31	8	20.0
Ependymoma	28	–	22	20	2	50.0
Medulloblastoma	44	1	42	38	4	47.7
Plexuspapilloma	5	–	4	4	–	40.0
Neuroma	96	44	95	88	7	31.2
Hemangioblastoma	22	1	21	8	13	22.7
Meningioma	309	21	261	259	2	57.2
Malignant lymphoma	32	1	30	29	1	65.6
Pituitary adenoma	187	4	173	166	7	2.1
Craniopharyngeoma	52	4	42	31	11	–
Epidermoid – dermoid cyst, teratoma	14	–	7	1	6	–
Other brain tumors	74	5	62	46	16	17.5
Metastases	260	15	241	222	19	81.9
Tumors of unknown histology	175	6	162	116	46	39.4
Total	2015	122	1828	1522	306	
%	100	6.1	90.7	83.3	16.7	50.1

The total amounts to 2015 tumors. 8 tumors are not identifiable by plain scans as they are not located within the range of cuts being examined

cerebellopontine angle region, CT is performed before and after intravenous contrast injection. If the result is negative, lumbar puncture is made. The patient's head is turned to the opposite side of the affected ear, relatively rapid lumbar injection of 5–6 cc gas follows; this protrudes into the pontocerebellar cistern to be examined and also enters the internal auditory canal. The patient is then brought to the scanner still keeping the lateral decubitus position. The patient's head is rotated about 45° with the gas-filled pontocerebellar cistern and the internal auditory canal upward. With proper technique, computed tomograms visualize the cerebellopontine angle. Tilting of the patient to the opposite side makes possible subsequent examination of the opposite cerebellopontine angle region. Intracanalicular as well as extracanalicular acoustic neuromas are distinctly demonstrated.

The method described is simple and of considerable diagnostic value. If the contraindications of lumbar puncture are considered, there is no risk to the patient. Some patients do complain of moderate headache, a tolerable side-effect.

CT Diagnosis in Newborns

Several papers have been published on intracranial hemorrhages in newborns. In our department my co-worker Dr. Ludwig has performed an extensive study on the value of CT in newborns in order to answer the following questions:

1. What kind of pathologic CT findings do newborns with pathologic clinical signs show?
2. Is there any correlation between the pathologic CT findings and the mode of delivery (spontaneous, vacuum or forceps extraction, cesarean sections)?
3. What percentage of clinically normal newborns exhibit pathologic CT findings.

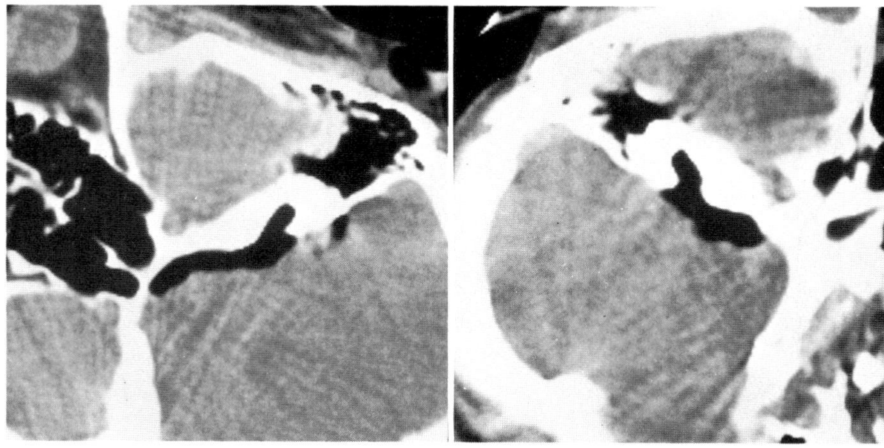

Fig. 1. Air-CT study of the right and left cerebellopontine cisterns. Normal case

Our examinations on 150 newborns were carried out between the 2nd and 10th day of age. One hundred and five newborns were admitted to the Children's Hospital because of clinicopathologic findings, and 45 newborns without any pathologic signs came from the Maternity Hospital as a so-called control group in order that we obtained normal CT images of newborns.

Apart from normal findings, our investigations displayed intradural, subarachnoidal, intracerebral, and intraventricular hemorrhages. It was found that 46% of the newborns with neurologic abnormalities had radiologic evidence of an intracranial hemorrhage, whereas only 6% of the clinically normal newborns had such a finding in CT. There was no difference in the frequency of bleeding in infants delivered spontaneously or with vacuum of forceps extraction. As expected, only in infants delivered by cesarean section was bleeding seldom found.

Follow-up examinations showed distinct atrophy after intracerebral hemorrhage with ventricular involvement, while after extraparenchymatous or isolated intracerebral bleeding only slight or no pathologic changes in the cerebrospinal fluid spaces were evident in CT.

CT in Tumor Follow-up Studies

It is pathomorphologically known that after radiotherapy or cytostatic therapy, brain tumors respond with growing of new vessels, necrotic changes, scarring, and regressive alterations. Accordingly, this tumor deformation must be represented in CT follow-up studies as both density and volume changes.

In order to cover all these changes definitely, my co-worker Dr. Kretzschmar has analyzed 125 CT studies in respect of density distribution and tumor volume. The results were compared to the success of therapy. The mean value of the Hounsfield units in the center of the tumor as well as in the surrounding parenchyma by means of histograms were determined.

In general terms, the statistical evaluation of the follow-up yielded the following results:

1. Volume changes are better parameters for the tumor reaction than density measurements. Successful therapy achieves volume resorption already at termination of radiotherapy or after the first cytostatic cycle, whereas the density distribution displays no significant change. In cases of therapy-resistant tumors, e.g., meningiomas or some gliomas, the volume remains stable although changes in density are evident.
2. It may be stated that not until 6 months after the end of radiotherapy may the maximum of tumor reaction be assessed. The tumor volume has reached its minimum at this date by the earliest. The density value then exhibits an increase or decrease, probably due to hypervascularization, vasodilatation, and glia reaction. Thus, the tumor density assimilates to the Hounsfield units of normal parenchyma. Recurrent or residual tumor growth then produces both volume and density changes.

These reactions occur more rapidly under cytostatic therapy; the regression, however, occurs for a shorter time.

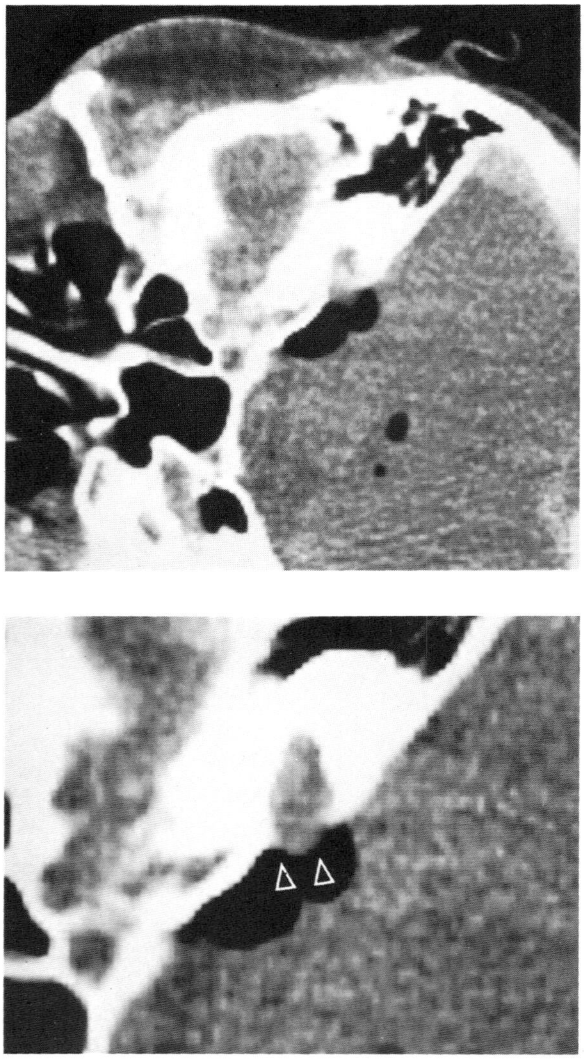

Fig. 2. Intra- and extracanalicular acoustic neuroma

3. In none of our 125 patients with cerebral tumors and without total extirpation of the tumor was complete remission achieved by radiotherapy or cytostatic therapy.

Within 4 years of the survey there was always evidence of measurable tumor residual elements or tumor growth. Tumor growth was sometimes very slow; so much so that in one of our CT patients suffering from a glioma of the corpus callosum we performed 21 controls within a period of 4 years.
It therefore appears necessary to orientate the success of therapy toward the CT findings instead of the survival time.

Table 2

Lesions of the orbit		520 cases
Benign tumors		145
Cavernous hemangiomas	25	
Meningiomas	47	
Tuberculum sellae		
Sphenoid wing		
Olfactory groove		
Meningiomas of the optic sheath	18	
Optic gliomas	21	
Neurinomas	9	
Lipomas	8	
Dermoids/Epidermoids	11	
Fibromas	5	
Angioleiomyoma	1	
Malignant tumors		107
Carcinomas, metastases	40	
Lymphomas	17	
Tumors of the lacrimal gland	14	
Melanomas	11	
Sarcomas	9	
Cylindromas	4	
Hemangioendotheliomas	3	
Hemangioblastomas	2	
Basaliomas	3	
Neuroblastoma	1	
Plasmoytoma	1	
Myoblastoma	1	
Histiocytoma	1	
Pseudotumors		30
Benign space-occupying processes		25
Mucoceles	13	
Abscesses	5	
Pyoceles	3	
Giant cell granulomas	2	
Cysts	2	
Malformations		30
Arteriovenous malformations	10	
Aplasia of the sphenoid bone	10	
Buphthalmos	6	
Fibrous dysplasia	4	
Endocrine exophthalmos		55
Myositis		15
Traumas		17
Hematomas, intraorbital	11	
Carotid cavernous sinus fistulas	6	
Histologically unverified		96
		520 cases

CT in Orbital Diagnosis

Table 2 which gives details of the numerous different space-occupying processes, inflammations, and malformations occurring in our patients in the region of the orbit, displays the high diagnostic value of CT.

How accurate is CT as compared with other diagnostic methods? Comparative studies between CT, ultrasonography, and roentgen tomography have been performed by several authors. All of them verified the high diagnostic accuracy of CT, which cannot be reached by any other method of examination.

This, however, applies only to the question: "Tumor: yes or no" and to the localization of the mass. As to the differential diagnosis of a space-occupying process in the orbital region, the predictability of CT is restricted. Even after intravenous contrast application the majority of cases show density increase which does not aid differential diagnosis. Malignant masses such as lymphomas or metastases exhibit the same increase in density as benign tumors, e.g., meningiomas or neuromas.

According to our experiences, in any case of suspected orbital tumor, ultrasonography should be carried out in addition to CT, since only this combination achieves optimum accuracy of differential diagnosis. One cannot distinguish between benign and malignant masses unless bone destructions are demonstrated by CT. Differentiation as to whether the tumor originates from the optic nerve or not is easy. Thus, differential diagnosis is limited to certain tumors, and is not definitely possible.

References

1. Kazner E, Grumme T, Lanksch W, Wende S (1977) Computed tomography (CT) and the operative indications for brain tumors. A cooperative study of three university hospitals. In: Proceedings of the VI. International Congress of Neurosurgical Surgery, Sao Paulo, June 19–25, 1977. Excerpta Medica, Amsterdam Oxford (International congress series 433). Neurological surgery, pp 28–36
2. Kretzschmar K, Aulich A, Schindler E, Lange S, Grumme T, Meese W (1978) The diagnostic value of CT for radiotherapy of cerebral tumors. Neuroradiology 14:245–250
3. Kricheff JJ, Pinto RS, Bergeron RT, Cohen N (1980) Air-CT cisternography and canalography for small acoustic neuromas. Am J Neuroradiol 1:57–63
4. Sortland O X-ray diagnosis of expanding lesions in the cerebellopontine angle. Meeting of the Nordisc Society of Radiology. Oslo, June 1978
5. Sortland O (1979) Computed tomography combined with gas cisternography for the diagnosis of expanding lesions in the cerebellopontine angle. Neuroradiology 18:19–22
6. Traupe H, Heiss W-D, Hoeffken W, Zülch KJ (1979) Hyperfusion and enhancement in dynamic computed tomography of ischemic stroke patients. J Comput Assist Tomogr 3:627–632
7. Wende S (1980) Die kombinierte Anwendung von Computer-Tomographie und Luft-Cisternographie bei Kleinhirnbrückenwinkel-Tumoren. ROEFO 132: 666–667
8. Wende S, Aulich A, Kretzschmar K, Grumme T, Meese W, Lange S, Steinhoff H, Lanksch W, Kazner E (1977) Die Computer-Tomographie der Hirngeschwülste. Eine Sammelstudie über 1658 Tumoren. Radiologe 17:149–156
9. Wende S, Aulich A, Nover A, Lanksch W, Kazner E, Steinhoff H, Meese W, Lange S, Grumme T (1977) Computed tomography of orbital lesions. A cooperative study of 210 cases. Neuroradiology 13:123–134

Computed Tomography of the Orbit

U. Piepgras

Universität des Saarlandes, Medizinische Fakultät, Abteilung für Neuroradiologie, Universitätskliniken, D-6650 Homburg/Saar

Introduction

CT scanning is an X-ray method that for the first time makes it possible to visualize directly the normal tissues and fluids as well as numerous pathological processes of the orbit with extraordinary precision [1, 2, 8, 12, 13, 18, 19, 20, 21, 24, 26, 27, 34, 35, 36]. The orbit and its contents are especially suitable for CT analysis as these are anatomical structures with sufficient differences in density. The retro- and peribulbar fat – with its extremely low density – acts as a natural negative contrast medium.

Methods

Since its introduction in 1972, CT scanning has undergone rapid further development. Progress in CT diagnosis of diseases of the eye and orbit mainly rests on the following factors:

1. Technical development of the equipment, with finer matrix, reduction of scanning times, reduction of the section thickness etc. has resulted in improved spatial resolution and image quality. It may be assumed that with CT equipment currently used for examination of the head the spatial resolution of a standard computed tomogram with a scan time of 1 min amounts to 1 – 1.5 mm [33, 37] for density differences of 10% (high contrast).
   With special stand-alone (independent) computer evaluation equipment the information obtained during examination and stored on discettes can be evaluated in detail (analog and digital processing) and further processing can be done. In this manner, once the patient has been examined, subtle quantitative density measurements, planimetry and thickness measurement of single areas in the object can be performed and profile sections (histograms) made.
2. Considerable progress has resulted from the elimination of the water mantle and enlargement of the gantry opening. This has made it possible to examine the head directly in marked reclination and corresponding angulation of the gantry, in addition to the transverse standard plane in the *coronal (frontal) aspect* [4, 10, 11, 28, 29, 30, 33].
   Direct visualization of the orbit in the sagittal plane in analogy with coronal examination by placing the head according to the technique described by Haverling and Johanson [9] and Wing et al. [38] can only be done with very large gantry openings and extremely lithe patients.
3. For pluridimensional visualization of the orbit and its contents *computer reconstruction* of the coronal and sagittal plane from the measurements in transverse sections is now possible. In the meantime the computer programs required and the stand-alone evaluation units have been developed to such a level that this important indirect technique can be used for routine purposes. For adequate imaging quality of the reconstructed sections the transverse standard CT has to be made with overlapping 5 mm slices in the object area of interest [6, 14, 15, 17].
4. More detailed information on the retro-orbital area is obtained by contrasting of the perisellar cisterns after intrathecal application of water-soluble contrast media (CT cisternography) [7, 11, 17, 33].
5. Undoubtedly, the principal factor in continued development must have been the marked increase in experience with CT and evaluation of CT scans of the orbit. It cannot be doubted that assessment of the individual case has become simpler and more reliable, since the number of pathological cases and combinations of findings described in the literature and personally observed has considerably increased.

Radiology Today 1. Ed. by M. W. Donner and F. H. W. Heuck

Results

Normal Findings (Figs. 1 – 3)

The improvement in spatial resolution, the possibility of obtaining coronal and sagittal sections in addition to the standard transverse cuts by direct technique or computer reconstruction, provides an exact visualization of the normal orbit in three-dimensional view. A very precise presentation of the normal orbit anatomy is given by Tadmor and New [28], Salvolini et al. [25], Vignaud and Aubin [32], Bacon et al. [3] and Jacobs et al. [11]. In the transverse CT the neuro-ocular plane [25] is the principal anatomical plane of reference (Fig. 1). This is characterized by three elements: the lens, the papilla and the N. opticus as far as the orbital opening of the optic canal. This section plane represents the equatorial area of the bulbus.
Dependent on the technical equipment applied, the kind and accuracy of examination, artifacts caused by metal dental fillings or movement and the patient's condition, CT reveals more or less exactly the following anatomical structures:

Eyelids
Anterior chamber/cornea
Lens
Orbital septum
Globe
Sclera
Optic nerve
Orbital fat
Extra-ocular muscles:
- lateral rectus
- medial rectus
- inferior rectus
- superior rectus
- superior oblique
- inferior oblique
- levator palpebrae

Lacrimal gland
Superior ophthalmic vein
Opthalmic artery
Bony walls of the orbit
Trochlea
Sphenoid bone
Optical canal
Superior orbital fissure
Sella turcica
Sinus cavernosus

Pathological Findings

In a discussion of the pathological processes of the orbital area a distinction can be made between diseases affecting primarily and exclusively one or both orbits and processes in the vicinity that start in peri-orbital structures and then involve the orbit and eye [22, 31]. The diseases of the orbit and peri-orbital area in which CT scanning at the current

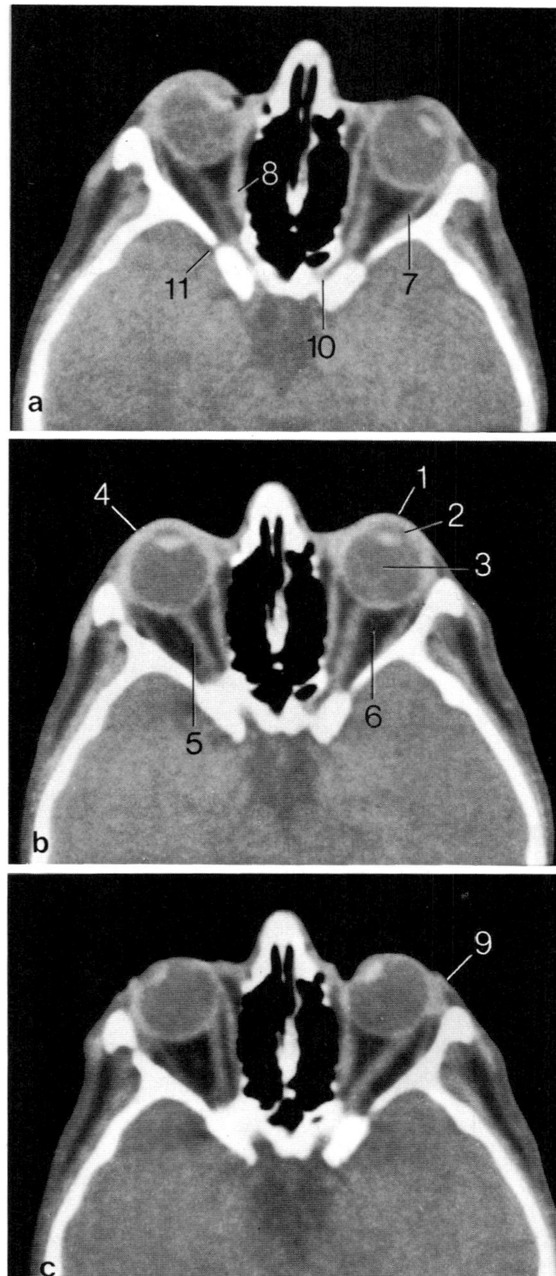

Fig. 1a – c. Normal standard transverse CT in the neuro-ocular plane of a patient looking **a** to the right, **b** straight on and **c** to the left without contrast enhancement. *1,* anterior chamber/cornea; *2,* lens; *3,* globe; *4,* sclera; *5,* optic nerve; *6,* orbital fat; *7,* lateral rectus muscle; *8,* medial rectus muscle; *9,* lacrimal gland; *10,* optic canal; *11,* superior orbital fissure

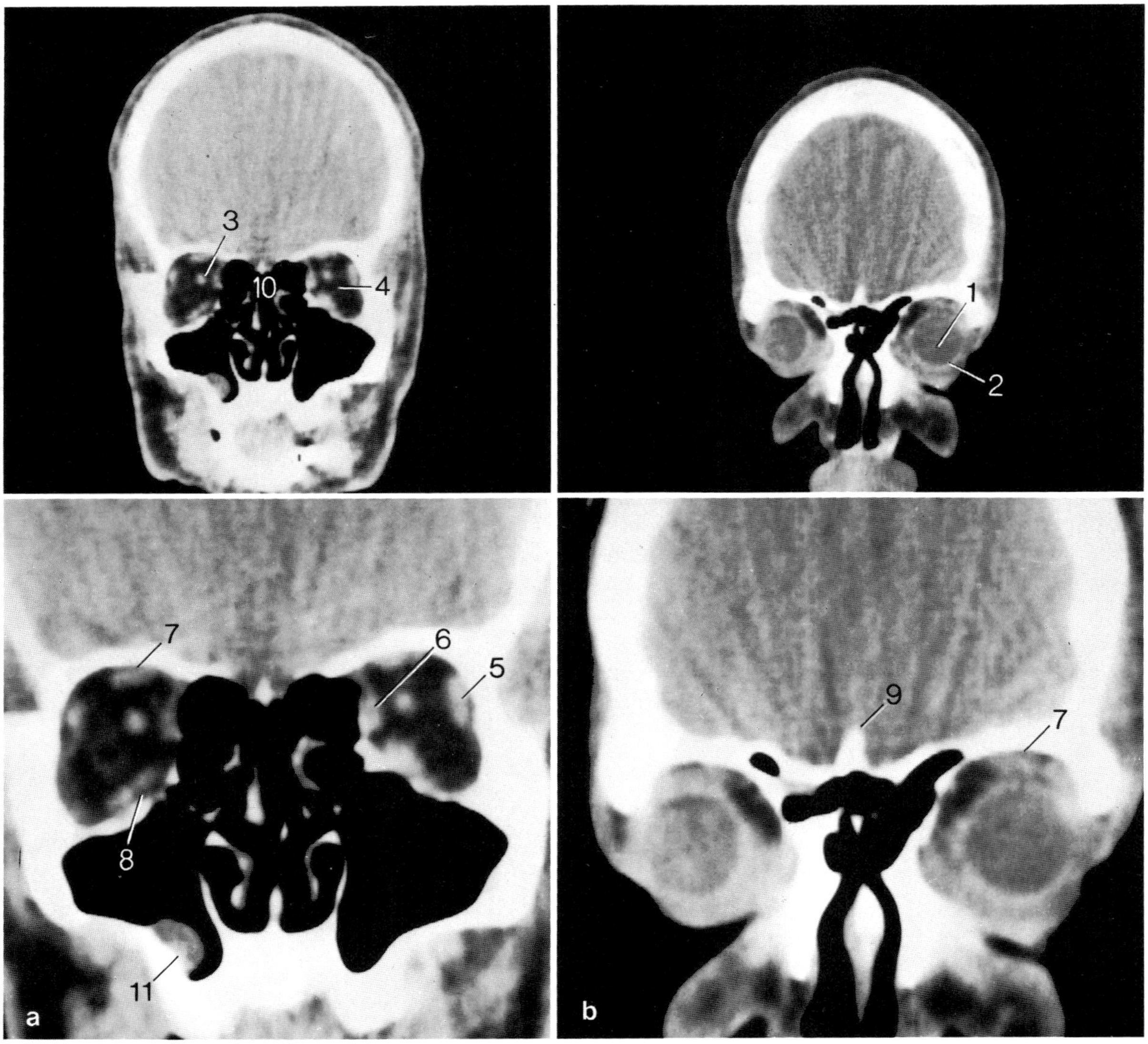

Fig. 2a, b. Normal coronal CT scan directly obtained by placement of patient's head and gantry tilting to an angulation between the scanning plane and the orbitomeatal line approximately at 70 – 90° (*Bottom:* enlargement, 1:2). Thickness of the slices: 5 mm (with a separation of 5 mm). Scanning time: 68 s. **a** Section behind the globe; **b** section through the globe. *1,* globe; *2,* sclera; *3,* optic nerve; *4,* orbital fat; *5,* lateral rectus muscle; *6,* medial rectus muscle; *7,* superior rectus muscle and levator palpebrae; *8,* inferior rectus and inferior oblique muscles; *9,* crista galli; *10,* ethmoid sinus; *11,* small polyp in the left maxillary sinus

stage of development yields fundamental or additional information are summarized in Tables 1 and 2. Fundamental discussion of all pathological processes mentioned is impossible and this review must be limited to some typical and important findings by way of example (Figs. 4 – 10).

Discussion

The cardinal point in CT diagnosis of the orbit lies in the possibility of directly visualizing space-occupying and other pathological processes of the eye, the bony orbit and peri-orbital area and to survey their topographic relationships to the neighbouring anatomical structures. Although diagnostic reliability has considerably increased as a result of technical developments and increased experience, CT remains limited with regard to identification of the histological nature of pathological processes of the eye and orbit. Although CT not infrequently suffices for a definitive, i.e. aetiological, diagnosis, complementary radiological examination such as plain X-rays, conventional X-

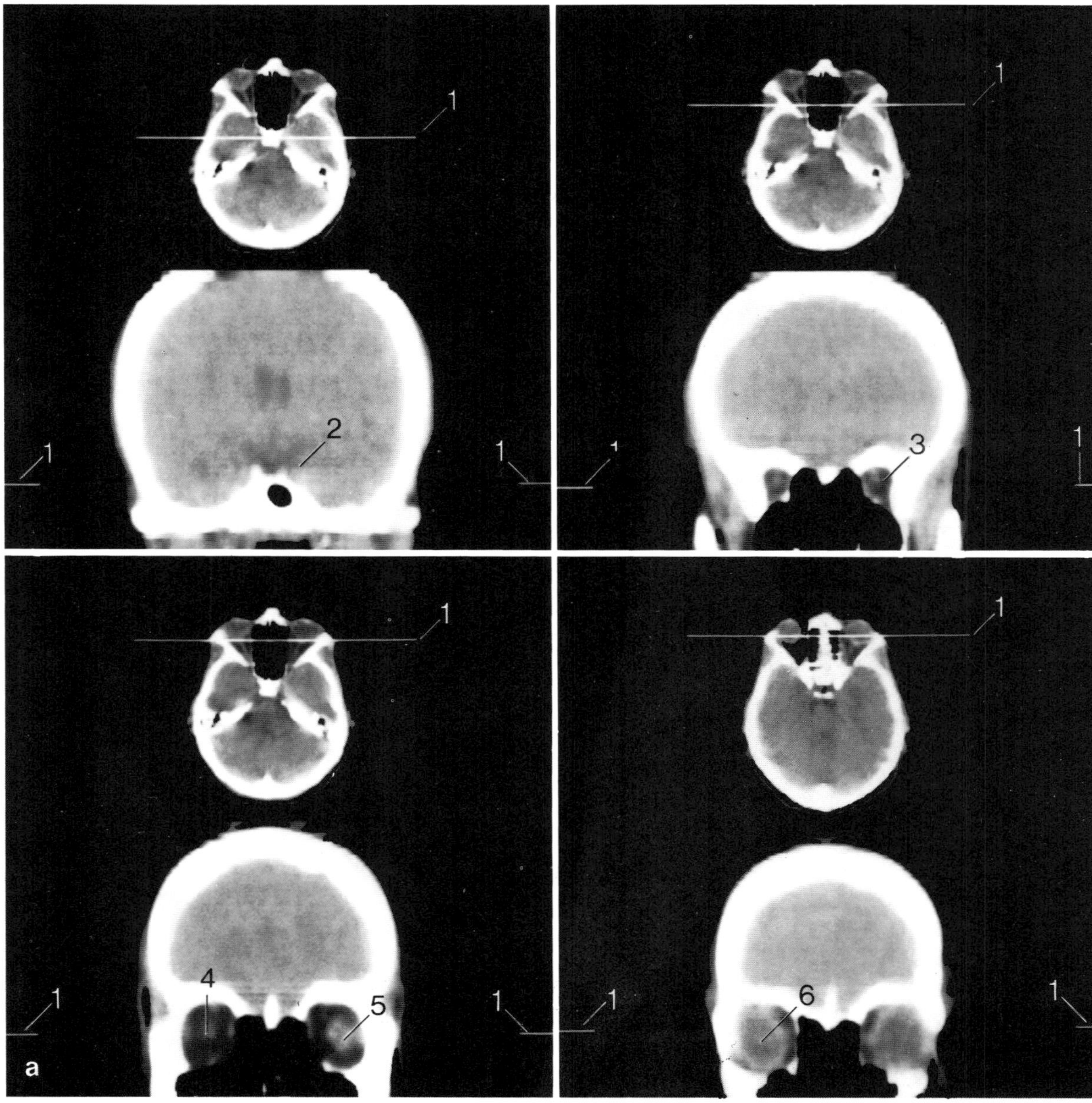

Fig. 3a, b. Normal **a** coronal and **b** sagittal CT scans of the orbits and the sella turcica, indirectly obtained by reconstruction (precontrast study). The transverse sections were carried out with an inclination of the scanning plane about 10° to the orbitomeatal line. The reconstructions were made from overlapping 24 transverse scans. A pair of slices is produced simultaneously in 68 s, each section being 5 mm thick. *1,* corresponding levels of sections (computer display); *2,* sella turcica and perisellar cisterns; *3;* optic nerve in the apex of the orbit; *4,* optic nerve behind the globe; *5,* posterior part of the globe with optic nerve; *6,* globe with sclera; *7,* lens; *8,* pineal body

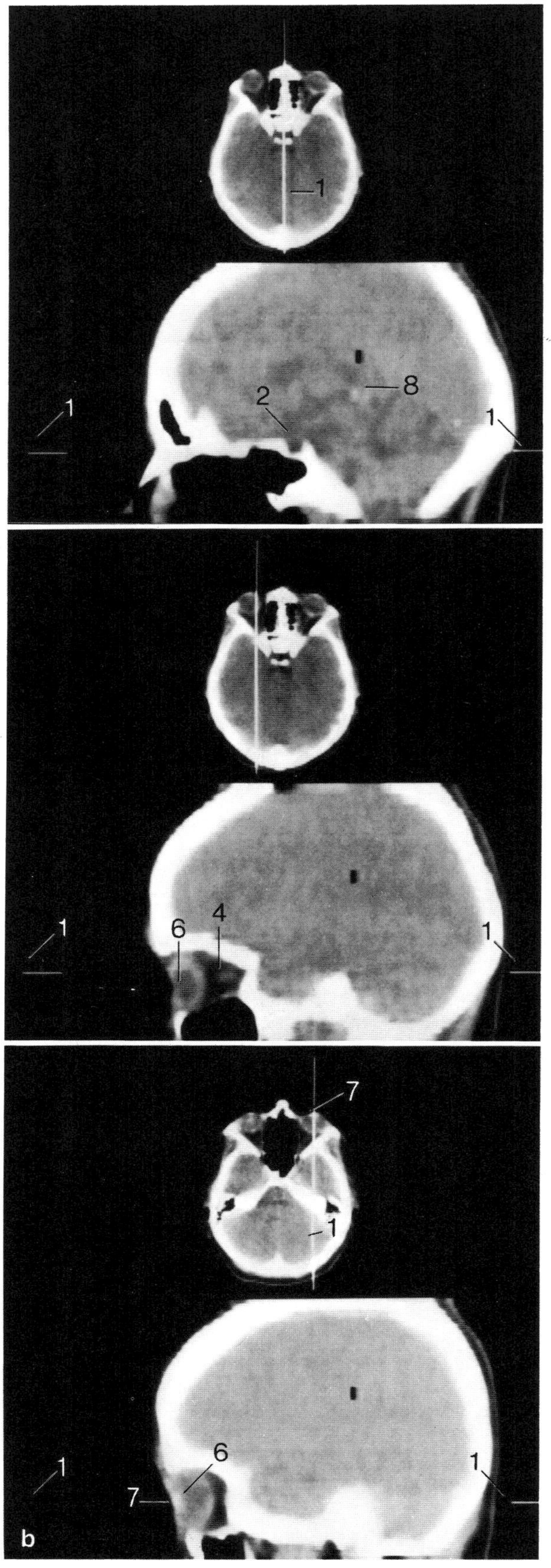

Table 1. Primary processes of the orbit and bulbus oculi

Congenital malformations

Hydrophthalmus
Microphthalmus
Aplasia of the bulbus
Aphakia
Ectopy of the lens (Marfan syndrome)
Myopia

Malformations with blastomatous or expansive component

Meningo-encephalocele
Dysplasia or aplasia of the sphenoid bone
Cavernous angioma
Arteriovenous angioma

Primary tumours

Dermoid/epidermoid
Tumours of the lacrimal glands
Retinoblastoma
Melanoma
Meningioma of the optic sheath
Neuroblastoma of the optic nerve
Glioma of the optic nerve
Neurinoma
Rhabdomyosarcoma and other sarcomas
Basalioma
Osteoma
Chondroma
Haemangiopericytoma
Lipoma
Fibroma
Myoma

Involvement of the eye in metastases and other systemic diseases

Metastases
Lymphoma, plasmocytoma etc.
Systemic diseases of the haemopoietic system
von Hippel-Lindau syndrome
Histiocytosis X

Inflammations

Orbital abscess
Pseudotumour of the orbit
Myositis
Inflammations of the bulbus integuments

Trauma

Fractures
Haematomas
Foreign bodies
Luxation and resorption of the lens

◂ **Fig. 3b.** Legend see p. 385

Table 1 (continued)

Vascular diseases
Phlebectasis/varicosis
Phleboliths
Spontaneous intra-orbital haematoma
Endocrine disorders
Endocrine exophthalmus
Sequels to surgery, trauma and injections
Enucleation
Eye prosthesis
Aphakia
Plastic plugs
Enophthalmus
Phthisis bulbi
Artificial bleeding

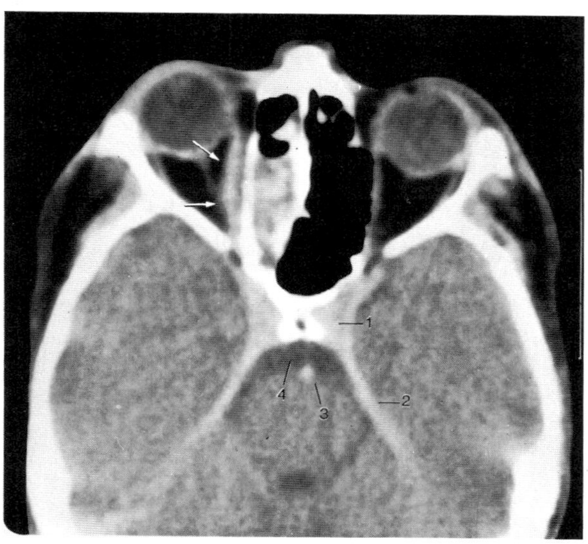

Fig. 4. Left-sided *ethmoiditis* with clinical and CT evidence of orbital involvement. A 5-year-old boy with low-grade fever, left frontal headache, diplopia and prominence of the left eye. Enhanced transverse CT reveals homogeneous increased density of the middle and dorsal ethmoideal air cells, mild exophthalmus and swollen medial rectus muscle (*arrows*) on the left. *1,* cavernous sinus; *2,* superior petrous sinus; *3,* basilar artery; *4,* interpeduncular cistern

ray tomography and scintigraphy of the brain and skeleton remain necessary in other situations for thorough diagnosis.

The indication for invasive contrast examination such as phlebography of the orbit and carotid angiography has been greatly limited by CT and is now essentially restricted – frequently as an additional or complementary method – to demonstration or exclusion of arteriovenous angiomas, carotid sinus cavernosus fistulae, thrombosis of the sinus cavernosus and large orbital veins, orbital varicosis and arterial aneurysms and to pre-operative analysis of the vascularization of tumours. In individual cases pneumencephalography remains necessary for the exploration of the chiasmic area, despite optimization of CT techniques.

Table 2. Periorbital processes with involvement of the orbit

Congenital malformations
Turricephalus
Dysostosis craniofacialis Crouzon
Fibrous dysplasia
Tumours
Sphenoid meningioma
Metastases
Sarcomas
Pituitary tumours
Glioma of the chiasma
Chordoma
Tumours of the paranasal sinuses and nasopharynx (carcinoma, chondroma, neuro-esthesioblastoma, cylindroma etc.)
Inflammations
Muco- and pyoceles of the sinuses
Orbital phlegmons from spreading inflammation
Myositis in ethmoiditis
Trauma
Carotid sinus cavernosus fistula
Complex craniocerebral trauma
Vascular diseases
Carotid aneurysms
Thrombosis of the cavernosus sinus
Spontaneous carotid cavernosus sinus fistulas

Combined application of ultrasound and CT is ideal in the diagnosis of diseases of the orbit and eye [2, 5, 16]. The two methods are supplementary in the localization and in assessment of the extent and specific diagnosis of pathological processes of the orbit, whereas echography of the retro-orbital area – in contrast to CT – has no diagnostic significance.

The limits of CT from the morphological point of view are the result of the limited space and density resolution. Some conditions that for the time being cannot be diagnosed by CT, or not with sufficient

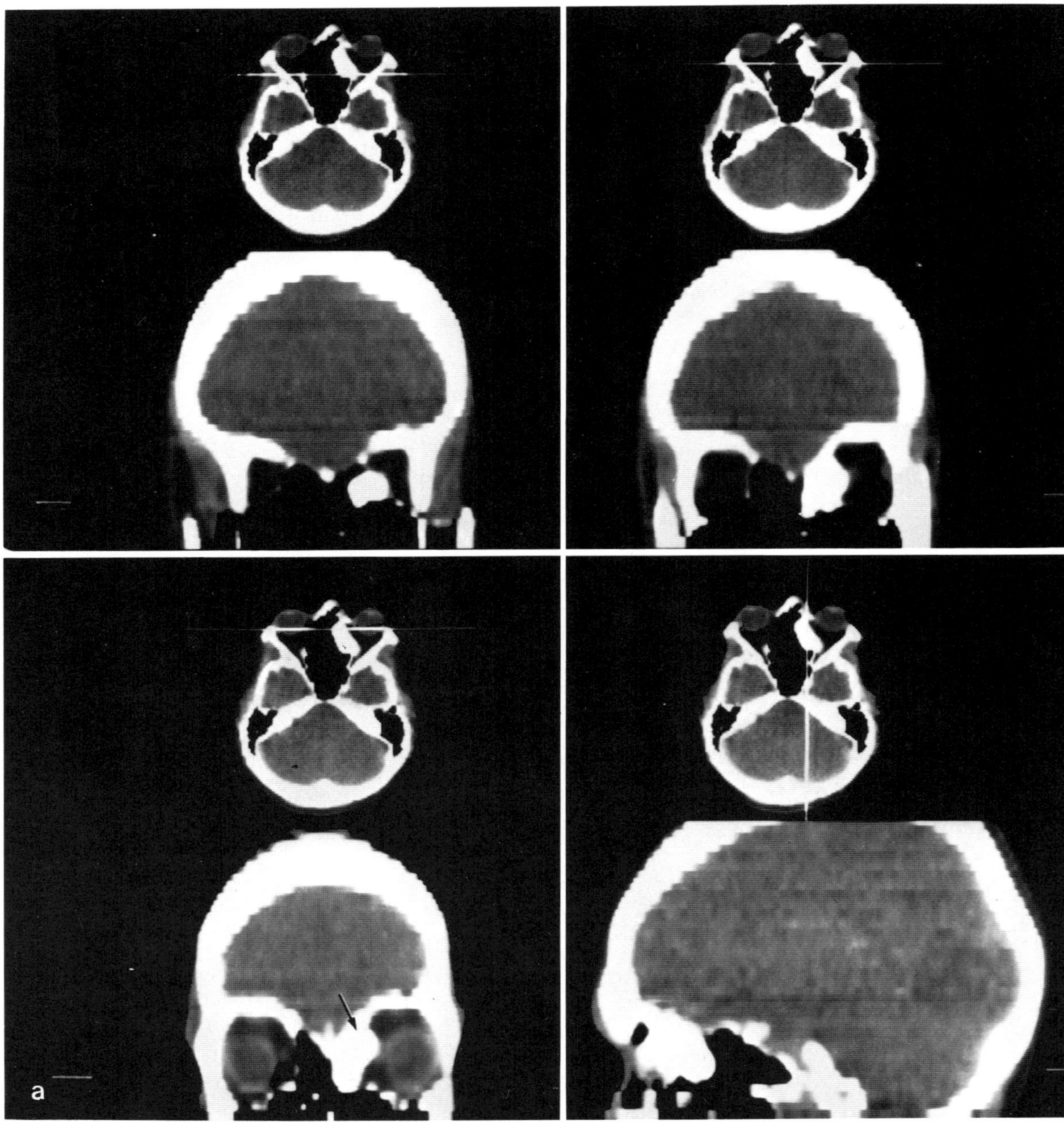

Fig. 5a, b. Right ethmoideal osteoma with large extension into the medial orbit. The tumour appears as a solid mass with densities of compact bone. The osteoma has gained considerable size up to the orbital apex. Coronal CT visualizes slight lateral and downward displacement of the globe (*arrow*). Threedimensional visualization by reconstruction of the coronal and sagittal plane (non-enhanced). **a** Reconstructed coronal and sagittal view; **b** transverse view

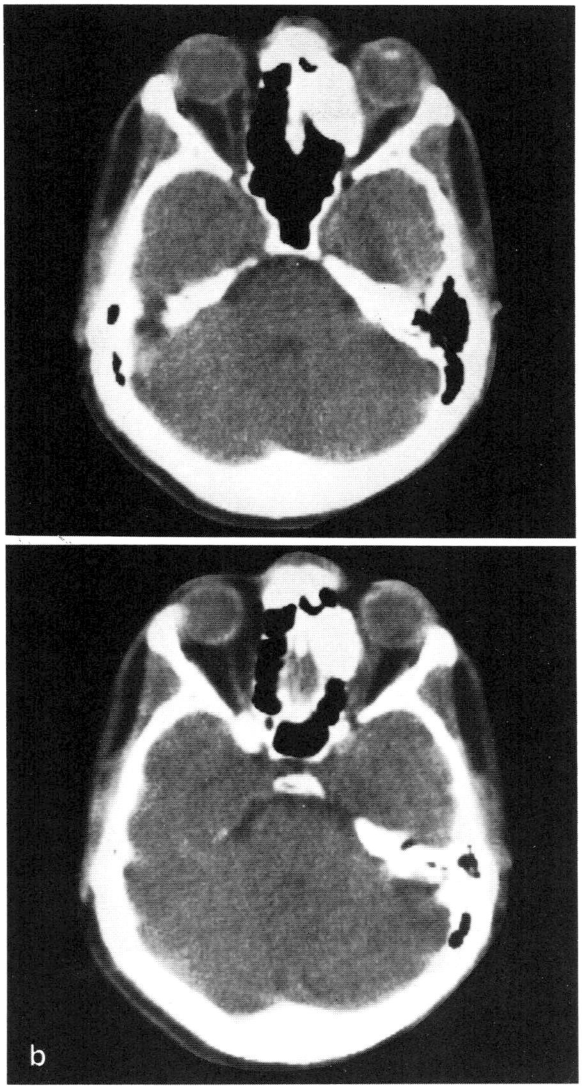

Fig. 5b. Legend see p. 388

reliability, are: retinal detachment, cataracts, neuritis of the optic nerve and circumscribed, flat, rapidly diluting and resorbed bleeding of the vitreous, bulbus and optic sheaths.

The radiation dose of the lens and the other structures of the eye depends on the scope of the examination and the position of the tube in the various pieces of equipment in relation to the eye. Figures quoted lie between 3 and 12 rads [11, 17, 23, 28, 29, 35]. The corresponding values of conventional X-ray examination – especially related to the lens – are considerably higher, so that the radiation exposure of the eye as a whole constitutes a relative limitation of the use of CT in the orbital area. It is necessary, however, to adjust the indications for CT scanning and conventional tomography carefully.

Summary

Computed tomography is the first X-ray method with which it becomes possible to demonstrate a large number of diseases of the eye and orbit, to localize them exactly and to demonstrate their effect on neighbouring anatomical structures. In the past few years, considerable progress has resulted from improvement in the equipment, from the possibility of three-dimensional visualization of the object by introduction of the coronal and sagittal planes of section via reconstruction and/or positioning of the head and from the general increase in experience. In the course of further development, the possibilities of specific diagnosis have increased, but complementary neuroradiological examination is still often necessary. A very high diagnostic reliability results from combined use of CT and ultrasound in the region of the eye and orbit.

References

1. Ambrose JAE, Lloyd GAS, Wright JE (1974) A preliminary evaluation of fine matrix computerized axial tomography (EMI scan) in the diagnosis of orbital space-occupying lesions. Br J Radiol 47:747 – 751
2. Aubin ML, Vignaud J (1978) Computerized tomography of the eye: a study of 62 pathologic cases. Neuroradiology 16:456 – 457
3. Bacon KT, Duchesneau PM, Weinstein MA (1977) Demonstration of the superior ophthalmic vein by high resolution computed tomography. Radiology 124:129 – 131
4. Balériaux-Waha D, Mortelmans LL, Dupont MG, Terwinghe G, Jeanmart L (1977) The use of coronal scans for computed tomography of the orbits. Neuroradiology 14:89 – 96
5. Bigar F, Spiess H, Gruber HU (1979) Kombinierte Anwendung der Computertomographie und Echographie in der Ophthalmologie. Klin Monatsbl Augenheilk 174:806 – 815
6. Delavelle J, Megret M (1980) CT sagittal reconstruction of posterior fossa tumors. Neuroradiology 19:81 – 88
7. Fox AJ, Debrun G, Vinuela F, Assis L, Coates R (1979) Intrathecal metrizamide enhancement of the optic nerve sheath. J Comput Assist Tomogr 3: 653 – 656
8. Gyldensted C, Lester J, Fledelius H (1977) Computed tomography of orbital lesions. Neuroradiology 13:141 – 150

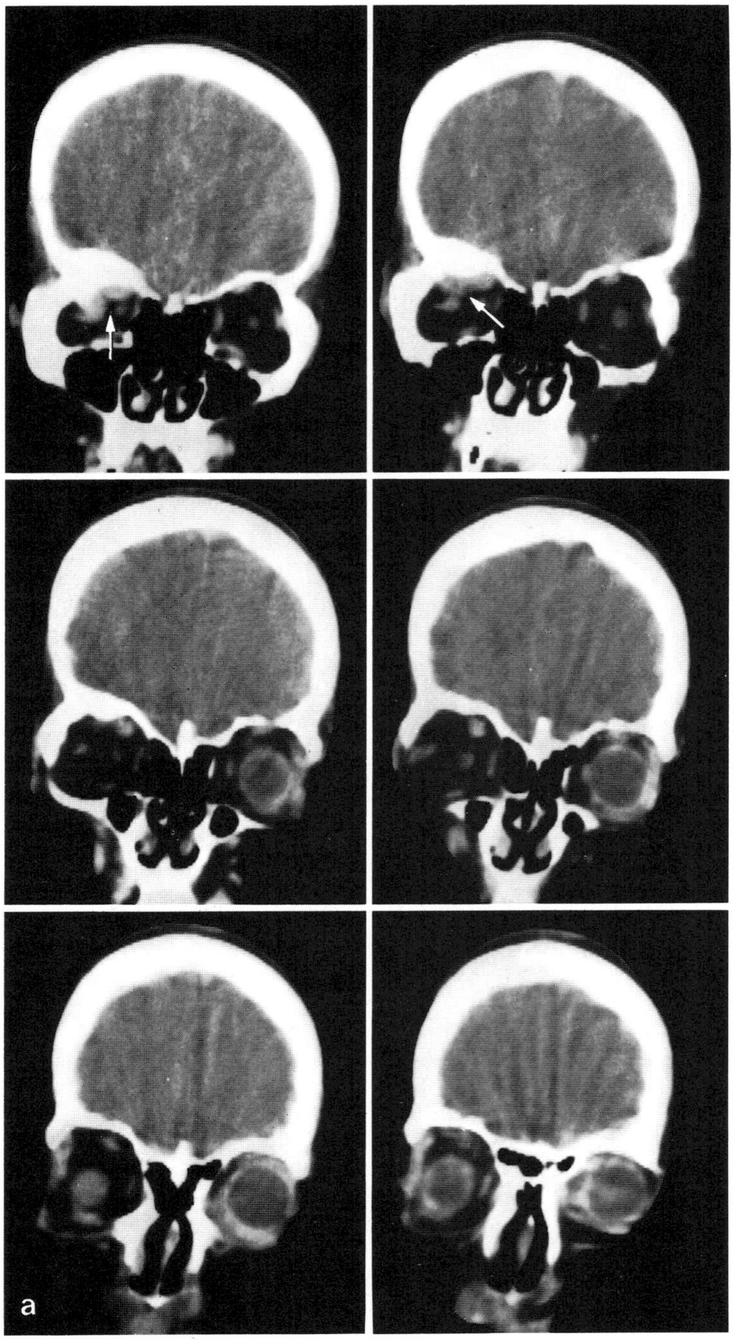

Fig. 6a, b. Left sphenoid wing meningioma with orbital involvement. Marked protrusion and depression of the globe. Medial displacement of the left optic nerve. The enhanced CT shows the thickened hypersclerotic sphenoid bone as well as the lobulated intra-orbital soft tissue portion of the tumor (*arrows*), which has penetrated the muscle cone. **a** Coronal view obtained directly by placing the patient in the prone, elevated chin position; **b** transverse view

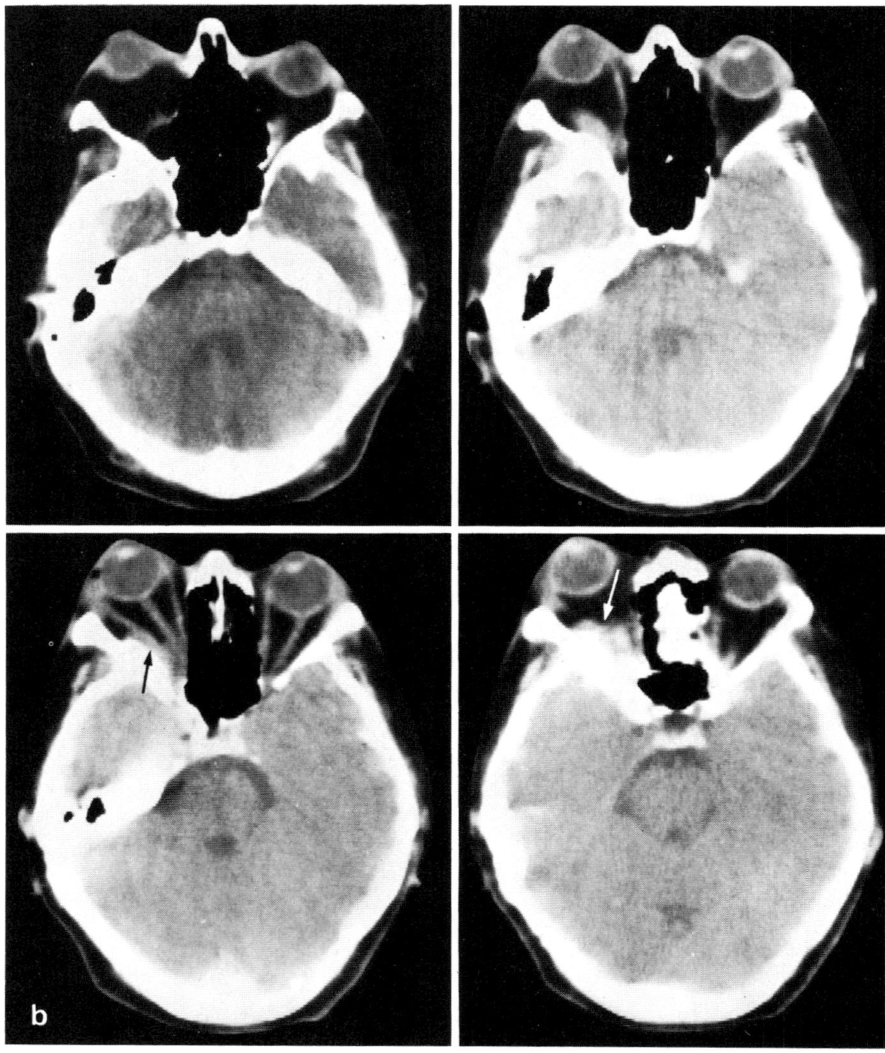

Fig. 6b. Legend see p. 390

9. Haverling M, Johanson H (1978) Computed sagittal tomography of the orbit. AJR 131:346 – 347
10. Huk W, Schiefer W (1978) Computertomographie bei Prozessen der Schädelbasis und der Orbitae: Kombinierte Anwendung von Horizontal- und Frontalschnitten. ROEFO 128:8 – 11
11. Jacobs L, Weisberg LA, Kinkel WR (1980) Computerized tomography of the orbit and sella turcica. Raven, New York
12. Kretschmar K, Wende S (1979) Möglichkeiten und Grenzen der CT in der Diagnostik zerebraler und Orbitaerkrankungen. Neurol Psychiatr 5:588 – 602
13. Lampert VL, Zelch JV, Cohen DN (1974) Computed tomography of the orbits. Radiology 113:351 – 354
14. Leonardi M, Barbina V, Fabris G, Penco T (1977) Sagittal computed tomography of the orbit. J Comput Assist Tomogr 1/4:511 – 512
15. Leonardi M, Fabris G, Penco T (1978) Etude tomodensitométrique tridimensionnelle de l'orbite. J Neuroradiol 5:327 – 331
16. Maier-Hauff K, Wilske J (1976) Correlation of A-scan echography and computed tomography of orbital tumors. In: Lanksch W, Kazner E (eds) Cranial computerized tomography. Springer, Berlin Heidelberg New York, pp 212 – 220
17. Manelfe C, Bonafe A, Fabre P, Pessey JJ (1978) Computed tomography in olfactory neuroblastoma: one case of esthesioneuroepithelioma and four cases of esthesioneuroblastoma. J Comput Assist Tomogr 2:412 – 420
18. Michotey P, Moseley IF, Aubin ML, Mouly A, Farnarier PH, Sanders MD, Aron D, Doyon D (1976) Apport de la tomographie axiale commandée par ordinateur en ophthalmologie. The contribution of computerized axial tomography to ophthalmology. J Neuroradiol 3:257 – 276
19. Mosely IF, Bull JWD (1975) Computerized axial tomography, carotid angiography and orbital phlebography in the diagnosis of space-occupying lesions of the orbit. In: Salamon G (ed) Advances in

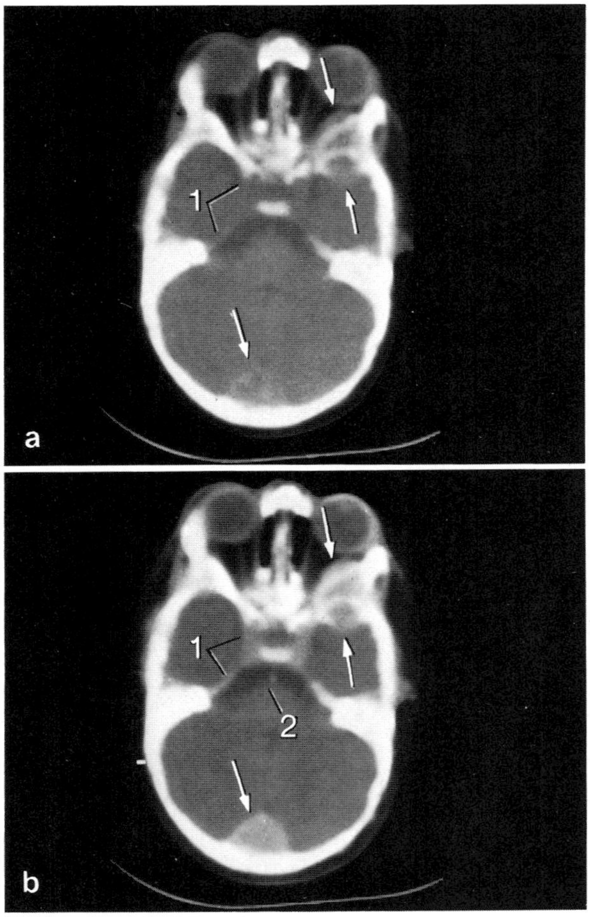

Fig. 7a, b. Right sphenoid wing and occipital *metastasis* (*arrows*) from neuroblastoma of the retroperitoneal space (1-year-old child) **a** without and **b** with contrast enhancement. Fusiform expansion and extensive destruction of the right sphenoid wing. The contrast-enhanced section (**b**) delineates clearly the intra-orbital and intracranial soft tissue part of the sphenoid metastasis. The occipital metastasis shows increased density after administration of contrast material. *1,* superior petrosus sinus; *2,* basilar artery

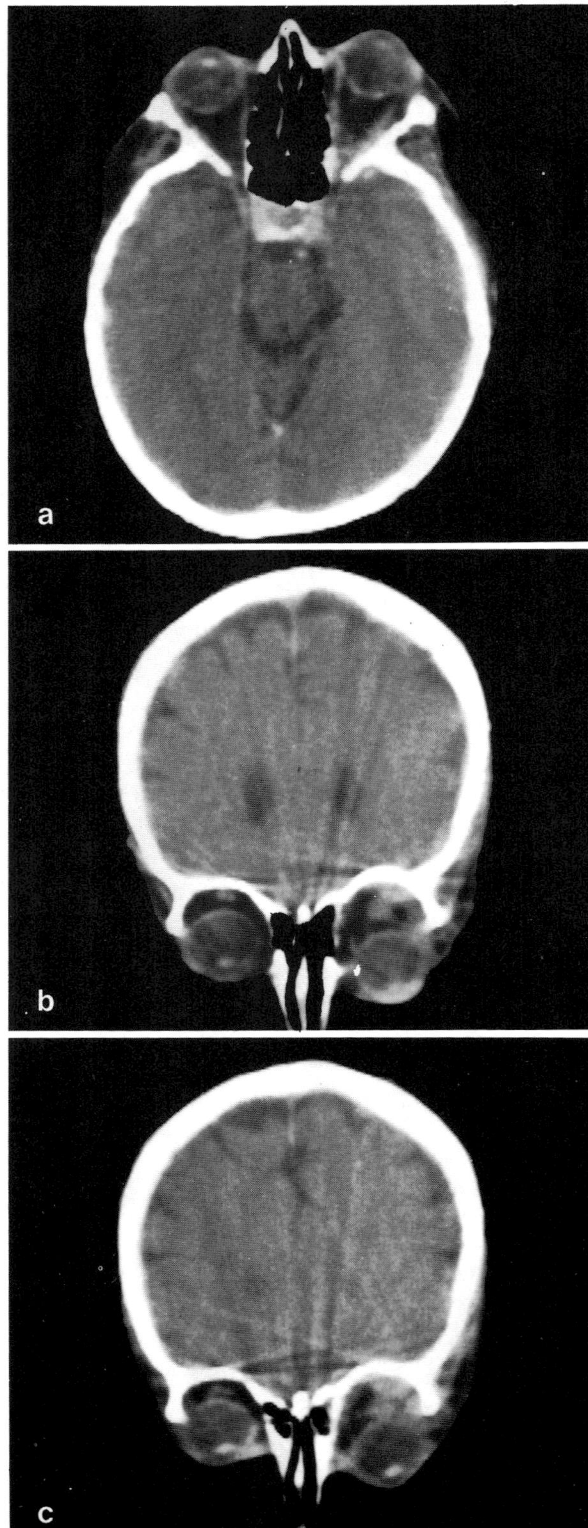

Fig. 8. a Transverse and **b, c** directly obtained coronal view of a *metastasis* (breast carcinoma). The inhomogeneous tumour is localized in the upper part of the right orbit and causes marked protrusion and downward displacement of the globe. The right temporal muscles are also involved

cerebral angiography. Springer, Berlin Heidelberg New York, pp 361–369
20. Moseley IF, Sanders MD, Claveria LE (1978) Diagnostic limitations of computerised tomographic examination of the orbit. In: Bories J (ed) Computerised axial tomography. Springer, Berlin Heidelberg New York, pp 52–62
21. Nadjmi M, Ratzka M, Wodarz R, Glötzner FL (1977) Bedeutung der Computertomographie für die Neuroradiologie. The significance of computed tomography in neuroradiology. Roentgen-Berichte 6:258–293
22. Naumann GOH (1980) Zusammensetzung des ophthalmo-pathologischen Untersuchungsmaterials. In: Doerr W, Seifert G, Uehlinger E (eds) Pathologie des

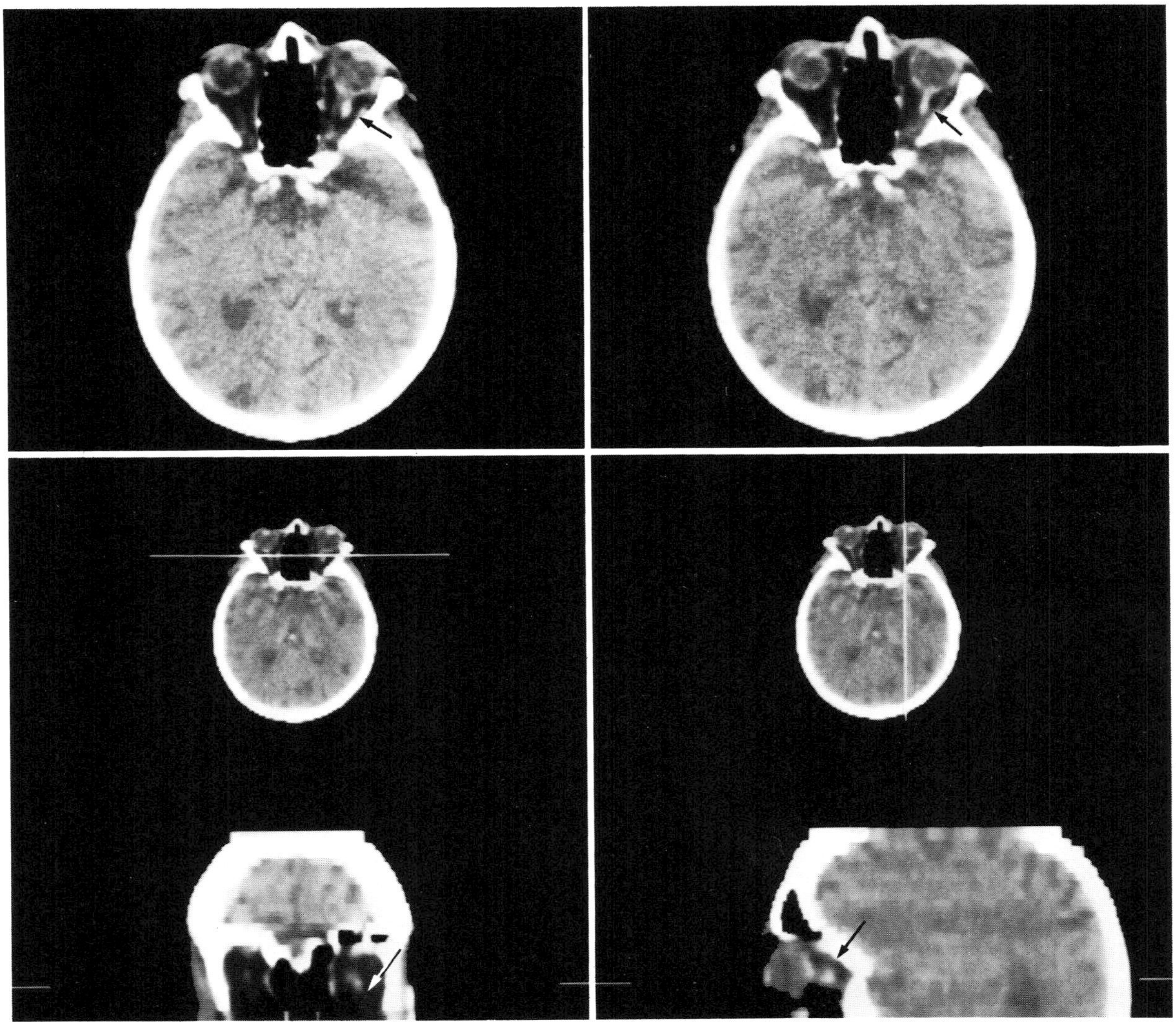

Fig. 9. Small, well-circumscribed *haematoma* in the right optic nerve sheath after intra-orbital injection of anaesthetic. The coagulated blood is distinctly delineated in the transverse view as well as in the coronal and sagittal reconstruction (*arrows*). Slight protrusion of right globe

Auges. Springer, Berlin Heidelberg New York (Spezielle pathologische Anatomie, vol 12, pp 50–56)
23. Nemec HW, Roth J (1976) Über die Strahlenbelastung des Kopfes, insbesondere der Augenlinsen, bei der axialen Tomographie mit dem EMI-Scanner. ROEFO 124:526–530
24. Nover A, Schmitt J, Wende S, Aulich A (1976) Computertomographie in der Ophthalmologie. Klin Monatsbl Augenheilkd 168:461–467
25. Salvolini U, Cabanis EA, Rodallec A, Menichelli F, Pasquini U, Iba-Zizen MT (1978) Computed tomography of the optic nerve: Part I normal results. J Comput Assist Tomogr 2:141–149
26. Salvolini U, Menichelli F, Pasquini U (1977) Computer assisted tomography in 90 cases of exophthalmos. J. Comput Assist Tomogr 1:81–100
27. Simon RS (1979) Möglichkeiten und Grenzen der Computertomographie in der Orbitadiagnostik. Röntgenpraxis 32:88–92
28. Tadmor R, New PFJ (1978) Computed tomography of the orbit with special emphasis on coronal sections: Part I normal anatomy. J Comput Assist Tomogr 2:24–34
29. Tadmor R, New PFJ (1978) Computed tomography of the orbit with special emphasis on coronal sections: Part II pathological anatomy. J Comput Assist Tomogr 2:35–44
30. Tadmor R, New PFJ, Davis KR, Roberson G, Taveras JM (1978) Computed tomography of the orbit with special emphasis on coronal sections. Neuroradiology 16:466–467
31. Thiel R (1980) Atlas der Augenkrankheiten. Thieme, Stuttgart

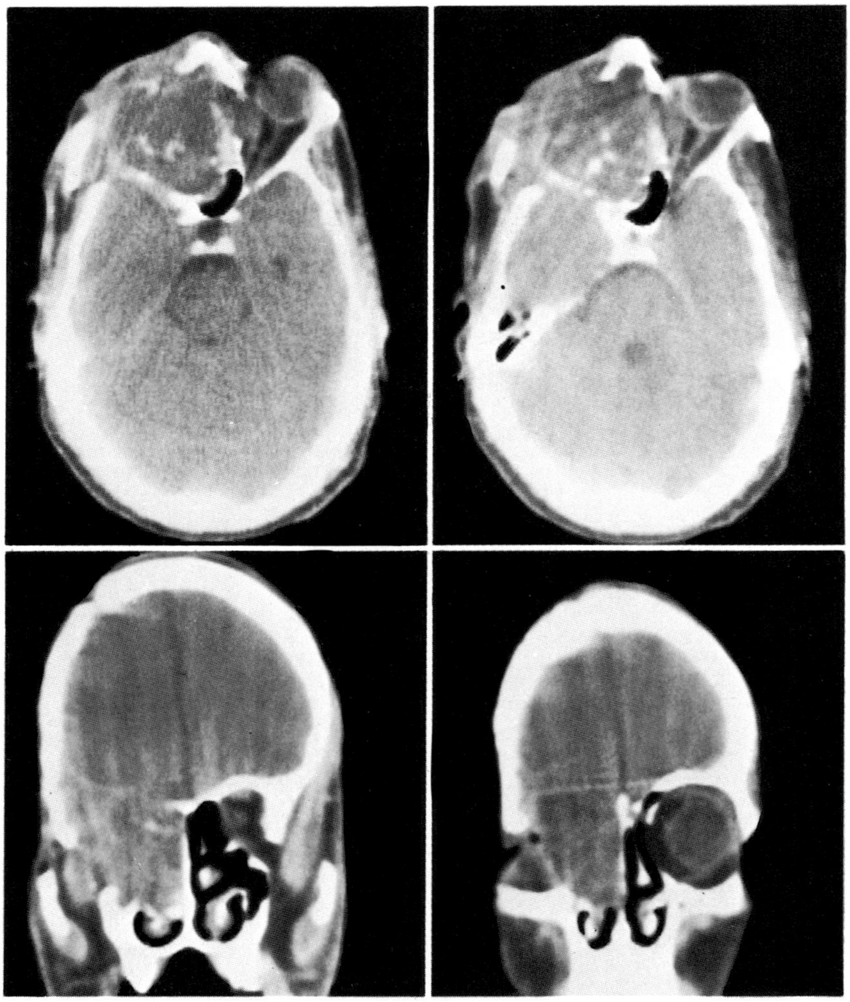

Fig. 10. Massive recurrence of a left *lacriminal gland carcinoma,* 4 years after ophthalmectomy. Transverse and direct coronal section visualize the enormous tumour invasion into the nasal cavities, the sphenoid sinuses and both orbits. Extensive bone destructions in the whole tumour surroundings. Irregular calcifications within the tumour

32. Vignaud J, Aubin ML (1978) Les coupes coronales (frontales) d'orbite en tomodensitométrie. Coronal (frontal) sections in computerised tomography of the orbit. J Neuroradiol 5:161 – 174
33. Vignaud J, Clay C, Aubin ML (1978) La tomodensitométrie en ophthalmologie ... en questions. J Fr Ophthalmol 1:675 – 686
34. Wende S, Aulich A, Lange S, Lanksch W, Schmitt EJ (1976) Computerized tomography in diseases of the orbital region. In: Lanksch W, Kazner E (eds) Cranial computerized tomography. Springer, Berlin Heidelberg New York, pp 208 – 211
35. Wende S, Aulich A, Nover A, Lanksch W, Kazner E, Steinhoff H, Meese W, Lange S, Grumme T (1977) Computed tomography of orbital lesions. Neuroradiology 13:123 – 134
36. Wende S, Kazner E, Grumme T (1979) Computed tomography of orbital lesions. In: Gerhardt P, van Kaick G (eds) Total body computerized tomography. Thieme, Stuttgart, pp 320 – 324
37. Wiggli U (1979) Computertomographie der Orbita. Klin Monatsbl Augenheilk 174:799 – 805
38. Wing SD, Hunsaker JN, Anderson RE, van Dyk HJL, Osborn AG (1979) Direct sagittal computed tomography in graves ophthalmopathy. J Comput Assist Tomogr 3:820 – 824

Angiography of the Brain: Therapeutic Aspects of Superselective Craniofacial Angiography

K. Voigt

Medizinisches Strahleninstitut der Universität, Abteilung für Neuroradiologie, Oslanderstrasse 22, D-7400 Tübingen

Introduction

The different types of arteriovenous haemangiomas and fistulae as well as tumours of the head, neck and face fed by the external carotid artery have in common that they may result in severe neurological deficits as well as in disfigurations of the craniofacial region and that they normally cause clinical and therapeutic difficulties [9, 10]. The development and further elaboration of superselective catheter techniques by the femoral route in order to demonstrate each single branch of the external carotid artery is largely owed to Djindjian [2]. Due to his and subsequent systematical investigations of the isolated vascular areas filled by each external vessel, the roentgenological-anatomical knowledge of the vascular supply of meningeal, osseous, muscular, cutaneous and mucosal branches as well as that of the intra- and extracranial skull base was emphatically enlarged [1]. Thereby, the technical and methodical prerequisites were simultaneously accomplished as regards the performing of therapeutic neuroradiological interventions by the systematic and exclusive occlusion of only those arteries supplying pathological lesions. Since there is still no general agreement on the management of patients with craniofacial vascular malformations and tumours, we decided to undertake our combined diagnostic and therapeutic neuroradiological treatment on a group of patients who had mostly already had a long course of disease or a bad prognosis with several failed therapeutic attempts. In the last 3 years we have embolised in our department more than 100 patients with different extra- and intracranial as well as spinal lesions. Since we have controlled the results of our embolisations by follow-up studies or operative and histological findings, we want to give an account of our material and methods in a group of 91 patients with lesions of the neck, face and head in consideration of a critical evaluation of the possibilities and limitations of this procedure from a clinical point of view.

Patients

The examinations were performed from January 1977 to March 1980 and included 54 female and 37 male patients aged between 7 and 80 years. In our material 41 patients had vascular lesions and 50 had different extra- and intracranial tumours. The different indications for embolisations are shown in Table 1. The vascular lesions mainly consisted of arteriovenous and capillary haemangiomas of the face (30 patients) and dural carotid-cavernous or carotid-tentorial fistulae (11 patients). In the patient group with tumours there were benign lesions in 43 cases (glomus tumours, fibromas), including 21 intracranial meningiomas, and 7 malignant tumours. In two patients with fibromas emergency interventions had to be made because of persistent mucosal bleedings in the region of the nose and throat. The different kinds of lesions and the post-embolisatory course are shown in Table 2.

Methods

All patients were investigated under general anaesthesia, except for those with arteriovenous fistulae, and with permanent control of the ECG.

Diagnostic Procedure. All selective and superselective angiographies were performed by the transfemoral route according to a combination of Djindjian's [23] and our own techniques [9]. In all patients with craniofacial haemangiomas and fistulae as well as extra- and intracranial tumours

Radiology Today 1. Ed. by M. W. Donner and F. H. W. Heuck

Table 1. Indications for neuroradiological interventions

Bleedings/hemorrhages	1) Traumatic or iatrogenic haemorrhages in the region of nose and throat 2) Tumorous bleedings in the region of nose and throat (angiofibromas, neoplasias of the maxillofacial area etc.) 3) Haemorrhages in systemic vascular disorders (e.g. Rendu-Osler's disease)
Tumours	1) Pre-operative diminution of tumour vascularisation (glomus tumours, angiofibromas, angioblastic meningiomas etc.) 2) Reduction of tumours before operation or after irradiation (meningiomas, malignant extra-/intracranial tumours of the skull base) 3) Therapeutic attempt in inoperable or elder patients 4) Palliative treatment to relieve pain (e.g. malignant tumours of the vertebral column and the spinal canal)
Vascular malformations	1) Pre-operative or permanent reduction or occlusion of shunts in arteriovenous and capillary haemangiomas of the maxillofacial area and spinal canal 2) Occlusion of traumatic or iatrogenic arteriovenous shunts 3) Curative treatment of dural carotid-cavernous or carotid-tentorial shunts
Special treatments	1) Combined embolisatory and pharmacotherapy of malignant tumours 2) Balloon catheter techniques for occlusion of internal carotid-cavernous fistulae 3) Intra-operative superselective angiographies and embolisations 4) Selective spinal angiographies and embolisations

Table 2. Diagnoses and number of lesions treated by embolisation

Diagnosis	Number		Post-embolisatory operation		Maximal post-embolisatory control (months)
Vascular lesions		41		19	
Arteriovenous angiomas	15		12		12
Capillary angiomas	9		6		16
Arteriovenous fistulae	11		–		24
Miscellaneous	6		1		6
Extracranial tumours		21		4	
Benign tumours					
a) Glomus tumours	6		2		22
b) Angiofibromas	5		–		16
c) Fibromas of nose and throat	3		–		18
Malignant tumours					
a) Sarcomas	2		–		24
b) Metastases	5		2		4
Extra-/intracranial tumours		8		2	
a) Tumours of glomus hypotympanicum	4		–		14
b) Tumours of glomus jugulare	2		–		18
c) Miscellaneous	2		2		10
Intracranial tumours		21		13	
Meningiomas	21		13		30
Total		91		38	

after selective angiographies of the internal and the main trunk of the external carotid artery, superselective probings and injections of each external branch feeding the lesions were performed successively. In the patients with dural carotid-cavernous or carotid-tentorial fistulae, selective angiographies of the internal and external carotid arteries and of the vertebral arteries were always performed in order to exclude or to demonstrate branches of these vessels supplying the shunts. Subsequently those branches of the external carotid arteries feeding the fistulae were examined by means of superselective angiography.

Therapeutic Procedure. All different kinds of pathological vascular and tumorous lesions (Table 2) were embolised by means of multiple injections of cut strips of Gelfoam and/or lyophilised dura into the feeding branches of the external carotid arteries. Thereby, the Gelfoam emboli had to be injected into the lesions themselves or as far and distal as possible into the feeding arteries in order to avoid opening of collateral vessels. The appropriate degree of embolisation could be jugded by intermittent contrast injections between each of the Gelfoam or dura administrations. After sufficient and satisfactory embolisation, control angiographies of the internal and external carotid arteries were performed during the same examination in each case.

Results

Superselective probings and angiographies of all external branches feeding the vascular and tumorous lesions could be performed in all but three patients, who are not included in this series. In two other patients, embolisation of a metastasis and a large glomus tumour invading the skull base resulted in severe complications with hemiparesis due to reflux emboli into the internal carotid arterial system which could be shown on the control angiographies. Minor complications of embolisation included transitory bradycardias in some patients during injections into the internal maxillary artery and the production of cutaneous necrosis in the facial arterial system in one patient. In all the other patients clinical incidents or neurological complications did not occur in any of the examinations.

Angiographic Findings and Results of Embolisation

In eight patients (three arteriovenous and one capillary haemangioma; three glomus tumours; one sarcoma) only subtotal embolisation of the lesions could be performed because there was early reflux of contrast medium into the internal carotid artery during the intermittent contrast injections between the actual emboli administrations. In the group of patients with capillary haemangiomas of varying extent, superselective angiographies without exception showed low-flow shunts in the mucosal and submucosal tissues. The post-embolisatory results and follow-up studies in these patients have already been published extensively [10]. A further 15 patients with shunt lesions had arteriovenous angiomas in the mucosae and muscle tissues mainly of the second and third trigeminal rami with pulsating deformations of the face (Figs. 1, 2), in which repeated operations had to be stopped because of dangerous intra-operative bleedings. After superselective angiographies and embolisations of those external carotid branches feeding the shunts (Figs. 3 – 5), distal occlusions and proximal stasis of the formerly feeders as well as remarkable reductions of the shunt areas themselves could be achieved so that these patients could be operated upon. In contrast to the patients with low-flow angiomas, however, even in nine patients with arteriovenous haemangiomas complete embolisations of all feeding arteries failed in the first procedure; therefore a repeated examination had to be done in order to occlude the remaining vessels. In three patients with arteriovenous malformations and in one patient with a capillary haemangioma, however, even the second attempt failed in occluding all pathological vessels.

In all 11 patients with dural carotid-cavernous or carotid-tentorial fistulae curative embolisations could be achieved by means of repeated Gelfoam and dura injections as has been already described [7, 8]. The long-term results (up to 2 years) of the embolisations showed no recurrence of any of the fistulae in these patients. In the group of 50 patients with different extra- and intracranial tumours, benign as well as malignant lesions were embolized. As a rule, however these embolisations were done as a pre-operative measure in order to facilitate surgical treatment in relatively bloodless conditions and without extensive loss of blood. Nevertheless, up to now embolisation as the only therapeutic measure was performed by us in six patients with large meningiomas which could not be operated upon (because of cardiac complica-

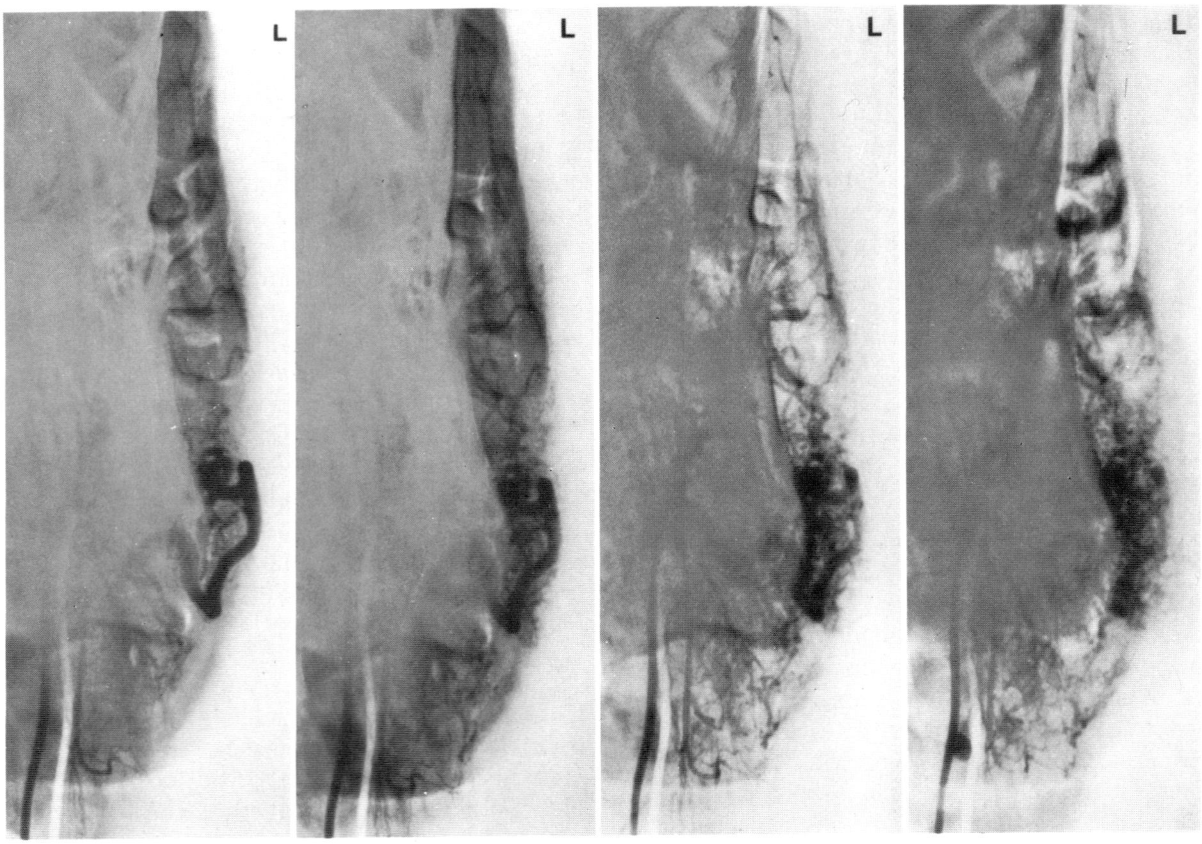

Fig. 1. Arteriovenous angioma of the left mandibular region. Demonstration of the increasing arteriovenous shunts with consecutive disfiguration of the soft tissues in tangential view

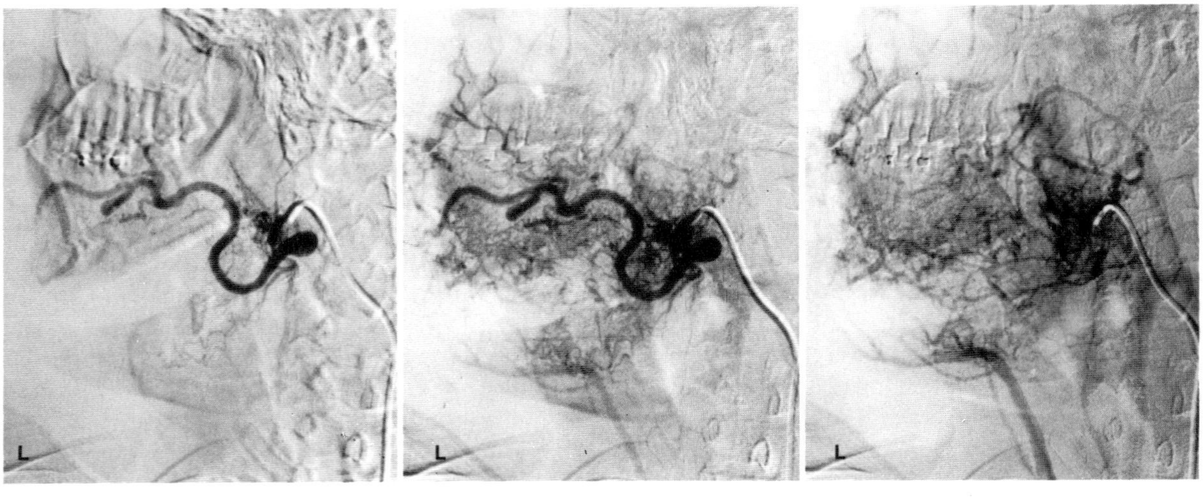

Fig. 2. Arteriovenous angioma of the left mandibular region. Demonstration of the dilated left facial artery, arteriovenous shunts and draining veins of the external jugular vein territory in lateral view (same patient as in Fig. 1)

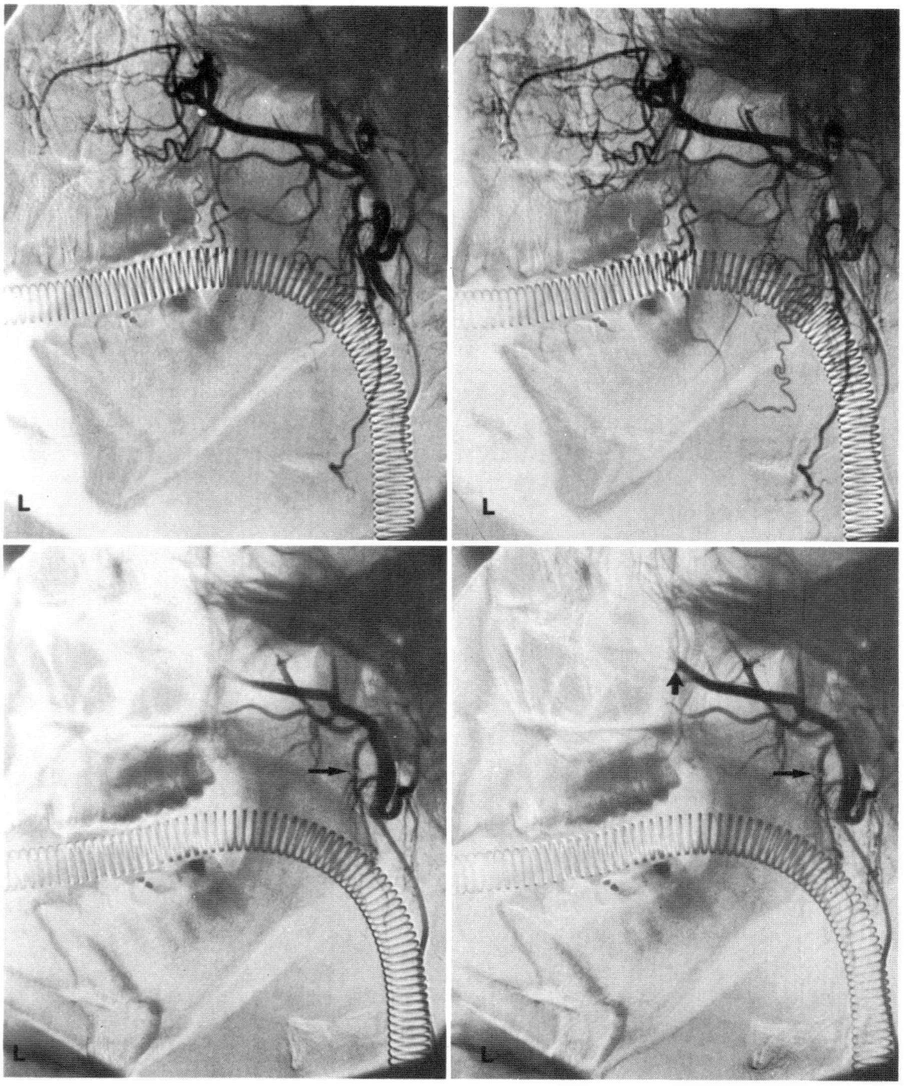

Fig. 3. Arteriography of the left internal maxillary artery before and after embolisation. Demonstration of multiple and dilated collateral vessels from the left internal maxillary artery to the facial artery before embolisation (*top*). After embolisation, distal occlusion (↑) of the internal maxillary artery, no filling of the former collaterals and demonstration of an embolus (→) (*bottom*) (same patient as in Fig. 1)

tions in the majority of cases) and all of which have now shown a favourable clinical course for more than 2 years due to central necrosis of the tumours only 4 weeks after the embolizations, as shown by CT controls [6]. As in arteriovenous angiomas in the group of vascular lesions, generally there were less favourable results in highly vascularised tumours. Thus, in four patients with tumours complete embolisations could not be obtained; and glomus tumours tend to recur between 6 months and 1 year even after superselective and angiographically complete embolisation. On the other hand, good palliative effects and a beneficial course of illness can be achieved by embolisation even in histologically proven malignant tumors, as demonstrated in the following patient: within 6 months after operation on a carcinoma of the oesophagus he developed a huge extra- and intracranial metastasis in the right parasagittal region; this metastasis even remarkably increased during irradiation, which was therefore stopped. Because of the size and high degree of tumour vascularisation (Figs. 6, 7) operative intervention was not undertaken, and the patient developed hemiparesis and urinary incontinence within 1 week. After that all feeding arteries (branches of the middle menin-

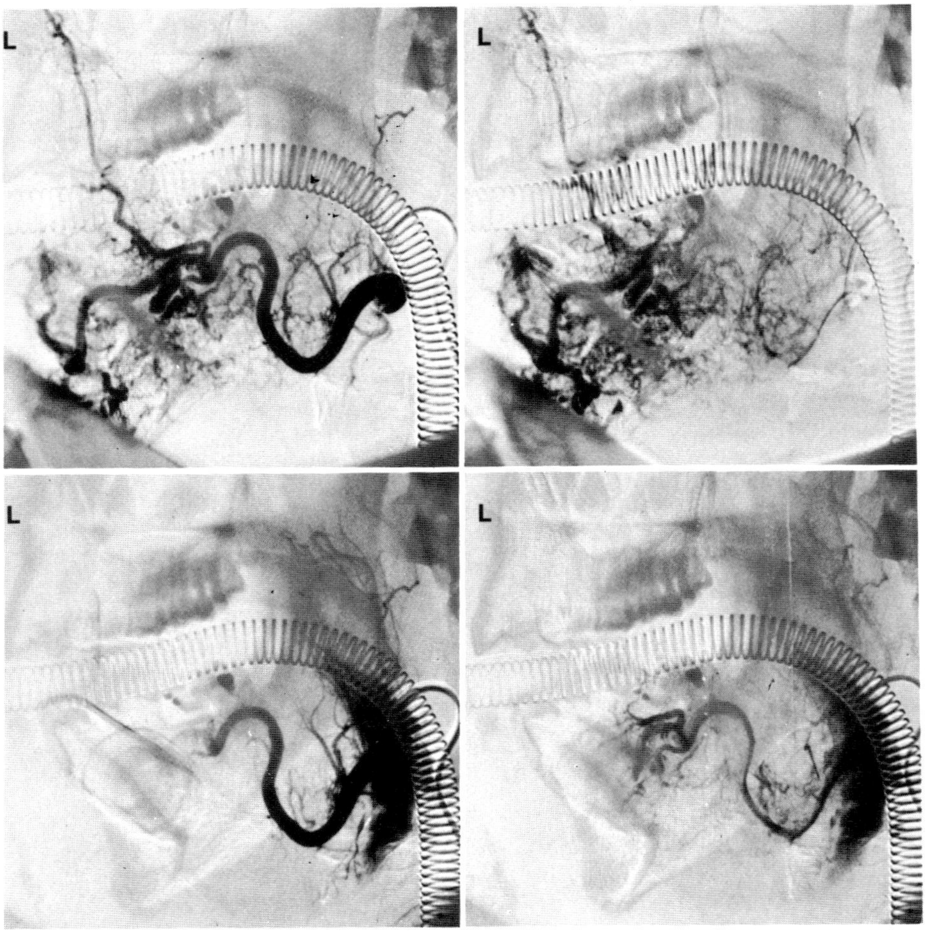

Fig. 4. Arteriography of the left facial artery before and after embolisation. Dilated and tortuous distal branches of the facial artery feeding the arteriovenous shunts before embolisation (*top*). After embolisation, distal occlusion of the branches and nearly stasis in the facial artery (*bottom*) (same patient as in Fig. 1)

geal, superficial temporal and external occipital arteries) of the highly vascularised tumour were superselectively embolized (Figs. 8, 9). Control angiography after these interventions showed a good embolisatory result (Fig. 10) and the patient was operated on without complications in a bloodless tumorous area.

Discussion

Since Djindjian's et al. [2] introduction of superselective angiographies of single branches of the external carotid artery by the femoral route this method of examination has been further developed to a neuroradiological therapeutic treatment with superselective embolisations of the feeding arteries in intra- and extracranial tumours and vascular malformations in the head, neck and spine.

According to the different vascular and tumorous lesions of our patient material we found diverse courses of illness and long-term results after embolisations. In general, in our opinion the embolisation procedure could be looked upon as a curative treatment in neuroradiology only for the dural carotid-cavernous and carotid-tentorial fistulae [7] as well as for the emergency treatment of persistent mucosal bleeding and some benign tumorous lesions [6]. Even in the six elderly patients with meningiomas who, because of medical reasons, could not undergo operations after the embolisations, we would have preferred surgical intervention despite their favourable post-embolisatory courses of illness (for more than 2 years up to now).

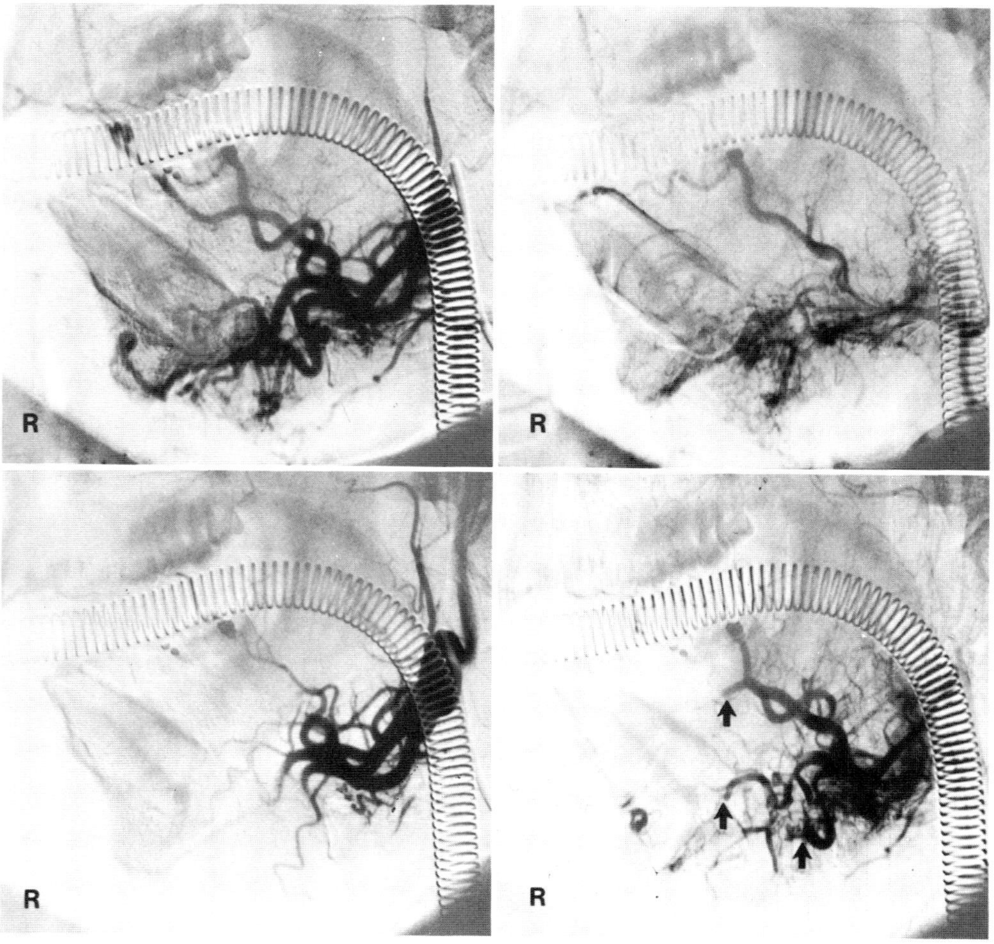

Fig. 5. Arteriography of the right facial artery before and after embolisation. Filling of the arteriovenous angioma from the contralateral facial artery before embolisation (*top*). Distal occlusion (↑) of the former feeders and stasis in the shunt area after embolisation (*bottom*) (same patient as in Fig. 1)

In external as well as in internal carotid artery – cavernous sinus fistulae many and varied operative techniques exist, but the therapeutic aim of surgical elimination of these fistulae from the cerebral circulation is at present an unsolved problem [5]. Moreover, dural carotid-cavernous fistulae are very likely to relapse postoperatively [3], because small and feeding distal branches of the middle meningeal arteries may be missed or not attainable during operation [4]. Therefore, superselective angiography and simultaneous embolisation of dural carotid-cavernous fistulae is proposed by us as the current therapeutic procedure of choice for the treatment of this special kind of vascular malformations.

In the majority of craniofacial haemangiomas as well as in highly vascularised tumours the neuroradiological procedure can only be regarded as a preparatory, preventive and palliative measure before surgical treatment. In our patients this kind and sequence of active medical treatment, with diagnostic superselective angiographies, simultaneous therapeutic embolisations and subsequent operations on the tumorous as well as deforming vascular lesions, were chosen and in the meantime have turned out to be appropriate and efficient in diminishing the intra-operative risks and the recidivity of tumours and in avoiding the common postoperative recurrence of the malformations by means of pre-operative elimination of the shunt vessels. From our experience in arteriovenous angiomas as well as in highly vascularised tumours, Gelfoam or dura embolisation scores only a temporally and locally limited success owing to the large shunt volumes and the new formation of collateral vessels. Therefore, shortly or directly

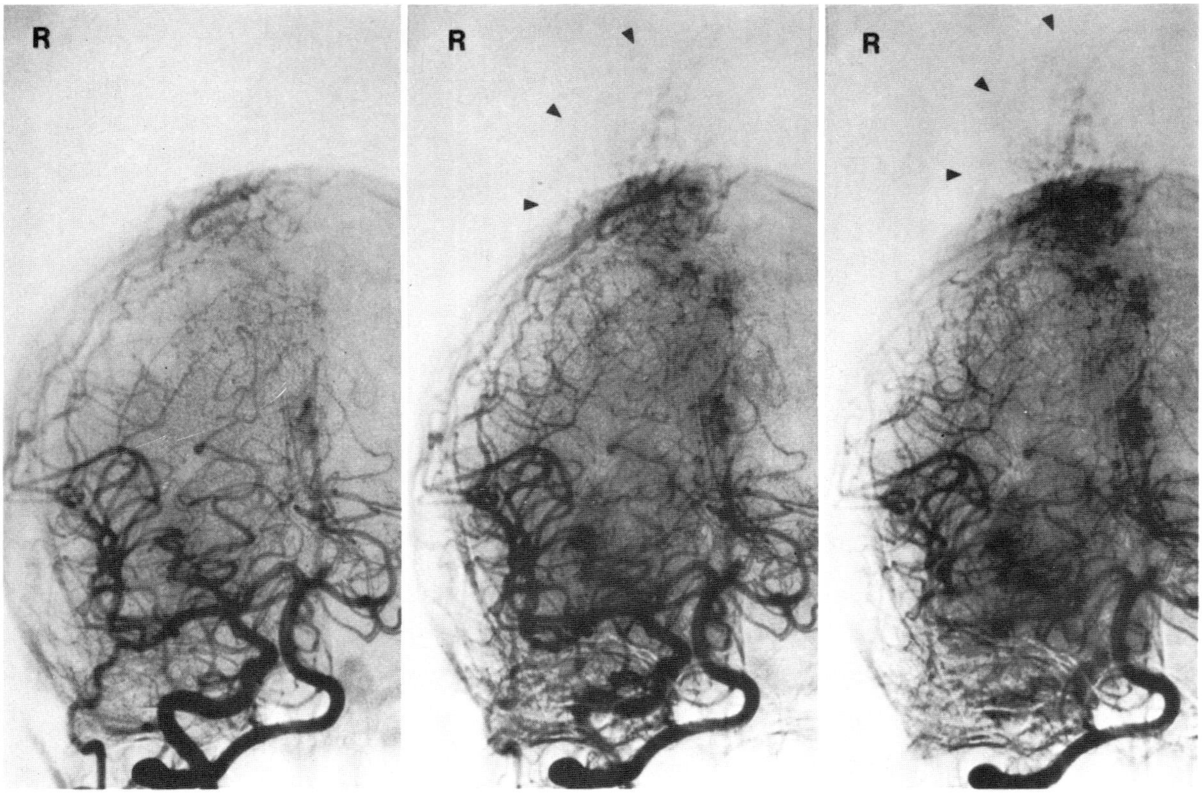

Fig. 6. Increasing opacification of a large intra- and extra-cranial metastasis. Demonstration of the tumour vascularisation in the right parasagittal region in AP view

after embolisation operative intervention has to take place, which is supported by the fact that it can be done in bloodless areas.

Summary

The technical and methodical procedure as well as the results and follow-up studies of superselective angiographies and embolisations with Gelfoam and lyophilised dura in 91 patients with different vascular lesions (arteriovenous angiomas and fistulae, capillary angiomas) and benign (glomus tumours, fibromas, meningiomas) and malignant tumours (sarcomas, metastases) in the region of the neck, face and head are described. The special indications for different neuroradiological interventions are discussed.

Due to the clinical findings and follow-up studies of up to more than 2 years, there were diverse palliative and curative results. Thereby, a uniform performance of the embolisatory interventions is contra-indicated. The arterial approach, the different catheter systems and the actual technical proceeding of the embolisations as well as the post-embolisatory point of time most propitious to operation has to be chosen according to the individual manifestation of the lesions and their anatomical and pathological conditions.

References

1. Djindjian R, Merland JJ (1978) Super-selective arteriography of the external carotid artery. Springer, Berlin Heidelberg New York
2. Djindjian R, Houdart R, Cophignon J, Hurth M, Comoy J (1971) Premier essais d'embolisation par voie fémorale de fragments de muscle dans un cas d'angiome medullaire et dans un cas d'angiome alimenté par le carotide externe. Rev Neurol (Paris) 125:119–128

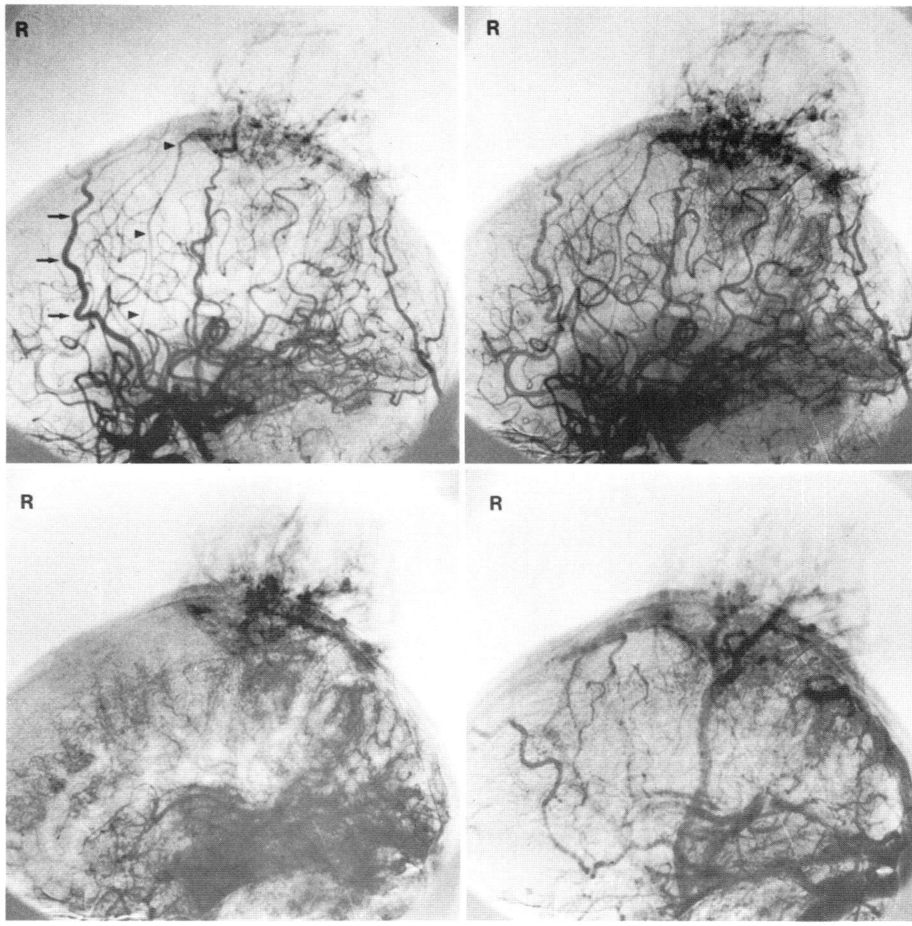

Fig. 7. Tumour vascularisation and feeding arteries of the metastasis. Arterial (*upper part*), capillary and venous (*lower part*) tumour vascularisation and feeding superficial temporal (→), middle meningeal (▶) and external occipital arteries in lateral view (same patient as in Fig. 6)

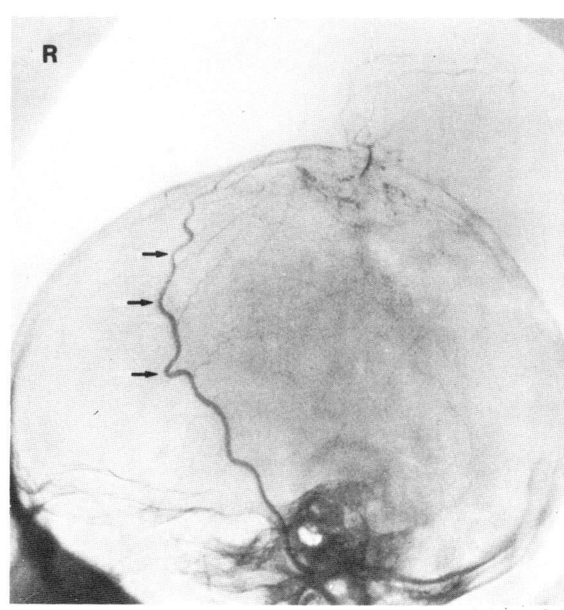

Fig. 8. Superselective arteriography of the frontal branch of the superficial temporal artery feeding the metastasis

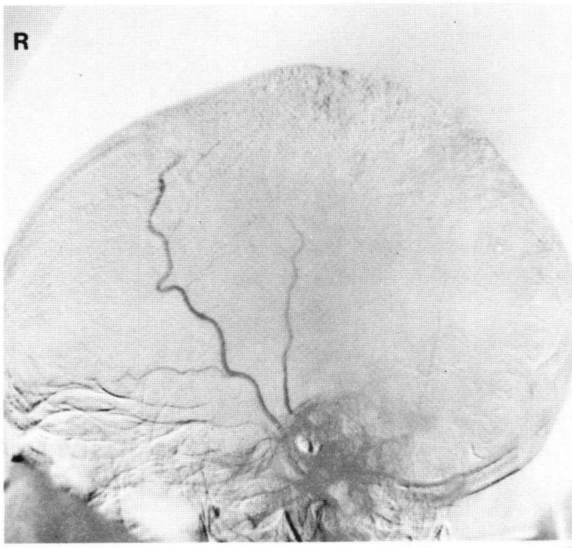

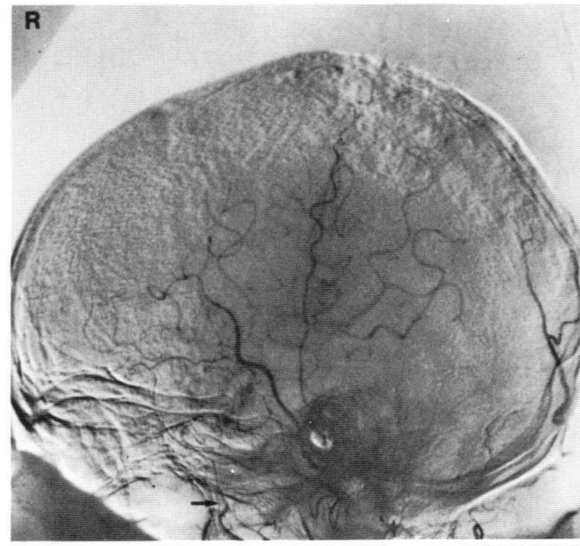

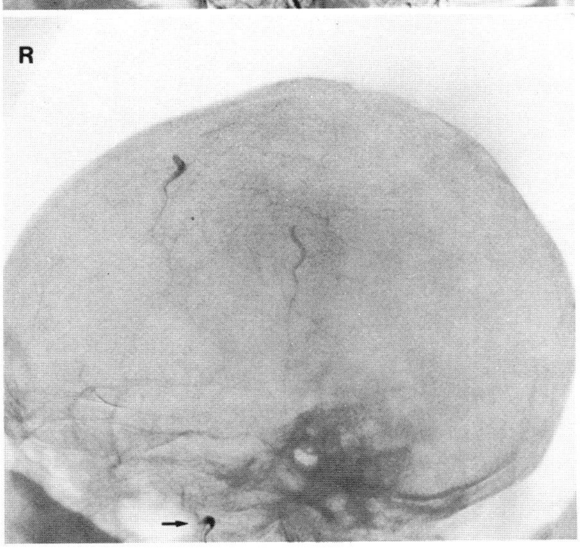

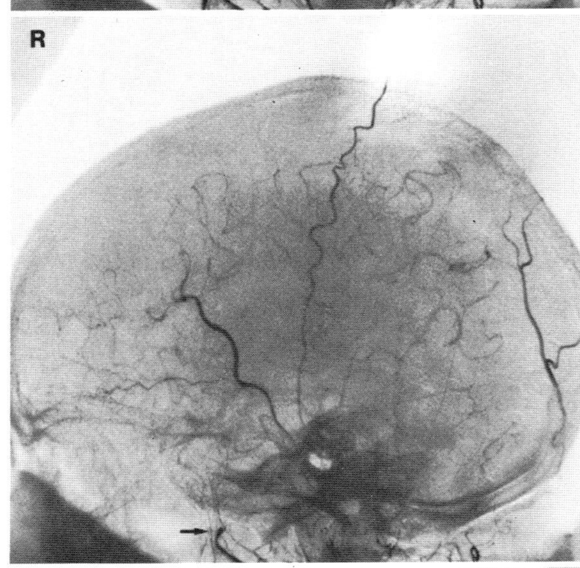

Fig. 9. Intra-embolisatory arteriography of the metastasis. Distal occlusion of the branches of the superficial temporal artery and of the internal maxillary artery (→) without filling of the formerly feeding middle meningeal artery (same patient as in Fig. 6)

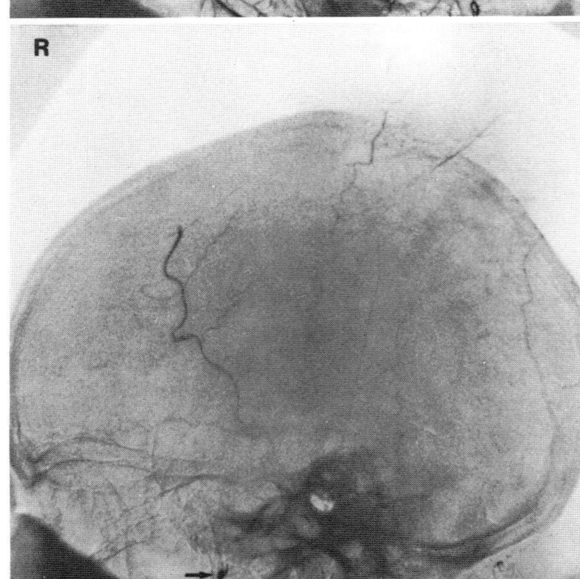

▶

Fig. 10. Post-embolisatory angiography of the metastasis. Distal occlusions and stasis of the formerly feeding arteries and lack of tumour stain

3. Edwards MS, Connolly ES (1977) Cavernous sinus syndrome produced by communication between the external carotid artery and cavernous sinus. J Neurosurg 46:92 – 96
4. Hilal SK, Michelsen JW (1975) Therapeutic percutaneous embolization for extra-axial vascular lesions of the head, neck and spine. J Neurosurg 43: 275 – 287
5. Lins E, Wappenschmidt J (1977) Transfemorale Embolisation einer Carotis-externa-Sinus-cavernosus-Fistel. Roentgenblaetter 30:621 – 625
6. Stoeter P, Reinshagen G, Voigt K (1980) Interventionale Neuroradiologie kranialer Tumoren bei inoperablen Alters-Patienten. In: Müller C, Wertheimer J (eds) Gerontopsychiatrie 7. Jansen, Düsseldorf, pp 259 – 268
7. Voigt K (1978) Neuroradiologische Diagnostik und Therapie von duralen Carotis-Cavernosus-Fisteln. Arch Psychiatr Nervenkr 225:359 – 377
8. Voigt K (1980) Selective embolization with the catheter technique in neck and face. Ann Radiol (Paris) 23:232 – 237
9. Voigt K, Djindjian R (1976) Superselektive zerebrale Angiographie. III Diagnostische Anwendung und therapeutische Möglichkeiten der Teleskop-Kathetertechnik im Versorgungsbereich der A. carotis externa des Menschen. ROEFO 125:214 – 218
10. Voigt K, Schwenzer N, Stoeter P (1978) Angiographic, operative and histological findings after embolisation of cranio-facial angiomas. Neuroradiology 16:424 – 427

Tomosynthesis and the First Clinical Results

M. Nadjmi and H. Weiss

Universität Würzburg, Kopfklinik, Abteilung für Neuroradiologie,
Josef-Schneider-Straße 11, D-8700 Würzburg

The procedure called tomosynthesis is a new radiological method which has been clinically tested in the neuroradiology department in Würzburg for some months. The investigation is based on the principles of classic tomography and not on those of computed tomography [1, 2]. The results can also be compared with those of the tomographic procedure with which we all are familiar. However, the main differences from classic tomography are that all the information necessary for the tomography of an object is obtained within the scope of a single exposition and that neither the X-ray tubes, nor the film, nor the patient are moved during this process. By means of this procedure the actual investigation, which takes a relatively long time in classic tomography, is reduced to seconds.

The procedure was developed in the Philips Research Laboratory in Hamburg. We first encountered this procedure in its laboratory stage, and in recent few years, close cooperation with the department in Würzburg made possible the development of a prototype of this equipment for neuroradiological investigations. This equipment makes possible tomography of the bone, angiotomography and to a certain degree tomography of myelography as well.

The technology and the principles of this method are as follows:

Imagine an object (O^i) which, for the sake of simplicity, consist of only two layers, a disc and a square (Fig. 1). We image this object with three immovable X-ray tubes (P) simultaneously and produce an image (O') on which three squares and three discs can be seen. Because of the distance between the disc and the square in the object, the distances from the shadows of the squares and the shadows of the discs to the middle of the film are different. With this procedure the actual tomography of this object is theoretically completed. We call this result a coded X-ray image, and in a second procedure we try to decode this image. This second procedure, whereby the presence of the patient is no longer required, is known as the decoding step. If we stay with our simple example of the disc and the square, the decoding step

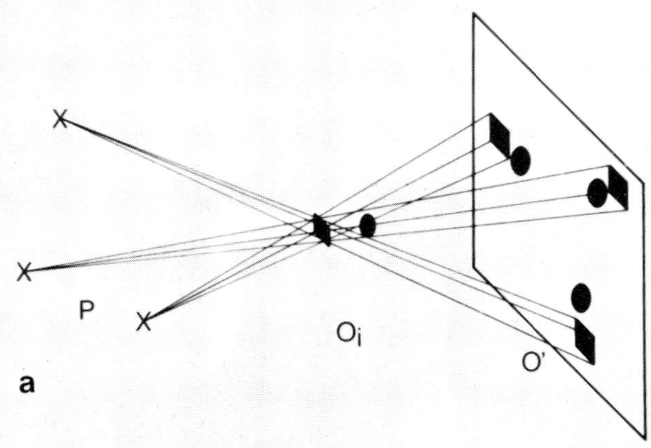

Fig. 1. a Recording step.
b Decoding step (see p. 407)

Radiology Today 1. Ed. by M. W. Donner and F. H. W. Heuck

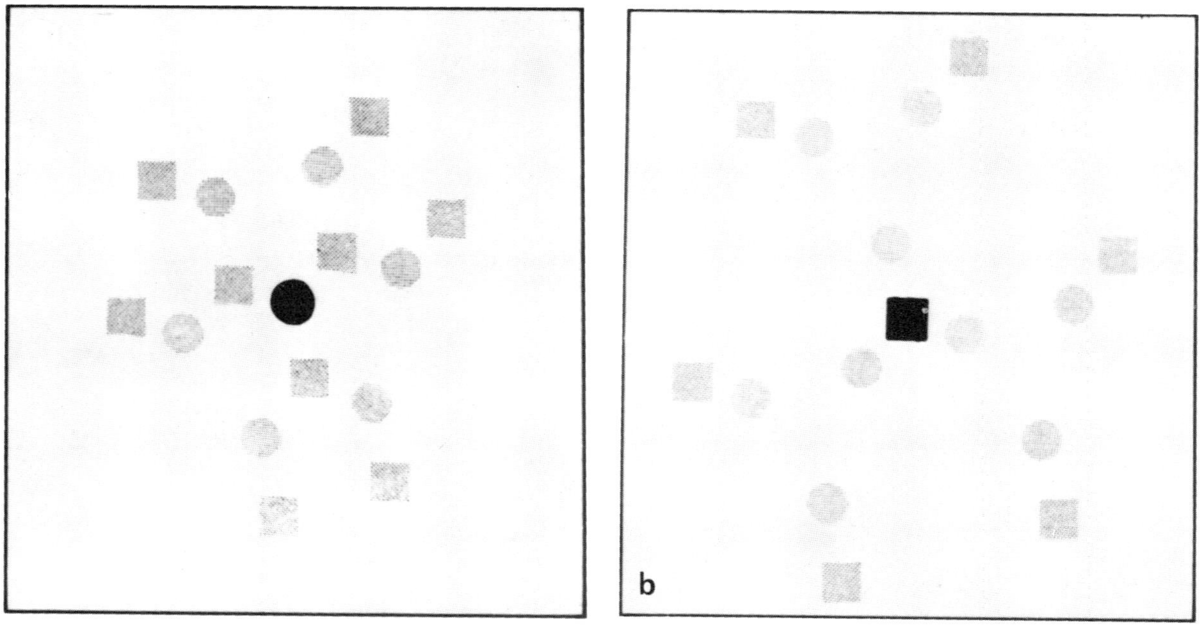

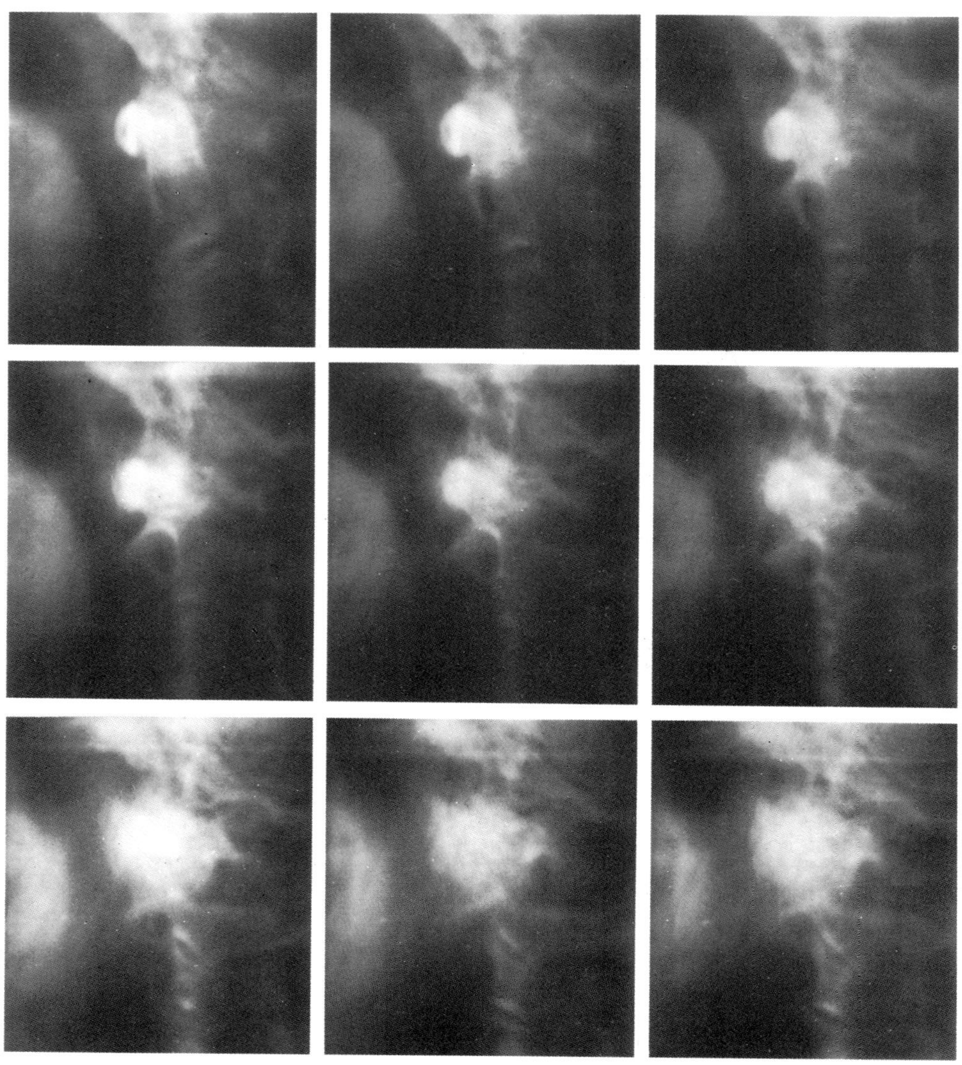

Fig. 2. Tomograms of the upper cervical region, mediosagittal and lateral, with the foramen transversarium

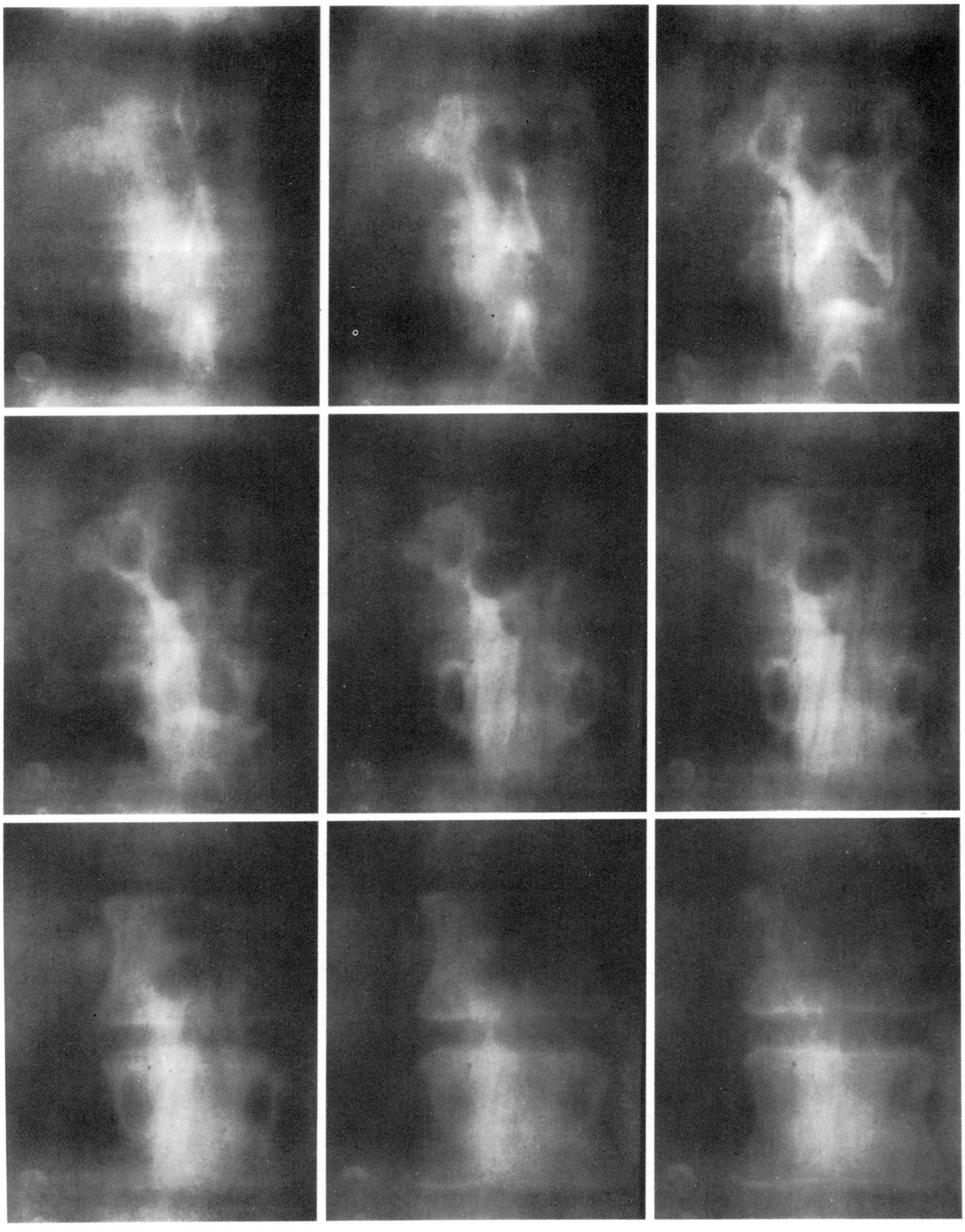

Fig. 3. Tomograms of the lumbar region in a lumbosacral myelogram with a water-soluble contrast medium. On the upper right are the bony structures, spinous processes and pedicles with pedicle roots. In the middle row is an intradural neuroma

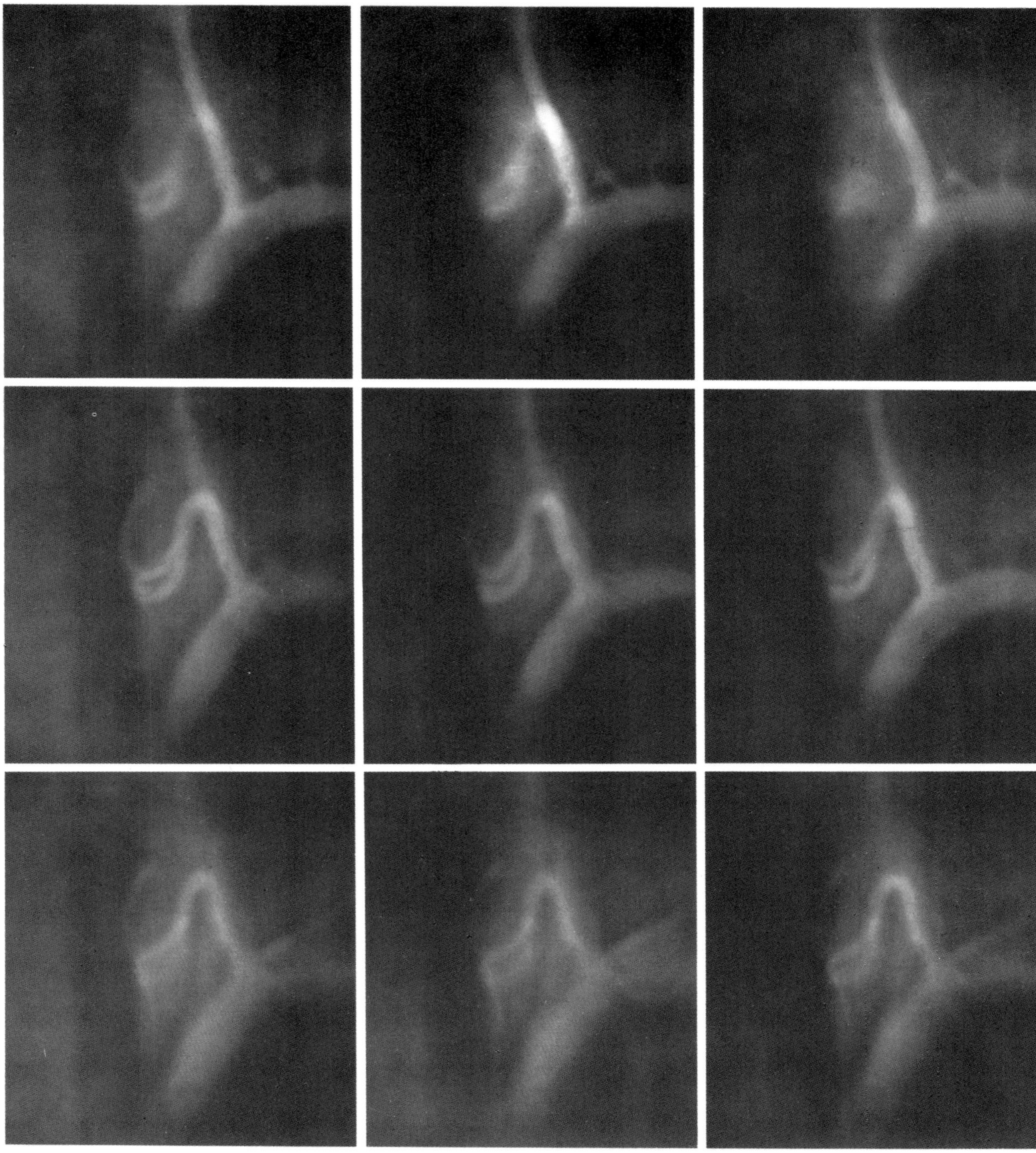

Fig. 4. Angiotomosynthesis of the left subclavian artery. Note the origin of the vertebral artery on the upper right and the thyrocervical trunk in the middle, both without superimposing on the other vessels

proceeds as follows: The coded image is projected onto a lens matrix with three lenses in the same position as the three X-ray tubes. The shadows which result with the lenses now contain nine discs and nine squares, whereby each time three discs or three squares are superimposed in the centre of the picture, thus forming a more intensive image. This is the precisely adjusted tomography of the disc or the square, whereas all other discs and squares are unclear and therefore artefacts.

In this example the layer chosen is three times more intensive than the artefacts, and when more tubes are used, the resolution is better.

The prototype of the equipment in Würzburg contains 24 X-ray tubes that can be flashed simultaneously.

Our main goal with tomosynthesis was to exploit the advantages of this method in cerebral angiography to the utmost. Long-lasting technical and experimental preliminary work was necessary. A special cassette was developed with which we could carry out serial angiotomography, which we call angiotomosynthesis.

Figures 2, 3 and 4 show examples of tomosynthesis of the upper cervical region, the lumbar region in a lumbosacral myelogram and the left subclavian artery in brachial angiogram.

References

1. Nadjmi M, Weiss H, Klotz E, Linde R (1980) Flashing tomosynthesis – A new tomographic method. Neuroradiology 19:113–117
2. Weiss H, Klotz E, Linde R, Rabe G, Tiemens U (1977) Coded aperture imaging with X-rays (flashing tomosynthesis). Opt Acta 24:305–325

CT Examination of the Spinal Cord: Overview

I. F. Moseley and P. Pullicino*

The National Hospital, Lysholm Radiological Department, Queen Square, GB – London WC1N 3BG

Technical Problems

Alfidi et al. [1] noted that "the spinal cord, its surrounding layer of epidural fat and the cerebrospinal fluid are distinguishable on CT scans. Whether this modality will prove useful in the study of spinal cord pathology or disc herniation remains to be seen." This open question does not appear to have been answered in the positive, since, although De Chiro et al. [12] reported some success with the diagnosis of syringomyelia, later workers were less sanguine [16, 17, 19, 23]. Several groups noted that the spinal cord could only be seen with any frequency in the upper cervical region [2, 3, 36], and Resjo et al. [39] commented that CT "yielded no significant findings in the spinal cord."

Oberson and Azam [32] analysed the results in a series of 83 patients, and commented that the spinal cord was "not discernible" in one-half, not sharply delineated in three-eighths and clearly recognised in only one-eighth. Nevertheless, they were able to detect cord pathology: three haematomas, eight cases of calcification, three cysts and four syrinxes. Although cord atrophy was "easily recognised," cord swelling, with consequent obliteration of the natural contrast of the subarachnoid space, was never detected. It is clearly unsatisfactory to assume that lesions which are shown by CT lie within a structure which cannot itself be identified. The appearance of a "pseudocord," represented by the lumbar theca below the termination of the cord itself (Fig. 1), was noted by Roub and Drayer [41].

What factors render the spinal cord so elusive? The crucial problems are contrast and spatial resolution on the one hand and elimination of artefact on the other.

Contrast Resolution

Contrast within the normal cord is effectively lacking, although occasionally a CT image will suggest the central grey matter. Thus, contrast within the spinal canal will depend on the epidural fat and the cerebrospinal fluid. The former, surrounding the

* Our thanks are due to EMI Medical Limited for assistance and to Miss Jill Cox for preparation of the manuscript

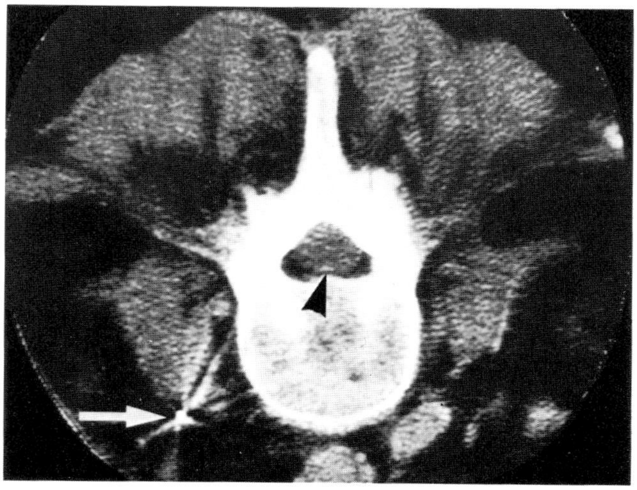

Fig. 1. "Pseudocord" – in fact the theca – in the mid-lumbar region (high resolution scan). There is contrast medium in the left ureter (*arrow*); a "pseudo-anterior spinal artery" is shown by the *arrowhead*

Radiology Today 1. Ed. by M. W. Donner and F. H. W. Heuck

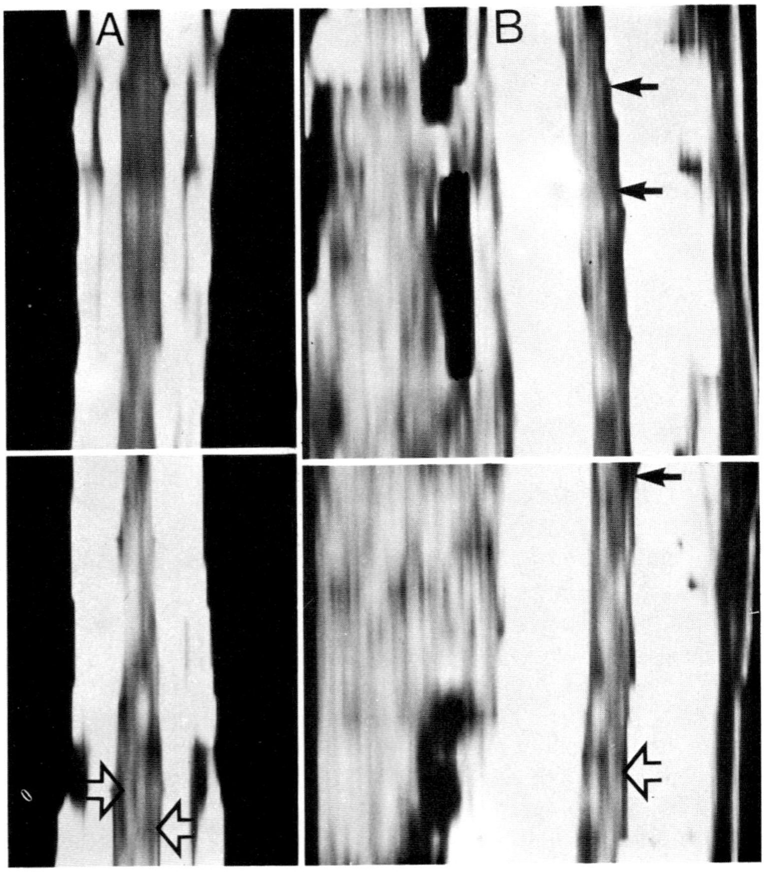

Fig. 2. **a** Coronal and **b** sagittal reconstructions of the thoracolumbar spine over 24 cm. The posterior epidural space is well seen (*arrows*), and there is an impression of the cauda equina (*open arrows*)

theca, gives rise to the "pseudocord" appearance referred to above; in the thoracic and cervical regions it may not be apparent to the observer that it *is* a "pseudocord" (Fig. 2). Experimental work led Isherwood et al. [24] to conclude that a subarachnoid space about 2 mm wide was necessary for visualisation of the spinal cord, which explains the observation that the normal cord is best seen in the upper cervical region, where the subarachnoid space is widest. The problem is complicated by the obliquity of the spinal canal and of the cord within it, which gives rise to partial volume effects. Every attempt should therefore be made (using gantry or table tilt and scanogram or scout film facilities, if available) to scan perpendicular to the cord at any given level [35]. Such a procedure will authorise the use of thicker (8 or 13 mm) sections, which will aid contrast resolution in some cases.

It should be noted that contrast resolution within the spine is probably impaired by the beam hardening effect of the relatively massive vertebral column. Some workers have employed programmes which attempt to correct for this effect [3], but without great success.

Godfrey Hounsfield suggested that low contrast areas might be rendered to greater effect if the data of several scans of the same area were used to reconstruct a final image, and if spatial filtering were employed. This suggestion was put into practice by D. G. King [15], using the high spatial resolution mode discussed below, to reduce noise levels to those of a conventional scan, and the technique has been used to investigate patients with suspected syringomyelia [5], with apparently successful results.

Repeated scanning of the same area has disadvantages. The first of these is the high radiation dose: Ethier et al. [15] stated that "several" sections were overlaid; if it can be assumed that at least four sections were required to reduce the noise level to that of standard scans [33], this would entail a dose of 17 rad/slice [28]. Secondly, any movement between sections would tend to degrade the final image. Even adding eight sections at the same level, in the anaesthetised pig, Isherwood et al. [24] found no significant gain in contrast resolution.

Spatial filtering, over 3 × 3, 5 × 5 or 7 × 7 pixel areas [15] can increase contrast resolution for relatively large objects, but reduces spatial resolution.

Spatial Resolution

This will depend on the individual CT scanner, and it would be invidious to make comparisons in such a review as the present one. Since radiation dose is proportional to the cube of spatial resolution (other factors being constant), improvements in the latter cannot be made simply by increasing the incident dose, which would rapidly reach unacceptable levels. Orwell et al. [33] described a method for increasing the spatial resolution of translate-rotate scanners without increasing dose rate, clinical applications of which have been described by Ethier and his co-workers [5, 15] and by Naidich et al. [29, 30]. The cervical cord has been shown more or less routinely by the use of this technique; the dentate ligaments and septum posticum, the nerve root sheaths and the ligamentum flavum are sometimes seen. Visualisation of the thoracic cord and cauda equina has been less reliable.

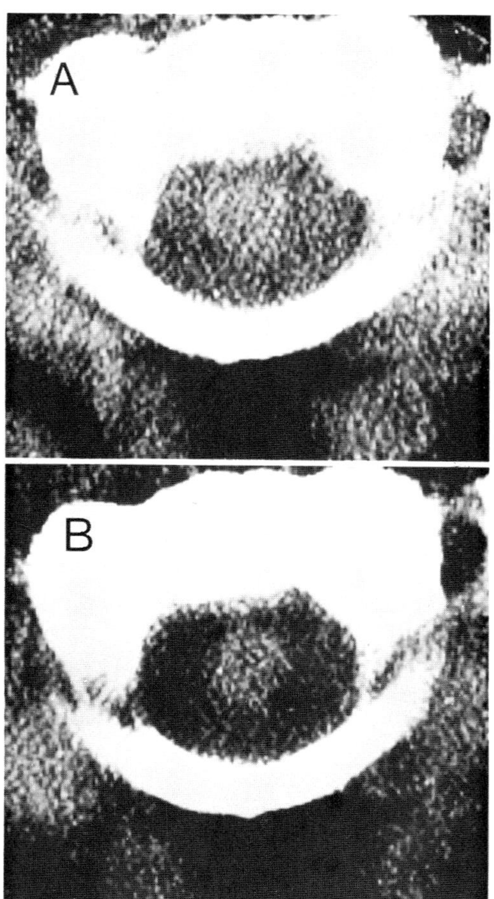

Fig. 4A, B. High resolution scans of cervical region, at same window factors. **A** Before and **B** after intravenous contrast medium. Note the higher contrast differential in **B**

Elimination of Artefact

Artefacts due to beam hardening and partial volume phenomena have been mentioned above. The most potent source of artefact in spinal CT is, however, movement: cardiac, respiratory, alimentary, involuntary and, in the case of the cervical spine, swallowing. Bowel movements can be suppressed by glucagon (0.5 mg IV every 20 min, to a total dose of 1.5 mg) [30], but the other types of movement are difficult to control without general anaesthesia – which may be one of the advantages of xenon as a contrast agent (see below).
It need hardly be added that iodised oil myelographic media, which may give rise to intense artefacts, should not be used in patients who may subsequently be studied by CT.
Given that the spinal cord represents a challenging area for CT, it may be suggested that reduction of movement artefacts is the crucial factor in successful imaging, since reports of work using fast scanners [21, 22] are encouraging; Naidich and his colleagues have recently claimed good visualisation of the thoracic spinal cord and of the nerve roots and sheaths using 3-s scans on the EMI 7070 [30]. The internal structure of the cord remains a blind spot [21].

Contrast Media for CT of the Spinal Cord

Contrast media which increase the differential in attenuation coefficients between the spinal cord and the surrounding structures have been administered by four paths: intravenous, intrathecal, intramedullary and by inhalation.

Intravenous Iodinated Contrast Media

As an extension of their use in cranial scanning, iodinated contrast media have been used in examination of the spinal cord. The epidural tissues, having no blood-tissue barrier, increase markedly in attenuation, and a smaller increase is seen in the cord; since the cerebrospinal fluid does not increase appreciably in attenuation, the contrast between it and the cord is thereby increased (Fig. 3). Pullicino [35] observed an increase of 10 H.U. in the attenuation of the spinal cord with a bolus injection of 30 g I, but Oberson and Azam [32] found that the visibility of the spinal cord was not significantly increased. Naidich et al. [29] noted improved demonstration of the cord and were able to visualise the normal anterior spinal artery in some cases. These workers were using a high spatial resolution programme; it had previously been stated by Di Chiro et al. [13] that "contrast enhanced [standard resolution] CT of the normal thorocolumbar spinal canal does not show detail of the normal intrathecal vasculature," although "structures which may correspond in position and appearance to the epidural veins" were occasionally seen.

It is generally agreed that intravenous contrast medium may make possible visualisation of intramedullary tumours [3, 20, 22, 31] although some workers have not shared this experience [2]. Spinal arteriovenous malformations have also been shown [13, 34], and contrast enhancement was reported in one case thought to represent acute demyelination [8]; a prior CT examination and a further study following steroid therapy were negative. Unfortunately, in this latter case, the published CT images are not adequate for satisfactory assessment.

Pullicino [35] recommended intravenous contrast medium as a routine measure when the spinal cord is being examined. It suffers, however, from the disadvantages of prolonging the examination, of promoting hyperpnoea and of its well-recognised toxicity. The modest rewards must be weighed against these factors. Intravenous media should not be used concurrently with intrathecal iodinated contrast medium, since the increasing attenuation coefficients in both cord and spinal fluid would be counterproductive. Concurrent use with inhaled contrast media may lead to problems of interpretation.

Intrathecal Contrast Media

Water-Soluble Iodinated Contrast Medium. It has been firmly established that of such contrast media currently available on a large scale, metrizamide is the only one whose toxicity is acceptably low (though not non-existent).

Post-radiculographic CT of the spine was carried out by Di Chiro and Schellinger [11] who noted that without further manipulation the contrast medium reached the thoracic region in 30–60 min and the cervical subarachnoid space in 60–120 min. These observations were extended by Isherwood et al. [23]: the attenuation coefficients of the spinal cord were observed to increase in the presence of metrizamide, a finding confirmed by Coin et al. [7] and Resjö et al. [39]. Experimental work by Isherwood and his colleagues suggested that this was not artefactual, but not all workers agree on this point [5].

There is no doubt that the outline of the spinal cord can be defined with great clarity using intrathecal contrast medium [32]. The normal appearances have been described by Thijssen et al. [46] (although these workers were unable to show the posterior or anterior median fissures in normal cases) and in children by Resjö et al. [39]. Intramedullary tumours have been usefully outlined by intrathecal metrizamide [2, 26]; indeed, Roub and Drayer [41] found that areas of low attenuation within the canal representing intramedullary neoplasms could not be distinguished from the subarachnoid space without opacification of the spinal fluid, and that the contrast medium was essential for delineation of the size and shape of the spinal cord. They were, however, using the same scanner as Hilal [22], who reported "consistent" identification of the subarachnoid space and of spinal cord tumours. Spinal dysraphism [38] and syringomyelic expansion of the spinal cord [16] have also been demonstrated using metrizamide. In the latter condition, visualisation of the Chiari malformation was improved from at most one-third without metrizamide to three-quarters when intrathecal contrast medium was used (Fig. 4). The effects of vertebral column and disc abnormalities on the theca can also be shown [7].

In syringomyelia, diffusion or direct passage of the contrast medium into the intramedullary cavity may be an added bonus with intrathecal metrizamide [10, 16, 27]. A similar phenomenon has been observed with oil contrast medium [12].

Other advantages of metrizamide are that the risk of arachnoiditis is very low and that it need not be removed. However, it is expensive, necessitates lumbar or cervical spinal puncture, and although relatively anodyne, is nevertheless neurotoxic and must be used with some caution. It has been noted above that it raises the apparent attenuation coefficients of the spinal cord by up to 30 H.U. [39]. This may result in a thin rim of cord tissue surrounding a large intramedullary cavity being concealed and mistaken for a large, low attenuation, possibly solid tumour [5]. Experimental work by Scatliff et al. [42] showed that some of the tissues found in dysraphic structures, e.g. fibrocartilage, may also be effectively masked when surrounded by metrizamide, although Dossetor et al. [14] found that the interstices of lipomas were well-delineated. Another disadvantage of any intrathecal (or intramedullary) contrast medium is that

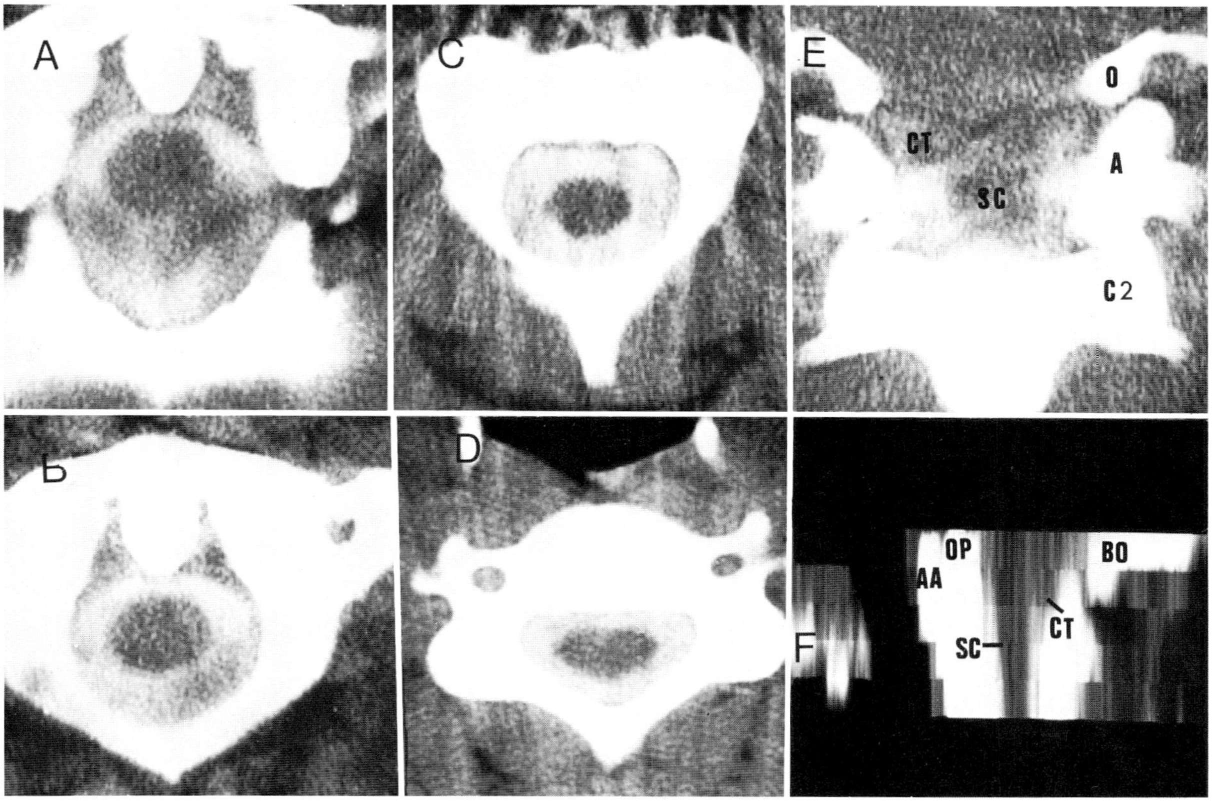

Fig. 4A–F. Chiari malformation in a young woman with headache provoked by intense physical excitement. High resolution scans with intrathecal metrizamide **A** at foramen magnum. The cerebellar tonsils are seen, behind the lower medulla. **B** At C1, the right tonsil is still visible. **C** At C2 and **D** C4, the spinal cord appears normal. **E** A coronal section and **F** a sagittal reconstruction both confirm the presence of tonsillar herniation. *A,* atlas; *AA,* anterior arch; *BO,* basiocciput; *C2,* second cervical vertebra; *CT,* cerebellar tonsil; *O,* occipital condyle; *OP,* odontoid; *SC,* spinal cord

some disturbance of the normal (or pathological) cerebrospinal fluid dynamics is inevitable [22].

If conventional myelography is to be carried out with metrizamide, there is a strong argument for extending the study by post-myelographic CT, on the grounds that the maximum information should be extracted from any invasive procedure. It must, however, be appreciated that certain aspects may be concealed rather than revealed by intrathecal positive contrast media.

Gas. The phantom studies referred to above [42] suggested that air may be the ideal intrathecal contrast medium for CT. Clearly, a very high contrast level can be obtained, although this may give rise to reconstruction artefacts. Oxygen was used in practice by Roub and Drayer [41], with satisfactory results; they had the advantage of CT apparatus with a tilting patient couch. In the absence of this facility, it may be necessary to use large quantities of gas, which very definitely robs CT of its non-invasive character.

Intramedullary Contrast Media

Endomyelography with gas, oil or water-soluble contrast medium may be combined with CT (Fig. 5). There is, however, little evidence that more information is gained than from conventional radiography. The invasive nature of the procedure is self-evident.

Inhalation Contrast Media

Currently only stable xenon is used as an inhalation contrast medium for spinal CT [36], krypton having proved less satisfactory. Xenon is absorbed three times as avidly by lipids as by aqueous tissues,

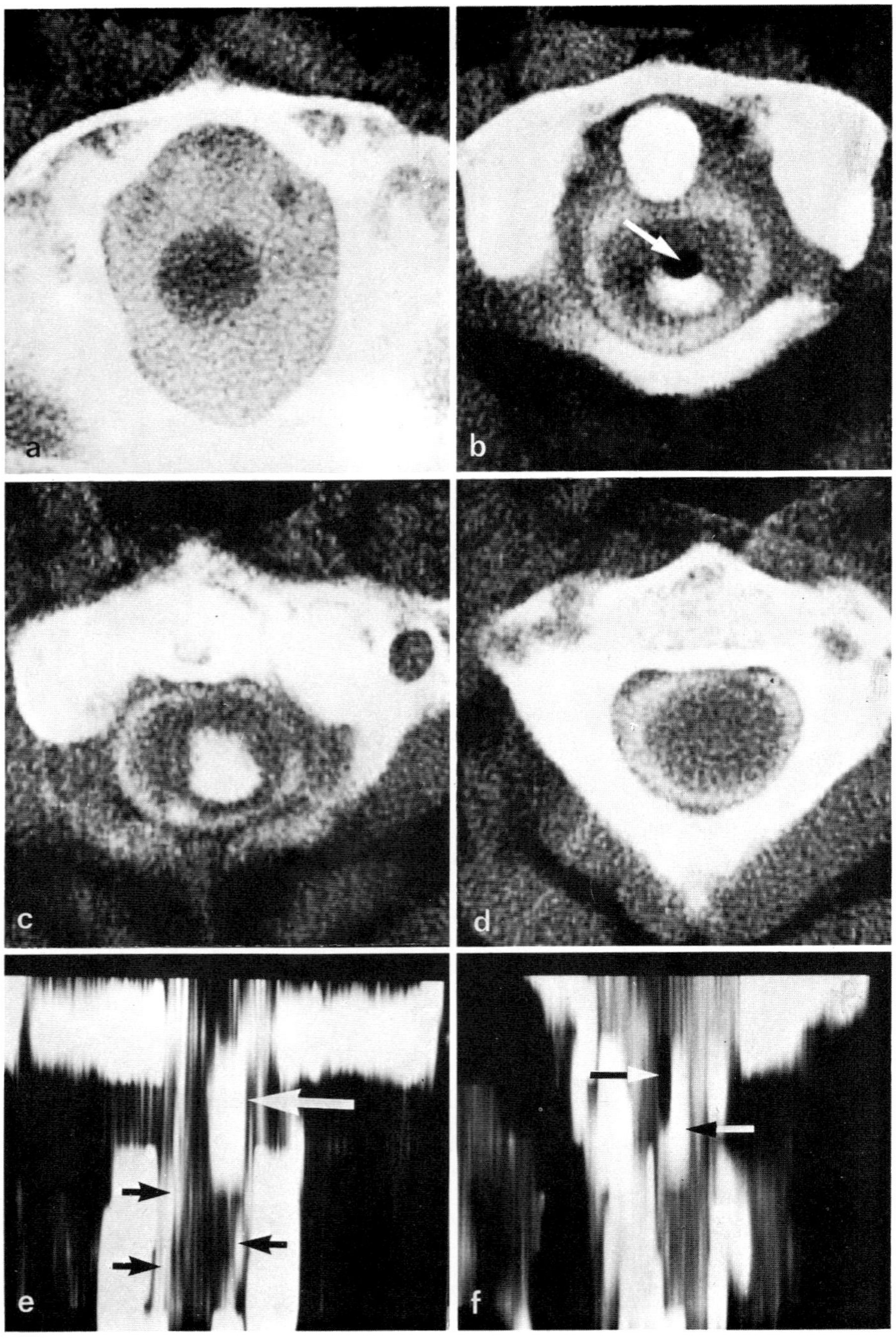

Fig. 5a – f. Syringomyelia with intrathecal metrizamide and water-soluble endomyelogram. High resolution scans. **a** At level of foramen magnum. The vertebral arteries are shown. **b** At C1 Note metrizamide and air bubble (*arrow*) in cord. **c** 10 mm lower. The cavity is eccentric. **d** 10 mm lower than **c**; no intramedullary contrast medium seen. **e** Coronal reconstruction. The eccentric cavity is seen (*long arrow*), as is the narrowed subarachnoid space (*small arrows*). **f** Sagittal reconstruction. The cavity (filled by air and metrizamide) is again seen (*arrows*)

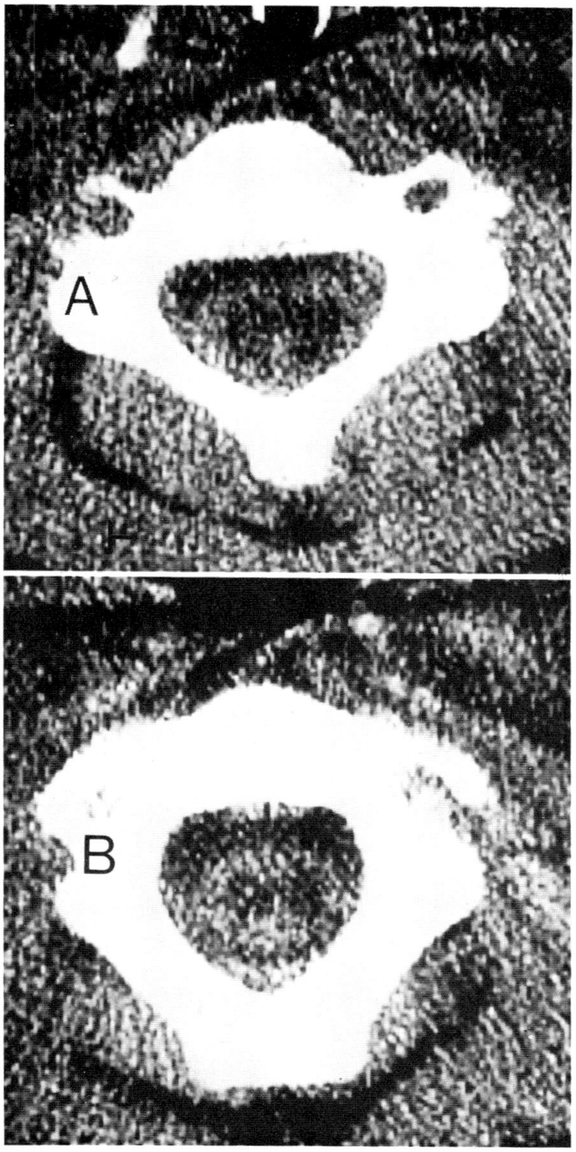

Fig. 6A, B. Syringomyelia. High resolution scans at same window factors **A** before and **B** after xenon inhalation. The cord and the central cavity are slightly more evident in **B**

and is therefore concentrated in the cord, increasing the contrast between neural and other tissues to a considerably greater degree than intravenous contrast medium. Pullicino et al. described its use in rendering syringomyelic cavities and cord atrophy more evident (Fig. 6) and in demonstrating that a large intramedullary tumour was most unlikely to be cystic.

A major disadvantage of inhaled xenon is that it is an anaesthetic agent, and its use requires the patient to be intubated. This latter fact can, however, be an advantage in difficult adults or children, particularly as the respiration can be arrested during scans. It is also very expensive to use, not only because of its high initial cost but also because it is labour and time consuming.

CT in Specific Spinal Cord Diseases

Syringomyelia and the Chiari Malformation

The largest corpus of literature on CT of the spinal cord concerns the diagnosis of syringomyelia. Attempts to demonstrate cavitation of the cord were given an initial impetus by the publication of a series of nine verified and nine unverified cases by Di Chiro et al. [12]. These workers were able to see a definite cavity within the cervical cord (containing oil contrast medium in two cases) in five of the nine verified cases (seven of whom had already been operated upon) and a possible cavity in two further patients. In the unverified cases, three definite cavities (one containing oil) and one possible cavity were seen.

It must be commented that in retrospect the quality of the published CT images suggests enthusiastic interpretation; indeed, Hammerschlag et al. [19] could not duplicate these results. However, Gonsalves et al. [18], working with the same type of machine as Di Chiro, published convincing images obtained in six of "a large number" of cases of confirmed syringomyelia and in one case of a post-traumatic syrinx, proven at necropsy.

Single cases or small series were reported by Scotti et al. [43], Balériaux-Waba et al. [3, 4], Handel et al. [20], Oberson and Azam [32] and Rinaldi et al. [40], but the first major contribution after that of Di Chiro was that of Forbes and Isherwood [16]. These workers studied 20 proven cases; in 8 cases the CT study was augmented by intrathecal metrizamide. The cord was seen poorly or not at all in ten of the 12 cases studied by plain CT, and no cavity was seen in the remaining two cases. In the metrizamide group the cord was well seen in six cases, and appeared expanded in three. A syrinx was visible in three cases (the contrast medium entering it in one). A Chiari malformation was indicated by the CT study in one-third of the plain CT and three-quarters of the metrizamide group.

Pullicino et al. [36] indicated that inhaled stable xenon facilitated the demonstration of the cord and of cavities within it, in both cervical and thoracic regions. They also used a high spatial resolution programme.

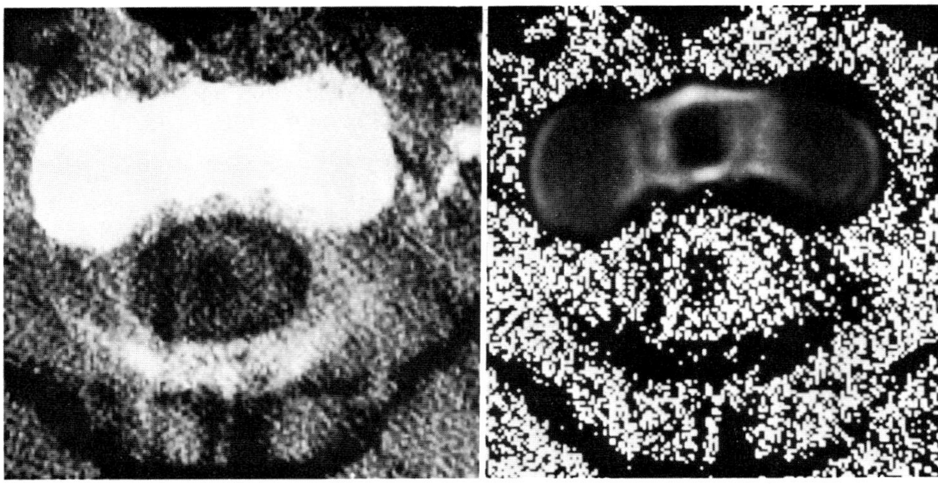

Fig. 7. Syringomyelic cavity at C2 level. *Left,* high resolution scan; *right*, CT numbers 25 – 40 EMI units highlighted. The cavity is again seen

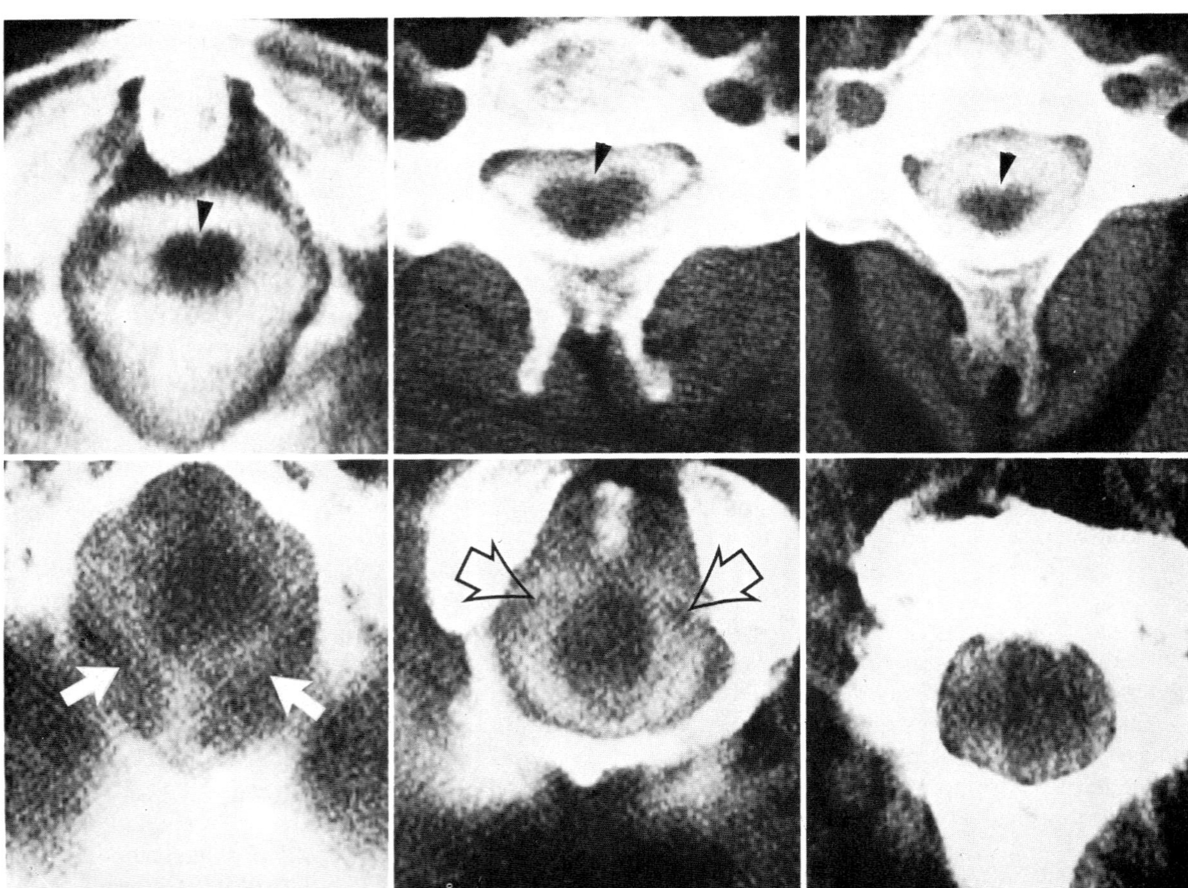

Fig. 8. High resolution scans of two cases of syringomyelia shown by intrathecal metrizamide. *Top row,* atrophic cord; note consistent demonstration of an anterior sulcus (*arrowheads*). *Bottom row,* cerebellar tonsillar herniation (*arrows*) and expanded cord; note vertebral arteries (*open arrows*)

The value of the latter, especially when combined with averaging of multiple slices and image filtration, was shown by Bonafé et al. [5] in a series of 32 cases, in every one of which a cavity was seen. Although incomplete CT studies or artefacts resulted in cavities being shown at only one level in four patients, more than half of the lesions were shown to extend over at least three vertebral segments. These workers described a swollen, round or "doughnut" cord shadow in ten cases, a cord and a cavity flattened anteroposteriorly in 13, a small cavitated cord in five, and a normal size, cavitated cord in four (Fig. 7). Myelography had been normal in eight cases. The C4 – 6 levels were affected in 90% of the patients, C1 – 3 in about half, and C7 – T1 in one-quarter. In keeping with the findings of Forbes and Isherwood, it was possible to demonstrate a Chiari malformation in only 10 of 21 cases in which the appropriate region was examined.

Hilal [22] showed a collapsed cord (indirect evidence of a syrinx) in "some cases" of the Chiari malformation (Fig. 8), while Crolla et al. (1980) [10] used CT to demonstrate metrizamide within a syringomyelic cavity following ventriculography.

Syringomyelia remains a difficult condition to diagnose by non-invasive methods, and although Bonafé et al. [5] list the features which distinguish a syrinx from other low-attenuation lesions of the cord, the unreliability of demonstrating by CT an associated Chiari malformation, which is important for surgical treatment, means that myelography remains indispensable at present.

Spinal Dysraphism

Dysraphism has also been the subject of a number of reports. Some workers have concentrated on the bony anomalies, particularly those of diastematomyelia [19, 47].

Four cases of this condition were described by Palmers et al. [34], in one of which the cord lesion had not been demonstrated by oil myelography; moreover, CT demonstrated a high attenuation "tumoral lesion" within the adjacent cord, which proved at operation to be a spongioblastoma. In another case of meningocoele, a possible low attenuation area was shown within the spinal cord.

Tadmor et al. [44] claimed to show without intrathecal contrast medium that splitting of the cord extended beyond the bony septum. Other abnormalities shown in six confirmed cases by James and Oliff [25] included an intraspinal lipoma (in at least four cases), and in a single patient, a thick filum terminale and a low termination of a cord fixed posteriorly (Fig. 9). (Lipomas, which may form part of the dysraphic syndrome or occur as isolated tumours, are considered further in the next section.)

It has been suggested by Resjö et al. [38], who carried out CT with intrathecal metrizamide in 25 dysraphic infants and children, that the low spinal cord seen in this condition is smaller and more rounded than the normal. However, with the recognised variations in attenuation coefficients of the neural tissue at CT, particularly with intrathecal metrizamide, the basis for the assignation of a given structure to cord or filum terminale must be questioned. These workers showed splitting of the cord in a number of cases, a feature missed at conventional myelography in almost half (Fig. 10). CT also showed neurenteric cysts in three patients and intramedullary dermoids in two.

Reservations about the use of metrizamide in dysraphism [42] have been noted above. Roub and Drayer [41], who used both metrizamide and oxygen as contrast media, commented on the value of CT as compared with conventional techniques in showing additional *extradural* anomalies; they insisted on the necessity for intrathecal contrast medium in assessment of the contents of the lumbar theca.

Resjö et al. [38] recommended plain films and CT with metrizamide for the basic radiological investigation of dysraphism. Many surgeons will need to be convinced of the adequacy of such a protocol.

Intramedullary Tumours

Delineation of intrinsic tumours of the spinal cord, particularly of their internal structure, has been particularly disappointing. Many workers have recorded negative results in proven cases of intramedullary tumours, or have merely shown low attenuation areas which could not confidently be identified as lying within the neuraxis [26, 31, 41] (Fig. 11). A report of "small foci of low density" within two ependymonas by Lee et al. [26] is difficult to assess without the original images. The same workers illustrated a clearly visible cervical ependymoma of high attenuation, which appeared to have fungated out of and to be compressing the cord. Abnormally high attenuation has also been described in cases of spongioblastoma [34], ependymoma, haemangioblastoma and medulloblastoma [2], while Aubin et al. [2] noted low attenuation in an astrocytoma, which was thought at operation to represent associated oedema. Since

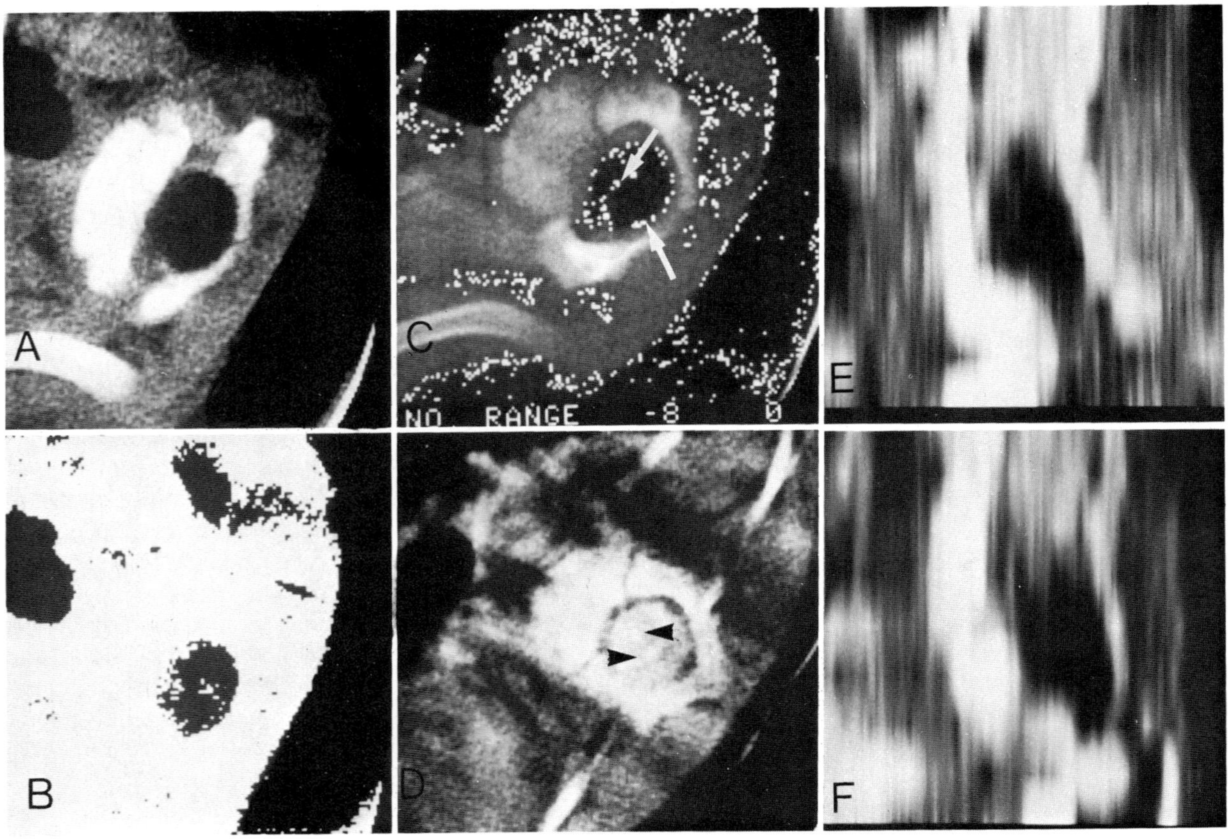

Fig. 9A – F. Dysraphism with intraspinal lipoma. **A** Lower lumbar region. A low attenuation mass expands the spinal canal; the posterior bony elements are dysplastic. (N.B. in **A – D,** the child is turned approximately 45° onto the right flank.) **B** As **A,** to show negative attenuation coefficients within spinal canal. **c** Highlighting of CT numbers – 8 to 0 EMI units. The "septa" and "capsule" (*arrows*) of the lipoma are of lower attenuation than water. **D** The lower thoracic spine cord is abnormally low in position, abnormally large and abnormally inhomogenous (*arrowheads*) **E** Coronal and **F** sagittal reconstructions of the lumbar region. The large cord is seen to end in the lipoma; the lower spinal canal is expanded

fat, which is of low attenuation, acts as a natural contrast medium, it is not surprising that there have been a number of reports of lipomas within the spinal canal [2, 14, 17, 22, 23, 25, 26, 31, 41]. These tumours may be wholly or partially intramedullary, although it is not clear in most of the published reports whether the relationship of the tumour and the cord was established by CT.

Conventional myelography would appear to be a more satisfactory method of identifying intramedullary tumours. CT could contribute to management were it to demonstrate whether tumours were clearly marginated or if they were cystic. Palmers et al. [34], and Zumpano [48] identified tumour cysts without the use of contrast media, the latter in a medulloblastoma, while no cyst was seen by Aubin et al. (1979) [2] in either of two astrocytomas found at operation to be cystic. Intramedullary "cysts" distinct from syrinxes were seen in three cases by Oberson and Azam [32], but whether these were neoplastic was not stated. Quencer [37], on the other hand, found intramedullary "lucencies" at CT in patients with masses which proved subsequently to be cystic in one case and solid in another. Similar changes were present in syringomyelia.

Intravenous contrast medium can render spinal cord tumours visible. This phenomenon has been reported in haemangioblastoma [4, 31, 32] and in astrocytoma [20]. Hilal [22] found tumour enhancement in "a large number" of patients; he also noted "consistent" detection of spinal cord tumours, but did not state whether this was pre- or postinjection.

Intrathecal contrast medium has been used to show expansion of the cord by intramedullary tumours [2, 26, 41] but has the disadvantage that contrast resolution within the cord is thereby reduced.

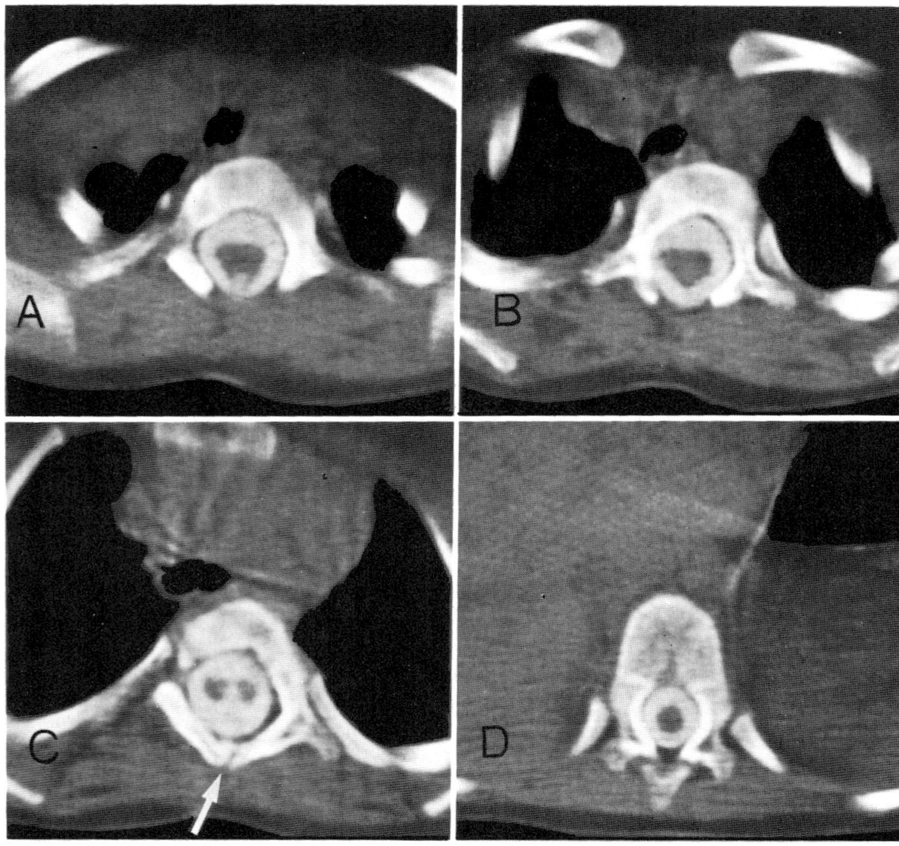

Fig. 10A – D. Diastematomyelia with extensive spina bifida. **A** Upper thoracic region. There is spina bifida and the spinal canal is expanded. The spinal cord is markedly dysplastic posteriorly. **B** Slightly lower. The cord appears less abnormal. **C** Mid-thoracic region. The cord is completely split, even though the spina bifida (*arrow*) is minimal at this level and no septum is seen. **D** Low thoracic region. The shape of the cord is relatively normal

Inhaled xenon, however, may be helpful in the distinction of solid from cystic tumours [36].
Thus, the current position would appear to be that CT as at most a very subsidiary role in the investigation of intramedullary tumours.

Other Conditions

Spinal Arteriovenous Malformations (Fig. 12). Abnormal vessels visualised after intravenous contrast medium were first described in one case with this condition by Palmers et al. [34]. Di Chiro et al. [13] subsequently published details of four cases: in two, abnormal inhomogeneity of the spinal contents before intravenous contrast medium was noted, with contrast enhancement (very marked in one huge lesion). The other cases were studied after embolisation or operatively verified spontaneous thrombosis, without positive CT findings.
In cases with a high degree of clinical suspicion of an angioma, it appears resonable to proceed directly from a positive CT study to angiography.

Demyelination of the Spinal Cord. A single case report by Coin and Hucks-Folliss [6] has been noted above. The possibility of demonstrating plaques requires further confirmation.

Spinal Trauma. Most reports on trauma have concentrated on the osseous lesions [8, 9, 45]. Improved visualisation of intraspinal fragments as compared with conventional techniques was claimed by Naidich et al. [29] and by Roub and Drayer [41]. The latter workers used intrathecal oxygen to localise an intraspinal block and showed a haematoma by CT. Oberson and Azam [32] found three

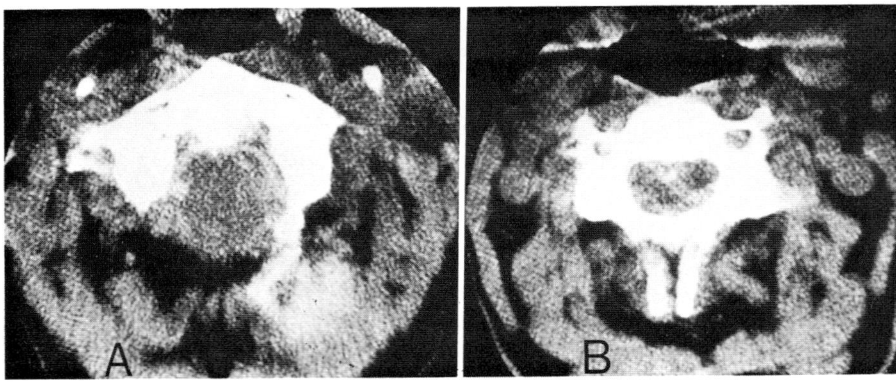

Fig. 11A, B. High resolution scans of previously operated cervical intramedullary tumour. **A** At C1 level; **B** at C4. The cord is expanded and of mixed attenuation; it is not possible to exclude cyst formation

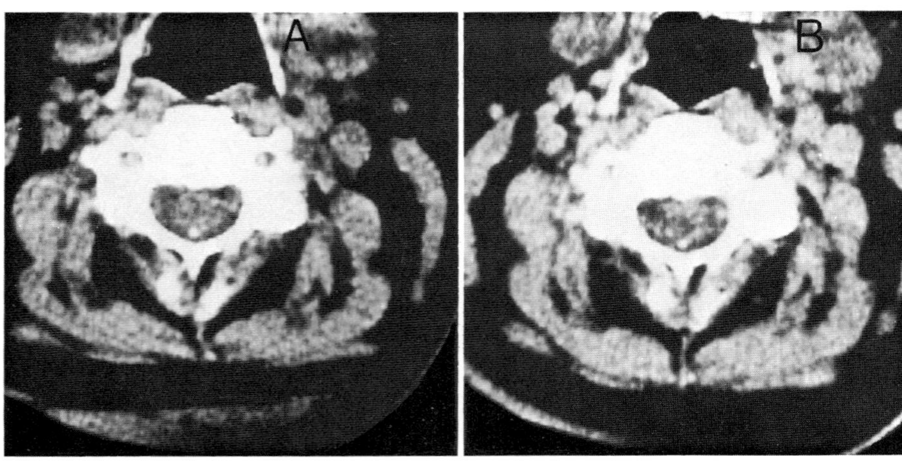

Fig. 12A, B. Presumed cervical arteriovenous malformation. **A** Before and **B** after intravenous contrast medium. There is abnormal spotty enhancement of the spinal cord

cases of intraspinal haematoma (but gave no further details), while Naidich et al. [29] were unable to show any evidence of intraspinal haemorrhage in high resolution studies of 14 patients. The value of CT in spinal trauma would seem to be limited not only by the quality of the visualisation of the spinal contents but also by the relevance of this information to management and prognosis.

Congenital Lesions. The effects of canal stenosis on the form of the cervical cord (as seen with intrathecal metrizamide) were described by Thijssen et al. [46], as was a presumed congenital malformation of the cord, with a midline groove posteriorly, in a case of congenital cervical fusion.

Conclusions

Despite the advances which have been made since 1975, it is clear that the use of CT to obtain useful information about the internal structure of the spinal cord cannot be regarded as a routine procedure of considerable value. It currently requires the highest developments of CT scanning and reconstruction techniques, but there is preliminary evidence that present day fourth generation scanners represent a real advance in this field of investigation.

Ideally, contrast medium administration would be unnecessary for spinal CT. Although it has disadvantages, the addition of CT to conventional metrizamide myelography would appear to give added information (in some cases) without added risk, but there is suggestive evidence that detail within the cord may thereby be obscured.

For the present, it would seem reasonable to investigate the spinal cord using available CT modalities, in an attempt to derive as much information as possible from a potentially non-invasive technique. It is, however, essential that clinicians should be aware of the technical and interpretative limitations of the method, and to this end it behoves the radiologist not to exaggerate its as yet modest achievements.

References

1. Alfidi RJ, Haaga J, Meaney TF et al. (1975) Computed tomography of the thorax and abdomen: a preliminary report. Radiology 117:257–264
2. Aubin ML, Jardin C, Bar D, Vignaud J (1979) Computerised tomography in 32 cases of intraspinal tumour. J Neuroradiol 6:81–92
3. Balériaux-Waba D, Babin E, Dupont M, Wackenheim A, Jeanmart L (1978) Computed tomography in lesions of the cervical spinal canal. J Belge Radiol 61:287–290
4. Balériaux-Waba D, Retif J, Noterman J et al. (1978) CT scanning for the diagnosis of the cerebellar and spinal lesions of von Hippel-Lindan's disease. Neuroradiology 14:284–244
5. Bonafé A, Ethier R, Melancon D, Belanger G, Peters T (1980) High resolution computed tomography in cervical syringomyelia. J Comput Assis Tomogr 4:42–47
6. Coin CG, Hucks-Folliss A (1979) Cervical computed tomography in multiple sclerosis with spinal cord involvement. J Comput Assist Tomogr 3:421–422
7. Coin CG, Chan YS, Keranen V, Pennink M (1977) Computer assisted myelography in disc disease. J Comput Assist Tomogr 1:398–404
8. Coin CG, Pennink M, Ahmad WD, Keranen VJ (1979) Diving-type injury of the cervical spine: contribution of computed tomography to management. J Comput Assist Tomogr 3:362–372
9. Colley DP, Dunsker SB (1978) Traumatic narrowing of the dorsolumbar spinal canal demonstrated by computed tomography. Radiology 129:95–98
10. Crolla D, Hens L, Wilms G, Van Den Bergh R, Baert AL (1980) Metrizamide enhanced CT in hydrosyringomyelia. Neuroradiology 19:39–41
11. Di Chiro G, Schellinger D (1976) Computed tomography of spinal cord after lumbar intrathecal introduction of metrizamide (computer-assisted myelography). Radiology 120:101–104
12. Di Chiro G, Axelbaum SP, Schellinger D, Twigg HL, Ledley RS (1975) Computerised axial tomography in syringomyelia. N Engl J Med 292: 13–16
13. Di Chiro G, Doppman JL, Wener L (1977) Computed tomography of spinal cord arteriovenous malformations. Radiology 123:351–354
14. Dossetor RS, Kaiser M, Veiga-Pires JA (1979) CT scanning in two cases of lipoma of the spinal cord. Clin Radiol 30:227–231
15. Ethier R, King DG, Melancon D, Belanger G, Taylor S, Thompson C (1979) Development of high resolution tomography of the spinal cord. J Comput Assist Tomogr 3:433–438
16. Forbes WStC, Isherwood I (1978) Computed tomography in syringomyelia and the associated Arnold Chiari type I malformation. Neuroradiology 15: 73–78
17. Gado M, Eichling J, Currie M (1977) The total body scanner in neurological disease. In: Du Boulay GH, Moseley IF (eds) First European seminar on computerised axial tomography in clinical practice. Springer, Berlin Heidelberg New York, pp 312–321
18. Gonsalves CG, Hudson AR, Horsey WJ, Tucker WS (1978) Computed tomography of the cervical spine and spinal cord. Comput Tomogr 2:279–293
19. Hammerschlag SB, Wolpert SM, Carter BL (1976) Computed tomography of the spinal canal. Radiology 121:361–367
20. Handel S, Grossman R, Sarwar M (1978) Computed tomography in the diagnosis of spinal cord astrocytoma. J Comput Assist Tomogr 2:226–228
21. Haughton VM, Syvertsen A, Williams AL (1980) Soft-tissue anatomy within the spinal canal as seen on computed tomography. Radiology 134:649–655
22. Hilal SK (1979) CT of the spinal cord with submillimeter fourth generation scanner. J Comput Assist Tomogr 3:567
23. Isherwood I, Fawcitt RA, Nettle JRL, Spencer JW, Pullan BR (1977) Computer tomography of the spine. In: Du Boulay GH, Moseley IF (eds) First European seminar on computerised axial tomography in clinical practice. Springer, Berlin Heidelberg New York, pp 322–335
24. Isherwood I, Antoun NM, Checkley D, Dovas T (1979) Experience with high resolution scanning of the spine. J Comput Assist Tomogr 3:566–567
25. James HE, Oliff M (1977) Computed tomography in spinal dysraphia. J Comput Assist Tomogr 1: 391–397
26. Lee BCP, Kazam E, Newman AD (1978) Computed tomography of the spine and spinal cord. Radiology 128:95–102
27. Manelfe C, Rascol A, Espagno J, Guiraud B, Mignard D (1979) Exploration des syringomyélies par myélo-cisternographie computerisée au metrizamide. 4ème Congres annuel de la Société française de Neuroradiologie. Société française de Neuroradiologie, Toulouse, p 175
28. Moseley IF (to be published) High spatial resolution computed tomography of the orbit and skull base

29. Naidich TP, Pudlowski RM, Moran CJ, Gilula LA, Murphy W, Naidich JB (1979) Computed tomography of spinal fractures. Adv Neurol 22:207 – 253
30. Naidich TP, King DR, Moran CJ, Sagel SS (1980) Computed tomography of the lumbar thecal sac. J Comput Assist Tomogr 4:37 – 41
31. Nakagawa H, Huang YP, Malis LI, Wolf BS (1977) Computed tomography of intraspinal and paraspinal neoplasms. J Comput Assist Tomogr 1:377 – 388
32. Oberson R, Azam F CT of the spine and spinal cord. Neuroradiology 16:369 – 370
33. Orwell C, Du Boulay GH, Kendall BE, Lloyd GAS, Moseley IF, Phelps P, Pullicino P (1980) High spatial resolution on the EMI 5005 and 7020 scanners. Xtract 8:2 – 7
34. Palmers Y, Baert AL, Marchal G, Coenon Y (1976) Computed tomography (CT) in affections of the vertebral column and spinal cord. J Belge Radiol 59:521 – 530
35. Pullicino P (1980) Computed tomography of the contents of the spinal canal. Ph. D. Thesis, University of London
36. Pullicino P, Du Boulay GH, Kendall BE (1979) Xenon enhancement for computed tomography of the spinal cord. Neuroradiology 18:63 – 66
37. Quencer RM (1980) Needle aspiration of intramedullary and intradural extramedullary masses of the spinal canal. Radiology 134:115 – 126
38. Resjö IM, Harwood-Nash DC, Fitz CR, Chuang S (1978) Computed tomographic metrizamide myelography in spinal dysraphia in infants and children. J Comput Assist Tomogr 2:549, 558
39. Resjö IM, Harwood-Nash DC, Fitz CR, Chuang S (1979) Normal cord in infants and children examined with computed tomographic metrizamide myelography. Radiology 130:691 – 696
40. Rinaldi I, Kopp JE, Harris WO, Reagan TJ, Murphy D (1978) Computer assisted tomography in syringomyelia. J Comput Assist Tomogr 2:633 – 635
41. Roub LW, Drayer BP (1979) Spinal computed tomography: limitations and applications. AJR 133: 267 – 273
42. Scatliff JH, Bidgood WD, Killebrew K, Staab EV (1979) Computed tomography and spinal dysraphism: clinical and phantom studies. Neuroradiology 17:71 – 75
43. Scotti LN, Marasco JA, Pittman TA, Feczko WA, Goldman RL (1977) Computed tomography of the spinal canal and cord. Comput Tomogr 1:229 – 234
44. Tadmor R, Davis KR, Roberson GH, Chapman PH (1977) The diagnosis of diastematomyelia by computed tomography. Surg Neurol 8:434 – 436
45. Tadmor R, Davis KR, Roberson GH, New PJF, Taveras JM (1978) Computed tomographic evaluation of traumatic spinal injuries. Radiology 127: 825 – 827
46. Thijssen HOM, Keyser A, Horstink MWH, Meijer E (1979) Morphology of the spinal cord on computed myelography. Neuroradiology 18:57 – 62
47. Weinstein MA, Rothner AD, Duchesnau P, Dohn DF (1975) Computed tomography in diastematomyelia. Radiology 118:609 – 611
48. Zumpano BJ (1978) Spinal intramedullary metastatic medulloblastoma. J Neurosurg 48:632 – 635

Subject Index